In 1970, I discovered that sunflower se[...] into indoor salad greens. As a result th[...] wheatgrass in a healthy living lifestyle, [...] part of the Hippocrates Institute program, [...] pea greens. I designed an inexpensive soilless garden system to allow kitchen gardeners to produce up to three pounds of delicious, organic full-spectrum salad greens per square foot, at less than $0.20 per pound. (It can sometimes be found in stores for as much as $32 per pound.)

For complete FREE details on setting up "Viktoras Indoor Gardens" in your kitchen, email viktorasretreats@gmail.com. (Please use "V Gard" in the subject line.)

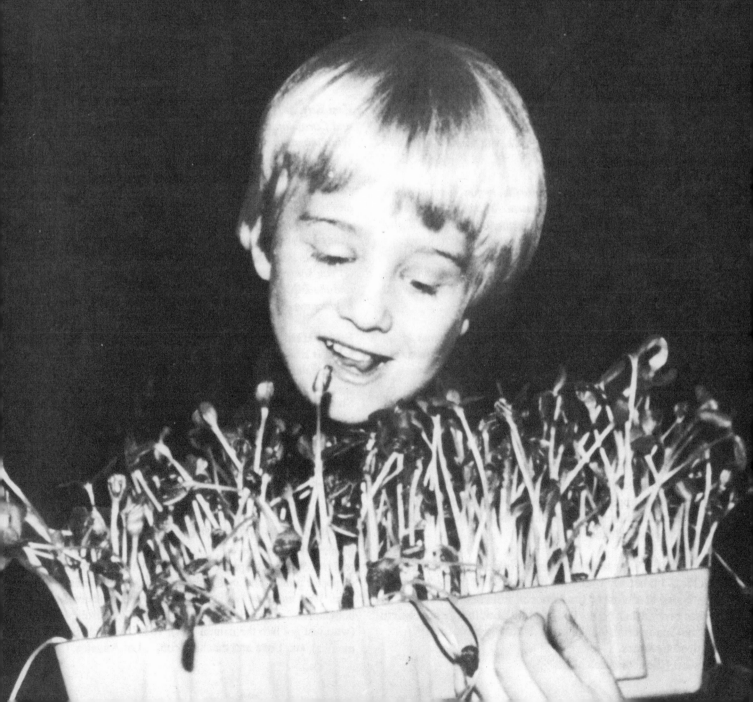

READERS COMMENTS ON VIKTORAS:

SPIN "Survival ... " is the "Das Kapital" of the modern raw food movement, outlining the forces of in science and history that lead inescapably to the un-cooked diet.. "I read the whole book that night. I stuck around him and fasted and learned all about live foods. . I became very raw, about 95%. I really love the lifestyle." (2/1999)

USA TODAY: " Victor kulvinskas, author of "Survival Into 21st Cen" warns that too many of us dining on chemical feast, pouring 'food into our poisons' and that 'real food that nourishes our body' is becoming virtually extinct" (Barbara Reynold)

www.Peter Max.com : "An inspired book".

Dick Gregory: "I got no problems, cause I got Brothers like Viktoras who balance out all the negativity on the planet. There is not another mind on the planet when it comes to nutrition that knows as much about the body with such integrity as Brother Viktoras. Don't know no book that talks as much as this "Survival In the 21st Century."

Rev. Ann Wigmore: " *I am forever grateful for your compan - ionship, assistance and contribution during the seven years we spend together in popularizing the wheatgrass therapy and tak - ing vision to reality the live food and enzymatic nutrition. Your holy book has been an important key to the new age and wholistic healing*"

Brian Clement *"Decades before trends began Viktoras pio - neered the progressive health movement. With Ann Wigmore he co-founded the* <u>Hippocrates Health Institute</u>.. *Viktoras will give you the information you need to move forward."* (<u>Director</u>)

Norman Walker: "Your contribution to humanity, with Rev. Ann Wigmore, will be forever remembered." (author, over 100 years young)

Gabriel Cousens MD *"Viktoras is extremely dynamic as he shares his vast insights and delicious recipes in those rare videos".* (Author; www.treeoflife.nu/)

David Wolf (*Nature's First Law*): *"Viktoras is an encyclopedia of knowledge. Seeing and listening to him speak is like reading a fascinating book"* (Author)

National Health Federation "Thank you. Viktoras Kulvinskas. for adding joy and health knowledge to our library Vow teachings, love and support will guide people to a better understanding of themselves and they will find truth in the wisdom of your pages." Stephanie Shane.

RESCUED: "Your teachings among others saved me from suicide.... i must say that your book survival in the 21st century is one of a blast of fundamental informations. it surpasses every other books i've read by now. it appears clearto me that many other books must definitely have been inspired by yours.
www.geocities.com/melenktus/

Rodale (Organic Gardening) *"Viktoras...fascinated the audi - ence with his ideas for healthier diet...I tasted 'sunflower let - tuce'...delicious."* Jeff Cox.

Ernest Krebs, Jr. D.S.C. (*Laetrile co-discoverer*) *"Valuable contribution to the literature of nutrition—Valuable addition to my library... Excellent reference."*

Ruth Rogers, M.D. *"This is the most informative and instruc - tive book on sprouts...One of the best health measures and treat - ments is raw foods, especially sprouts."*

Dr. Bernard Jensen. N.D. (*iridologist*) *"Thank you very much for the book. I certainly am enjoying it and 1 appreciate your mentioning me. All best for your success."*

Mr. and Mrs. V.E. Irons(*Vice Chairman: Board of Governors. National Health Federation*) *"are very much impressed with your book, Survival. Will you quote a price on a minimum of 10 books?"* Please let me know and we will place the order from this office." C.W. Dahlin.

Ken Key. Jr. (*Founder and president of Living Love Center and Cornucopia Institute*) *"Thank you for the copy of Survival. What a beautiful job you've done."*

Uri Geller (*Master of psychokinesis, telepathy, clairvoyance*) *"They are some of the most informative books I have ever read on the subject."*

Mary Latane (*87-year-old youth*) *"Cleansing from holiday spree is making me see how much God loves his Son. Want to let you know your splendid book. Survival Into the 21st Century, and the Bible are my guide lights. Thank you for being you and helping me."*

Bosley Hiss *"What a holy book you have written. Words fail us, but it is so beautifully done — the Aquarian Bible of the Age. You have created something the world needs."*

Stanley Bass, D.C. *"Your Survival is most stimulating, an ency - clopedic and bold attempt at a whole integrated look at Man and the Universe. I recommed it to my patients."*

Beatrice Hunter Author *"This is a useful, well-researched booklet, well worth the investment."*

VEGETARIAN WORLD"Dear Viktor — "Survival" is the greatest! I'm working on
reviews of it for the paper (Vegetarian World)...prospective card or poster publishers...symposium on longevity... interview for East/ West and new age journals... new age bookstores... college bookstores... major New Age spokesmen like Airola, Roszak (who just got into the natural diet), Tom Laughlin (Billy Jack movies), etc. Love and thanks, Scott, , Los Angeles, CA

SURVIVAL
in the
21ST CENTURY

PLANETARY HEALERS MANUAL

—

By

Viktoras Kulvinskas

Introduction: Dick Gregory

Front Cover: Peter Max

Back Cover and Art: Jean White

—

Book Publishing Company
Summertown, Tennessee

Published in the United States by
Book Publishing Company
PO Box 99
Summertown, TN 38483
(888) 260-8458   www.bookpubco.com

Printed in Canada

ISBN 978-1-57067-247-7

16 15 14 13 12 11 10   9 8 7 6 5 4 3 2 1

POLICY STATEMENT ON THE USE OF INCLUSIVE LANGUAGE

The authors are aware that language used generally (words such as "man" or "brotherhood") unconsciously excludes women. While they believe that the use of exclusive language is representative of the predominantly patriarchal male-oriented historical and social context from which we are emerging, they are nevertheless dedicated to achieving androgynous consciousness. To this end, they are making all feasible attempts to utilize inclusive language in our publications.

"We shall be one person."

Pueblo Indian

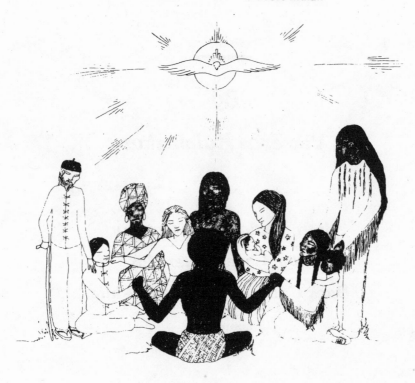

Disclaimer
The information in this book is presented for educational purposes only. It is not intended to be a substitute for the medical advice of your health care professional.

Book Publishing Co. is a member of Green Press Initiative. We chose to print this title on paper with postconsumer recycled content, processed without chlorine, which saved the following natural resources:

BOOK PUBLISHING COMPANY

93 trees
2,589 pounds of solid waste
42,650 gallons of water
8,855 pounds of greenhouse gases
30 million BTU of energy

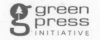

For more information, visit <www.greenpressinitiative.org>. Savings calculations thanks to the Environmental Defense Paper Calculator, <www.edf.org/papercalculator>.

How to thrive in the Now and after the 2012 era with a sustainable mind of enlightenment

The paradigm of hope

"And in those days the children shall begin to study the laws,
And to seek the commandments. And to return to the path of righteousness.
"And the days shall begin to grow many
And increase amongst the children of humans
Till their days draw nigh to one thousand years,and to greater number of years than (before)
was the number of days.
"And there shall be no old people
Nor one who is not satisfied with one's days,
For all shall be as children and youths.
"And all their days they shall be complete and live in peace and in joy..."
(The Book of Jubilees, xxiii: 26-30, vol. ii, p. 49, Essene Scroll)

"Be Green or be Mulched."
~ VIKTORAS, 2012

Out of chaos...stars are born.
~ Friedrich Nietzsche, Essene Scroll

A house with a light...never attracts thieves.
~ Buddha (c. 500 BC)

"Materialistic science will receive a deathblow...one by one,
facts and processes in Nature's workshops are permitted to
find their way into the exact sciences, while mysterious help
is given to rare individuals in unraveling its arena."
~ Madame Blavatsky (c. 1888-1897)

The Earth is defiled by its people; they have disobeyed the
laws, violated the statutes and broken the everlasting
covenant. Therefore a curse consumes the Earth; its people
must bear their guilt. Therefore Earth's inhabitants are
burned up, and very few are left.
~ Isaiah 24: 4-6

Dear Friend and Reader,

You have a few years' window of opportunity to transform your holistic body in alignment with Mother Earth - Father Sun and the cycles of the Grand-parent Milky Way Galaxy that dictates the 100,000 year earth cycles that will reach the cusp on winter solstice of 2012, give or take a few years. To dodge the cosmic bullets, plagues and earth changes, you need to be instinctual and strong. You will have the powers and guidance if you are mostly raw, alkaline, vegan, green-oriented, fully holistic, and in service to higher good. Above all, do not be attached to life; all experiences are good with a cosmic attitude. No fear—just do good, enjoy the ride and wait for further instructions from the creator. Pray and meditate; all will be made paradisically perfect.

No...the drama is not a Disneyland production, for the script was read eons ago by the Mayans, who viewed the timeless galaxy in their sacred, astral bodies fueling the physical with cosmic raw alkaline essence. They encoded in their calendar and myths.

You already know that OLD age is over. Mother Earth is about to renew herself of the parasitic, acid, enzymeless, toxic Tamasic and or Rajasic humanoids initiating an era of the Satwich Ahimsa Age of Harmony.

Be prepared for chaotic decimating Earth Changes, as we, the survivors, transition from Competitive Colonial Capitalism into a Partnership of the Paradise Paradigm of Possibilities. Fueled by the Living Raw Lifestyles that are truly sustainable, we continue to usher and manifest within a culture of ageless, healthy and joyful naturalists.

The vision was born over two "scores" ago in dreams while fasting. They are now in a state of accelerated manifestation. More and more of the leaders, as well as media, acknowledge my contribution. In vision, I was not alone. I partnered with other great souls who similarly had "close encounters of the third kind" as they saw the need to prepare for "the day after tomorrow." And to heal and save as many earthlings as possible.

Brother Viktoras (viktoras4u.com, viktorasretreats@gmail.com)

Quotes about Viktoras

"Viktoras has been a mentor to me since long before we first met...but when he did meet me and tasted my food he said, 'You must teach this to chefs...every chef in the world should know how to make this food like this. It should be on every menu...and you're the one to do it.' Of course, I couldn't say no. So within two weeks Living Light Culinary Arts Institute was born. It was an Institute of One, but I knew I would grow into it...and I did. I can thank Viktoras for that, because, if it hadn't been for him I might not have taken that leap of faith. I thought, if he says I should do it...I should do it. So I want to thank him. He is a pioneer of the Living food Movement. In fact, we think of him as the Father of Living Foods. Lithuanian Raw Mystic is what we also may call him, writing *Survival In The 21st Century*, offering a comprehensive survival strategy to 2012 and beyond. A visionary, Educator, Researcher, Raw Food Chef and Author, Viktoras has mentored many of the key people in the Raw Food Movement!!"

~ Cherie Soria, founder of the first raw culinary school, rawfoodchef.com, 2009 Raw Festival

"I don't even know if I can find the words to say how important Viktoras Kulvinskas is to the scheme of things in the raw and living foods field. We affectionately call him the Godfather of Living Food. I can assure you that I would not be here today...my wife would not be doing her work...Hippocrates Institute would not exist...without Viktoras. He's not only one of the most brilliant people I know in my life, and I know a lot of really brilliant people, but he's also equally compassionate and that combination is rare, that one has as big a heart as they have a mind. He has had many people recover from disease because of his compassionate words. Probably...if you put several of us together...Viktoras has done a better job than we have!! I want you to really just listen with your heart. We're blessed to have Viktoras come teach our Health Educator Program at Hippocrates several times a year. And what I always tell the health educators just before he comes is...you may not always understand intellectually what he is saying...but if you open your heart and listen to what Viktoras is saying...that is the gift you're going to get from him!!"

~ Dr. Brian Clement, director of the number one rated spa, hippocratesinst.org, 2009

"My friend Viktoras K. is one of the most impressive speakers I have ever seen on stage. He says that he does not prepare for his speeches and that he simply lets God speak though him and I believe him. Vik is somebody who really has something to say and his way of communicating his message is unique, effective and very, very impressive. If you ever have the chance to learn from somebody who really knows what he is talking about, you need to read Viktoras' publications, but most of all please experience him live. He will change your life! With gratefulness and deepest respect for Viktoras, his work and our friendship."

~ Dr. Leonard Coldwell, DrLeonardColdwell.com

" 'Survival...' is the 'Das Kapital' (classic economy theory) of the modern raw food movement, outlining the forces of science and history that lead inescapably to the uncooked diet. I read the whole book that night. I stuck around him, fasted and learned all about live foods. I became raw, about 95%. I really love the lifestyle."

~ SPIN, Feb 1999

More Links from Viktoras

Beyond the recognition by the leaders in consciousness, as above, we were inspired by Biblical truths and the most ancient of wisdom, especially the *re-birth* of The Raw Revolution that was initiated two generations prior. This was done on a "grass" roots level, person to person, by two Lithuanians who are also the co-founders of the now world famous Hippocrates Health Institute (hippocratesinst.org). Please notify us that you are attending and let them know that I, Viktoras, sent you!

Eat your basic Super Food Essentials every day: LivingRawSuperFoods.com

Now, you can Google up most diseases and find clinical treatments with enzymes, alkaline juices, and/or raw foods.

According to Joseph Mercola (a leading opponent of vaccination, especially as related to the swine flu fake), "Raw food is clearly one of the keys to maximizing your health." (See mercola.com.) The suffering masses are waking up saying, "We're not going to take it anymore."

Check out healthfreedomusa.org—change.org is also very good.

We can now be armed with free cyberspace knowledge, as well as fed by the research of "Cultural Creatives" and "Paradigm Shifters," as well as from those on a "grass" root level, initially led by downloading the timeless Akashic Wisdom. In addition, with another beautiful mainstream document, the best-selling book *The Wellness Revolution: How to Make a Fortune in the Next Trillion Dollar Industry*, self-awareness blossoms supreme, leading the charge with "Whole Food," the next organic, fast food apple.

Because of the Internet, adopting a whole food, vegan diet, low cost with door to door delivery (greenpokadot.com/survival), is simply a mouse click away.

Also, isn't it time you broke your cooking pot, pan, and fire addiction and joined the Raw Solar Revolution to enjoy living in Paradise? There simply is no future after 2012 for dead food fuel. It is exciting to observe the growth of veganism and the raw food lifestyle. I envisioned forty years ago it would take two generations for our society to adopt this. A large medical association (PCRM, pcrm.org) did research to show that not only is a well-chosen whole food vegan diet adequate, it also revealed that any other diet is contrary to health.

The largest nutritional study ever conducted, The China Study (thechinastudy.com), concluded "humans have not had long enough evolution time to adapt to consumption of flesh food."

Check out Dr. Leonard Coldwell at drleonardcoldwell.com. Also, check out his book *The Only Answer To Cancer*.

We also recommend Emotional Freedom Technique (emofree.com) on how to heal yourself with tapping.

I can now, with certainty, declare by 2012 all Earthlings will be Vegan, and most will be raw. No, I am not smoking grass—although I did have a cup of *wheat*grass* juice. The old, unnatural ways will be cleared by Mother Earth as she initiates a healing crisis of rebirth. This will be evident to the innocent as volcanic pimples, flu, fevers, remineralization of our farm lands, tsunamis, and hurricanes, as a skin scrubbing of the earth's surface. Also, we will have induced fasts for the enlightened being via famine, triggered by unusual global weather conditions. To top it all off, only the green-consuming life forms will be able to handle the December 2012 electromagnetic solar radiation created by sun spot hurricanes and the zodiac zone that we will have entered, scientifically noted for intense radiation.

You are about to participate in the grand cosmic script that may seem like a tragedy; however, it is a purification process that repeats itself every 26,000 years, bringing the surviving humanity into the thriving millennium. Living for a thousand years will be within everybody's reach. With perfect health, ageless bodies, and a psychic connection to all life forms, we shall thrive in a harmonious era, where astral travel and the journey of the soul will free us of all time and space constraints."

Our knowledge has started the countdown to the "11th Hour" which was preceded by the "fictional" *The Day After Tomorrow* as the masses are having serious "Crude Awakenings." There is no time to waste before we hit 2012. The web site suprememastertv.com speaks in over 20 languages: go veg, be green, and save the planet (or rather ourselves). This message reaches over two billion viewers daily.

More enlightenment tools can be delivered to your door, available through viktoras.hubhub.org

To further educate how the old genre deals with peoples' energy go to zeitgeistmovie.com, as well as the documentaries *Endgame* and *Fall of the Republic* by Alex Jones. In the video *Small Change*, see how peoples' lives can be a extinguished for a "Small Change" (http://video.google.com/videoplay?docid=7866929448192753501).

The web has helped provide us the freedom to be One. Raw food will make us be As ONE, like cells of the One Planet Entity. No more competition, only co-operation.

Some find the deeper reality too frightening. There are so many of what we once called "challenges" in this world, that we can now perceive as opportunities for growth. Toxic fluoride in our water...aluminum in the air from chemtrails released in the sky...mercury aplenty in vaccines, as well as pesticides and genetically modified organisms in the "food" supply. It's like the Four Elements being attacked by the Four Horsemen!! Water...Air...Earth and the Fire of Spirit all being truly compromised by only one mutual horse they ALL ride called our Night"mares." Let us not forget how powerful our mind is. In the process of cleansing our bodies with optimal foods and strengthening our immune systems with the best nutrients and minerals available, the focus of our thoughts and our ability to manifest love and light should not be underestimated. The false flags and fear mongering by mainstream media will not interfere with the claiming of our birthright essence as inheritors of the Earth!!

I strive to help people by providing the simplest, cheapest methods to wellness, slimness, freedom from addiction, and being naturally happy with guidance to assist all into their natural power.

Embrace the gift of the Internet and sources of alternative news.

Love in Service,

Brother Viktoras (Viktoras4u.com, viktorasretreats@gmail.com)

Sun Healing

One of the greatest energies on the planet is the sun. All life forms are changed by harvesting its gift. The ancients knew of its unlimited and vast potential. The Egyptians, Greeks, Mayans, and Native Americans, to name a few, had great respect for and honored deeply the treasures the sun brings both within and without. Humanity, for the most part, has become detached from this blessed concept. Modern education tells us, "Don't look at the sun...you'll go blind"..."Don't stay in the sun...you'll get cancer." Over time, the sun has become something we are taught is dangerous and our "enemy," yet science also tells us that some amount is beneficial and gives us a source of Vitamin D. As all plants need the sun and absorb its energy to transform and grow into its essence via photosynthesis, we are no different. Most can agree that our brain is like a super computer, an incredible "battery" of consciousness for the human vessel. We also know that our eyes are a powerful extension of our brain. We have the ability to receive and give a great deal power through our eyes. All emotions of self and others can be perceived, as they relay the incoming messages to our brain. Therefore, while it is a detailed and delicate science, we know that through solar gazing we can charge our brain and soul through looking directly at the sun during sunrises and sunsets. Most of us have some memories, as well as pleasure, of seeing the sun as it rises and falls, creating its amazing array of colors. If we imagine our brain as our personal computer and our eyes as a kind of solar panel that charges and stores its energy source, we become aware of an intuition that all life forms hold. It's important to know that it is directly through our eyes alone that we can most optimally take in energetic photons to feed our cells and inner space. With this information, a whole new (yet old) method of spiritual empowerment is revealed!! Make the time to do a little research to explore the timeless treasures of sungazing, an ultimate source for the physical realm (solarhealing.com).

If you are in the position to do so, tools like a solar-powered generator would be very useful (mysolarbackup.com).
Systems that produce pure water out of the air are also a very wise investment (ecoloblue.com).

You are being introduced to an extrapolation of the best of all the teachers and students who participated with me in this great experiment (also found at survivalinthe21stcentury.com). It has reached many millions of readers world wide, as well as the outreach program that Rev. Ann Wigmore and I started over forty years ago at Hippocrates, rated as the number one educational health spa in the world, where I have been active most my life.

Ask the Universe, "How can I serve?" When one does this, we start to see opportunities in how our authentic self can be creative. It's not about "saving the world," rather it's about being a reflection of the beautiful emerging paradigm.

Thought forms that are coming from a sense of connection are far more powerful than those that come from a place of separation.

So it's about those individuals who are holding the space of infinite possibilities, vibrating at that higher level, that will erase and neutralize the mass of "lower" thought forms. We indeed hold the living template for all that will emerge in our next stage of evolution. We can easily see that the media is frantically reporting their propaganda from old and dying realm of belief systems.

Now we can ask ourselves, "Are we giving more than we are receiving?" What does your "Spiritual Credit Card" look like? When we give more than we receive, we build up our line of credit with the Universe. We accumulate interest with the cosmos that goes much further than any bank! When we give to ourselves and others, the Universe takes notice, and without question it will not let your good credit build up too high before it starts blessing you tenfold for your unconditional investments!! So when you give, be prepared for what you ask for, because the Universe may answer you at any given time. Perfect Love, the Consecrated of God does so claim her beloved birthright!!

Make greens for yourself or your favorite cause, such is the path of Planet Earth.

Dis-ease knocked at the door; a raw foodist got up to answer it, and no one was there.

Love In Service   *We Are One* ALL Is Love*
Rev. Viktoras
(viktoras4u.com)
For further enlightment, please read the Introductions from 2002 and 2006.

Private Health Consultation with Viktoras - Scheduled by appointment

Consultations are available with Viktoras in person, by phone, or by email, as well as lectures and retreats. Please write viktorasretreats@gmail.com.

OVER HALF MILLION COPIES SOLD
48th Updated Printing

Rediscover from Ancient Memories and Genetic Inheritance the Simplicity of Life Food and the Healing Powers of Grasses

From the world-famous University of Texas System Cancer Center, research analyzed in the *Report to the Physicians of Texas Newsletter* and *Science Digest*, concludes:

"When Dr. Chiu-Nan Lai and her colleagues applied extracts of wheatgrass to certain cancer-causing chemicals, the activity of the chemicals diminished radically, by 99% in some instances." See pages 296-7.

At Linus Pauling Institute of Science and Medicine, founded by the two-time Nobel Prize recipient, Dr. Arthur Robinson did a two-year study which was written up in *Barron's*, the national financial weekly.

"Raw fruits, vegetables, wheatgrass and vitamin C caused a remarkable 35-fold decrease in cancer incidence." See page 299.

At Hippocrates Health Institute, Dr. Ann Wigmore, founder and recipient of a recognition award from the Nobel Prize Foundation for work on the regeneration of human cells and tissue, states:

"The most thrilling experience I can recall was to see cancer cells taken from a human body and thriving on cooked food but unable to survive on the same food when it was uncooked."

Here's What They're Saying About Our Books

National Health Federation "Thank you, Viktoras Kulvinskas, for adding joy and health knowledge to our library. Your teachings, love and support will guide people to a better understanding of themselves and they will find truth in the wisdom of your pages." Stephanie Shane.

Rodale's Organic Gardening "Viktoras...fascinated the audience with his ideas for healthier diet...I tasted 'sunflower lettuce'...delicious." Jeff Cox.

Ernest Krebs, Jr. D.S.C. (Laetrile co-discoverer) "Valuable contribution to the literature of nutrition...Valuable addition to my library...Excellent reference."

Ruth Rogers, M.D. "This is the most informative and instructive book on sprouts...One of the best health measures and treatments is raw foods, especially sprouts."

Dr. Bernard Jensen, N.D. (Noted iridologist) "Thank you very much for the book. I certainly am enjoying it and I appreciate your mentioning me. All best for your continued success."

Mr. and Mrs. V.E. Irons (Vice Chairman, Board of Governors, National Health Federation) "are very much impressed with your book, *Survival*. Will you quote a price on a minimum of 10 books?" Please let me know and we will place the order from this office." C.W. Dahlin.

Ken Keys, Jr. (Founder and president of Living Love Center and Cornucopia Institute) "Thank you for the copy of *Survival*. What a beautiful job you've done."

Uri Geller (Master of psychokinesis, telepathy, clairvoyance) "They are some of the most informative books I have ever read on the subject."

Mary Latane (87-year-old youth) "Cleansing from holiday spree is making me see how much God loves his Son. Want to let you know your splendid book, *Survival Into the 21st Century*, and the Bible are my guidelights. Thank you for being you and helping me."

Bosley Hiss "What a holy book you have written. Words fail us, but it is so beautifully done — the Bible of the Aquarian Age. Truly you have created something the world needs."

Stanley Bass, D.C. "Your *Survival* is most stimulating, an encyclopedic and bold attempt at a whole integrated look at Man and the Universe. I'm recommending it to my patients."

Beatrice Hunter "This is a useful, well-researched booklet, well worth the investment."

Personal Healing Testimonials

Prostate and Weight Loss: "I was full of pills, antibiotics and a catheter...I continued the therapy and after 12 days lost 30 pounds and removed the catheter...No operation necessary." See page 239.

Hypoglycemia: "Lightheadedness, headaches, fatigue, depression, senility, 13 years of tranquilizers...After natural therapy I take no pills...I have unlimited strength." See page 242.

Menstruation: "The greatest value of your book was lifting my worry about the cessation of my period. After detoxification diet, all symptoms of menstruation ceased within 6 months." See pages 35 and 243.

High Blood Pressure and Grey Hair (Age 77): "While drinking wheatgrass, hair began to turn to original black color...High blood pressure gone down." See page 245.

Teeth, Pyorrhea (Age 29): "Doctors suggested teeth extraction. After trying wheatgrass, puss gone, front teeth tight and body odor cleaned up." See page 246.

Cancer: "Thirty-day cobalt treatment leading to pain and bleeding and hourly evacuation necessary....After wheatgrass, bowel movements became normal and pain ceased." See page 246.

Arthritis (Age 68): "Sufferer goes on wheatgrass 42-day fast and clears up protein deficiency, muscular attrition, liver disturbance and osteoporosis of the spine." See page 238.

Paralysis and Shattered Disk and Non-Functioning Elimination: "According to doctors, by now I should be capable of lifting, painfully, a few pounds. Instead, in the desert I had to carry 90-pound rocks to put inside my tent to fasten it down in the 100 m.p.h. winds.... I can do all the yoga postures, even handstands." See page 303.

INTRODUCTION
2/22/2002

"Sit down before a fact as a little child, be prepared to give up every preconceived notion, follow humbly wherever and to whatever abysses nature leads, or you will learn noth - ing."   Thomas H. Huxley

"Almost always (persons) who achieve these fundamental inventions of a new paradigm have been either very young or very new to the field whose paradigm they changed."
   Thomas S. Kuhn, "The Nature of Scientific Revolution"

"An important scientific innovation rarely makes its way by gradually winning over and converting its opponents. What does happen is that its opponents gradually die out and that the growing generation is familiarized with the idea from the beginning."   Max Planck, Theoretical Physicist

"Yesterday is history, tomorrow is a mystery, today is a gift, that's why they call it the present."   Author Unknown

I am writing in light of September 11. With wars and rumors of war swirling around us, it's my conviction that the message of Survival In the 21st Century is even more relevant today than when it was first released over a quarter a century ago. As much of the world is mesmerized by the intensity of earthly affairs I am here to offer hope, vision and action. I believe our best hope lies in reawakening our body's natural instinctive capacity for self-healing; strengthening our minds connection to universal intelligence and reconnecting our soul with the divine essence of love within us.

In 2002, in light of the world-situation, the flow of world events may seem beyond our control, yet as micro-gods-in-drag (disguised as human beings) we still possess tremendous collective power to unite with other kindred souls to make a real difference. One may not have a direct line to the behind-the-scene decision-makers, however on an individual level, only oneself may prevent the preparation of one's bodily temple.

I believe all things are ultimately working out for the best, yet that doesn't mean there will not be challenges to overcome. Whatever does happen, let us pray we'll have the wisdom and courage to follow our highest light when our character and soul's integrity are tested. It's my belief that we are being tested here and now.

In the process of conveying this, I may at times sound pessimistic or alarmist. Other's may see me as an "internal alarm repair specialist in action." Hence, inspite of a strong desire to express my insights and feelings about the ongoing "violence", I will step back. For that too shall pass. One does not need to become a "victim of changes". Truly, I am an idealist and an optimist, for I believe nothing can extinguish the immortal divine spirit in humanity. So...my non-stop mantra for these challenging times is:

"Love is my intention and now with my attention......love grows and grows and grows."

Place your attention on love and it will multiply. Place your attention on life and you will become more a-live.

Health Held Hostage, a Media Hype

Nowadays, many of us are so caught up with the day-to-day demands of "making a living", the excuse is that we've lost touch with how to live in tune with our natural instincts and intuition. The insidious effects of this ceaseless external assault keeps us in a perpetual state of frenetic business "in emergency mode" making it difficult to connect with the infinite source of inner wisdom and outer harmony. What makes it even more difficult for one to get back in touch with our authentic needs is that 8 out of 10 Americans are "chemically altered" due to prescription drug use. The result is a drugged-out, weakened populace experiencing unprecedented levels of chronic "dis-ease." In fact, the so-called "health care system", more accurately referred to as the disease management system, is itself responsible for 4 out of every 10 casualties...5 times more people each year than the toll caused by auto accidents. Case in point: One would think that when doctors went on strike, mortality rate would go up for lack of medical care, right? However Dr. Mendelsohn tracked mortality rate statistics when doctors went on strike and found ...rates decreased significantly! Taking personal responsibility for your health, is the only cure' for the "dis-eased" illusion.

Survival into the 21st Century continues to be a best-selling health classic because it presents a new paradigm of nutrition that shows people how to effectively detoxify, heal and rebuild the body temple, all while living in modern society. Sure, its longevity as a popular book had something to do with its home-grown charm: funky hand-written diagrams and lay-out, hip visionary artwork and quirky photos, but what mattered most were the foods themselves, the high-enzyme, easy-to-digest whole foods our modern culture had almost forgotten. However millions of years of cellular programming in us did not forget. So when a new health generation got the chance to taste these incredible, edible living foods, a love affair was born and a new movement was launched.

Germination was at first slow, but in each decade following Survival's release we witnessed the sprouting up of more and more living food healing centers, raw food support groups, gourmet "no-cooking" culinary schools, raw websites and a host of vacation resorts around the globe.

Dietary Recommendations to Ward Off Internal Toxicity

At the time of the initial release of Survival, the general dietary direction I recommended was to eat progressively lighter high-energy foods such as fresh squeezed wheatgrass, green drinks and vegetable juices, indoor baby greens, sprout salads and fruit. One would eventually reach a level of internal purity that would not only enhance the ease of metabolic functioning, but also enable living fooders to tap into more subtle life-energies found in sunlight and air.

Without proper guidance, however, some people became "spacey", lost too much muscle mass and generally became too vibrationally sensitive in relation to their surroundings. I'm not completely dismissing this direction in dietary evolution...there's a time and a place for everything.

The awareness of mother earth's birth changes...her methods of cleansing, healing and growth, are all around us in many consciousness raising forms. Nuclear power plants, "ill" municipal water supplies, anthrax, infected livestock and other various methods of mass chemical saturation, just to name a few. So here's some updated nutritional advice for these turbulent times, gleaned from my nutritional counseling experience over a span of 30 years. Many people I counsel have already come a long way in their dietary evolution since their years of eating the Standard American Diet (SAD). In fact, a significant number of people have arrived at a primarily cooked vegan diet even before we have our consultation. Becoming a vegan takes a tremendous burden off the environment and oneself, yet the diet itself has drawbacks. Although many offending foods have been eliminated (animal food, dairy products), the typical starch based vegan diet doesn't supply sufficient quantities of enzymes/full-spectrum-minerals and other delicate nutritional co-factors that are destroyed by cooking. To compensate for the cumulative effect of enzyme-deficient food over a lifetime, I recommend a transition to at least 80% uncooked foods "the more raw, the better". This change can be accomplished at your own pace, unless there's an existing health problem that can be helped by a more accelerated transition to living foods. The ease with which you move toward eating a higher percentage of raw foods depends on many factors: psychological make-up, living situation, work environment, constitutional strength, etc. That's why nutritional counseling is considered an art as well as a science. In addition to living foods themselves, I almost always recommend the daily intake of certain food concentrates such as plant-based enzymes to make up for past enzymatic losses. Blue green algae for the full spectrum of nutrients, as well as the introduction of oral pro-biotic cultures (acidophilus, bifidus, and many other beneficial microbes) nourishes a healthy, non-toxic gastrointestinal tract and creates protection against Anthrax, Salmonella and Campylobacter,Staph, Botulism, etc.

Make sure to eat enough live plant protein each day. I've seen too many raw fooders deficient in essential amino acids. Eat the kind of protein that has its enzymes still intact. Sprouted grains, soaked seeds and nuts are the highest sources of high quality, enzyme-rich protein. They can be consumed in fermented form as well. Eat plentiful amounts of green and blue-green foods. Blue-green algae from Klamath Lake, Oregon, wheatgrass juice, sea vegetables such as dulse, nori, wakame: organic green salads, vegetable juices and well-selected therapeutic herbs and

spices also play a prominent role in my design of individual dietary programs. In addition, over the last 5 years or so, I advise many people to cut back on the quantity of fruit they consume, even carrot juice, as these sweet foods aggravate compromised immune systems and those suffering from candida yeast problems, chronic diseases and/or staph infection.

As far as "cleansing diets", I'm all for them, however, as I alluded to above, I have one caveat: As you're bound to lose some muscle mass in the process, make an effort to rebuild as soon as possible. For if you get too skinny and yinny (spacey) you'll become too sensitive to environmental pollution as well as any psychic and physical discord around you. More specifically, I don't advise permanently losing more than 10-15% of your recommended weight for your height and body build during any single cleansing period. But if your weight does take a nose-dive, an exercise program which includes some form of resistance training (i.e. heavy lifting or weight training), in conjunction with, a diet of sprouted grain/soaked seed and soaked nut with other super foods will speed muscle mass recovery at rate of about pound a week.

If You're Not Aging, You're Youthing

There's an evolutionary step beyond periodic internal cleansing which I call "youthing." It's the actual reversal of aging. To be able to become physiologically younger even as you chronologically get older, you'll need to increase your level of enzyme supplementation as well the quantity of enzyme-rich superfoods you eat. That's not all.. "youthing" entails living in alignment with each and every component which contributes to health, such as mental poise, sufficient rest, sun, meditation, fresh air, pure water, etc. Many a health expert and famous nutritional author have consciously or unconsciously minimized the importance of one or more of the above health essentials and paid dearly in the form of premature aging or early death. Aside from the renewed sense of youthfulness you'll feel, a no-cost, lowtech way of tracking your youthing progress is to monitor changes in your iris through the diagnostic science of iridology. Healing lines and the disappearance of lesion marks on the iris are signs your body is rejuvenating. Consult the iris diagnosis map on page 197 in Survival if you're interested in the details of the wonderful healing going on inside you.

In summary, the way of the living food lifestyle is a path toward freedom, inner joy, strength, youthfulness, clarity of mind and the blossoming of the
heart. Be true to yourself and trust you'll be guided at every step.

Ten (More) Commandments for Thriving in the 21st Century

1. Heal thyself, first and foremost. All else follows from this. Charity starts at home. True self-love, (not narcissism) precedes love of others. If possible, find a supportive

group of kindred souls who are also working on themselves. Pick your friends and work conditions wisely.

Do your best to put into practice what you read in Survival, as well as other self-help books, videos and CD's. Become active in community service. Trust your intuition and instincts to where life leads you. Network with others by attending raw food events and any life-positive direction to which you're guided. Also wise is to drink lots of pure, clean water.

2. Everyone Gets To Play An Instrument in the Divine Symphony of Life

If you're a musician, sing songs that spread the message of love. In our culture, music is even more influential than the written word. I feel that by creating a major musical-dance-media event with a theme of "Back to Nature, healing with the planet and all Life forms, compassion and a return to simplicity... ", the live food community can create a visibility and a forum for sharing this natural, practical, economic way of life. Music is the language of the heart which will draw one to the vision of universal growth. I have outlined a format for events of this nature because I feel the time is now to "expand our sound". Please feel free to contact me if you are involved in the media and/or music industry.

If you're a money manager, support ecologically friendly investments. If you're a health practitioner, recommend high-enzyme live foods. In whatever way you can, use your energies in service of helping others. Any support they receive from you will help them get more in touch with their soul's internalized spiritual guidance system. Once they connect, they'll be better able to experience the beauty of life on earth and help others in the process.

3. Get with the Net

There's now a spin-off to the saying, "Think globally, act locally." It's "act locally, internet globally." The Internet is one of the most incredible networking/informational tools of the New Millennium. If you're not yet familiar with using the technology, relax, all you need is a little encouragement and guidance. Simply find a friendly person to introduce you to the basics of how to "surf the net, send and receive e-mail, or do an information search, etc.

If you're financially challenged and don't have your own computer...public libraries, friends, associates, storefront Internet cafes are other ways to get into cyberspace for little or no cash.

It's easy to receive free e-mail service you can access almost anywhere on earth. All you need is a telephone line and a computer that's online. A good first step is to get your own free e-mail address. This can be done on any online computer wherever you may be. Examples of free e-mail services are "www.hotmail.com" & "www..yahoo.com." There are many others. In addition to the above basics, cyberspace chat-rooms (people at computers in different locales communicating with each other in real time) can accelerate both your personal growth as well as the healing of the planet. There are chat-rooms of every description, as well as, every type of club and support group under the sun.

4. Love the Children

Many of our dreams for a better world may not occur in our own lifetime. We may plant the seeds of the future, but it will be our children and our children's children who will tend them to harvest. We need to nurture the children now so that they'll be able to nurture our dreams in their realities.

Your service of children may find expression in raising your own biological family. Or it might take the form of actively seeking out troubled youngsters or orphaned children who need mentoring and positive role models. Although we may feel many children need our help, guidance and love, all children truly come to earth in the role of helping and guiding others. There is a unique group that several contemporary writers call "Indigo children." These special souls come down to this earthly dimension at this critical time in history equipped with extra-ordinary soul-qualities, amazing intuitional and psychic abilities and often genius-level intelligence. It's predicted Indigo Children will join the more progressive segment of our present population whom sociologists call the "cultural creatives"...people of all walks of life, political persuasions and socio-economic levels who share a common constellation of life-positive values. Together, they will form the necessary critical mass of light-workers that will lead humanity into a new Golden Age of peace and higher consciousness. So make yourself available to the children: Spend time with them. Teach them. Learn from them. Believe in them. Love them and let yourself be loved by them. "Let the children guide you".

5. Hope Is A Molecule

Feelings of optimism and high oxygen levels in the bloodstream are correlated. Reducing internal toxemia has been shown to reduce attention deficit disorder, increase mental focus and allow us to relax into deeper meditative states. There's a bio-molecular foundation to optimizing physical, psychological and spiritual growth. Our thoughts, feelings, words and deeds are building blocks for the type of molecules we create on a moment-to-moment basis.

Purifying and strengthening physical functioning transforms the old you into a more conscious vehicle for the expression of divine love and infinite creativity. Once sufficiently purified physically, it will be easier, as the Bible says, to be as mindful of what comes out of your mouth as what you put in it! When an animal is slaughtered, it releases a "fear" endorphin into it's bloodstream. When one ingests that animal product...one eats "fear".

Fear is a molecule, as well. By self-introspection and witnessing our thought patterns, we can halt the manufacture of fear-based molecules in favor of endorphin-like carrier-molecules of love and bliss.

When you find yourself emotionally out of sorts, pull up your short-term memory files of recent internal self-talk (thoughts you said to yourself in your head) that doesn't feel right to you. Then take the time to listen for corrective guidance and you'll surely be shown how to "make things more in tune."

If your introspection continues to bring up hidden fears, decide whether these fears have any basis in reality. If so, it's possible you can prevent or reduce the likelihood of any real uncomfortable situation manifesting. Think of concrete action steps you can take instead of worrying about or being afraid of what may happen in some imagined future. What we concentrate on, we create. Take these positive action steps and then move on. Do not linger in a state of fear. If somehow you still cannot completely shake off all of the fear...sing to yourself, either out loud or internally, "I am love, I am love, I am love..."

You may also want to focus your attention on your breath: Breathe in, hold your breath, then breathe out and relax. Repeat again and again. Simply watch your thoughts float by until you are closer to an emotionally neutral, unattached state. We have the power to shift our thoughts, words and deeds in the direction that will make us feel safer and more in touch with what makes us and others in our life, happier. And if you feel you still need additional professional help to become clear of unpleasant holdovers from the past, by all means seek that special person to assist you.

6) Please do not judge yourself

if you make mistakes or sometimes backslide on your resolutions. Remember, every saint had his or her checkered past and every so-called sinner has his or her bright future to look forward to. Just as you fell many times when you were first learning to walk, be patient with yourself if you break your word or repeat again what you said you weren't going to do. If you fall short of your intentions, simply pick yourself up and gather up more resolve and courage to do better next time. I'll say it again, concentrate on where you want to be and eventually you'll get there.

7) Death is an illusion, life is eternal.

Fear of death is considered the number one stress in people's lives. The idea that your essential self is the soul may or may not be something you believe in at this point in time. It's my conviction that all souls will at one time wake up to know, from direct experience, that we are more than our personality, roles and sense-based input. If you take the fast-tract to inner and outer transformation as laid out in Survival, your spiritual awakening to the reality of soul may occur even sooner than later.

You may even learn to master the secrets of physical life-extension and be able to live a long, long time. Eventually, you may decide you've learned the lessons of this present incarnation and be able to make a fully conscious physical exit...gracefully moving in and out of various dimensional energies as a "spirit-soul."

8. Cycles of Time

Countless past civilizations have existed on this earth for many millions of years. Carbon-dated fossils show human footprints walking side-by-side with dinosaurs, contradicting the official party line held by academic anthropology and archeology. From time immemorial and even today,

spiritually awakened teachers have been reminding us that life on earth goes through cosmic evolutionary cycles of destruction and re-creation. At the end of each grand cycle of the past, whole civilizations and their eco-systems have been dismantled by flood, fire, earthquake and other earth changes as the flower of human progress is once again blessed to start over again in the compost of stone-age conditions.

One example of this was the fall of Atlantis, which many believe was a much more advanced civilization than our own. We won't go the way of Atlantis, however. The good news...is that after the transitional period of political and social upheaval we're in the throes of now...prophecy predicts there will not be another "fall". A new Golden Age is being born in which a collective "change of heart" will be our saving grace. It will be done... and you are one of the players in the New Millennium.

9. The Healing Balm of Forgiveness

Embedded in the word "forgive" is the word "give." Give from the heart selflessly and live in communion with your divine self, the source of love, through deep meditation. Forgiveness is born out of compassion, not only for others, but also for oneself. When forgiveness is awakened in your heart, grudges and grumbling towards self and other disappear as night-shadows at dawn. Living without judgment in the "co-creative now", you'll feel the ecstasy of being in tune with the power of Unconditional Love. When you have true self-love for yourself, you'll effortlessly be able to forgive.

10. Meditating on Your Divine Self

Having a human incarnation is a wonderful opportunity to realize the ultimate beauty of existence: Self-knowledge and spiritual illumination. As a human being, you've been given the gift of the hardware (human body) to access the ultimate software program..."the Infinite Bliss within you."

As you have a body right now, do not miss out on this golden opportunity to meet the Divine Beloved within you. At your own pace, create a comfortable atmosphere to address whatever issues are keeping you blocked from experiencing your true nature.

Resist the common temptation to escape into the oblivion of "sense enjoyments" for loitering at the level of the three lower chakras may burn one out sooner than later. There are many types of meditation. To access the eternal "beyond time and space" part of your being, you must first learn how to relax without falling asleep.

Here's a universal form of meditation which you may wish to integrate into your current spiritual practice: Assume any comfortable position in which you can relax your body, and bring your attention just above and between your two eyebrows, located in the center of your forehead.

With eyes closed, look gently ahead of you, as if you were looking into a television screen about 7 or 8 inches directly in front of you. Don't strain your physical eyes as you gently gaze into the middle of whatever you see. You may see swirling darkness, lights of different colors, bright white or golden light, the sensation of traveling through a tunnel or even flying through inner space. If you just see blackness, look into the middle with more attention and light will eventually sprout forth. Whatever you see and experience, know it is not being seen by your physical eyes but by the subtle faculty of the soul's inner sight. The spiritual center of perception is called the "3rd eye", "the single eye", 'the inner eye" and many other names in different spiritual traditions.

This inner Light is actually emanating from higher dimensions of reality beyond the physical universe. This light is keeping us alive. Even the life-energy found in living foods are a transmuted form of this same non-physical light.

At one point, you'll also hear an Inner Sound, which can be thought of as the "flip-side" of this Inner Light. This Inner Sound is not being heard by your physical ears but by the soul's intrinsic ability to hear. This Divine Melody itself has been called "Om", "the Word", "Music of the Spheres", "the Voice of Silence", "Holy Sound", "Tao', and many other titles.

Like the Inner Light, this Inner Music is reverberating from the inner planes of creation beyond the physical realm. Both the Light and the Sound can transport the soul to its True Home beyond the physical, astral and causal planes to the realms of Pure Spirit. Meditating on the Inner Light and Sound is a way of experiencing your soul directly. All the answers to life and the universe are present in these two primal manifestations of the God/Goddess principle. Ask and it shall be given, seek and ye shall find. In your asking for guidance, you may be led to a spiritual Master who will escort you into inner space, help you throughout life, even at the time of your rebirth.

Paradise Found

After the publication of Survival, I traveled to several continents to spread the message of living foods and higher consciousness. During this time, only a few people really knew the extent of my own health challenges. I naturally sought to keep my personal health issues confidential, not wanting my students, clients and the people buying/reading my books to know I had chronic migraine headaches associated with high acidity and low enzyme levels. I also had a lot of emotional "demons" from my youth that I carried into my adult life. When I discretely sought the advice of colleagues and other health practitioners, I often didn't follow through on their wise counsel.

So you could say I've been one of the slow learners to my own health advice! However, when I was 50 years old and I was sick and tired of being sick and tired, I finally got serious about getting rid of my persistent headaches and other signs of imbalance.

I created an individualized program for myself and began to experience more positive results. My program consisted of: frequent small meals, eating only when stomach was really empty, food concentrates of enzymes and Super

Blue Green Algae, drinking plentiful amounts of toxin-diluting water, sufficient rest, yoga, meditation, chiropractic adjustments, weight-lifting, cultivating right relationship with significant others, learning better communication skills to express my needs and sharing more love with others and with myself. When I finally approached my own health holistically, on ALL levels, only then did I begin to feel the buoyant joy of what it feels like to be healthy in body, emotions, mind and spirit.

So be honest with yourself and see where you can be more in alignment with the laws of the universe. Seek the help and support you desire to be reborn. Come from your heart by living a life of truth and love. Discover your gifts and share them with the world. Everyone can find ways to serve, even if one is physically disabled and can't even get out of bed. How? By warmly expressing your gratitude to those who serve you! Paradise is within you and me and everyone. We can and will bring this paradise out into the world with visualization, meditation, focused intention and right action. We will do it... i believe in us.

In closing, let me state the eternal truth that love can travel beyond the limitations of earthbound time and space. Although we may not as yet have met physically, as you read these words I send you my love, without conditions, directly from my heart to yours. Can you feel it now? Take it in deeply and go out and spread your own love with others.

Love in service,
We are One,
All is Love
Enzymatically Yours

Rev. Viktoras Kulvinskas MS

www.youthing101.com - includes free newsletter
Viktoras, PO 2853,, Hot Springs, AR , 71914

"And in those days
the children shall begin to study the laws,
And to seek the commandments.
And to return to the path of righteousness.

"And the days shall begin to grow many
And increase amongst those children of humans
Till their days draw nigh to one thousand years, and to greater
number of years than (before)
was the number of days.

"And there shall be no old people
Nor one who is not satisfied with ones days,
For all shall be as children and youths.

"And all their days they shall complete
and live and peace and in joy ...

(The Book of Jubilees, XXIII: 26-30, Vol. II, p 49)

Dear Ones (2006),
It is time to prepare for no time. Not many are! Are you the one?

Mayan calendar ends 2012. By then we will have reached the critical mass (10% of the population) for a consciousness paradigm shift In this new Millenium, the birth of the psychic (Indigo) children, with 99 th monkey effect, will initiate the surviving Earthlings to experience at-onement.

At-onement is a time of psychic connection between all beings. It is similar, to the co-operation, that exist between the cells in your body, likewise we will have co-operation between all earthlings. Lies and deceit will be extinguished in all relations. Co-operation, care and sharing will be the basis for all transactions. The Garden of Eden life will evolve into manifestation, within pockets of the 'no age' civilization.

Change is not pleasant, especially when it could be very turbulent. Weather the de-population will be due to plagues (as predicted by so many psychics, as well as in the conservative Readers Digest 11/99) or due to chemtrails or man initiated catastrophes or some other earth change phenomena, it is a certainty. Separations from strangers and loved ones is hard. One needs to be in the awareness, that the departed are going back to safe zone for further education. Also, you will see many of them again, as your family of close reincarnates. You can definitely anticipator the surviving Earthlings, will be those who are aligned with Mother Nature - as was predicted in my book Survival in the 21st Century, over 35 years ago.

The survivors, will be on a green whole organic food oriented diet, within a rainbow of color, where blue/purple plays a key role in the vibrationally opening of the higher centers, and making the Earthlings connected and communicating on a psychic level, while being aligned with their darhma (life purpose) and the creator of us all.

The ingesting of greens will protect you from the intensity of the Zodiac and solar (as well as man made) radiation. Actually, you will feel energized by this radiation, which will be destructive to all those who are not biologically prepared. On a predominately (at least 80%) enzymatic raw plant based nutrition, one will, within a period of several years, overcome all diseases and become invulnerable to the energy of the changes. Ones consciousness will reach high level of intuition, thus just like all wild life forms, one will be psychic and one will migrate from the areas of danger, months or even years ahead.

Most people are brain dead due to lack of oxygen, ie they are anemic. With technology consuming oxygen four times faster than created by the life forms, the oxygen level of planet have dropped radically. The only solution to oxygen starved brain, more greens in diet, (especially wheatgrass and blue green algae) which will heal anemia and lead to maximum levels of oxygen transport. Thus the dormant 95% of the brain will once again be fully functional.

The future looks bleak, for most earthlings. The Georgia Monuments - written in eight most widest read languages - The intent by those in 'power', is to reduce world population to 500,000,000
http://www.crystalinks.com/gaguidestones.html

Let these be a guidestone to an age of reason.
Georgia Monuments " Maintain humanity under 500,000,000 in perpetual balance with nature.; Guide reproduction wisely - improving fitness and diversity. Unite humanity with a living new language. ; Rule Passion - Faith - Tradition - and all things with tempered reason. ; Protect people and nations with fair laws and just courts. '; Let all nations rule internally resolving external disputes in a world court. ; Avoid petty laws and useless officials. ; Prize truth - beauty - love - seeking harmony with the infinite. ; Be not a cancer on the Earth - Leave room for nature."

One of the daily evident signs of future doom is in our sky, the chemtrails, reflecting, on part of the non-sustainable global hierarchy, an attempt to slow down the greenhouse effect. They believe that through daily spraying all the world population centers with a metallic cocktail of polymer threads embedded with 'biological material' (among them is mold retardant) they can protect the toxic masses.

http://www.carnicom.com/
http://www.willthomas.net/Chemtrails/How_To_Stop_Chemtrails.htm;
http://www.willthomas.net/Chemtrails/chemtrail_video_download.htm
http://www.lightwatcher.com/chemtrails/smoking_gun.html; http://www.holmestead.ca/chemtrails/waynehall.html

"The question of why polymer threads embedded with 'biological material' have been found in residues from aerosol spraying, the insider (given the pseudonym 'Deep Shield') explained that 'since the suspended particles eventually do settle into the lowest part of the atmosphere and are inhaled by all life forms on the surface, there is an attempt to counter the growth of mold by adding to the mixture mold growth suppressants, some of which may be of biological material.'

Deep Shield acknowledged the potential of the aerosol spaying to cause sickness: 'Some people are more sensitive to the metals, while others are sensitive to the polymer chemicals. It is true that people will get sick, and some will die. The World Health Organization has carried out most of the relevant studies. Some have said the ill effects will be minimal, along the lines of a million or so, while others have found the numbers to be far higher – 3 or 4 billion. The Accepted Estimated Casualties (from the World Health Organization) is 2 billion over the course of six decades. The majority will be either the elderly or those who are prone to respiratory problems.'

Emphasizing the 'globalist' aspects of the operations and the need to 'ensure the chemicals are not tampered with' Deep Shield claims that 'they are mixed and sprayed over random nations. This means that chemicals produced in the USA have a good chance of being sprayed over Russia. Russian planes may be seen in US skies, but so too will US planes be seen in Russian skies. The canisters are sealed in a third nation that has no idea where its canister is going. All of this is to ensure that the shield is not used as a weapon. Non-participant nations are sprayed by participant nations, who must spray in order to get enough material to maintain their nation's shield. It is understood that not spraying is as much a military offense as shooting at the planes.'

One implication of this spraying of non-participant nations by 'participant nations' is that, following the defeat of Saddam Hussein's Ba'ath regime in Iraq, all of the Middle East – possibly including Israel, where spraying has started in recent months – is now being sprayed from bases in Iraq.

According to Deep Shield ordinary commercial aircraft are involved in the particulate scattering operations and are not diverted from their regular flight paths. 'But the combined resources of the nations of earth are not enough to allow constant spraying. Though we have achieved a high level of technology, there is a great surface area that needs to be covered nearly daily. Large sections of ocean are all but ignored. The remaining land masses are more than what can be covered efficiently.

Far from seeing his work as something to be proudly publicized, Deep Shield sees the existing secrecy as necessary to maintain public calm for as long as possible: 'The Earth is dying. Humanity is on the road to extinction. Without the shield, mankind will die off within twenty to fifty years. Most people alive today could live to see this extinction take place. This means that an announcement of the situation we face boils down to telling every man, woman and child on earth that they have no future, they are going to be killed. People
would panic. There would be economic collapse, the production and movement of goods would collapse. Millions would die in all cities on earth. Riots and violence would reduce civilian centers to rubble within days.'

The secrecy of the sunscreen project was justified to him, Deep Shield says, on grounds of national security. 'All those who know are expected to remain silent. All those who suspect are either faced with trying to prove the virtually un-provable or are faced with good enough reasons to remain silent. I would assume that this situation is worldwide and this could be considered as one of the dangers of the project. I can see why there is a desire to repress the information, not that spraying is taking place but the face that we are facing a period of human history which might be the end of civilization."

The past systems, as well as present used in population control
http://educate-yourself.org/nwo/nwopopcontrol.shtml   and the future
http://educate-yourself.org/mc/mctotalcontrol12jul02.shtml
http://www.geocities.com/lord_visionary/thegeorgiaguidestones.htm

<u>How strong are we. We are god/dess like and can survive</u>
1. Fire walking - as well as Daniel and other Essenes in the Ovens, or lion den untouched. We transcend the reality, by state of thoughts and feelings and beliefs.
2. The explosion at the Union Carbon India plant (1985) - folks who did the 'fire ceremony" were untouched by the deadly gas.
3. Hiroshima - a Christian Monastery, within the circle of death, totally unaffected and the monks who watched the event in their service, were totally unharmed..

Attitude and belief systems. Combine EQ within IQ under the spiritual   at-onement and we can change ourselves as well as handle any crises.

Love in the light, We are One, ALL is Love All Ways ---- Viktoras
<u>The Future Looks Bright</u>
Originally written in Hebrew, fragments of twelve manuscripts were discovered among the Dead Sea Scrolls. The Book of Jubilees dates itself to the time of Moses and was possibly written by him. Jubilees is a polemical pseudepigraph featuring an Angel of the Presence, whom it portrays as addressing Moses on Sinai, " predicting the future". The work reveals secret laws that Moses kept from Israel at the time of the original revelation. Only now, says the book, can these secrets be known.... see the End of The 2-22-2002 Introduction
- The Book of Jubilees, XXIII: 26-30 For more, visit,
Viktoras4u.com   viktorasretreats@gmail.com

DEDICATION

To my mother, whose love, courage and assistance made this original work possible. To my father who influenced my life in many subtle ways to pursue the path of truth. To my wife Youkta, whose dedication and love, as well as her wisdom and focus on the path of truth, has kept me in the light. To all my readers, who encouraged me.

SPECIAL THANKS

Katharine Clark, a dear friend, inspiration and leader, who made it possible the printing of this edition.

ACKNOWLEDGMENTS

I am indebted to the many friends who cooperated in the creation of this book. My deepest thanks to Hermine Hurlbut who worked with me over the years as an editor, experimenter and helper in the structuring of the book. I am grateful to Joan Newman for her reading, suggestions and editing. My thanks to Louis Acker who kindly shared his manuscripts on Yoga; to Christine Goursky who assisted in compiling the section on Color; to Ken Keyes, who inspired me with his radiant lifestyle for allowing me to include the chapter on happiness from his book; to Johnny Lovewisdom for his spiritual dietetics.

I thank Jean White, who gives joy and life to the sacrificial paper with her art images for sharing her visions with us. My gratitude is extended to David Base and Margaret Geiger who did the Zone Chart of Reflexology and to Ed Jordan who introduced me to and assisted me in the technology of publishing.

My thanks to Professor Hilton Hotema and Dr. Raymond Bernard of Health Research Publications for their writings on longevity, sex and diet. I am grateful to Professor Edmund Bordeaux Szekely for permission to quote the many inspirational passages from the "Essene Gospel of Peace" and to Dr. Jensen for allowing quotations from his excellent book on iridology to be reproduced. I thank Dick Gregory for his friendship and inspirational lifestyle proving the possibility of the fruitarian path. Last, but greatest in importance I thank Dr. Ann Wigmore who founded the Hippocrates Health Insitutute in Boston, Massachusetts and who continues her work and teaching on natural living.

Furthermore, I acknowledge my indebtedness to the forerunners of the new culture who greatly influenced me both in person and through books thereby helping me to ascend from disease and ignorance: L. Hamilton, H. G. Bieler, Adele Davis, M. Kushi, H. Shelton, T. De La Torre, J.H. Tilden, E. Krebs Jr., N. W. Walker, B. Hunter, W. H. Fitzgerald, A.C. Guyton, and A. Ehret.

I want to thank the personnel at the Harvard Medical Library and the Massachusetts Institute of Technology Library for assistance and permission to use the facilitities for research. A word of deep thanks to the many brothers and sisters who asked me questions, shared their secrets and offered me guidance. Also, my special thanks to clients, friends and far away acquaintances who experimented with me in the many phases and aspects of natural healing and diet.

My silent thanks goes to the angels and elves for guidance in the writing and publishing of this book especially for their assistance in format design, layout and paste—up. Also, I am highly indebted to the staff of Casle Publications, especially to Robert Phinney, Bob Ryan, and to Brenda and her assistants who made the printing of this book possible.

Within the context of the book, I have attempted to give credit to the sources of the quotations and various ideas which have been incorporated into the text. Because of the extensive number of reference sources cited and the difficulty experienced in contacting the authors in order to obtain quotation privileges, I want to thank all of them here for making it possible to extend the boundaries of human knowledge through the sharing of their discoveries.

TABLE OF CONTENTS

Book VI, HOW TO BE HAPPY.

BOOK VII APPENDICES

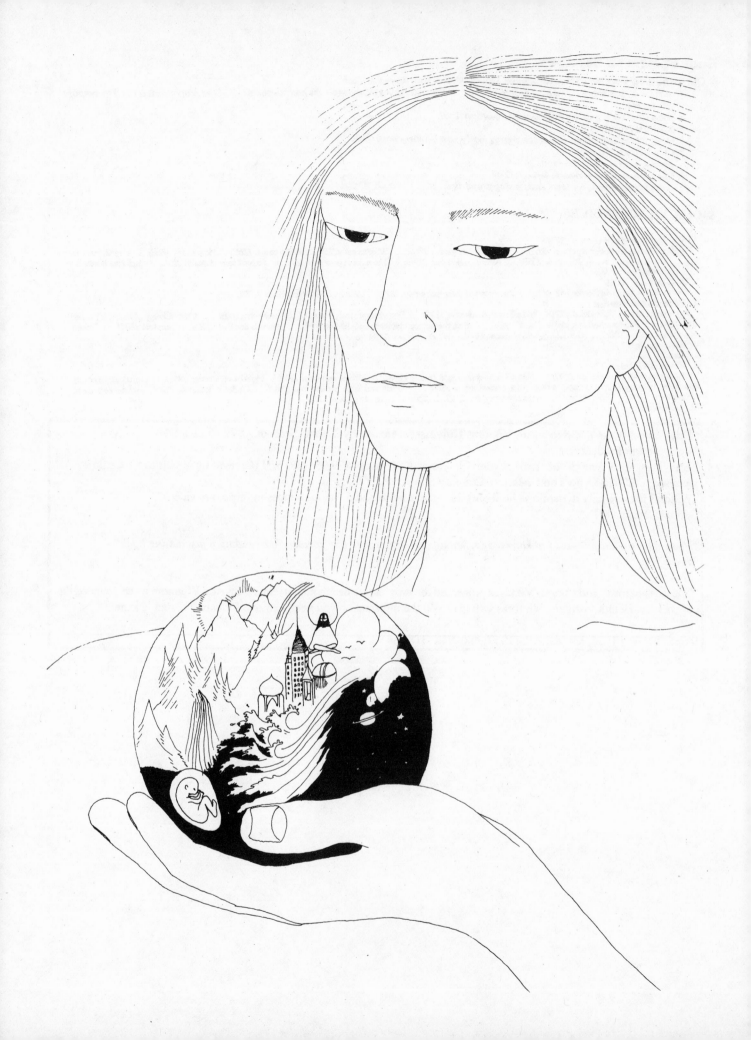

INTRODUCTION

Brothers and Sisters,

What you all fixin' to do about what's comin' down so fast? Have you figured out yet what they're doin' to you — how they're manipulatin' your body through the food you eat and the medicine you take; manipulatin' your mind through what you read and watch on t.v.; manipulatin' you through schools and churches so you ain't got no mind to say "boo"? "They" is the CIA — FBI — One World Government, a handful of greedy, power hungry white men fixin' to see that no one feels joy, happiness and peace within. Take a good long look at this land of the free and home of the brave and how it's directed by them. They pitted the white folks and black folks against each other and sat back to watch that movie. They got you with the t.v. What's on Saturday mornin' for your children? Cartoons, right? Wrong. They got yellin' and fightin', threatenin' and thrashin', violence and murder right in your livin' room. Where's the love and friendship valued so highly in this land? Then for the big folks they got the six o'clock news — only 'stead of cartoons they got what looks like real pictures of real folks doin' the same thing! They got the educational system together to teach you how to make a livin'. Y'all know how to make a livin', but how come y'all don't know how to live?

With all of what you got, are you happy? You got no cavities from usin' toothpaste, security from buyin' that life insurance, protection from fire, a car to drive your kids to and from wherever, frozen t.v. dinners cause you're too busy watchin' soap operas to get it together and there's Kentucky Fried Chicken on the weekend or when guests unexpectedly drop in and walk over your shiny waxed floors. There's hamburger extenders for mothers who want to feed their family the best while living on a shoe string budget. Course, it don't matter its full of saw dust and sugar. Or maybe it'd be safer to eat the shoe string: good bulk for tired Americans. So tired they need laxatives to dump out everything they dump in?

Ever read the labels on food packages? They think so little of your intelligence they list all the stuff they put in your food to kill you! You see twelve words you can't pronounce and you eat it anyway. All them chemicals, preservatives, sugar and poisons they add to food — that ain't nutrition, that's behavior modification! America is the number one hoarder of money, land, natural resources, and food. We eat more food more often than any other nation, and then carry it around inside for seven weeks, seven months, seven years, seventy years. That's why you all stink. Your armpits, your bad breath, they're tellin' you that you stink from what you eat! From what's rottin' inside of you.

Take care of your bodies — Please! Try living seven days with no sugar. NO SUGAR. Try seven days with no poisoned, sprayed—with—insecticides, pesticide—laden food. See how you feel. You'll learn somethin' about bein' chemically manipulated when you give your body one weeks rest from all that poison. Remember to pray a lot too. When you start fixin' to take care of yourself by deprogrammin' from the poisoned robot manipulation, freedom will flourish throughout the world.

Tune into the God Force locked inside your head! The only thing they can't manipulate is your spiritual power. They can poison the water — you can distillyour own and drink pure water; they can spray all the fruits and vegies — you can grow your own sprouts and plant unradiated seed now, for fresh food and healthy seed for next year's planting. Throw out the t.v. and tune into universal channel of love. Wear natural fibers — cotton and wool — and let your body breath. You can start askin' lots of questions in your prayers and listen for the answers. They can cut off your arms and legs, blind you, and make you sick, but even the most powerful physical force on the planet cannot TOUCH your spiritual power. Choose your way: Absence of death or the presence of life.

There's a handful of us out there committed with our lives to make this world work right, cause we believe it can be. If I had to give up my life in the mornin' I got no problems, cause I got brothers like Viktoras who balance out all the negativity on the planet. There's not another mind on the planet when it comes to nutrition that knows as much about the body with such integrity as Brother Viktoras. Don't know no book that talks as much as this-"Survival Into The 21st Century". There's a whole lot of folks out there who love what you're doin', Viktor, and a whole lotta folks out there is gonna be alive when the mess comes down because of you. Whole lotta folks love your book "Love Your Body" cause that, friends, is what it is all about! Look after your bodies, your minds, and your spirits — please! You got 62,000 miles of blood vessels in your bodies — understand the beauty and mystery of its needs and its life force that keeps on keepin' on. Treat your body right — you deserve it. Do light exercise, walk, breathe through your nose, stretch your muscles, preserve your sexual fluid, eat right — no chemicals, no sugar, no processed government food. And pray!

Get up early one morning, look yourself in the mirror, realize what you see — there ain't another you in the entire universe. That should let you know you are somethin' special. Regardless of what you think of yourself, you are somethin' special, so treat yourself special. Take a load off your mind. Give up all hatred, violence and anger — carryin' that around hurts you and everybody else. YOU CAN TURN IT AROUND. Get in touch with yourself from the place of protection within you and let go of fear. Love yourself and one another. That's what it's all about. Nothin' else. I love you. God Bless. And peace be with you Always!

March 1, 1981
Bristol, Rhode Island

Dick Gregory

PREFACE

Dear Brothers and Sisters: We are living in a most challenging age. Love is the only reality that can resolve the dilemma of our time. Materialism is dead. It has been composted by today's youth to fertilize the seed of love and spirituality. Materialism has served its purpose. The ugliness and suffering about us have made us more appreciative of tenderness, beauty, grass and trees. Psychedelic drugs have weakened us to our overwhelming need to experience spiritual reality.

"February, 1962, ushered in the Aqarian Age — the age of light. This light is a power that can construct or destruct." The transition from the era of Pisces and materialism into the sign of Aquarius and spirituality is the stage for current events. Each passage of an age has been attended by drastic alterations in the spiritual, philosophical, psychological, social, economic and scientific structures of humanity.

Abuse of nature's laws is bringing about a major ecological healing crisis of the earth. One does not make superior wine in the dregs of an old cask. Nature will eliminate congestion in order to establish the original purity of earth. The world will become an insane asylum and war will be its therapy. Misuse of the sexual functions and over—population will be cured by famine and pestilence. Darkness from air pollution will be filtered out through the lungs of billions of asthmatics, victims of lung cancer and respiratory disorders, so that the light of cosmic radiation may once again play on our bodies and nourish our consciousness.

Do not be troubled by unhappy events predicted. They will all come to pass. We are not evolved enough to circumvent the tragedies induced by cosmic cycles. Suffering will rejuvenate the spiritually dormant who will learn of the oneness of all in God through love.

The next several years are crucial to our survival. Do not expend energy complaining about environmental disasters. Work toward a change. Unloving thoughts and internal body pollution from an unhygienic diet are far more devastating to health and well—being than external environmental factors.

If you are not getting anywhere — stop, don't try. Be where you are. You have to start somewhere, so start by seeing yourself as you are at this second.   Maybe you're a slob, eat like a pig, are lustful, take drugs, cheat. steal, procrastinate, are filled with little secrets and lies — and more. No one could love you, if they only knew. So what?

Accept yourself. The past has been good, for it has brought you to this moment of consciuosness. The Kingdom of Heaven is within; it can be unlocked through self—love. Then it becomes very easy to love others. Everything becomes easy. Nothing can hurt you.

God has a plan. There are no accidents. Don't complain about seeming badness. Get into God's trip. Listen in silence. God is calling all of us.

Everything is going according to the cosmic plan. In our present patriarchal world the desire to control Nature has created the conditions on this planet — poisonous chemicals, pollution, war, murder, famine, plague. and the rape and devaluation of women.

Chemicalized and junk foods, liquor and Madison Avenue conditioning have made us sick. Likewise, they have made us pause to question our pop—a—pill—for —what—ails—you culture. These poisons are sacred. They have been our teachers. Bless them and thank them.

Intellectuals heard about the Indian Yogis who were in superhigh states. We americanized their highs and tripped out into a beautiful color, cybernetic nature and became non—violent on pot and LSD. These were short highs. So the drugs were dropped in the pursuit of the 24 hour—a—day high of the Yogis. Let us bless the drugs for introducing us to the heaven within.

Pollution has its blessings. It has forced many away from an unnatural city life to the vibrant healthy life in the country.

The insecticide manufacturer, the AMA, the FDA and the mad bomber are working together very hard with the saints. and with you and me, to purge ourselves of the thousands of years of materialism in order to speed the emergence of the most beautiful age. We have to purify ourselves, hence the path of suffering and death for many. especially for those who fail to discover through suffering the laws of Nature and of God. Those who have become aware of these laws and are living by them have already influenced many. More and more of our brothers and sisters are purifying their bodies through diet and exercise, raising their consciousness through loving acts and meditation, and planting the seeds of blooming themselves.

YOU CAN SURVIVE. The spirit is timeless. In this book, I present ways to survive and prepare for the new world to come. Be not dismayed when you seem to be alone in the pursuit. Remember, "Few are chosen". Your close friends and family may ridicule you. Let them not offend or provoke you. Love them just the same — do not fight back. Teach others by your example, not with empty words. "You shall know them by their deeds."

The coming deluge will herald a civilization based on the universal timeless teachings of the ancient masters and the disinherited healers of history: women. Survivors will be few — no more than ten percent of the earth's population. They will be conscious of Nature's laws and of the corrective measures evoked by disobedience. From the dying age of intellect and materialism, a new cosmic marriage will occur. Spirit and intellect will sit side by side upon the throne of world unity. Theological speculations are gasping their last breath. The religious care but little for dogma and metaphysical games. The new earthlings want to experience spiritual realities. They are drawn to philosophies that blend body, mind and spirit under a single cosic view. The new religious orders have large followings and you can find them everywhere — Krishna Consciousness, Meher Baba, Kirpal Singh, Zen, Macrobiotics, Yoga, Bah'ai, study of the Ancient Masters, the search for and discovery of woman dieties, and many others too numerous to mention.

In a few generations, death will come by choice; sex as we know it today will have disappeared: the majority of earthlings will be breatharians; people will travel at will by astral projection; the mind will be once again purified and tuned in to function on the extra sensory level; people will become co−creators with God; and the world be ruled and united by the power of love. The individual will have no needs other than the desire for self−perfection and the fuller attainment of consciousnessas. A Greek philosopher has said, "Worship the Gods, if you must; but your first duty is to find out who and what you are yourself". Know yourself and you will know all. "The kingdom of Heaven is within." You are a microcosm of the macrocosm. Your body is built of an infinite number of molecular planets which are inhabited by an infinite number of beings no less conscious than yourself. You are God. Be good to yourself.

Be conscious. Alexis Carrel, Nobel Prize winner, asserts that today's individual uses only one millionth of his or her brain cells. We have the greatest adventure open to us as we devote ourselves to the exploration and application of this nerve cell labyrinth that places the powers of the universe at our disposal. In the Bible, it is clearly expressed that we are created in the image of God − all perfect, all powerful, all knowing, all present: it is up to us to claim our birthright.

For those who seek this path, this book contains useful information on how to start the awakening of dead bodies through rejuvenation regimes, how to obtain nourishing food inexpensively, and what physiological changes one can anticipate as one activates dormant cells. You can rebuild your body. It is built to live indefinitely. Every cell in your body is replaced in one to seven years. You can be young at any age.

I present to you alternatives, not unqualified ultimatums. To remove the confusion from dietary philosophies, I have examined Kosher, vegetarian, macrobiotic, sproutarian, fruitarian, aquarian, and breatharian paths in the light of scientific documentation and spiritual qualifications.

This book is designed to reach the inner being on the level of simplicity. It is the first real challenge to the concept of a high protein diet and the alternative most frequently suggested, a high starch diet. This book represents five years of preparation which involved two years of background study at the Harvard Medical Library, intensive self−experimentation, and, as co−director of the Hippocrates Health Institute, Boston, Massachusetts, observation of the rejuvenation of many people who I guided into the live food diet.

The guidelines in this book will not be restrictive. You will naturally gravitate toward dietary changes if you let your body guide you. Heightened discrimination of taste and smell as well as enduring vitality will assure you of the Truth as you simplify your lifestyle. The hygienic path will give you more freedom and time to participate in the non−destructive pleasures of living.

Never settle for less than complete compatability of your best knowledge and practice. As you grow, new teachers will continue to appear, each one leading you toward self understanding and the bliss that comes from living in the universal love consciousness.

This is a most exciting time to live, a time of cosmic high. Cataclysms of global scope have been foretold for the near future by many prophets and seers. Powerful astrological forces will soon come into play: a planetary alignment is forecast for 1984; it will be preceded by the Jupiter/Uranus alignment of March, 1983. Such alignments have historically coincided with widespread cataclysmic activities, and in this specific age, could lead to great earthquake and volcanic activity, which are likely , in turn, to trigger a nuclear holocaust of N−power plants and stored weapons, as well as fires and explosions from stored chemicals, gases, and other toxic substances.

We can work to create harmony or be careless and lose the billions of years of earthly evolution. The Bible includes many stories where planetary disasters were offset by the cooperative action of a dedicated people . A life oriented toward prayer, love, fasting, and service can so help to alter the vibrational field of the planet such that the gravitationally induced cataclysm will not occur. The renowned clairvoyant and prophet Edgar Cayce has said emphatically that the actions and the applied morality of a people can temper or sometimes postpone or avert disaster.

The most important work an individual can do to prepare for planetary survival is:

− chew daily on wheatgrass: absorbed immediately in the mouth, it will afford protection against pollution, radiation, chemical carcinogens, and emotional depression (see text for additional details).
− love yourself and others unconditionally.
− increase body consciousness through continuous dietary transition as body sensitivity demands changes towards higher purity. A diet of at least 80% raw food , with emphasis on the rejuvenating indoor greens and sprouts is essential to counteract the planetary contamination effect.
− work hard to improve the planet and stay detached from the results
− remember daily in prayers and meditation that we are perfect, have been perfect, and will continue to be perfect as we live in a world that allows our evolutionary perfection to manifest through the daily challenges presented by the Divine.

We are given a chance to reap the fruits of action born in love of life. Thoughts dominated by love precipitate loving acts. Love is what everyone wants. The giver is always loved. Two people loving create the oneness of spiritual consciousness. The more there is of loving the less fragmentation and the more oneness. We must be positive in our acts. Praise, never condemn. It will bring perfection and harmony in every soul. The body will be healed by eating with love and living in love. The life of today is just a moment in eternity, a continuation of our many rebirths on earth, our passage to the next adventure of spiritual evolution, if only we dedicate ourselves to service, love and non−attachment.

Go out to your brothers and sisters. Ask nothing. Give everything. Lovingly accept what is offered. Love when nothing is offered. Sing in praise for a chance to serve, not because others need help, but because you may become one with them. In helping you are helped. All have something to teach.

But in your desire to serve, don't lay your trip on anybody. It's all right for us all to be different even though we are one -the cop, the politician, the soldier, mother, father, pacifist, and general - in God. Raw foodism is good, but love your brother and sister who eat meat - that is their trip; if they want to be balanced on salted rice, they are right. Don't argue, don't create a disharmony of hate by trying to force your way.

Just give. Give. Give. The more you give, the more you have. You are enriched when you give up material possessions. This uncovers spiritual richness and contentment with "nothing" which becomes everything when immersed in the radiance of loving and living in the moment.

We must work with the universal principles of nature. To return to the Garden of Eden: detoxify the body; move to or create a more natural environment; work with the earth; establish a spiritual life-style; create in each succeeding generation more perfect beings. As the sunshine returns, let us promise that neither we nor our children will ever forget our true Mother.

In a few generations, every child will be a genius housed in the body of an Atlas or Athena. And they will be beautiful, surpassing all our standards. What is considered a miracle today will be, in the new era, a common occurrence. We will learn, as did the ancient ones, to work will the laws of Nature in harmony with the rhythm of love.

Love is the utterance one felt, feels, will feel when one is in Christ (Buddha . . .) Consciousness. The flood of euphoria will heal every sickness in your body. Your face will be the sunshine in every heart. You will heal with a glance. You will know everything . . . and nothing.

Love is the music of the universe. It needs no language. Stones understand it, birds sing it, and the universe vibrates to it. Love feels good because it is real — it unites us into one Godhead.

As you read this book, I invite you to explore the mysteries of the human body, spiritual potentials and strange powers of the mind. I share with you the path of natural living which I have learned from many teachers, from personal experimentation and from the experiences of thousands of brothers and sisters who have shared their visions.

Be joyous! New men and women are returning armed with their souls. Let us dance in the timeless bosom of the universe filled with the darkness of light that thundeers the OM ecstacy.

Peace and love in our time.

2002 MESSAGE TO THE READERS

I wish to express my appreciation to all the wonderful friends that I have made through the book. You have been my inspiration, my teachers and my greatest allies. You are the people who are transforming the planetary choices and reconnecting the society & culture back to the natural. A century of peace is at hand. The best way for getting the full benefit of this book, is to read the introduction to feel the new Millenium impact..

The information in this book is not intended to be prescriptive. In spite of the safety and simplicity of the programs suggested for persons suffering from chronic debilitating conditions, for optimal results and for additional guidance, the author suggest that all should consider to be under supervision of health care practitioner, who is versed in enzymatic nutrition, cleansing and detox, crises management and withdrawal symptoms under dietary change. Considering that the everyday environment of the individual, is what created the debilitating conditions, the author feels most people would do well to go for at least a three week program at one of the live food centers. If need extra guidance, may emal to viktoraslive@yahoo.com.

The book makes no claim as to offer a cure for aches and pains, colds or chronic conditions, like cancer, diabetes, arthritis or heart disease. Instead, the book offers you a way intune with Nature's Laws which leads the body to activate the natural inner healing systems, that leads to the return of the body, to its healthy homeostasis.

The natural systems that support healing may not be in accord with the established consensus of the medical profession. The book nor the author profess to diagnose, treat or prescribe any treatment for disease. The information is made available to all those who wish to investigate all known methods of healing. In time of sickness, approach an enzymatically versed health practitioner, for support and guidance. Be prepared to get self diagnosed, as needed by the medical system, then find the best solution, from all the wonderful resources that exist at this time. In case of an accident, it would be wise to use the highly advanced skills and technology of the medical community while working with your chiropractor and other health care practitioners.

The 25 years, since the publishing this book, I have received tens of thousands of successful stories, of the power of the methods, as found in this book. It continues to inspire another generation of youth.

The healing section of the book is written in layman's language. The technical papers cited should be consulted by doctors to evaluate the full potential of the ideas and data.

The publisher can assume no responsibility for improper application or interpretation of the Laws of Nature contained in this manual. No guarantee is implied and all actions pursued as a result of the material contained herein are all the sole risk of the reader. However, we feel that the benefits accruing from such procedures and practices far exceed the consequences of the use of medicine and poisons for therapy. Right nutrition is the key for providing the diseased body with the needed building blocks from which to rebuild itself, with optimal material and minimal stress.

Love in Service

We Are One
All is Love

SURVIVING THE APOCALYPSE

"Go out from her, my people: that you be not partakers of her sins, and that you receive not of her plagues."   Apoc. 18:3

"Blessed is he that readeth and they that hear the words of this prophecy and keep those things which are written therein; for the time is at hand."

"Hada , Hada spread your wings and fly this place
Before the storm begins.
Your face and body are not to suffer harm;
Hada, Hada spread your wings and fly this place."   — Franklin Davis —   THE GOOD FAIRY, in Spanish

"Follow me, and let the dead bury the dead."   Matthew 8:22

"I wish there were some wonderful place called the Land of Beginning Again." —Lois Fletcher— LAND OF BEGINNING AGAIN

". . . EVERYWHERE AT ONCE, ON EVERY PLANET, EVERY WORLD, GOVERNMENTS WERE TOPPLING, CITIES WERE CRUMBLING, WHOLE POPULATIONS WERE RAGING INSANE THRU THE RUINED STREETS, THE TORN COUNTRYSIDE; THE FABRIC OF CIVILIZATIONS WOVEN THRU PAINFUL AEONS HUNG IN TATTERS ON THE RACK . . .

VOICES OF THE FRENZIED INSANITY SHRIEKED FROM NEWSPAPER HEADLINES, RADIOS, TELEVISION TUBES, THE WHOLE NETWORK OF COMMUNICATIONS WAS POPPING, BURNING, FIZZLING IN A MINDLESS HYSTERICAL RELEASE OF ENERGY THAT WAS PURE UNADULTERATED PANIC . . .

'. . . "I SEE THE CRIPPLED PRESSES GASPING LAST BLACK WORDS OF DOOM AS THE INK POTS GO DRY AND PHONE WIRES FUSE TO THEIR INSULATORS, TORN AND BROKEN THREADS OF SPEECH STREWN ACROSS DYING AMERICA . . .'

VOICES OF WONDER SAT AND WATCHED IN CAVES OR FROM THE SHELLS OF BOMBED OUT BUILDINGS. MEN WHO HAD WAITED FOR THIS DAY, MEN WHO HAD KNOWN IT WAS COMING . . . THE WHOLE PERVERTED MESS, FALLING INTO ASHES, A FEW LAST SPASMS OF NUCLEAR HYSTERIA, THEN NOTHING . . . JUST A LIGHT WIND IN THE EMPTY TREES, AND A DUST AND SAND WHIRLING IN THE SILENT STREETS . . ."

—Tom Veitch
from the LUIS ARMED STORY

"These changes are coming, not at random and in chaos (which will be a product of such changes for a time), but these changes are coming of a planned, orderly, spiritual, creative force, that will bring about better conditions for the survival of man as a spiritual being, in harmony and peace with his world, with himself, and with his maker...See?...The purpose of many will be changing, and the emphasis will be put in many different places. Those who resist too much change shall be blown down in a heavy wind...then let the spirit lead thee. Let these changes which   must come take thee gracefully."

Seasons of Changes, Associations of the Light morning.

(Heritage Pub., Virginia Beach)

"Repent ye, for the end of the world is nigh." These seem to be words uttered by some crackpot prophet of doom — they provide a good source of amusement. Harvard Lampoon's parody on LIFE featured a special on "The End of the World," taking a long, last look at the Planet Earth before it dissolves in 'cobra-cola'. Each time a new deadline predicting the end of the world is bypassed, many laugh, saying, "look, we are still alive! Ha, Ha." Then they swallow an assortment of courage pills to tranquilize their nerves facing, by the same token, the prospect of lids closing slowly and mysteriously on their self-made coffins.

The Bible warns of "famine and pestilence." The native of our synthetic jungles, vision blinded by a full stomach, dismisses such forecasts as 'scare messages.' The electronic lips of microwave tom-toms fill the air with words — crime, sex, power failure, violence, rape, drugs, government corruption, inflation, cancer, food shortages, flood, drought, war, disease — as they mesmerize the public into a stupor of the 'norm'. The new native does not know life or death. The new native is insane.

"The mills of the Gods grind slowly, but they grind exceedingly well." Long before Jean Dixon and Edgar Cayce, many prophets were describing events that would occur in our generation – the generation that would see "all things come to pass." Christ said in Matthew 24:6-7, "And ye shall hear of wars and rumors of wars. See that ye be not troubled, for all these things will come to pass. But the end is not yet. For nations shall rise against nations and Kingdoms against Kingdoms. And there shall be famines, pestilences and earthquakes in diverse places."

A Yorkshire woman named Mother Shipton, who was born in 1488 and died in 1561, made this prophesy:

"Carriages without horses shall go,
And accidents fill the world with woe.
Around the world, thoughts shall fly
In the twinkle of an eye.
Under water, men shall walk, shall ride,
Shall sleep and talk.
In the air men shall be seen, and
Covered by hail and snow.
The world to an end shall come
In nineteen hundred and ninetee-one."

The dramatic end to this age will come as a result of one or several of the many triggering mechanisms which we have built into our national life-styles. It could be depression, energy failure, epidemic, war, famine, earthquake, ecological disasters.

We have become enslaved via a debt of 440 billion dollars to the international bankers. We pay out over 20 billion dollars to them yearly in interest. Furthermore, the money made from land speculation, plus unearned interest rates has produced an inflation spiral. Politicians, the military, the medical profession, pharmaceutical firms and the Mafia further contribute to inevitable economic disaster. The poor are becoming poorer slaves. The rich are becoming richer masters. The last depression was planned and controlled. The coming one is going to be total anarchy.

The key signs of oncoming depression or runaway inflation are: a) prime interest and discount rate of Federal Reserve Banks accelerating rapidly – this curtails business expansion and increases shortages of all essential matterials; b) the more vehemently the administration insists that the economy is sound, the more certain you can be of the opposite; c) shortages of food, fuel and goods; d) rapidly rising gold prices.

As mistrust in the economy increases, there will be a run on banks, which will be forced to close on a national level. Since banks hold only twenty percent of the currency needed to back up savings, withdrawal will be impossible. Banks will burn. The lower classes and poor folk who bank are not suicide-prone like the middle class of 1930. Cities will turn into infernos of violence. This will happen over a period of a month.

Spaceship earth is running out of energy and food. There are 3½ billion people on the earth now and the population grows 2 percent annually. Although India increased it crops of food grain, it also increased its population. There are 70 million more Indians to feed since the mid-60s when India began to increase its production. We see this year the pictures of starving live-stock and children in India hit by the monsoons, and those in Africa who are victims of drought.

When the major crisis comes, as nature rebalances herself, the United States may well be the last nation to be hit. But there are already many signs, such as the shortage of gasoline.

Biologist Barry Commoner said at the AAAs convention in Boston in 1970 that it is already too late to stop the population from reaching the eight billion limit the world can support. We will help to feed the world at an estimated figure of about $41 billion a year. "This investment, together with operational costs, would require a sum probably in excess of $10,000 billion in all."

Even if we have this money, there is no new place to plant. Virtually all the land which can be cultivated with known or easily forseeable methods is under cultivation.

Raymond Bouillenne, professor of Botany at the University of Liege, Belguim, according to UP, March 10, 1962, (released by the American Association for the Advancement of Science) says,

"Mankind is gaining 120,000 mouths to feed each day and losing 20 million acres of food-producing land each year . . . We are in the throes of an apparently irreversible reduction of the surface of cultivable land. The area of such lands has decreased by an estimated 20% in the last 100 years. Of the 40 billion acres remaining, at least 20 million disappear irretrievably each year . . . Man the destroyer having wiped out hundreds of animal species is well embarked on a course which threatens his own kind with extinction."

Others fantasize that although land agriculture cannot possibly take care of our food needs, we still have endless resources in the sea which can be tapped so that we can populate the earth until people are jammed, insane, like sardines in a can. They forget that the oceans are civilization's cesspools.

General William H. Draper predicts that in another thirty years, six to eight billion people will be fighting to live on a planet that is not adequately feeding half the number.

Jose de Castro, Director of the World Association for the Fight Against Hunger, and former director of FAO, stated: "Of the sixty million deaths recorded annually in the world, thirty to forty million must be attributed to malnutrition." (Black Book of Hunger).

Thomas M. Ware, Head of the Freedom from Hunger Foundation, testified before a Senate subcommittee: "Very few grasp the magnitude of the danger that confronts us . . . The catastrophe is not something that may happen; on the contrary, it is a mathematical certainty that it will happen."

At a Senate Government Operations Subcommittee hearing from several Nobel Prize Winners on hunger, Dr. Albert Szent Gyoraui of Marine Biological Laboratories at Woods Hole in Massachusetts, stated that a time will come when "men will kill one another and eat one another."

It is already to late. William and Paul Paddock succinctly stated their case in FAMINE – 1975! (William Paddock is a plant pathologist and agronomist; his brother is a retired foreign service officer). As far as they are concerned, "The people are already here who will cause the famines. Birth control techniques are for the future, they cannot affect the present millions of hungry stomachs."

We have altered dramatically the weather pattern of the globe. By displacing the forests with concrete cities and farmlands, we have created shafts of hot air above such regions so that the temperature rarely drops low enough to lead to condensation of air moisture into raindroplets – hence drought   is the way of the south and west coast of the USA. The cool air of the east condenses on metallic particles spewed from a thousand factories and precipitates. Excessive rains have ruined many of the eastern crops. If these natural forces should destroy enough of the grain crop, the USA will be in a state of FAMINE. Likewise, famine will affect all other countries which are dependent upon our crops. Since 1970, we have lost a major portion of the mung bean, wheat , rice, alfalfa and hay crops.

FOOD IN YOUR POISON

"If you poison us, do we not die?"   Shakespeare

Although Americans are eating more, (in spite of shortages and high food prices), they are receiving less nourishment. Real food, for the most part, is virtually unknown. Most Americans don't care. Their attachment to food is emotional and induced by advertisement. They load their shopping carts with a variety of colorful, unnutritious, plastic foods, saturated with synthetic ingredients. "Oh! But it tastes so good," they exclaim as they endlessly cram their stomachs, but remain unsatisfied.

To help produce our food, farm factories use DDT, Benzene Hexachloride, Lead Arsenate, Calcium Arsenate, Parathion, TEPP, Aldrin, Chlordane, Lindane, Toxaphane and other poisons. In 1951, the quantity of pesticides produced in the United States (274,840,000) was sufficient to kill 15 billion human beings – approximately six times the population of the world[1]. Sales continue to mount.

More and more people are becoming conscious that both shelved and perishable products in the supermarkets can contain a wide array of poisons. The mass media, even as they glorify such products, announce that they are embalmed with over 3,000 questionable chemicals.

The average consumer as defined by scientific literature and popular publications is a phenomenon of the 20th century, with no antecedent in history. There was a time when no one dined on poisons and called it lunch. Food producers are deliberately supplementing the diet with food additives of a toxic nature at the rate of over three pounds per year for every person in America [2].

A stranger in our land, reading labels, might wonder whether American food is too fresh. Almost every package has something added to preserve freshness; BHT, sodium propionate and a host of other preservatives.

After a fresh imitation dinner, a dizzy spell, difficulty in breathing, or a peculiar feeling in the stomach is very common. Some even think it is love when the pulse rate increases and they become feverish. Others turn to the 'imitation life box' for relief from their distress. Every other commercial, served at the rate of 60 doses per hour, encourages food habits that lead to disease or prescribes a potion to alleviate food-induced illness. They lull us into the belief that it is all right to sin as long as we turn to the right product for forgiveness.

Most shoppers in 1970 anticipated the removal of cyclamates from the market. They may instead discover that the fine print on the label warns that the additive may be dangerous to one's health. Yet this chemical is capable of inducing cancer, and recent tests show that calcium and sodium cyclamate can induce chromosome breakage in the human leucocyte in vitro [3] and in rat spermatogonial cells in vito [4]. Its effects are very similar to a type of chromosome damage reported for LSD [5] as well as caffeine [6] when used in large doses.

Likewise you are cheering the projected ban of DDT in 1973. However, California still permits its use on onion, pepper, citrus and alfalfa crops. Six major pesticide companies have decided to fight the government drive to end all but essential use of DDT. Because they have appealed, the question will be turned over to a scientific panel for a ruling; in the meantime they continue to market DDT [7]. You may discover that instead of removing the DDT, manufacturers will combine it with a catalyst which can make DDT less toxic within six hours of application [8], but the studies fail to let us know whether the catalyst is poisonous. Even if it is eventually removed from the American scene, DDT manufacturers will lose only 30% of their market, for they export 70%. We will be importing DDT from foreign countries via air, water and food.

Pesticides are washed into streams and lakes, where they poison the inhabitants to create conditions for the "last Spring" which will follow the 'Silent Spring' of Rachel Carson. In Clearlake, California, where gnats were controlled by pesticides, it was noted that the residue level in plankton was ten parts per million; 2690 parts per million in carnivorous fish; and 2134 parts per million in fat of fish-eating birds (9). If people eat these fish, or any other animal product they further concentrate in their own bodies the chemicals that appear in the animal flesh.

There has been an enormous increase of hepatitis since the introduction of pesticides (10). W. Coda Martin, M.D. reports (11): "It is now believed that the greater number of hepatitis cases may be caused by DDT on the leaves of green vegetables." Other contributing factors are increased pollution in air and water, plus drug use which places a great burden on the liver.

Dr. Knight wrote (12): "It is conceivable that rapid weight loss in animals or humans storing large amounts of DDT could release enough into the blood stream to cause symptoms of acute poisoning. Clinically this seems to occur   "

The United States Public Health Service conducted a survey. They chose 113 volunteers, and took fat samples. 111 of the volunteers, had deposits of DDT in their fat samples ranging from 0 to 68 parts per million, averaging 6.4 ppm. As little as 3 ppm has been found to inhibit heart cytochrome oxidase.

Medical World News for March 14, 1969 reported a Miami University investigation which showed that terminal cancer patients, chosen at random were found to have a high concentration of pesticide residue in liver, brain and fatty tissues. A recent experiment in Hungary reported that the low doses of DDT in the diet of mice produced a high incidence of leukemia in the third generation (13).

These studies do not stop the manufacturers and food producers from introducing stronger poisons each year. The nation's drug manufacturers warned that New York state legislation, which requires written 'informed' consent from a patient given experimental drugs, will seriously impede medical research in New York City (14). The chemical industry is not required to obtain our 'informed' consent in order to medicate our food, air and water. Certainly they do not know the short or long term effects.

An article (15) headlined: "Are Cancerous Chickens Edible?" Yes! People will eat anything. "If tumors are detected on the wing of a bird, the wing could be cut off and used in products like hot dogs and the rest of the bird sold as cut-up chicken — all supposedly without posing a threat to human health."

There are at least 30 known animal diseases which are transmitted to man through mammalian meat (16). Trichinosis is the most widespread example. It affects every sixth person in America; many believe this percentage is even higher. About 5% who are infected, die (17). Salmonella infection, most often traced to animal foods, afflicted at least 20,000 Americans in 1966. The FDA reported 69 known deaths from it in 1967 (18).

The odds are four to one that the next beef steak you eat will come from an animal which has been speeded to the slaughterhouse with the aid of antibiotics and potent hormones (19). Stilbesterol is a female sex hormone used to increase the weight of beef and chicken. The practice of injecting stilbesterol under the skin of the animal was discontinued in 1959 after ten years of approval by the FDA, finally they discovered that residue of the hormone appears in meat.

One farmer used stilbesterol pellets and paste for his chickens. Consumption of this meat caused his four year old son and two year old daughter to develop enlarged breasts and his wife to experience the menstrual period twice a month (19).

Presently, farmers may add the hormone to animal feed. "Today about 80% of the cattle feed marketed, has been treated with stilbesterol." Brazil, which is a big meat eating country, took to fish when charges were circulated that men were being feminized by stilbesterol. Presently, over 20 countries refuse the import of American chicken and beef.

Stilbesterol is recognized as carcinogenic by the National Cancer Institute. It has been shown to cause cancer in mice, guinea pigs, dogs and rats. According to the Federal Act (158): "No residue of additives should be found in edible portions of the animal after slaughter." However, stilbesterol residues were detected in 15 out of 558 samples.

Even minute amounts of estrogen, another female sex hormone, can produce noticeable effects. Three young boys and one girl were using an ointment and hair lotion containing estrogen. They showed signs of darkening of the areolas of the breast. The girl developed pubic hair and vaginal bleeding (1).

It is well known (21) to chemists that subjecting organic compounds to high temperatures produces complex polycyclic compounds by pyrolysis. Several carcinogenics are included in this group of compounds. A benzopyrine (carcinogenic) content, as high as 50 micrograms per kg was found in some instances. It seems to arise from pyrolysis of fat when cooking food. The amount produced increases with increased fat content and longer and closer exposure of the food to the flame. Benzopyrine is found also in all smoked foods. The relatively higher incidence of gastric cancer in Northern Russia and Iceland has been related to the large quantity of smoked fish eaten by the inhabitants of these regions. In a review (22) of cancer-causing properties of benzopyrine, it was found to be quite high in salami, salmon, bacon and provola.

Eating heated fats may be deadly. Animals fed cooked fat die prematurely said Dr. R. Kurkella, University of Helsinki (Zusammen faassiender Vortrag mit Literaturangaben 1968, No. 3 , 57-65). Research have discovered that the more fat a person eats, the shorter will be the life span (246, 247).

Meat, the most perishable (and most expensive) of all foods is also one of the most tampered with. To see exactly how meat is produced one should read the Animal Machine (23) by Ruth Harrison. It is the story of animal factories, where animals may live out their lives in darkness, immobile in steaming pen from birth to death, fed by conveyers containing drugs, antibiotics, tranquilizers, pesticides and hormones. For the best written article on the same subject write to Karen Messer at 308 E. 89th St. New York 10028 for "The Meat On Your Table Comes From Living Creatures."

After an animal is slaughtered, or dies from disease, it is shipped off to the processing house. The meat is doctored up, for the benefit of the gullible public, with aesthetic beautifiers, stink reducers, taste accentuators, color additives, drug camouflagers, nutritive enhancers, bleaching agents and death certificate. No corpse gets such a face lift by the embalmers and with good reason, for the corpse is soon buried, whereas salami, hotdogs, bologna, and chicken may sit on the shelves for months.

Meat is colored red with sodium nicotinate otherwise it would turn yellow-gray. Uneven or excessive application can result in severe sickness, even death. However when such incidents occur they are seldom diagnosed correctly.

At the Congressional Hearing on Meat Inspection (24) it was reported that the sausages, ham, hamburgers, and the hot dogs you eat, may be filled with hog blood, cereals, lungs, niacin, water, detergents and/or sodium sulfide.

The FDA refuses to recognize tests conducted by Dr. Patrick Riley at a London Medical School, where it was shown that BHA, a widely used preservative is carcinogenic. This preservative appears in luncheon meats, such as salami, bologna, and pressed ham, canned meats, peanut butter, canned chicken and other foods. Senator Alan Cranston commented in 1970 that "perhaps they (FDA) consider food processor's interests more than people's interests."

A typical associated press release occured around Thanksgiving 1969: "U.S. finds pesticide in 90,000 turkeys in toxic levels." A few years ago cranberries were found to be unfit companions to the turkey. In Massachusetts alone (25) during a more active month for health inspectors, 250 tons of meat were seized because it was contaminated. Such meat is quite often resold as 4-D meat: dead, dying, disabled or diseased. The winter of 1969, Boston had a month long scandal over the pollution in the slaughter houses of Massachusetts. Someday we are going to be civilized enough to be concerned over the killing and torture that goes on in the same slaughter houses.

ONLY TEN PERCENT of the meat adulterated with pesticides and chemicals, or contaminated with filth and diseased organs is condemned by food inspectors. The other 90 percent gets through to the unsuspecting consumer, so claims Leray Houser of the Health Education and Welfare Department (26).

"In 1965, a total of 711 firms suspected of producing harmful or contaminated consumer products refused to let the FDA conduct inspection . . . the FDA does not have subpoena authority either to summon witnesses or authority to require firms to divulge pertinent records." (2)

A very striking observation about the quality of animal products comes from the lips of the Health, Education and Welfare Secretary, Robert H. Finch, who FEARED THAT WE WOULD BECOME "A NATION OF VEGETERIANS" if there were strict enforcement of pesticide residues in red meat, dairy produce, eggs, fowl and fish (27).

Today we are faced with an external environmental crisis. We can control the inner body environment through good diet, pure water and joyful, positive thoughts. To procure good organic food economically, cooperation is a must. Let us, brothers and sisters, work towards becoming "A NATION OF VEGETERIANS" UNDER A HAPPY GOD, LOVING ONE ANOTHER AND ENJOYING THE EARTH TRIP.

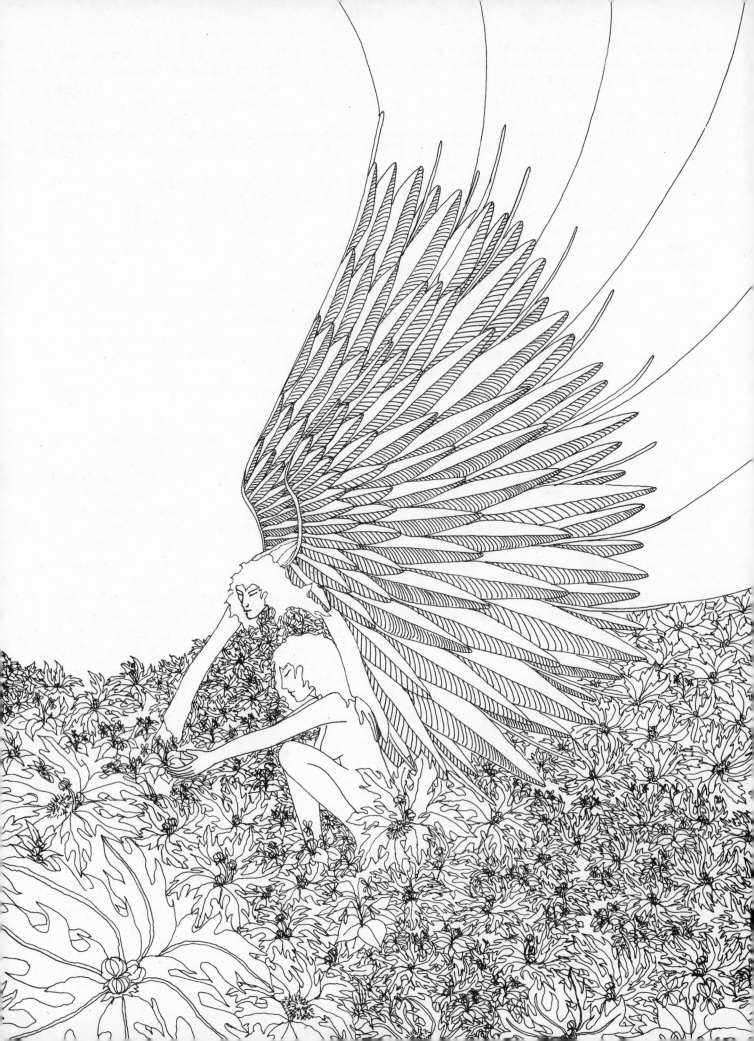

FOOD HUNTING

To serve   survival needs, the wise hunter will pack up   family and belongings, wave the smog goodbye, and set off an a safari to the nearest open farming country. Such a step is extreme for the average concrete-glass-brick caveman. Hence one has to direct one's instinct for organically grown 'game' within the city or through the mail. Presently such survival foods are scarce.

There are, however, growers who harvest such food, "produced on remineralized soil, rich in humus and biologically composed natural fertilizer, without the use of synthetic agricultural chemicals, dust or spray." We call this "organic" or "natural" produce.

To obtain organic produce, start the hunt in the Yellow Pages under the heading "Health Foods" or "Nuts and Seeds". Usually you will find several listings, contact them first. Find out what live foods are available locally. For additional information read local underground ecology papers, commune directories, bulletin boards at occult book stores; request information at Yoga centers and at talk shows.

At the store, purchase only those products marked "organic" or "natural". Read the labels; some health food stores carry foods with perservatives and synthetic additives.

For instance, a company might pick "Mountain Top Organic Juice Inc" for its label. The word "Organic" has nothing to do with the content in the bottle. If the label does not specify "organically grown," then you can be sure that it is no different from the commercial variety expect more expensive. Many farmers who claim to grow organically without insecticides are using compost from non-organic vegetables and commercial cow manure. Some individuals have reported toxicity reactions from eating food grown with this type of compost.

Today, because of heavy pesticide residues, pesticide fallout from neighboring farms, contaminated water and air pollution, it becomes next to impossible to grow food totally organically. This should not discourage you from using organic foods, for they are nutritionally superior. Even when organic food is not ideally grown, the contamination is many times less than in a commercial product.

Generally you are sure of finding organic seed, nuts, dried fruit, honey, sea kelp and oil. An increasing number of natural foods also carry fresh organic fruit and vegetables.

If organic food is not available locally, put in a special order. Purchase in bulk. For example, order a 25 pound bag of carrots, a 40 pound crate of apples, or a bushel of citrus fruit. Do not strive for variety; it can be expensive. It is far better to have apples one month and oranges the next. You will never tire of naturally grown produce. Limit your list to a few staples such as carrots, seed, and salad ingredients. At home, you can grow a variety of greens and sprouts from seed in less than eight days.

If your area has no natural food store, and if you are unwilling to take on the operation yourself, contact one of the local independent grocery store owners, and let him or her supply you. Tell the owner why you want organic produce — no poison, better taste, more nutrition. Tell the owner of sources: suggest that he or she display organic produce next to chemicalized produce and let people choose. The store owner can start with non-perishable staples and work up to fresh produce. The food should be advertised as free from additives or poisons. Once the store owner starts getting natural produce, let your friends and neighbors know where it is available. In Boston a large food chain, Star Market, has an organic food section.

It is much less costly to order directly from an organic food distributor. To cut transportation costs and make the operation economical, you need at least six families to place their organic food orders together. During my 6000 mile journey on Shiloh Farms' produce distribution route, I noticed that many health food stores were started by the desire of one family to obtain quality food. Once the operation gets under way, the size of your organic buying club will grow as fast as the word spreads.

In group purchasing you place an order by mail. When shipments exceed one hundred pounds, delivery by air, rail or truck can cut transportation cost by at least 50% of the cost of parcel post. On orders of 2000 pounds or more, there is a 33% air freight reduction. Use a combination of Yellow Pages, the list in the Appendix of this book, the Organic Food Directory (Rodale Press) and bulletins from local health groups in the search for organic food distributors. Write to several of them, sending a list of the kind and quantity of produce you would like to order monthly. Request an estimate of shipping charges. Once you receive answers to all inquiries, inform your group. Choose a dealer who has the desired produce at reasonable cost and who is close enough to keep your freight charge low. Put the order together, collect the money and make the transaction.

COOPERATIVE BUYING FOR LOW PRICES

As your buying club grows, you may wish to start a cooperative. Presently there are over 37,200 cooperatives nationally, ranging in service from group health plans to nursery schools, from credit unions to health foods. They affect at least 30 million consumers. The co-op is an economic tool created to serve the needs of both the individual and the community.

To start an organic food co-op you will need members and a non-profit charter. You may become better acquainted with the co-op concept by requesting free information from National Cooperatives, Inc., 343 South Dearborn Street, Chicago, 4, Illinois.

Produce is sold at the current market price. Records are kept of each member's purchases. At the end of the year, the cost of the operation is deducted from the receipts. The money saved is either refunded to members proportionate to the amount of individual purchase or reinvested in the co-op. Since there is no middleman, the individual is able to obtain quality produce at a greatly reduced cost.

Every community already has hundreds of health-minded individuals who are looking for quality foods. Publicize the organic co-op in your neighborhood advertisers and through the local vegetarian or hygienic groups. Let your friends and neighbors know. Very soon you will have at least a dozen interested persons.

At the first meeting you should discuss the purchase fund, source of produce, choice of foods, place of distribution and the number of group orders per month. Enlist volunteer workers. You will need someone who has had bookkeeping experience to keep records of the financial transactions.

Since the group will have to send money with the order, you will need an initial investment. It is a good practice to open a checking account in the name of the bookkeeper. Collect the initial sum decided upon by each member. Give a receipt for the investment. This will entitle the member to purchase up to that figure on each order. Hence, if J. Smith deposits forty dollars into the account, he will have the right to a maximum purchase of forty dollars on each order. The co-op investment will limit the size of the group purchase. Upon receiving the food purchase, each customer will have to pay the cost of the order to maintain in the checking account the initial investment of the group. An alternative is to have the customer mail the cost of the purchase with the order. This would eliminate the need for an initial investment.

Begin with a small variety of produce. Become acquainted with the problems of the operation. As the group's trust in the co-op increases, the members may be persuaded to consider an investment in a communal backlog of non-perishable seed — at least one hundred pounds for each man, woman and child. One never knows when a tremendous food shortage due to a strike, drought or famine will develop.

Initially the perishable staples may be oranges, celery, carrots, beets, apples, and onions. Find out when the desired produce is in session in different locales. By ordering a large quantity, transportation costs can be cut in half. In addition, many growers allow a discount on group orders. You might consider asking independent health food stores to join you in the purchase.

In placing the group order, select one member to compile the individual orders. Regular dates of the month should be set to call the members to request that their orders to mailed to the co-op. On the assigned day, members who did not mail an order should be contacted to make certain they did not intend to order. A tally of the orders should be taken to ascertain that none of the members exceeded the size of their initial investment or the amount of money sent with the order. Then place the order with the dealers. On arrival of the shipment, notify members so they can pick up the produce. For large orders where storage space is lacking, immediate pick-up is recommended. Those who did not send money with their orders should pay at the time of pick-up.

When members of the co-op are planning a car trip, it would bring the co-op substantial savings if a van or station wagon were used to pick up organic produce en route. Planning is of prime importance. Before vacation time, write to dealers to find out what is available. Send the order to the farmer informing him of the approximate time of your arrival.

First choice should be non-perishable staples — one ton of seed can be readily loaded into a van. Be certain to reduce the speed of your vehicle.

Second choice items should be the semi-perishables — apples, carrots, beets and other tubers, squash, citrus, mangoes, papaya. A further saving might be obtained by picking the produce yourself. You can use canvas and wet newspaper to protect fruit and vegetables from the sun.

When the produce arrives you will need a temporary storage space where members can pick up the goods. Choose a centrally located home with a cellar, sunporch or garage, readily accessible to all co-op members. A room can be adapted for long term storage of seed, apples, tubers and citrus by installing a used air conditioner to provide a low temperature. An inexpensive insulator can be installed in the room to cut down heat entry.

COOPERATIVE LIVING

The cooperative can also be used as a vehicle for investment through collective purchase of land or a farm, near, yet distant enough to lose the consciousness of the city. This land can become a healthful recreational center where members can work toward establishing a financially, self-sustaining, organic farm. From working in the sun, open air, in a community spirit, with a sense of fulfillment and achievement of unity with nature, you will improve in appearance, develop a trimmer figure, enjoy new health, tranquility plus nights of sleep and relaxation. Your children will become oriented toward nature rather than drugs and abuse of the body. You will be helping to create a generation based on a solid foundation of health.

With investment in a greenhouse, you will be supplying vegetation for your co-op all year round. Such a project will be self-supporting and health-promoting. All members of the co-op can participate in the work on the farm. Once you have experienced this tribal living, under a self-governing structure, you will never want to live any other way.

PREPARATION FOR SURVIVAL

Now seems a good time to prepare materially for cataclysms predicted. Members of the cooperative can sell their city property and with the proceeds buy land at least one hundred miles from major cities. It might be wise to choose an area least desirable to others — mountains where agriculture is next to impossible for most people. The Essenes chose the Dead Sea area where nothing grew and the water was salty, yet they established a highly advanced esoteric society by applying nature's simple laws. Stay away from major geological earthquake fault lines, nuclear power plants, airplane routes, farming regions, cities, power lines, mining — any evidence of civilization. Keep in mind the predictions of psychics.

If you keep your body pure, you will be sensitive to God's angels as they serve you and direct you to safe areas. Eventually, after the disaster, you will be able to settle in a high altitude tropical paradise.

Those who have free time will be able to start building. For a northern retreat, it would be good to build special, hidden reinforced concrete underground storage areas for water, tools, books and enough food and seed to tide you over until you are able to start farming.

In your retreat you should include for storage a substantial supply of seeds for your vegetable garden. In the future world seeds will be of more value than money. To make life easier be sure to have garden tools such as shovels, spades, forks, rakes and hoes in storage. For indoor gardens store up trays, glass jars, gallon cans, liquid and/or powder kelp fertilizer and peatmoss. A stainless steel distiller (which can be operated on electricity as well as wood stove) and/or a water purifier is a must for survival. A manual grain mill when adjusted for fine grind will enable you to use it as a blender for greens; a juicer for grass, weeds and sprouts; a grinder for sesame and sunflower seeds to make yogurt; and as a juicer for shredded carrots or beets.

You might consider storing the following amounts of food for each person: 50 lbs. unhulled buckwheat seed, 100 lbs. wheat, 25 lbs. mung beans, 25 lbs. unhulled sesame seed, 50 lbs. navy beans, 30 lbs. honey and 1 quart of liquid kelp (see Appendix). Seed should be stored in a cool, dry place. Take special precautions against rodents. The senses of wild animals are very keen; they can present a hazard to your food supply.

Keep on hand gardening tools, bikes and repair kit, short wave radio, axe, building tools, numerous nails, saw, hand drill, books on gardening, building and education, and warm, durable clothing and bedding.

If you are unable to start growing food before famine becomes acute, at least get your land cleared and composted. Dig a well for water.

Keep your funds in Canadian banks. Their checks can be used in the USA. Canadian banks probably will fail a month later than USA banks. When American banks fail, spend all your Canadian currency to purchase additional food, tools and books for storage.

Robert Preston makes the following recommendations about finances: "Do not keep money in a savings and loan or bank. Leave only enough money in your checking account to pay your bills each month and that is all   ...   convert most of paper currency into a ready reserve of from $250 to $1,000 in silver coins ... Junk silver coins ... are sold generally in $1,000 quantities. They are silver coins that have been gleaned from all the coins in circulation ... These coins may be purchased through a local coin dealer or a coin exchange."

The author further suggests that you keep your silver storage a secret. Don't store it all in one place. Build hiding places buried in concrete. Tell location to all family members. He also feels that for those with large sums of money, the most secure investment is silver buillion. For those who want silver in small units such as an ounce.

If possible, move onto your land before a crisis comes. When you see the city totally falling apart — food rationing power failure, gasoline shortage, no sun, only continuous smog, bank failure, guerrilla warfare — leave the area. You may use an automobile, but always carry a bike. Pray that you don't have to evacuate in winter. While fasting, on a racing bicycle, you will always be able to cover at least 600 miles. In the event you are not able to reach your land, you may reach a wilderness area where food can be found. You can travel clear across the world using only wild grass juice for power.

To prepare for hasty evacuation of an area affected by plague, drought, widescale insanity, revolution, ecological disaster, thermonuclear war; keep on hand a racing bike (or endurance to walk long distances while fasting), world road map, sub-zero sleeping bag, backpack, 1 gallon distilled water or portable lightweight water purifier, 2 pounds of sproutable mung and alfalfa seed, compass, book on edible weeds.

Perhaps the most important preparation for any disaster is to purify your body and to practice Yoga: exercises, meditation, the art of breathing, so that you will be strong, healthy, clearheaded, able to face any situation with equanimity. You will learn the art of bodily survival and lose all fear of death.

Prepare your body to fast for at least 15 days without any cleansing reactions; be able to live on very little food, such as weeds; practice the art of breathing until you learn to live on fewer breaths. Learn to feed yourself with colors. We live and eat colors. Color meditation can provide a satisfying, energygiving meal (See Breatharianism).

If it becomes necessary to neutralize radioactive fallout and other poisons, you may drink at least two ounces of wheatgrass juice mixed with water daily. (Any meadow grass will do). Exert minimal effort to minimize breathing.

Do not plan to use weapons to defend your property. It is best to have little and to need little. When others assail your area, fast. Eat only enough to stay alive. Always look like a scarecrow. Ask them to join you in fasting and prayer. During fasting you will be protected from plague and disaster. Be loving.

DIVINE NECTAR

One of the greatest secrets of the military training in survival is the fact that a person can use ones own urine for nourishment. The 3 - 5% toxins within urine are quickly filtered out within the intestinal tract and act as laxatives. With 4 days of urine drinking, the taste becomes almost like water. It is rich in enzymes, minerals, vitamins and some amino acids. One can live for a minimum of a month on solely urine. This has been tested by miners trapped in a cave, where it took 35 days to excavate. Their health actually improved. With this knowledge you never have to panic, as you can always travel on your own liquid and any grasses available in fields to an area of safety. Much has been written in the books of the oldest natural healing practices of the Ajervedic system and the body liquid was called the "divine nectar". For more information on this subject and it's therapeutic and survival usage, read "Water of Life", Armstrong, Nutribooks, Provo, Utah and Shivambu Kalpa, Pauls D. O., Orthobionomy, 5502 MacDonald Avenue, El Cerrito, California 94530.

1. HOW TO PREPARE FOR THE COMING CRASH, Robert Preston $2.00. Wake Up Pub Co., P.O. Box 150, Provo, Utah
How to prepare for survival.
2. FAMINE, CAN WE SURVIVE? $1.00. Ambassador College, Pasadena, Cal.

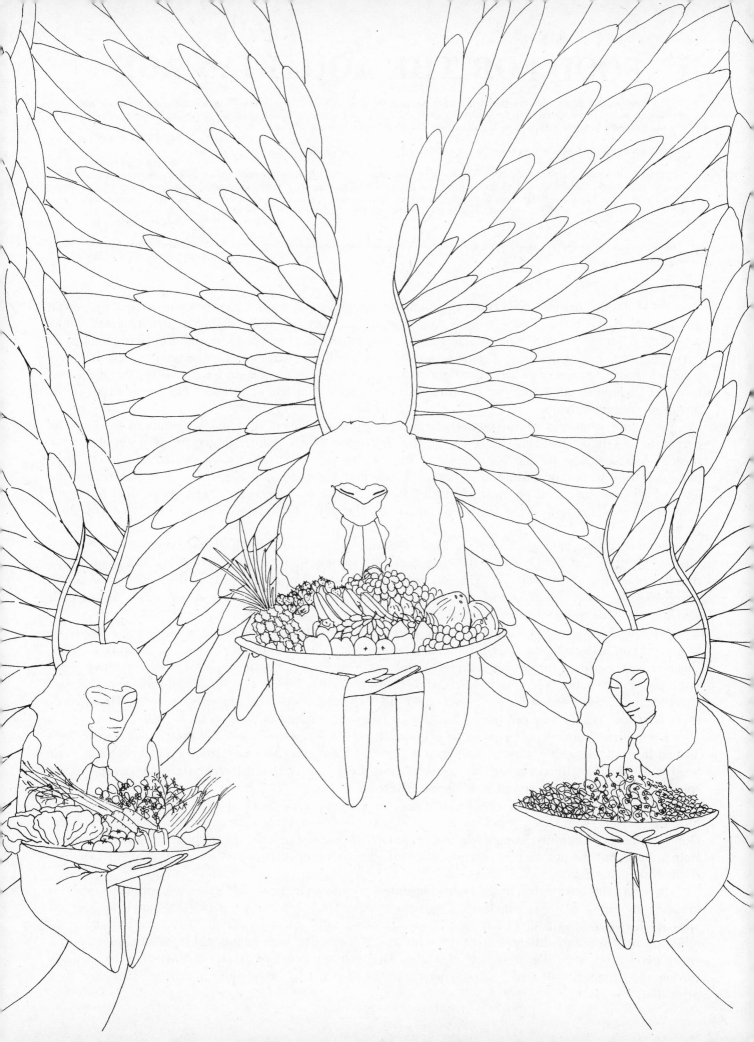

FOOD FOR THE AQUARIAN AGE

"A new subrace began to enter the earth's plane around 1932 because of a change in astrological influences, and we are admonished to insure better products for a better people . . . You expect a new root race. What are you doing to prepare for it? You must prepare food for their bodies, as well as their minds and their spiritual development."

CAYCE READINGS 5748-6, 470-39

"The food of the future will be fruit and seed. The time will come when meat will no longer be eaten."

BAHA'I WRITINGS

"The food which is agreeable to different men is of three sorts . . Men of sattwa like foods which increase their vital force, strength and health. Such foods add to the physical and mental life. They are juicy, soothing, fresh, and agreeable. But men of Rajas prefer foods which are bitter, sour, salty, hot, pungent, acid, burning. These cause ill health, and distemper of mind and body. And men of tamas take a perverse pleasure in foods which are stale, tasteless, rotten and impure. They like to eat the leavings of others."

BHAGAVAD–GITA

"It is my view that the Vegetarian manner of living by its purely physical effect on the human temperament would most beneficially influence the lot of mankind."

— ALBERT EINSTEIN, Dec. 27, 1930

Food is the earliest addiction, the basic prejudice, starting with the newborn's first mouthful, continuing to the grave. Food is more controversial than sex, politics, religion or drugs. Many people feel their whole life-style is put to a test and is discredited if you refuse, on philosophical grounds, to eat certain food at their home. People generally have no instinctual or rational basis for their diet; as a result they can become very emotional about it. The average person has no idea what is natural food or how to maintain good health. Doctors know a great deal about disease but very little about health-promoting nutrition.

"You are what you eat." Today there are many philosophies of diet, many choices of food and its preparation. I have examined the diets from many perspectives. Value judgement is reserved for the reader. Astrologically we are all different; this predisposes our body to choose certain foods. In a natural setting we would instinctually choose foods that provide just the right energy vibrations for the level of consciousness and physical adventure we would like to experience. "The stars impel but don't compel". The divine will of the individual supercedes the stellar limitations. You become what you want to become.

After you purchase good organic food, the way you use it will determine whether you will be "happy, healthy and holy." The diets suggested in this book are listed in progressively health-improving order from heavy, dead foods to light, sunshine, juicy foods. Improving your diet gradually will lessen psychological, social and physological discomforts associated with change. As you progress on the path you will see betterment in your health and life.

With each stage of advancement, a new spiritual and mental diet will be adopted – a new life-style. It enters you naturally; do not resist change. A person who is addicted to alcohol, cigarettes, drugs, sugar or coffee will go through withdrawal symptoms when he reduces or stops the intake of the poison. Similarly the supermarket food addict who stops (or cuts down) the intake of poison-embalmed, non-organic (dead) food will go through mild drug (wrong food) withdrawal symptoms. They are of short duration, lasting no more than a few days; sometimes, as long as two weeks.

Don't fight your vices. Learn to love yourself and they eventually will fall away. Don't make food an end in itself. Be gentle. Don't be a proud vegetarian. Love everyone. Construct a diet as good as your head can tolerate without losing the joy of living. Everyone is at a different stage along the infinite spiral of experience and everyone's needs are different.

You chose your body for this incarnation, for working out Karmic debt and for the introduction of more perfect, complete vibrations into your eternal divine aura. Listen to your own inner voice. Don't condemn. Your first commandment should be to know yourself, the second to become yourself. Help others, but do not thereby destroy yourself. We are all on the journey of enlightenment together. Right food can aid you.

Persons who have eaten meat, highly seasoned gravies, extremely rich cakes and preserves; cannot immediately relish a plain, wholesome, nutritious diet. Their taste is so perverted that they have no appetite for a wholesome diet of fruits and vegetables, sprouts, juices and seed. They need not expect to relish at first food so different from that in which they have been indulging. If they cannot at first enjoy plain food, they may fast until they can. That fast will prove of greater benefit than medicine, as the abused stomach will find that rest which it has long needed. Real hunger can be satisfied with a plain diet.

Those of you who are not yet ready for natural foods, (unless you use an abundant supply of mixed sprouted seed, rejuvelac, ferments and fresh organic juices), may benefit from vitamin supplements (especially A,B-complex, C,E), grain germ oils, kelp and other sea vegetables for the complete mineral spectrum. Avoid all protein supplements; they are never an answer to health. Nearly everyone eats too much protein. If you have difficulty digesting protein foods, pancreatic enzyme supplements may help until digestion improves. With starch meals, a papaya base with mylase can be helpful. You may sip a half cup of papaya and mint tea to aid digestion.

Do not try to skip too many steps in the order of diets. I have seen youth, because of enthusiasm, go directly into fruitarianism but, after one week, return to bread and cheese. To make a complete transition into live foods might take years; to feel balanced on a fruit diet from one to five years. If you have a hard time keeping your head together, do not be afraid to binge; but go back to the path and become more disciplined.

Better to indulge in cooked green vegetables or tubers than to overburden yourself with raw nuts, grains, seed or dried fruit. I have witnessed people at the Institute who, after a six day wheatgrass juice fast, have gone out to eat lobster or fried bacon, eggs, toast and coffee. Some have become violently sick, and, were it not for the use of zone therapy, they may not have survived. After indiscriminate eating, you may anticipate on the second to fifth day, the discomforts of cleansing reactions. After a binge, you may benefit from zone therapy, leaving the electric light on during sleep and digestive enzymes. The following day pursue a vegetable juice regime or a dry fast. After the transition to a good diet, you will feel less and less desire for unwholesome foods.

As your body becomes healthier and cleaner, it will tolerate less and less of the foods which in the past seemed agreeable. If you have been on a raw food diet for some time, a meal of cooked food or animal products could induce nausea and diarrhea. Your body will become like that of a healthy child, immediately rejecting unsuitable food. Habitually eating bad food weakens your body so that it cannot reject such foods, and, after many years, may award you with a chronic ailment.

Do not vacillate greatly between a predominantly cooked and a predominantly raw food diet. Although the dietary hierarchy is introduced with Kosher foods, everyone may instead start with a vegetarian diet.

NUTRITIONAL FALLACIES

"Man eats solar vibrations trapped in nutrients. Enzymes, protein, vitamins are temporary energy traps; under the action of enzymes in the body, energies are released for building and maintenance of the human body. Some individuals get the necessary nutrients via sun and color; most via food."

Viktoras Kulvinskas, LOVE YOUR BODY

Food can provide energy and stimulation, cleanse the bloodstream and build an efficient body. Many people who are adopting a vegetarian diet may cling to prevailing concepts of dietary needs. Do not be misled by requirements listed in nutrition tables.

During the early stages of dietary transition, when the volume of food is decreased, the metabolism osmotic pressure between the digestive tract and the tissues surrounding it will also be decreased. In a toxic congested body, the mucous linings of digestive tract and blood vessels are greatly reduced in permeability. This can produce temporary signs of deficiency of some nutrients in the bloodstream. This is not cause for concern. The missing nutrients will be replenished as membrane permeability is reestablished.

Even when nutrients which orthodox dieticians consider essential are missing in your food, they are supplied to you as needed, provided you are moderately detoxified, from other sources: biological transmutation (141), air and sunlight (see Breatharianism), the metabolic nutrient pool in the lymphatic system which contains recycled cells, and from nutrients created by friendly bacteria inhabiting the intestinal tract.

VITAMINS

VITAMINS are found in nature's foods. Each food color indicates a different nutrient content. Eat sprouts, fruit and vegetables of varying color; nibble on some grass, expose your body to sunlight. This will supply all your vitamins.

VEGETARIAN SOURCES OF VITAMIN B-12

VITAMIN B-12 is considered the anti-pernicious anemia vitamin. There is widespread belief that meat is the primary source of this vitamin. But where does the herbivorous cow obtain vitamin B-12? Dr. Spencer and Dr. Prevest (34) state that "the ultimate source of all nature's vitamin B-12 in the world is bacteria." Vitamin B-12 is manufactured by the friendly bacteria in the animal's intestinal tract. This is true for all vegetarian animals including the human being.

At a vitamin B-12 conference (152) it was stated: "The need for vitamin B-12 is difficult to demonstrate in some species, particularly in ruminants, owing to vigorous bacterial synthesis in the rumen or alimentary tract. . . . Pernicious anemia appears to arise not from shortage in the diet but from impairment of the ability to absorb vitamin B-12."

Putrefactive bacteria destroy friendly bacteria thus inhibiting synthesis of vitamin B-12 .Putrefaction in the intestine is caused by ingesting cooked animal protein, bad food combining, overeating of any concentrated protein food, chemical additives and medicine.

Drs. West and Hillard (35) showed that a high protein diet increases vitamin B-12 requirements. Other studies (71) demonstrate vitamin B-12 to be heat sensitive—normal cooking can destroy up to 89 percent. Hence those who rely on cooked meat as a primary source of vitamin B-12 are more likely to develop pernicious anemia.

'Vitamin B-12 has been found (152) in significant amounts in nature in fermented materials" (like yogurt). In studies on vegetarian humans, Dr. Wolfgang Tiling discovered the synthesis of vitamin B-12 in the intestines of children who were on a soy milk diet (151).

Clinical and experimental animal studies have shown that pernicious anemia (36) can be successfully treated with chlorophyl. I believe that chlorophyl destroys putrefactive bacteria in the intestine and helps to reestablish the natural bacterial flora which manufacture vitamin B-12.

To insure the active production of vitamin B-12 by intestinal bacteria, vegetarians should limit protein intake, watch food combinations and observe the other hygienic rules.

SUN VITAMINS

One should spend at least one hour daily outdoors. Walk or run on grass, along beaches, swim in nature's waters, climb mountains, visit fields and forests. Breathe deeply. Even in winter, you can sunbathe. Build a two foot high windbreak. For more sun intensity, incorporate a sun reflector. Even at 25 degrees F., sheltered from wind, naked in mid-day sun, one will feel very warm. Sun and fresh air are the two most important ingredients in one's diet. Sun does not cause skin cancer, though it may act as a triggering mechanism. During sun bathing, as much as six pints of fluid can be expelled through the skin in a day. If the fluid contains carcinogens, skin cancer may possibly develop. Cancer of the skin is impossible on a hygienic low protein vegetarian regime.

The skin of dark races filters out a great spectrum of sun rays. They originally inhabited sundrenched areas But living in the north in deficient sunlight, eating processed sunless foods, those who have abused the body longest and most intensely may develop the sunlight deficiency disease of sickle cell anemia.

WHO NEEDS HIGH PROTEIN DIET

PROTEIN – Perhaps the most predominant food fallacy is the high protein intake (40 to 100 grams daily) usually recommended. Protein in excess of our needs is not utilized by the body.

There are several factors which greatly diminish availability of dietary protein. If we use meat as our source of protein, cooking destroys at least one of the essential amino acids needed for building enzymes and healthy tissue. Cooking can destroy 40 to 85 percent of the available protein in most food.

Most cooked food enters the stomach at a temperature of more than 104 degrees; this heat destroys some of the gastric enzymes needed for digestion. Liquids served at a meal delay protein digestion by reducing the concentration of gastric juices. Serving a concentrated protein food at the same meal with fats, sweets or starches further inhibits digestion because each of these foods requires different digestive juices. When too large a quantity of concentrated food is eaten at a meal, much of it remains undigested. Many people cannot digest meat because of deficiency in pancreatic enzymes, bile and hydrochloric acid.

Practically all pain, pathology and cell destruction is known to be due to high blood acidity which results from excess intake of protein, especially acid-forming animal proteins. However even vegetable protein such as seed, when eaten to excess can cause toxicity.

Dr. C. L. Elvehjem in "Amino Acid Supplementation of Cereal" warns that twice the daily requirements of certain amino acids in food leads to toxic cell disturbance (29). Dr. Bieler states that one of main sources of overacidity in the body is an excess of amino acids which disturbs the nitrogen balance (30).

"All deaths are due to progressive acid saturation." (Cee W. Crile, M.D.) The acid condition generated by a high protein diet, destroys body cells, hence new ones will have to be built.

If there is a heavy coating of mucus in the digestive tract and deposits of waste in the blood vessels, protein (amino acids) is poorly absorbed and largely unavailable to the cells. For these reasons much of the protein we eat passes from the body, or is stored in tissues as waste.

The degree of a person's physiological degeneration can be determined by the amount of protein needed to maintain normal weight. High protein needs indicate that organs, blood and lymph system are clogged with mucus. Large protein intake creates an osmotic pressure in the digestive tract high enough to force the amino acids through even badly congested cell walls.

The short term beneficial effects of a high protein diet can be attributed to the following factors. Most people are protein starved. The cells are deficient in protein because the whole interior of the individual from the digestive tract to the finest capillary, as well as cell walls, are coated with extraneous mucus, hardened fats and layers of inorganic mineral deposits which interfere with the transport of amino acids into the interior of the cells.

The intake of high protein foods (especially without starches) increases the osmotic pressure of the amino acids: this sets up the pump mechanism for the increased amino acid transport into the cells. Health improves. Furthermore, there is the stimulating effect one gets from protein, since uric acid, a waste product of protein metabolism, has a structure almost identical to caffeine. Likewise, in the case of individuals who are on a cleansing diet, protein foods stop further detoxification, hence eliminating the feeling of weakness that is associated with cleansing.

Lastly, in diseases such as toxemia of pregnancy, which is a cleansing "sickness", a high protein diet has been effectively used in stopping or preventing the development of the process of detoxification.

The long term effect of a high protein diet is always bad. It leads to an accumulation of the waste products of protein metabolism, thus acidifying the body. For example, the human liver and kidneys combined have a limited capacity to excrete only about 8 grains of uric acid in 24 hours. However, one pound of meat can generate as much as 18 grains of uric acid. Hence, some uric acid will be left in the body from any one meat meal which will accumulate to produce the disease of gout, rheumatism or the complications of arthritis.

Very similar statements can be made about the megavitamin-mineral therapy. Here the results can be impressive and immediate. However, the disease still has a dietary basis and unless the individual pursues an improved dietary regime, the junk foods will eventually have their effect. Furthermore, no supplement can supply all the factors that are found in raw, living foods. Likewise, the human body was not structured for a fragmented nutrient intake; vitamins work best not alone, but in conjunction with other vitamins, minerals, enzymes and amino acids as found in food from nature. It is interesting to note that in his studies Dr. Kohler found it to be impossible to create a dietary supplement which utilized all the known dietary factors, equal in benefit and growth rates, to that which one finds in grasses. (167, 37)

The real solution to diet is to clean out the body. This increases the permeability of body linings, skin and cell walls, thus permitting easy transport of nutrients. A detoxified individual can eat very little of simple foods such as sprouted seeds and fruit and maintain excellence of health, strength and intellectual acuity.

IS COMPLETE PROTEIN POSSIBLE OR NECESSARY?

Protein from vegetable sources is composed of ratios of the various amino acids different from those found in the human body. Protein in domestic animals raised for food consumption while alive, has almost exactly the same amino acid composition as those of the human body. However, the dead animal protein is greatly damaged when cooked and the amino acid ratios are destroyed (see: Cooking Effect on Food) thus making cooked meat as different in amino acid composition and ratios as the vegetable sources. This raises a question: How does one get a complete protein intake adequate for body maintenance and growth?

Most people maintain health and adequate protein intake from a mixed, varied diet. The deficiency of an essential amino acid in one protein in the diet can be supplemented by adding another protein which contains the missing amino acid.

However, there is no need to eat a complete protein mixture at any one meal. What is more important is your amino acid intake for the day, the week or the month. An individual may never have a complete protein at a single meal and still show no signs of protein starvation.

If on Monday your lunch was deficient in lysine (an essential amino acid) yet 5 days ago you had a meal which was high in lysine (the excess of which was stored in liver and other body cells) then the deficiency in today's meal will be compensated by the liver releasing the stored lysine to give the bloodstream all the essential amino acids for the building of cells, enzymes and hormones.

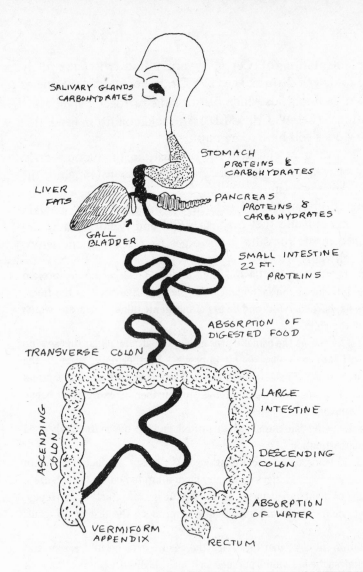

SALIVARY GLANDS
CARBOHYDRATES

STOMACH
PROTEINS &
CARBOHYDRATES

LIVER
FATS

PANCREAS
PROTEINS &
CARBOHYDRATES

GALL
BLADDER

SMALL INTESTINE
22 FT.
PROTEINS

ABSORPTION OF
DIGESTED FOOD

TRANSVERSE COLON

ASCENDING COLON

LARGE
INTESTINE

DESCENDING
COLON

ABSORPTION
OF WATER

VERMIFORM
APPENDIX

RECTUM

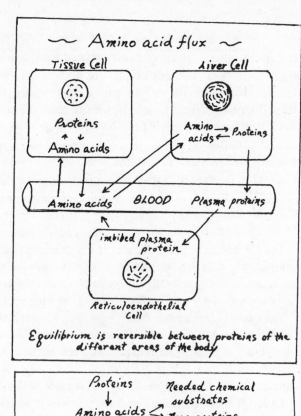

~ Amino acid flux ~

Tissue Cell   Liver Cell

Proteins   Amino → Proteins
  ↑↓   acids
Amino acids

Amino acids   BLOOD   Plasma proteins

imbibed plasma
protein

Reticuloendothelial
Cell

Equilibrium is reversible between proteins of the
different areas of the body

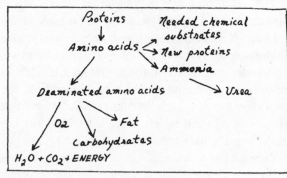

Proteins   Needed chemical
  ↓   substrates
Amino acids → New proteins
              → Ammonia
  ↓
Deaminated amino acids → Urea

        O₂   Fat
          ↘   ↗
        Carbohydrates
$H_2O + CO_2 + ENERGY$

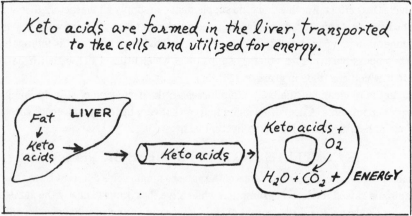

Keto acids are formed in the liver, transported
to the cells and utilized for energy.

Fat   LIVER
  ↓
Keto
acids → Keto acids → Keto acids +
                              O₂
                         $H_2O + CO_2$ + ENERGY

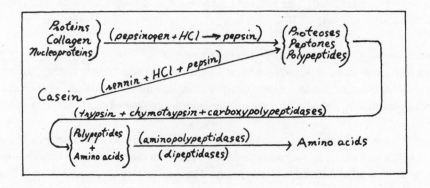

Proteins
Collagen   (pepsinogen + HCl → pepsin)   Proteoses
Nucleoproteins   Peptones
                                                Polypeptides

Casein   (rennin + HCl + pepsin)

              (trypsin + chymotrypsin + carboxypolypeptidases)

Polypeptides
    +   (aminopolypeptidases)   → Amino acids
Amino acids   (dipeptidases)

"All cells synthesize far more protein than is absolutely necessary to maintain the life of the cells. Therefore, if amino acids are needed elsewhere in the body, some of the cellular protein can be reconverted into amino acids and then transported in this form . . . The reconversion process is catalyzed by enzymes called kathepepsins that are in all cells. The quantity of protein in a cell is determined by a balance between their rate of synthesis and their rate of destruction . . . By this [see diagram] constant interchange of amino acids the protein in all parts of the body are maintained in reasonable equilibrium with each other. If one tissue suffers loss of protein, many of the proteins in the remainder of the body will soon be converted into amino acids which are transported to the appropriate point to form new protein." [119]

The liver acts as a buffer in case of an excess of protein in diet. When there is a high amino acid concentration in the blood, a large proportion of the amino acids is absorbed by the liver cells and formed into small proteins. When there is a deficiency of certain amino acids, the liver (as well as other body cells) will release the missing amino acids, if it has them in storage.

"After absorption through the intestinal mucosa, the amino acids pass into the capillaries of the villi and then the portal blood, flowing through the liver before entering the general circulation . . . All the different amino acids are in the blood and extracellular fluid in small quantity . . . because on coming in contact with cells they are absorbed very rapidly." [119]

"Amino acids are in a state of continual flux from one part of the body to the other. If the amount of amino acids in the cells of one area falls too low, then amino acids will enter these cells from the blood and will be replaced by amino acids released from other cells." [119].

The digestion of protein starts in the stomach. It is broken down into proteosis (smaller combinations of amino acids than protein) and polypeptides (still smaller) by pepsin under the action of HCL acid. After entering the small intestine, it is further split by trypsin of the pancreatic juices into amino acids.

EATING VEGETARIANS
MIGHT BE HARMFUL TO YOUR HEALTH

I, for my part, wonder of what sort of feeling, mind or reason, that man was possessed who was first to pollute his mouth with gore, and allow his lips to touch the flesh of a murdered being; who spread his table with the mangled forms of dead bodies and claimed as daily food and dainty dishes what but now, were being endowed with movement, with perception, with voice.

Plutarch

It is only by softening and disguising dead flesh by culinary preparation that it is rendered susceptible of mastication or digestion, and that the sight of it's bloody juices and raw horror does not excite loathing and disgust.

Percy Shelley, Vindication of Natural Diet

THE CANCER IN MEAT

MEAT — It is not loving to kill. To eat meat is generally unnecessary and unecological. It takes 50 to 100 times more land to produce meat than it does to produce its equivalent in vegetarian food. Animal feed contains DDT, pesticides, hormones, stilbesterol, antibiotics, tranquilizers. Diseased animals are slaughtered and sold to the public. Moreover, meat is not a healthful food. Fatty meat is high in cholesterol. The waste products of protein metabolism are acid (uric) which accumulate eventually precipitate in tissues as crystals. Meat tends to putrefy in the colon, producing toxic waste which speeds the metabolism and causes degenerative diseases, leading to premature death.

Dr. John Berg (154) of National Cancer Institute reported at the American Cancer Society Conference that heavy beef eating is related to high incidence of cancer of colon and rectum. Dr. Earnest Wynder, president of the American Health Foundation felt that beef (also eggs, dairy products and foods containing saturated fats) should be incriminated as cancer-promoting.

Dr. Ernest Wynder, president of Am. Health Foundation, told a symposium sponsored by Boston American Cancer Society and the Greater Boston Medical Society that dietary fat and animal protein combine with bacteria in the gut to form acids linked to tumor formation. Now he said the evidence shows links also between these fats and cancer of the breast, pancreas, kidney, ovary, and prostrate as well (Boston Globe, Dec 5, 1974, p. 49).

Cancer immunity is built on a low protein, non processed diet. These observations were made by Dr. Robert Good, University of Minnesota, from his studies of aboriginal children and animals (161).

Rich protein decomposes in the stomach into poisonous ammonia, which in turn produces nitresamines. Biochemist, Dr. Lijinsky said: " . . . they are among the most potent cancer causing chemicals known." Furthermore, Dr. W. J. Visek (New York State College of Agriculture and Life Science of Cornell University) states: "The presence of ammonia increases susceptibility to virus infections, which are known to cause cancer in animals and are suspect in man."

Other studies showed tryptophane, an essential amino acid, which is about twenty times more concentrated in meat than in fruit, to be carcinogenic in the urinary tract (33). In the press, Nov 25, 1962, it was reported that Dr. Richard Gordon of Monsanto Chemical Co, St. Louis discovered that "an acid called tryptophane causes growth and aging." By excluding tryptophane from their diet, Gordon kept animals youthful and active without any signs of aging in excess of normal lifespan. Introduction of tryptophane resulted in the appearance of normal aging.

Dr. A. Voisin states (153), "The formula for tryptophane is very close to that of indole-acetic acid, which is a growth hormone in plants. This hormone can be produced by plants from tryptophane."

THE HEART DISORDERS IN MEAT

In the USA, heart disorders are the largest cause of death. Hardening of the arteries, according to Dr. Paul White, affects even two-year-old children. All related studies point to the culprit—fat and mineral deposits in arteries—which places a heavy strain on the heart.

In the past, hardening of the arteries was believed to be caused by high cholesterol foods from animal sources (162). A more recent study by Dr. John Gainer (163) showed protein to be the major contributing factor. He demonstrated that even a slight increase in blood plasma protein can reduce oxygen transport in blood by as much as 60 percent. It has been shown by a Danish researcher that oxygen-deficient atmosphere (like smog-filled cities) induces atherosclerosis. Dr. Gainer observed that rabbits on high cholesterol diets had thicker blood vessel walls than those on normal diets; rabbits on protein-rich diets had thicker blood vessel walls than those on high cholesterol diets.

Oxfred Muller, the inventor of the capillary microscope showed through experiments the benefit of a vegetarian diet in heart related disorders. He states (231):

> "The influence of a vegetarian diet presents itself in this way: The capillaries strech out and their convolutions become straightened out. We thus can see that this form of nourishment caused a certain unburdening of the peripheral section of the blood vessels while the purely meat diet seems to represent a heavy burden."

A study by Annand (220) and another by Yarushalmy and Hilleboe (221), showed in various countries that the higher the level of vegetable consumption, the lower the level of heart disorders.

Annand found that (220) vegetable protein exerts a powerful protective action against arteriosclerosis in animal experiments. Groen et al, (222) also Morse and Overlay (223) in their study found that vegetable protein lowers the cholesterol count.

A low fat diet, maintained for a period of up to 3 years, failed to lower either the mortality or morbidity of patients suffering from arteriosclerosis (224) whereas after a period of only 4 to 5 weeks a diet high in fresh vegetables caused a significant reduction in this affliction (225).

LEAUKEMIA IN MEAT

Leukemia is the overproduction of white cells to fight the blood toxemia associated with breakdown in protein metabolism. The Russian, Dr. Kouchakoff, discovered that when cooked meat is eaten, white corpuscles in the bloodstream increase tremendously following the meal. They are there to fight an infectious condition. Furthermore, leukemia is always associated with an extremely high amount of uric acid in the blood. This can come from only one source—dietary intake of concentrated protein (animal products and seed). Lancet and Polish Medical Journal report Dr. Kalikowski's studies where low protein diet was used, in conjunction with high alkaline solutions, to cure leukemia: "favorable effects in ten out of thirteen children with leukemia . . . a strikingly fast disappearance of blast cells in bone marrow was noted compared to controls." One of the reasons given for lack of complete success was that they had not yet devised an optimal diet (31).

THE SCHIZOPHRENIA IN MEAT

"I am a heavy eater of beef, and believe it does harm to my wit."   Twelfth Night

Drs. J. Wurtman and F. D. Fernstrom (M.I.T.) reported in Science Magazine that high amounts of tryptophane in the blood reduces serotonin, which controls creative brain activity.

More people in the USA are hospitalized and treated for the condition of "schizophrenia" than for the total cases of cancer, diabetes and heart disorders. As this "condition" has been variously and inadequately defined as well as used to categorize many who have been put in mental hospitals without recourse to their civil liberties and the law, we do not take this term literally as such and have indicated this by quotation marks. In Russia, Dr. Yuri Nikolayev of Moscow Research Institute of Psychiatry has fasted 20 to 40 days psychiatric patients to health. His work showed that "schizophrenia" is a form of protein toxemia. He states that his starvation therapy has been useful in treating eczema, metabolic disorders, bronchial asthma, hypertension, gallstones, tumors, hardening of the arteries, as well as "schizophrenia". Prior to the fast the patients were given a cleansing diet; following the fast the patients followed a vegetarian diet if they did not want the sickness to return. Today, Dr. Allan Cott, M.D., is using a modified version of Dr. Nikolayev's therapy in New York City for the treatment of "schizophrenia."

(164)

LOW PROTEIN DIET IS THE HUMAN DIET.

The Biblical self-fertilizing hermaphrodite Adam and other parthogenic individuals were definitely non-carnivorous. Their dietary needs were spelled out specifically "And God said: Behold I have given you every herb bearing seed which is upon the face of all the Earth and every fruit yielding tree; to you it shall be for meat." This fare of Melthusalah times called for no complicated preparation only what came directly from a tree or plant.

It is difficult to see how the early man who had neither claws nor fangs, nor the fleetness of foot to catch prey, could have been anything but the frugivorous animal which Charles Darwin and Julian Huxley maintain he was.

In Darwin's "The Descent Of Man" he shows a very close relationship between the fruitarian anthropoid apes and man both in structure and function. It would be a remarkable thing that all the primates, with the exception of man should be frugivorous.

A very definite remainder of the true dietary needs of man is the first food that he would ingest, had he been raised naturally, mother's breast milk.

A comparison of equal weight of breast milk and fruit shows (237) that mother's milk has the calcium content of an orange; sodium value of a cantoloupe; potassium count of blueberries; magnessium weight of an apple; iron composition of red currants; copper of figs; phosphorus of lemon; chlorine of pineapple; sulphur of tangerine; vitamin A of plum; B1 of grapefruit; B2 of banana; calorie of pears.

The protein content (237, 238) even of ambivorous human mother's milk is between 1.0 and 2.4 percent, average value of 1.4 percent. This small percentage supplies the baby all the essential amino acids, protein, during the period of most rapid growth and maturation. Grown humans don't have a need for such high value of protein once they have stopped growing. Excess to the dietary needs will result in fat and ill health.

There are many examples of heavy meat diet producing robust and apparently healthy individual. It was Dr. L. H. Newberg of Ann Arbor University who found that when he fed large quantities of meat to test animals, they grew bigger and more alert than other animals on a vegetarian diet. But three months later, these animals contracted kidney damage and died while the vegetarian animals lived healthily and happily (239).

It has been shown tryptophane, an essential amino acid of the protein complex, in high enough concentrations, when ingested continuously over a period of time, can result in urinary cancer. The average content (237) of tryptophan for 20 listed fruits is one twentieth of the value found in round medium fat beef.

The range of protein content for fruit was (237) .4 to 2.2 percent, which is approximately the range of protein in human breast milk. Meat is 10 to 24 percent protein, and is unsuitable food for man. Grains, nut and seeds are 10 to 50 percent protein and unless sprouted, which reduces protein concentration, are unsuited foods for humans.

The comparison (240) of protein content of milk of classes of animals is worthwhile.

FRUITARIAN	ANBIVOROUS		CARNIVOROUS	
Man 1.25 — 2.7	Guinea Pig 8.55		Dog	10.1
Monkey 2.3	Rat	8.7	Cat	11.1
	Swine	14.98	Russian Wolfhound 10.6	
		& 7 .	Pointer	9.2

From common sense we would anticipate the concentration of protein in human mother's milk to be much higher than in a mother cat if the size of the organism produced was the main criterion. Human protein needs come closest to the protein needs of the fruitarian monkey. Big, strong bodies are built from fruit protein, as any gorilla would prove to you.

One of the most famous Anatomists, Professor Baron Cuvier in his "Lecon d' Anatomie Comparative" as quoted by Shelly in his essay entitled "A Vindication of Natural Diet," he says:

> "Comparative anatomy teaches us that man resembles the frugivorous animals in everything, the carnivorous in nothing . . . It is only by softening and disquising dead flesh by culinary preparations that it is rendered susceptible to mastication or digestion, and that the sight of its bloody juices and raw horror does not excite loathing and disgust . . .
>
> "Man resembles no carnivorous animal. There is no exception, unless man be one, to the rule of herbivorous animals having cellulated colon. The orang-outang perfectly resembles man both in order and in the number of his teeth.
>
> "The orang-outang is the most anthropomorphous [man like] of the ape tribe, all of whom are strictly frugivorous. There is no other species of animals which live on different foods in which this analogy exist."

Even fruit can be a source of protein Dr. Hilbert (33) describes the complex structure of an orange: "We now recognize 11 amino acids . 17 carotenoid pigments, of which 4 have vitamin A activity, and 11 flavanoids . . . the flavoring constituents of the oil are no less than 28 in number, of course there are many others yet to be found."

Consider the following table from PSYCHO-PSYSIOPATHY (241) by Dr. T. De la Torre.

	CARNIVORA	ANTHRAPOID FRUIGIVORA AND FRUITARIAN MAN
Teeth	Incisors are underdeveloped; molars are long, sharp and pointed.	Incissors are well developed. Molars for crushing and grinding.
Jaw	Up and down motion for tearing or biting.	Equipped for grinding motion.
Saliva	Acid saliva geared to digestion of animal protein; lacks ptyalin, a chemical which digests carbohydrates.	Highly developed system; alkaline saliva adopted to the digestion of sugar and starch. Oblong in shape, complicated in structure, convoluted with duodenum.
Stomach	Simple, round sack which secretes ten times more hydrochloric acid than that of vegetarian, proportionately.	
Intestine	Three times the length of the trunk.	Twelves times the length of the trunk.
Colon	Short and smooth, designed for prompt evacuation, not digestion.	Long and involved; digestion takes place in it.
Liver	Far more active than in fruigivora. Eliminates proportionately 10 to 15 times more uric acid.	Capacity to eliminate only the uric acid produced by the organism itself.
Hands	Claws for tearing flesh and for killing.	Fingers adopted to pluck fruit.
Skin	Do not sweat through skin. Excrete excess moisture through bladder and controls body heat by rapid breathing. No pores.	Sweat through the skin to lose excess moisture and to control body heat. Has pores.
Urine	Acid, offensive in odor.	Alkaline, with inoffensive odor.
Eyes	Sideways.	Forward.
Tongue	Rasping.	Smooth.
Mobility	Go on all fours.	Walk upright.

The human being requires minimal dietary protein as obtained from sprouts, grasses and fruit. The protein composition of the body is in a constant state of change, with proteins constantly being broken down and resynthesized. Tissue protein breakdown and dietary protein contribute to a common metabolic pool of nitrogen from which amino acids are withdrawn for rebuilding tissue protein and for the formation of new protein for growth. There is a great deal of recycling of protein.

Nutritional Experiments (32) by W. Lintzel showed that plant proteins are more efficient than animal proteins in maintaining the nitrogen balance in adults. His experiments showed that smaller quantities of potato and rye grain protein were required than protein from milk, egg or meat.

The human being needs the eight essential amino acids found in a complete protein. A protein is complete if it can maintain a healthy body. The strongest animals—the ox, elephant, horse—live on a diet of grass. The gorilla can maintain life on the protein provided by a diet of fruit: oranges, bananas, mangoes. The human being's digestive system and physiological makeup is identical with that of a gorilla; hence people can maintain themselves on a diet of fruit.

Furthermore, on a low protein vegetarian diet, according to studies by Drs. Oomen and Hipsley, the natives of New Guinea had in their intestinal tract bacteria, clostridium refringes B, which supplied a major proportion of protein, by creating amino acids from nitrogen inhaled with air.

Once the body is cleansed, its tissues regenerated, cell wall and membrane permeability reestablished, then .5 (or less) to 10 grams of protein daily are adequate. Under such conditions, the low protein diet (which is non-acid forming) does not destroy cells, and there is minimal new cell building.

MINERALS

MINERALS — We are told that we require a large quantity of alkaline minerals, especially calcium. Actually, they are needed to neutralize acid waste products derived from metabolism of the typical high sugar, high fat, high starch, high protein diet. The higher the ingestion of phosphorus, the more calcium we need. Meat and grain are very high in phosphorus. On such a diet, without calcium from milk, dolomite, dulse, sesame seed or fresh fruits and vegetables the body would sicken and die from acidosis. A vegetarian diet, low in starch and protein, provides just enough alkalinity to neutralize the acid waste products of metabolism. The greatest aid to metabolising calcium and alkalinizing the bloodstream is sun-radiated air and water. Vegetarians who maintain a diet high in cooked minerals especially calcium, sometimes develop arthritis (deposition of excessive mineral in the tissues) at an early age. Stones in the kidney and gall bladder are the result of a high inorganic mineral intake.

CALORIES

CALORIES – Another fallacy is the recommendation of at least 2400 calories per day just to stay alive. (See: Liquitarianism; Overeating.) This energy would be required only for metabolism of the typical high protein, high starch, cooked diet. Waste resulting from such a diet clogs the body, impairing normal function. Layers of sludge and fecal matter in the colon diminish absorption of nutrients, causing loss of energy. Arteriosclerosis (affects most Americans over 20) and clogging of fine capillaries demand additional energy to maintain a high blood pressure for circulation. Thickening of the blood with the waste products of protein and starch metabolism (mucus), builds resistance to its flow, again requiring increased energy for its circulation

Energy comes from the combustion of fuel. This requires oxygen. Most lungs are so filled with mucus and air pollutants that they are utilized to only one sixth of their capacity. Very low oxygen intake means incomplete combustion of food, which must be eliminated at further expense of energy.

Dr. R. W. Gerard writes: (40) "Body is not a particularly efficient machine from the energy point of view. The transformation of chemical energy in food into actual work involves a considerable waste of fuel. The human body is only about 30 per cent efficient, ranging from 20 to 40 per cent. About three times as much energy is consumed in the form of food as comes out in the form of physical work."

Only the inefficient use of energy in a toxic body demands a high caloric intake. In turn, a high caloric intake induces a toxic body which uses energy inefficiently.

CONDIMENTS

CONDIMENTS – Spices and salt were the ingredients the ancient Egyptians used to embalm the dead. Modern dietetics helps to start the embalming process early in life via salad dressings. It results in dry, pale skin, shrunken tissues, white hair, hardened liver and arteries. Natural oil is difficult to digest. Heat-treated or processed oil, or that derived from animal sources is next to impossible to metabolize. Generally it deposits out in arteries to hinder circulation and prevent passage of nutrients into cells. The best source of oil is whole seed, nuts, olive or avocado. The best oil comes from olives, avodaco or sesame seed–always request unfiltered, virgin, cold pressed. Keep refrigerated.

Fats are stored in tissues for later use or oxidized to carbon dioxide and water. Fat is unaffected by the saliva and only slightly affected by gastric juices. If we coat any food with oil, much of the food remains undigested until it reaches the intestine where bile can dissolve the oil.

On a fruitarian diet, carbohydrates are converted into the fats needed by the body. The fat-soluble vitamins (A, D, E, K) are created by the cells as they interact with sunlight.

DEADLY DAIRY

DAIRY PRODUCTS – We are the only animal who continues to drink milk after weaning. Pasteurized dairy products are very mucus-inducing. Cataract, respiratory disorders, arthritis, arterial degeneration, allergy commonly result from eating pasteurized dairy products. Pasteurized milk is as deadly as meat, yet so many vegetarians take this path of slow suicide (30,73,167,251-258).

Dr. Annand, in a ten year study, proved conclusively that heated milk is a primary contributor to all forms of heart disorders (38).

Dr. G. O. Kohler, et al, (37) in a study "Relationship of the Grass Juice Factor to Guinea Pig Nutrition" observed that animals died within 5 weeks of respiratory complications (mucus) when placed on a diet of pasteurized milk and orange juice. However, when grass juice was added, it provided enzymes to metabolize the mucus. He states: "Animals receiving mineralized milk, orange juice, and grass juice grew at a good rate and no abnormalities were observed. When the grass juice was omitted the animals died."

STIMULANTS

STIMULANTS is any substance which speeds body metabolism. When one starts the change from processed, low quality foods and stimulating poisons, the eliminative organs start expelling medicine, stimulants, pesticides, excess bile, tissue deposits and mucus, gas in cells, cementing material from stiff joints. One goes through symptoms of a withdrawal of stimulation–slower heart rate, decrease in nervous energy (with apparent mental stupor). Less energy is available for physical activity.

Stimulants must be avoided at this time. They do not give any more energy than a whip applied to a sick work horse. In the human body, a "death struggle" ensues to throw off such a chemical. Under stimulants we must include cigarettes, teas, many herbs, coffee, sugar, cocoa meat, medicine, spices, alcoholic beverages, pepper, salt. How do they affect us?

The introduction of a pathological amount of food and waste material causes the body to increase its rate of metabolism. One of the waste products of protein metabolism is uric acid, which is a purine (like caffein), a known stimulant. Withdrawal from animal protein makes one feel weak for several days.

Coffee, tea, cocoa have a somewhat alkaline reaction. Their residue combined with uric acid and other colloids is precipitated out as crystals (urates), which may be deposited out in tissues to cause rheumatism, arthritis and kidney stones.

Spices, condiments and alcohol act as irritants to delicate cell walls. They stimulate increased flow of body fluids and can effect sensations of false hunger. Eventually, they cause thickening of cell walls.

Stimulants can create a desire for excessive sexual activity, which increases production of sexual fluids, drawing minerals and other nutrients from teeth, bones and other tissues for their manufacture. This speeds the aging process and the eventual wasting away of teeth, hair, vital organs and reserve energy.

A diet heavy in grain and meat and stimulants such as alcohol, tobacco coffee, give the adult a pickup for a moment. Yet notice the happy state and quick energy of the child who eats natural sugar—fruit.

HOW TO GET STONED ON WATER

Many doctors and nutritionists still recommend drinking six to eight glasses of water daily. Is this wise? According to government figures over fifty percent of tap water fails to meet minimum standards. The purification process for tap water introduces twenty to sixty new chemicals into your drink. Sodium fluoride (rat poison) acts as an enzyme inhibitor, causes or intensifies allergies, kidney-liver-thyroid-bone damage, may affect the newborn and cause mottling of teeth. Chlorine (bleach) destroys cells and ages the body prematurely. Additives and pollutants in water are one of the causes of toxemia.

The "pure" water that one may drink from spring, lake, river, well or running stream is one of the major factors in producing the cemented joints of arthritis; gall and kidney stones hardening of the arteries and the brain.

Throughout our lives, we build up inorganic sedimentary deposits in tissues, blood and lymph vessels and eliminative organs of the body. At birth the baby is about 75 percent water; by the time it reaches age thirty, the percentage of water in the body is about 55 percent. Where did the water go? It was displaced by the accumulation of precipitated minerals.

It is physiologically impossible for your body to assimilate inorganic minerals in building healthy tissue and blood. Calcium carbonate (lime) and other minerals will cement your body. Were it not for the activity of the eliminative organs, most people, by the age of forty, would accumulate enough cement in their bodies to become statues.

Distilled water, although preferable to other water, has a slight tendency to leech calcium and other nutrients from teeth, bones and cells. To prevent leeching, expose water to sunlight for several hours, and/or use colored drinking glasses. Or soak dried or fresh fruit (or vegetables), seed, (alfalfa, wheat, fenugreek) or crushed grass overnight, to introduce nutrients into dead distilled water and convert it to live juice. Such water will help to flush out accumulated poison from bloodstream and cells.

When obtaining distilled water, be sure that it does not come in plastic bottles. The plastic imparts a plastic taste. Do not buy chemically distilled water. Find a source which uses stainless steel and glass distilling apparatus. Get a complete analysis of the water, whatever the source. Most companies are happy to provide this information.

Drinking water is completely unnatural and is necessitated only by a concentrated acid-forming diet. Our natural foods, fresh fruits and vegetables, contain at least ninety percent energy-charged tasty fluid. This is all the water we need.

ROUGHAGE AND NATURES PREDIGESTED FOODS

After detoxification ingestion of nature's predigested foods (sprouts fruits juices) will increase vitality. You will be minimizing the following digestive tasks: starch digestion (three hours), protein digestion (four to six hours), fat digestion (six to ten hours), mixed digestion (four to twenty-four hours to empty the stomach) and pasteurized milk digestion (twelve to forty-eight hours).

Dr. Abrahamson states (41): "In digestion all the carbohydrates are converted into sugar. Fifty-six percent of the proteins also are converted into sugar, but only ten percent of the fats." The body has to go through a great deal of work to convert starch and complex protein into sugar. It is far better to get more natural sugar in the form of fruit and less from concentrated foods.

Your body has no need for starch or fat; they can be supplied by sunlight and sugar from fruit and vegetables. There is no known nutritional value in cellulose. For toxic individuals eating processed foods, cellulose acts as an intestinal broom, insuring daily removal of waste. As purity is increased, the size of the internal organs decreases; very little bulk is required to have a good daily bowel movement. The slightly acid pH of sweet fruit, and up to one gallon of fluids from fruit or juice, will insure daily elimination. When one is totally detoxified, daily elimination is not all that important, since most metabolic waste products can be excreted by the skin and kidneys.

Juicing eliminates most of the cellulose. Most raw juices contain enough protein to build healthy bodies. Juice is digested and assimilated in twenty minutes. In vibrant individuals, it is evacuated in two hours. However, it takes ten to twenty hours to eliminate a vegetable meal; two to twelve hours a fruit meal. A mixed non-vegetarian meal takes one to five days.

You will need less sleep; fruitarians sleep one to four hours; raw food vegetarians, three to six hours; cooked and mixed diet, six to twelve hours. If you eat little, use live food, and fast at least six hours between meals, your digestive tract will spend a great deal of time resting instead of working so hard to eliminate excessive food. You will become stronger, more beautiful, witty, spiritual and happy.

MUCUS CLEARED UP

Mucus is found in the lungs, gonads and the intestinal tract lining. Its function is to protect the delicate tissues of the body from the external corrosive irritable fluids and gases.

In the gastrointestinal tract you will find glands which produce mucoproteins that can resist the action of almost all digestive juices. They form a thin film on the intestinal tract to protect the mucosa. The mucus (or mucoproteins) is a clear slimy fluid that can neutralize either acids or bases. Mucus acts as a lubricant that assists the passage of food along the digestive tract.

The mucus secreted in the mouth acts primarily as a lubricant for easy swallowing. In the stomach, where the largest amount is secreted, the mucus prevents the stomach walls, which are made of protein, from being digested. In the absence of mucus, an ulcer hole would be formed in the stomach walls within a few hours. A large amount of mucus is also secreted in the duodenum and along the rest of the small intestine to neutralize the HCL acid and pepsin found in the chime (predigested food) newly arrived from the stomach.

A diet of high proteins and processed foods causes the secretion of strong digestive juices. As a protective measure, the body increases tremendously the activity of the mucus secreting glands. The mucus interacts with the digestive juices (and/or some of the harsh dietary factors) and precipitates out as an undigestable complex mucoprotein. The excessive amount of these mucoproteins congest the system. The intestinal lining is densely covered with villi which are imbedded with many blood capillaries and lymphatic vessels. The lymph system has openings large enough to accommodate the entry of some of the mucoprotein, plus some of the complex partially digested proteins.

The mucoproteins build up extensively and go through some dehydration and hardening, congesting the lymph vessels and introducing poor protein distribution and some localized starvation. The mucus build-up causes serious interference with oxygen exchange, biological functions and food digestion. The degree of mucus build-up can be observed in the iris by noting the degree of cloudiness and the extensiveness of the "lymphatic rosary"

The condition is reversible. A diet which excludes foods that are processed and/or high in protein and/or fat is best. When one eats fruit, sprouts and indoor greens — food in which protein is in the predigested form of amino acids and enzymes — one greatly assists the body to correct the diseased condition. Fasting, when advisable, and juice regimes are the fastest ways to clean up the lymph vessels. If a long fast is not desirable, to speed the cleansing of the mucus linings the following program is advisable. Repeat it as often as needed.

To begin, skip the evening meal. Instead have juice with a mild herbal laxative. Before bedtime, take one or more enemas. If you wish, follow it with a grass juice implant. (Evacuation on this program might not occur until the second day, giving you a temporary feeling of fullness. You can expect worms, putrefactive strings, solid particles, stones and /or ropes of mucous, unimaginable in size and quantity.)

Material needed: fresh juices, seed grinder and one pound of psyllium seed. One can use the psyllium drink upon arising and on retiring in conjunction with a cleansing diet or one can go on a 3 to 7 day cleansing juice regime as described below. To prepare the drink, finely grind one cup of the psyllium seed. Place a heaping teaspoon of powdered seed into jar. Add one cup of juice, tea or water, cover tightly. Shake for about ten seconds. Drink immediately before it turns into jelly.

Juice regime: For the first three days start the day with one cup of hot peppermint papaya tea (or any one of your favorite herbs). During the day take five psyllium drinks about every two or three hours apart. Each time drink an additional glass of water. Take a fruit or vegetable juice one hour later. In the evening take several enemas. If possible, follow with an implant.

For the last three days, continue the program, except for the evening meal you may have a vegetable or fruit salad. Use enemas as needed and implants as available. On the seventh day resume eating mucus lean solid food.

A cleansing regime can bring on conditions which are conventionally called diseases such as colds, flu, boils and skin rash. Abstain from solids, drink plenty of fluids, rest and persevere (see Crises). People quite often feel they are on the wrong regime. The healing process is not necessarily pleasant.

OVEREATING AND ELIMINATION

"If we keep food going into our stomachs only once every 24 hours or 48 hours, and do not get the foolish idea that this cannot be done, then we can train our stomachs to eat once a week and our stomachs will not call for food more than once a week, we could live as long as Methuselah"

ELIJAH MUHAMMAD,   HOW TO EAT TO LIVE

"You will not give even an hours rest to me your stomach. Day after day, every hour you keep on eating. You have no idea how I suffer, O trouble making ego. It is impossible to get on with you."
Osborne

"Enter only into the Lord's sanctuary when you feel in yourselves the call of his angels, for all that you eat in sorrow, or in anger, or without desire, becomes a poison in your body. For the breath of Satan defiles all these. Place with joy your offerings upon the altar of your body, and let all evil thoughts depart from you when you receive into your body the power of God from his table. And never sit at the table of God before he calls you by the angel of appetite.
Rejoice, therefore, always with God's angels at their royal table, for this is pleasing to the heart of the Lord. And your life will be long upon the earth, for the most precious of God's servants will serve all your days: the angel of joy."
Jesus, THE ESSENE GOSPEL OF PEACE

"He who is slave to his stomach seldom worships God."
SAADHI

"It is better to go to the house of mourning than to go to the house of feasting."
ECCL. 7:2

"The way to eat a lot is to eat little, that way you live long enough to be able to eat a lot."
Anonymous

"God places the sin of gluttony in the same catalogue with drunkenness. So offensive was this sin in the sight of God that He gave directions to Moses that a child who would not be restrained on the point of appetite, but would gorge himself with anything his taste might crave, should be brought by his parents before the rulers of Israel, and should be stoned to death. The condition of the glutton was considered hopeless. He would be of no use to others, and was a curse to himself. No dependence could be placed upon him in anything. His influence would be ever contaminating others, and the world would be better without such a character; for his terrible defects would be perpetuated. None who have a sense of their accountability to God will allow the animal propensities to control reason."
ELLEN G. WHITE [23]

"Blessed art thou, O land, when . . . thy princess eat in due season, for strength, and not for drunkenness."
ECCL. 10:17

JAMES 5:16

"Confess your faults one to another, and pray one for another that ye may be healed."
MARK 11:24
"Therefore I say onto you that things soever ye desire, when you pray, believe that ye receive them, and ye shall have them."

Eat little, be happy, love everybody and earthly joy will follow. Most of us know all that is needed to make us perfect and to give us and our children eternal youth and happiness. Why do we lack will power to put knowledge into action? Will is of divine origin and is easy to execute when all our actions are in tune with God's will. The fall of the human being from the plane of God-consciousness, and degeneration to weak will, came from eating forbidden food (all seed and animal substance), which upset the balance of endocrine secretions necessary to psychic power, will power, constancy. Food stimulants replace the spiritual love currents which electromagnetically activated tropical fruitarian man and woman. Therefore, when you wish something, stop to consider whether your body really needs it.

During dietary transition the hardest task will be to cut down on the size of meals. Most doctors recognize that overeating is the greatest killer.

Dr. Exton-Smith (155) for example points out that his own experiments have shown that the diet promoting fastest growth both hastens maturity and shortens life. The optimal diet is that which produces a slow rate of growth and that which produces a slow rate of growth and late maturation, "You can have every confidence that a feeding regimen that results in a thin child who matures slowly will produce a healthier, longer-lived adult."(156)

Some of the major causes of overeating are forced feeding in childhood, anxiety, unnatural diet, spices, poor mastication, enlargement of the stomach from past feasts.

The image of self is very important. It develops, in the most subtle way, from the pre-natal period onward. A poor image of self creates anxiety, which is discomforting. This leads to a course of action to reduce discomfort. Since anxiety is mainly a mind-emotion activity, anything that reduces the energy level in the brain will also reduce anxiety. When you eat, the vital forces of the body become centralized in digestion. Many people even feel sleepy if they eat too much. The awareness of self and its contrast with the ideal self is lowered; thus anxiety is relieved. When you were a baby, mother relieved your anxieties by giving you food. When older, you try subconsciously to duplicate the experience.

No matter how difficult your childhood may have been, it is not too late to change the self-image. Read books in the field of positive thinking. (see Appendix: Spiritual and Psychology Books). The inspirational writings from great spiritual texts have even more to offer. Participate in meditation, sensitivity and encounter sessions. Discover the cause of anxiety and make every effort daily to overcome it. Unless the cause of stress and anxiety is discovered and eliminated, prolonged tension can cause mental and physical exhaustion.

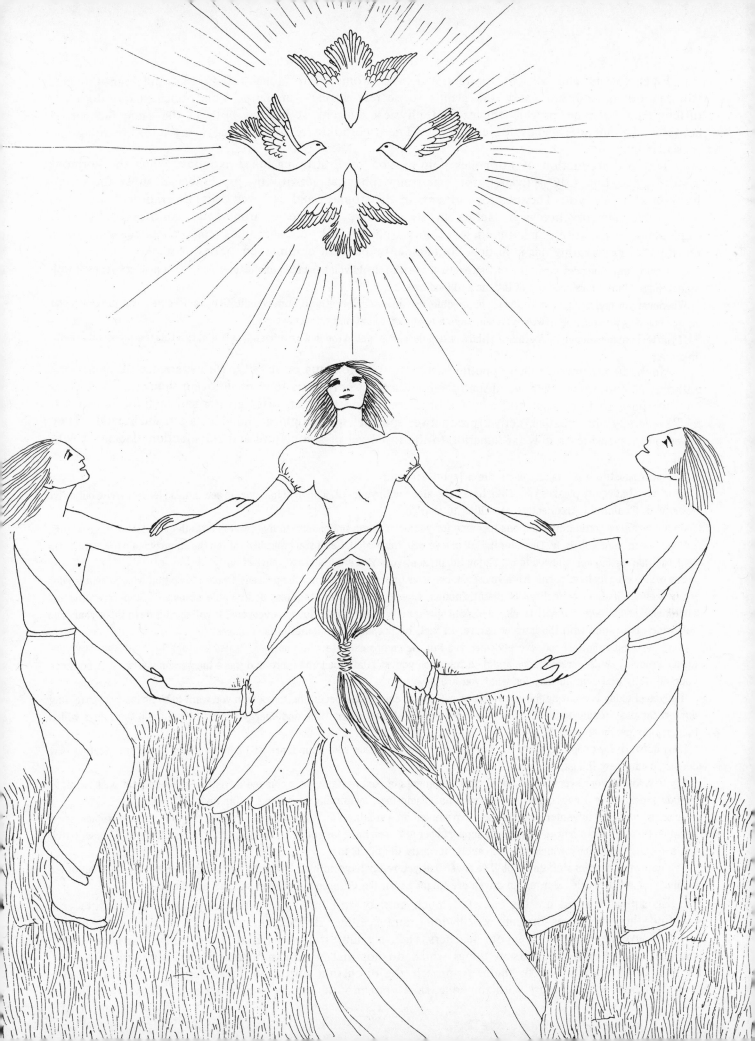

Psychologists and ancient masters and wise women have long known that unloving thoughts towards others and self cause the glands to secrete strong stimulants. Your subconscious does not differentiate between psychic threats and physical dangers. It handles both in the same manner. It activates the ductless glands for emergency. The secretions create increased heart rate, breathing and muscular tension.

This overproduction of hormones poisons you by destroying inner harmony. When the hormone system is continuously activiated for emergency physical activity by psychological stress the excess hormones can age you. They destroy nutrients in the stomach and can even cause ulceration.

Beside the psychological factors in stress, there are the environmental contributors such as unpleasant occupation, inharmonious colors, noise, lack of sunshine, cold climate, indigestion, constipation, overeating, air pollution, contaminants found in clothing, cosmetics or soap.

In "Desiderata" the poet says:"Nurture strength of spirit to shield you in sudden misfortune. But do not distress yourself with imaginings. Many fears are born of fatigue and loneliness.. .."

Whenever you feel tired, rest. If this is not possible, do some deep breathing, some meditation; take some fresh juice or a cup of ginseng or gotu-cola; otherwise, you will have a tendency to eat and to overeat.

If you feel anxious, lonely, experience failure or hopelessness; get in touch with a friend; talk it out; if this is not possible, write in a diary.

Much of our uncontrolled appetite is the result of toxemia or anxiety. We experience discomforting withdrawal symptoms when we abstain from addictive "poisonous food or unloving thoughts."

We have to find a substitute for feasting, something that can offer greater satisfaction; don't feast, fast. Generally the creative, active, productive, spiritual, philosophical individuals are small eaters. They have found pleasure that is far superior to the low level of stimulation and stupefaction associated with food.

The best substitute is making one's life a joyful adventure.

Find out what really pleases you. Take time to be alone with yourself. This will help you to see things clearly. Write out a five year plan. Evaluate it frequently; be willing to change.

Join a group or community that has meaning for you or create a philosophy to live by. Become the creator of the real you.

Visualize the new you daily. Discover it. Fall in love with this vision. Let it start taking a role on the stage of your life. S/he is the real you that was never allowed to be. Enjoy the present you. You can recreate yourself daily.

See where your feelings spring from your past, negative experiences and not the present. Choose to do that which creates good inner feelings instead of feelings of dissatisfaction. Check all your acts against a desirable standard. Stop repeating old addictions. Eventually you will develop a blissful spontaneity that radiates love to everyone. It will spring forth from your true self which is in tune with the laws of nature. In fact, be prepared for some initial failures.

Don't persecute yourself too severely when you fail. Be compassionate with yourself. Praise yourself for your successes and keep on moving. With perseverance and determination you will daily become more and more the person you want to be. Love yourself daily and continuously for what you are now.

The you of today is creating the you of tomorrow. Spend energies in becoming the person you want to be instead of struggling against the past images and addictions. The more good you do, the less time and energy you will have to do the things which hinder your personal growth.

Look outward for people to share the adventure of life with. Don't let your fears and hang-ups stop you from meeting new people, trying new things, new diets.

Try to rekindle your secret childhood dreams, moments of past ecstasy and achieved adventures. These past wishes might include a desire for a new career, travel, spiritual disciplines, swimming or sailing to far away islands.

To bring into being adventure into the new, experiment on a small scale. For example, if you desire to live in the tropics, try a vacation there, find out how to marginally support your self, learn the language of the country you wish to go to. This will give you a feeling of security which you can apply towards the big leap.

Evaluate your current situation. You'll discover that you really have nothing to lose by becoming the new you. Seek out other similarly attuned people. Sharing an adventure might mean the difference between success and failure.

Egosim and greed are the cause of much anxiety and hate. From the study of laws of nature you will find the few things that are worth doing and keeping. Be discriminating; like what is worth liking, but love everyone for all are your teachers, each a manifestation of God. Don't judge, be here in the univeral now. Yield to others in things which do not matter. On important issues, communicate your feelings to those who evoke them. Approach the discussion with love; it will result in mutual psychic growth. When you are angry with someone, shut your mouth, silence your mind and let love flow in.

If daily, you feed you mind with optimism, constructive thoughts, and only useful, loving information, it will speed you to health and God consciousness. Every physical pain leaves emotional scars, likewise psychic blows are physiologically integrated as body ailments. Emotional cleansing, as well as physical detoxification can be a painful process. You have to be honest. Know thyself. We must flush out emotional blockages with a fast of love and self-discovery. The reward will be innocence and joy.

To lessen anxiety temporarily, choose a challenging activity. A simple task such as cleaning a room, washing dishes, fixing a machine, building a fence, yoga, dance, song, or exercise can be very therapeutic. Psychic energy is converted to physical activity. It temporarily diverts you from the threadmill of negative emotions. After finishing your task, you have strengthened your self-concept by having something visible of which to be proud.

Some who have failed over the years to control their appetites, have found success and were healed when they recognized that they were possesed by disincarnate souls, seeking worldly pleasures. Jesus said "Nothing shall be impossible for you thru fasting and prayer." Knowing the cause of one's glutteny, pure thoughts and words can be used to send spirits away. They will leave you when through fasting you take away the sensual pleasure.

If you are trying to control your diet, do not keep in the house specific food, drink or spices which you wish to avoid. When you feel anxious you will indulge in them. Afterward, feeling guilty because of lack of discipline, you will eat even more.

Ambivorous Anonymous.

Some techniques have been found to assist an individual during the dietary changes.

Try an imaginary binge. Eat with your mind to your stomach's content all the naughty foods you are trying to avoid. Think about how the food tastes, feels and smells. Feel your stomach expanding, your consciousness diminishing and youth fading.

Recall the details of how you felt after a feast. Visualize the kind of disease a congested body can cause. If you still have vigor, analyze the tempting piece of pie, cake or pizza. You'll see all the mucus it will generate in your body, the tooth decay it will cause. See the composition: lots of calories, foodless starchy white flour, hydrogenerated fat, lung destroying pasteurized milk, cancer causing artificial flavorings, nerve wrecking color additives. Ask yourself: How was the pie grown? Was it on a tree, a bush, or was it created by a human being in a laboratory?

Keep a diary of your daily eating habits. Time, quantity and choice of food should be entered. What were the motivating psychological reasons for overeating: punishing someone, anxiety, avoidance. Were you tired and eating for stimulation? Are you hypoglycemic? How did you feel before and after the meal? Enter daily your weight. Where did you eat? Was it straight from the refrigerator, a can or a restaurant? Did you leave many temptations of naughty foods around the house?

Before you begin eating you generally still have some sanity about your dietary needs. On a plate in the kitchen serve as much food as you think you should eat. Take the plate to the dining room. Do not go for seconds or nibble after the meal. Remember, "One extra mouthful will be too much and a hundred will not be enough." Sharing food with others, eating slowly, chewing food throughly, being quiet in peaceful surrounding will reduce overeating.

Start each meal with a prayer, chant, or meditation. Ask the Omnipresent Spirit for aid in self-mastery. Think about the strength and health the food is to give you. Visualize yourself in the beautiful body you can gain by self-mastery. Do not read, listen to the radio or watch television. Concentrate on the Omnipresent as you chew throughly your simple fare. It is best not to indulge in conversation while eating, but if you have company, limit discussion to friendly love exchanges, no disputes. Only pleasant thoughts encourage good digestion.

Have few preferably unseasoned, selections at a meal. Each new food creates its own hunger by chemical stimulation. One food at a meal reduces a minimum the craving for large fare. Meat satisfies one kind of hunger. If it is followed by bread and butter, new cravings are created and must be satisfied. There is no limit.

Many people eating an inadequate diet, continue to experience hidden hunger even when their stomachs are full. This craving is a sign that the diet lacks certain food vibrations. Unless they are supplied, the individual will develop visible symptoms of deficiency. If hidden hunger remains unsatisfied, the eventual result of ignoring this survival mechanism is chronic disease and death.

To overcome this craving, include in your diet some grass or raw, fresh vegetable juice, a mixture of sprouted alfalfa and mung beans, sea vegetables and sun. Chew on the grass between meals. Hidden hunger will quickly disappear.

ONLY THE SKINNY WILL SURVIVE

Unless you change your life-style, you may anticipate the "vengeance of the gods", In the Puranas, (Ancient Hindu Scriptures), the food god complains to Lord Vishnu, the sustainer of the Universe, that people misuse him a great deal. To this, Lord Vishnu replies: "Those who eat too much, you must eat them up, for that is the only remedy."

The warning of Lord Vishnu was vividly demonstrated in 1927 when the late Dr. Clive McCay of Cornell University made his classic dietary experiment. He doubled the life span of rats by halving their food intake. This would be equivalent to 140 years in human terms(248, 249, 250).

Professor Huxley extended the life span of worms by a factor of 19 through periodic fasting. In orthodox geriatric studies, it has been found that a slim body, due to little eating and excellent elimination, is an essential factor for reaching the century mark.

The U.S. National Academy of Science made these recommendations for diet among people above age 55; For males, 2,400 calories with 65 grams of protein; for females, 1,700 calories, with 55 grams of protein. According to a U.S. Department of Agriculture study, Americans of all ages consume a daily average of 3,300 calories with 100 grams of protein, 157 grams of fat and 380 grams of carbohydrate.

The countries which have the highest number of centurians, by American standards are starving to long life. In a survey of 55 adult males in Hunza, Pakistani nutritionist Dr. S.M. Ali found an average caloric intake of 1,923, with 50 grams of protein, 36 grams of fat, and 354 grams of carbohydrate. Meat and dairy products constitute only 1-½ percent of the total . Similarly, Guillermo, Vela of Quito found the daily diet of the elderly of Vilcabamba to average 1,200 calories, 37 grams of protein, 12 to 19 grams fat, and 200 to 260 grams of carbohydrate (160). On this meager diet, many a centurian covers 30 miles of rough mountain terrain in a 24 hour period.

In the USA, there are men who have applied the wisdom of under-eating for optimal endurance. Park Barner (199) lived on fruit and vegetable juices for the week before a 52 mile marathon race. He fasted for 24 hours preceding the race. It was reported "not only did he finish without having his energy run dry; he ran almost a half hour faster than his previous best for 50 miles."

"Under-eating" can increase our physical endurance, clear our heads and give us long life. In times of crisis, when famine is a reality, more people could be fed on less, giving everyone a fair share of the planet's harvest.

LOSE WEIGHT NOW!

Some individuals even when following a relatively good diet fail to lose weight. The problem stems from extensive amount of mucus throughout the body. This produces poor circulation. With the fat unaccesable there is very little weight loss. However, once the mucus is reduced the weight loss is speeded up.

The second factor which diminishes weight loss is a disorder of the gall bladder, especially if one has stones in this organ. Many individuals, after pursuing a vegetarian regime for at least one month have successfully passed stones in fecal matter through the following regime:

For three days, one stays on a liquid diet of apple juice and/or lemon drink. Enemas should be used. On the fourth day, one takes every two hours one to two ounces of raw organic olive oil mixed with four ounces of lemon drink. Drink a total of 6 to 12 ounces of olive oil.

The initial quick weight loss that many individuals experience is often the result of water loss when one excludes salt and other poisons from one's diet.

In weight reduction programs no mention is ever made of the central role the endocrine glands play.

Thyroxine secreted by thyroid glands control the rate of metabolism of all cells. Hormones secreted by the adrenal cortex regulate reabsorption of sodium by the kidneys (which may cause water retention) and also regulate some aspects of carbohydrate, fat and protein metabolism. Insulin, from pancreas, regulate fat and carbohydrate.

Ovarian degeneration or overactivity as might occur after marriage, bring on the sudden fattening of the body.

Regeneration of ductless glands can be brought about through non-toxic diet, continence and zone therapy stimulation of the glands.

TRANSITION TO KOSHER FOOD

Kosher dietary is the first civilized approach toward making eating a science in harmony with the physiology of the body. Moses saw that his followers were not ready for live food, hence he introduced correct food combinations and a selective diet.

"Bread in the morning and meat at night." (Exodus 16:8). Do not mix heavy starch and heavy protein at the same meal. Bread requires alkaline, meat requires acid digestive juices. Violating this rule results in constipation, putrescence, flatulence, indigestion and eventually cell starvation.

Another common error is eating honey (molasses, sugar or sweet fruit) with starchy or protein food. Starch digestion starts in the mouth. The taste buds recognize the sugar and send messages via the brain that pytalin (starch digestant) should be excluded from the saliva. Hence, starch (bread, cereal, sprouted grains) digestion does not get started. Sugar digestion takes place in the small intestine. The sugar mixed with starch or protein remains in the stomach much longer than it would if it were eaten alone, resulting in a fermentation (starch and sugar) process producing alcohol, or in putrefaction (protein and sugar) (Dr. Shelton, Food Combining Made Easy). Combining acid fruit (tomatoes, berries, oranges, sour apples, sour grapes, lemon) with starch also interferes with its digestion. Ptyalin is inactiviated by acid. Take fruit and starches at separate meals.

Milk is highly alkaline, high in fat content, hence it can slow digestion when combined with other protein foods. Too, drinking fluid with starch (or protein) dilutes and weakens the action of gastric juices in the stomach causing poor starch and protein digestion. Milk tends to form a large curd in the stomach, which can take up to 48 hours to eliminate. Or it can surround other foods with curd, isolating them from gastric juices. If milk is used, it should be taken raw and alone. Goat's milk is easier to digest than cow's milk.

Many people are suffering from protein, calcium and many other mineral starvation because of bad food combinations or bad food sequence at a meal. In nature, we almost never find protein from seeds, greens or nuts mixed with any acids. As a contrast, nature offers protein in predigested form, such as is found in fruit, where it is mixed with fruit acids.

In our stomach hydrochloric acid is secreted for the digestion of protein, calcium and other minerals. However, when acid fruit is eaten the digestive process excludes the secretion of hydrochloric acid; otherwise, a diet of fruit plus internal body acids would lead quickly to the development of ulcer or acid burn in the stomach. In fruit digestion, alkaline secretions are released.

Persons who eat fruit first or fruit and protein combination will develop protein and mineral deficiency in the long run. During the transition period, especially if you have a good digestion, you may use fruit as dessert: i.e., eat a meal rich in seeds or nuts and greens first, follow at least 30 minutes later with acid or sub-acid fruit (this includes lemon, tomato — unless it is the yellow non-acid kind — pineapple, apple cider vinegar). For a salad dressing, sprinkle lightly with sea vegetables, olive oil (or lecithin granules) and a dash of brewers yeast.

Beside food combining, Moses instructed his people in choice and preparation of meat. Fear, at death, floods the animal's body with strong hormones which poisons. Moses told the Jews to drain the carcas of blood to remove these hormones, germs and toxic waste. Animals that eat filth — all scavengers such as pig, eel and lobster — were prohibited from the diet. If diseased, the animal was unfit to eat.

You may start the transition to a better diet by excluding gradually all of the following non-foods: sugar, pasteurized dairy products, white bread and bakery products, all carbonated drinks, hamburgers, hot dogs, alcohol, cigarettes, snack foods, canned or processed foods, salt and strong condiments, vinegar, coffee, ice cream, candy, fried foods, chocolate and large fish (tuna, swordfish).

You may eat plenty of raw and cooked sprouts and vegetables, some Kosher (or organic) meat, such as chicken, and white fish and yogurt. Cut down on the size of meals and adhere to the food combining chart.

If you persist in eating bread, toast it dry and dark to reduce the mucus-forming (see Fasting) property peculiar to fresh bread. It will then provide enjoyment with minimal body harm. Eat it with avocado and sprouts.

Drink liquids at least twenty mintues before the meal; none with the meal. Eat starch (or sweets) and protein at separate meals. Eat raw before cooked food. If digestion is very poor, you may want to try juices and blended fruits or vegetables for several days to give the digestive organs a partial rest. In addition, you may do zone therapy in areas related to digestion and expose the body to red light for at least thrity minutes directly after a meal to increase the vitality of the digestive organs. If necessary, you

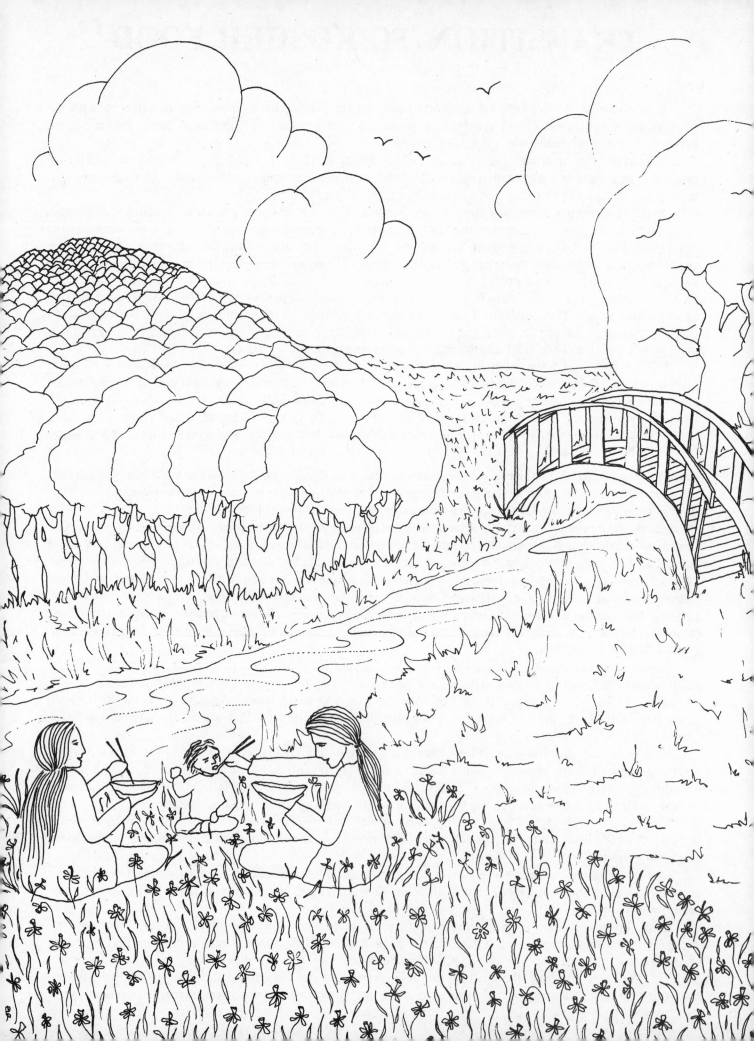

may use digestive enzymes. If hungry in between meals, drink herb tea, vegetable broth, vegetable or fruit juice. At least twice a week eat vegetables (cooked or raw) only.

The following schedule may help you into your new way of eating:

Morning: Immediately upon rising, a few Yoga asanas (or exercise). Deep breathing and meditation (or prayer). Close your eyes, press the eyeball with moderate pressure, if sore it indicates that the stomach is not emptied. In that event, for a happier day, skip breakfast or do a stomach wash (see Fasting). Do zone therapy. If the eyes feel good upon pressure, take lemon juice or rejuvelac. Before leaving for work, take fruit juice, fresh or dried fruit (soaked overnight or steamed), or steamed millet cereal or sesame yogurt with tomatoes or apples.

Lunch: Sprout or vegetable salad (carry the dressing or seed yogurt in a separate container), or ground seed, or fruit, or bread with a spread of avocado and sprouts. Take a fruit break instead of coffee, but only if hungry.

Supper: Vegetable and sprout salad with either baked vegetables or meat or fish. Occasionally try a fruit salad for an evening meal.

Evening Snack: Fruit, citrus juice or tea.

If anyone asks you about your food habits, just say, "doctor's orders". "Who is your doctor?" "Moses, of course."

If several hours after a meal you experience tiredness, gas, burping, nausea, aching in the eyes or lower back or any other discomfort, it may indicate that you have broken health rules (see Appendix).

If you have had no experience with fasting, skip breakfast at least once a week. After a month of improved diet, fast on fruit or water one day a week. Initially fasting is not so important.

VEGETARIAN AND MACROBIOTIC

"Since the ultimate cause of every illness is violation of the order of the universe through ignorance or arrogance, supreme medicine inclines toward the patient and sometimes lengthy technique of philosophy and education, rather than the quick "cure" by injection or amputation. It teaches man how to release his own innate ability to achieve sound judgement. Disease and illness in the philosophy of Zen Buddhism prepare and dispose man to receive the perfect health and happiness that only supreme medicine has to offer."

SAKURAZAWA NYOITI
(You are all Sanpaku)

"Formerly men had no fire but ate all their food raw. At that time they did not need to die for when they became old God made them young again. One day they decided to beg God for fire. They sent a messenger to God to convey their request. God replied to the messenger that he would give him fire if he was prepared to die. The man took the fire from God, but ever since then all men must die."

(Darasa, Dada, p.121 myth #49 in African Myths & Tales ed. by Susan Feldman pub. by Dell publ. co. 1963)

Today many studies have been published about vegetarians. The medical profession has observed that vegetarians enjoy superior health, outlive flesh eaters and have chronic disorders appearing less frequently and much later in life (42, 43). Dr. L. Avioli, director of endocrinology at Jewish Hospital, St. Louis, declared that vegetarians suffer less osteoporosis than people who eat lots of meat and have a high protein intake (150).

A classical study of 18 years duration was reported in the Australian Press. Sixty offspring of American soldiers were adopted by L. O. Builiz. They were reared vegetarians in the open country without innoculation or drugs. The diet consisted mostly of raw organic vegetables and fruit. For the last fifteen years dairy products were excluded. They never ate any meat or eggs or fish. Doctors examined the children periodically. Their conclusion was that these children were the healthiest in the world. They attributed the childrens' good health to their unusual diet (44).

Dr. Robert S. Harris of Massachusetts Institute of Technology, at the International Conference (226) on Vitamins in Havana in 1953, declared: "Both the vegetarian type and carnivorous type of diet can adequately feed people. It does not matter whether the calcium comes from milk or tortilla, whether iron comes from meat or tapala, whether niacin comes from wheat or rice, as long as these nutrients are available."

However, we see that it does matter where our food comes from. A cadaver is not the same as tapala; one will maintain health, the other will lead to disease. However, it does point out that scientists are willing to give status to the vegetarian diet which is practiced by about 80 per cent of the world's population.

The most brilliant thinkers and spiritual leaders: Buddha, Jesus, Pythagoras, Plato, Socrates, Ovid, Seneca, Plutarch, Swendenborg, Tolstoy, Rousseau, Voltaire, Milton, Shaw, Newton, Wagner, Bacon, Russell and many others heard the call of Nature and God: "Behold I have given you every herb bearing seed which is upon the face of all the earth, and every tree in which is the fruit of a tree yielding seed; to you it shall be for meat " (Genesis I 29). And it is becoming more and more accepted that in the great Taurean ages of matriarchy, people were vegetarians.

Every major city in America has a vegetarian restaurant and food center. Many are giving up killing animals and self with the prevalent dietary tradition. This is in tune with the majority of other earthlings who are vegetarians.

One of the most popular vegetarian paths is the macrobiotic. There are many advantages to this life-style. It leads one to develop a cosmic view and to study practical philosophy with the emphasis on Eastern culture. One discontinues using meat, processed foods, sugar and honey. Instead one eats a balanced diet of organic grains, vegetables, seed and some local fruit. Table salt is replaced by minerals from sea vegetables and sea salt. Harsh spices are replaced with fermented derivatives of grains.

Improvement in health and the apparent therapeutic effects of this diet can be attributed more to food excluded rather than to food included in the diet. A macrobiotic (like others on New Age food) has gotten away from the typical American practice of a high protein meat diet, bad food combinations, two pounds of sugar weekly, twenty-two pounds weekly of processed foods (white flour, fat, sugar, carbonated drinks), at least twenty pounds of preservatives per year, pasteurized dairy products, coffee, medicine. If one eliminates these items, one's health has to improve.

However, this diet is not optimal as a permanent diet for those who seek the ultimate in health, long life and spiritual growth. The short term effects are good, however the long term results have many disadvantages. Cereals are mucus-inducing and eventually constipating. Many adults and children on a high starch grain diet must turn to the handkerchief, which is completely unknown among detoxified raw fooders.

COOKED STARCHES

When living under unnatural city conditions, one obtains a very limited amount of sunshine and oxygen. The mucus-forming nature of grains reduces further the entrance of oxygen into the lungs. Furthermore, the sun rays that were trapped in food by plants, are destroyed in cooking, making them unavailable to the cells. Many of the most precious elements are found in the fragrance of cooked food; they are totally absent from cooked food itself.

Tubers and grains contain a high concentration of starch and mineral salts. When subjected to heat (cooking) the minerals are rendered insoluble and may be deposited in body tissues. Starch improperly combined with other foods, or when not well chewed can ferment in the stomach, producing alcohols injurious to health. Unsprouted grains are highly acid-forming, legumes even more so. They cause an acid condition in the body which may result in hardening of tissues and loss of bone-teeth calcium.

Feeding children a diet rich in starch is unwise. Henry Bieler, M.D. states (30) that "starches and fats are always poorly digested during the first year of life. After that, if there remains any degree of indigestion they should not be given." Dr. Hay writes(174)that the introduction of starch foods before teeth are formed results in acidity, bilious attacks, lack of appetite, sour vomit, irritability, bed-wetting. Nature does not provide enough ptyalin for their digestion until teeth are formed. If grain were a perfect food, it would not give a child indigestion.

SALT

Grains don't taste good without salt. Why? They are not a balanced food. The high concentration of potassium phosphate requires additional sodium for balance. If potash accumulates in the tissues, it causes irritation of the muscles and paralysis of the nerves. It is very toxic in the bloodstream. Interaction of potash and soda (salt) converts both elements into less harmful chemicals .The attempt of the body to achieve chemical balance makes starch-eating animals and humans crave salt.

Dr. Murphy states (46) that excess salt may cause a waterlogged condition which may lead to deafness and impaired sinus function. Quite early in clinical studies (47) it was recognized that salt disturbs cell mineral balance which can lead to cancer. Dr. Seeger observed (48) also that excess salt is a factor in cancer. A study (49) by the World Health Organization demonstrates that the level of consumption of salt by the Japanese relates to the frequency of stomach cancer.

A salt free diet was found by Dr. De Snoo (118) to be valuable in the prevention of eclampsia. Many other authors strongly advocate the reduction of salt (120, 121) when toxemia of pregnancy is feared.

Excess use of salt will preserve the individual just as it preserves plums, fish and other briny preparations. Doctors recognize that such practice can lead to hypertension.

Dr. L. K. Dahi, an authority on salt, advises (50) us to eliminate the use of all salt. Most of us consume 16 grams or more of salt per day. At most we need no more than five grams daily, he tells us, a quantity which can be supplied from natural foods.

Other authorities believe one gram is closer to the body's needs. In an article (51) "Body Fluids—A Major Medical Problem," J.D. Ratcliff wrote: "This year some 200,000 Americans will drown—not in oceans, streams or pools, but in their own body fluids. The cause is often congestive heart failure, as big a killer as cancer."

He says heart failure is often the result of excess body fluids which the organism retains to reduce concentration of the poisonous salt in the tissues and bloodstream. He states: "When diseased hearts are unable to pump enough blood to the kidneys, those organs fail to excrete the body's surplus fluid and it congests tissues. Feet, leg and ankles swell with retained water, a gallon or more may accumulate in the abdomen or chest—an ounce of salt in the body will trap and hold three quarts of water."

Dr. L. White et al (28) from studies on animals expressed: "added NaCl resulted in markedly increased water intake, food intake, and weight gain, less adrenal hypertrophy, larger tumors and increased hydration of the carcass."

CITY VEGETARIAN DIET

To avoid complications from improper food combining during the early stage of transition to the vegetarian diet, it is best to avoid all sweeteners. This will have the further benefit of more moderate cleansing reactions (see Crisis). Go light on grains—better are the cooked starchy vegetables—eat little of all seed. A touch of sea vegetables or fermented, aged seasoning from grains and legumes (miso, tamari) will provide salty taste.

During the transition you may have periods of cravings for specific natural wholesome (not necessarily optimal) foods—raw cheese, avocado, egg, garlic, hot pepper, fish, for example. Use them or equivalents sparingly in the purest form available. Cravings generally indicate a dietary need. These desires will disappear as health improves. Use plenty of juices and sprouts. Never eat more than enough.

Daily Diet

Breakfast: Vegetable or fruit juice, or soaked dried fruit, or fresh fruit in season or seed milks.

Lunch: Vegetable or grass juice 20 minutes before meal. Complete meal sprout salad (see Recipes), 1 to 2 cups. If chewing is a problem, blend the salad. Serve with soaked seasame and sunflower seed or ½ cup sesame-sunflower seed cheese or perfect dressing (see pg. 258) or with a little virgin cold press olive oil (wean off it, all oils stress body) and kelp/dulce.

Supper: Juice 20 minutes before meal. Sprout salad with olive oil (optional), kelp and other compatible vegetables. Iron pot meal or baked patato, yam, butternut squash, parsnip or other tubers - one cup or less.

Evening Snack: Celery or grass juice or herb tea.

Raw food vegetarians who are addicted to highly concentrated foods—seed, nuts, oil, avocado—live not much longer than meat eaters. It is far better to replace such foods with cooked low protein meals, especially in wintertime city conditions, maintaining at least an 80 percent raw food diet. Tubers or squash when baked or cooked in an iron pot, will satisfy the desire for heavy foods. They are far less a burden to the digestive and eliminative organs than high protein or fat food.

VEGETARIANS (233)

"Vegetarianism has been advocated and practiced by many of the greatest philosophers, scientists, leaders, and others, including Emerson, Thoreau, Buddha, Plato, Socrates, Pythagoras, Origen, Diogenes, Cicero, Herodotus, Porphyry, Sir Isaac Newton, Voltaire, Shelley, Pope, Plutarch, Ovid, H.G. Wells, Maeterlinck, John Wesley, Scott Nearing, Dr. Annie Besant, Field Marshal Lord Montgomery, Sir Stafford Cripps, Air Chief Marshal (RAF — "Battle of Britain") Lord Dowding and Lady Dowding, Louisa May Alcott, Vinoba Bhave, etc.

On the lighter side, in the entertainment world, the ranks of vegetarians have included such stars as the late George Arliss, Dennis Weaver, Clint Walker, Samantha Eggar, Dick Gregory, Susan St. James, Candice Bergen, Melanie, and many others.

In the field of sports, a vegetarian regimen has long been known to help build endurance. Among the athletes who have lived and/or trained as vegetarians are swimmer Johnny Weissmuller, Olympic multiple-gold-medal winner Murray Rose, "Flying Finn" runner Paavo Nurmi, wrestling champ George Hackenschmidt and "Mr. America" wrestler Gene Stanlee. Jack McClelland and Bill Pickering are famous channel swimmers who are vegetarian; in 1956, Pickering won fame by swimming the English Channel faster than anyone in history.

The Vegetarian Cycling and Athletic Club has held as many as 40% of the National (bicycle racing) Road Records, although their members comprise a small percentage of the racers. In 1963, vegetarian Ron Murgatroid swept a series of 15 out of 15 bicycle events in Great Britain.

In football, a 1970 article on former Oakland Raiders linebacker Chip Oliver (said to be "one of the finest young prospects in football") noted that he played better after switching to a vegetarian diet. And the annual race — ON FOOT — to the top of Pike's Peak was recently won two years in a row by a vegetarian.

No serious vegetarian would claim that by adopting his way of living one will automatically become an instant superman, or increase one's I.Q. by 50 points. But we should examine WHY so many thoughtful, intelligent, compassionate people become vegetarians."

ONE HOMOSAPIEN WELL DONE PLEASE

"It is in the cooking pots that your love in inflamed; it is in the kitchen that your faith grows fervid; it is in the flesh dishes that all your hope lies hid . . . who is held in so much esteem with you as the frequent giver of dinners, as the sumptuous entertainer? . . . Consistently do you men of flesh reject the things of the spirit. But if your prophets are complacent toward such persons, they are not my prophets." TERTULLIAN (77)

THE TEMPERATURE OF YOUR FOOD AFFECTS YOU

Anyone living in a northern climate, not only experiences the extreme range of seasonal temperature variation from nordic to tropic, but also tries to internalize these conditions by eating cold, frozen as well as heated, spiced foods. The consequence of extreme temperature range is apparent on the surface of the body. The face and hands age much more quickly than the covered portion of the body, which does not experience such seasonal variations. The unexposed skin of a seventy year old appears no different than that of a twenty year old. It has been protected. The same phenomenon operates internally. By eating extremely hot or frozen foods, one destroys oneself from within. After 20 to 60 years of such abuse, old age seeps in.

Franz J. Ingelfinger, M.D., authority on gastroenterology and editor of the New England Journal of Medicine in a study (52) of the civilized digestive tract, describes a dilemma similar to that of the Ancient Mariner dying of thirst while immersed in water. A person may starve while ingesting from the horn of plenty because the stomach cannot absorb the nutrients it contains. He says: "For want of an enzyme, a sugar is lost; for want of a sugar, salty fluid is lost; for want of such a fluid, much food is lost; and for want of the food, the patient is lost." Why? Because of the destruction of enzymes and of the stomach lining by hot, seasoned foods.

Doctor Ingelfinger reassures us: "complete shutdown of the absorptive process doesn't occur very often. Partial or near-total malabsorption, however, is quite common, and classically expressed in a disorder variously known as celiac disease, non-tropic sprue, idiopathic steatorrhea and celiac sprue." He examines the pathology of celiac sprue. "Under a hand lens, the normal mucosal lining of the small intestine resembles the myriad tentacles on the underside of a starfish; in sprue, it (small intestine) looks like a tanned pigskin. The villi are gone. Where the lush masses of fingerlike projections usually sway in dense profusion, the terrain in sprue is quite flat except for the pock marks that indicate the opening of persisting crypts." (See Page 218).

Dr. Conn McCluskey points out that constant irritation of the throat and tongue by hot foods and beverages, as well as alcohol can bring about cancer of the throat and tongue. He says: "If one is prepared to test the temperature of liquids which seem cool enough to drink by dipping the little finger in them and holding it there, it can be a shock to discover that the finger may actually by scalded. How much more must the delicate mucous membranes (of the mouth and throat) suffer." (The Lancet, 12, 29, 1973)

A recent study on enzyme destruction in body because of hot liquids consumed found that the intake of drink at high temperatures is positively associated with mucosal abnormalities in the stomach. A team of British doctors (**Lancet,** 9:56) interviewed 155 patients with gastric biopsies.

At the conclusion of the interview, each was given a fresh cup of boiling tea. When the patient drank the tea, its temperature (of the tea) was taken. The results: 2 out of 13 patients who drank tea below 122.5 F. showed any gastric enzymatic abnormalities, but those who drank tea above 137.5 F. showed disorders at the rate of 14 out of 18.

Hot foods and irritant spices produce this 'tanned pigskin.' You can prove this to your satisfaction. Every time you eat cooked food or drink hot fluids, pour the same amount on an area of your skin. Keep the hot material there until it cools to body temperature. Then you will sympathize with your suffering tongue, stomach and small intestine. You will notice that the skin turns initially pink, then red; after many applications, the skin cells take on the appearance of age. Then scars form. No less occurs in your digestive organs.

A microscope reveals the "intestinal roast" in more detail. "The normally slender, columnar epithelial cells with their regularly shaped and evenly placed nuclei are replaced by a ragged row of uneven cuboidal cells with distorted, haphazardly placed nuclei. Under the surface epithelium the crypts are still there. But they penetrate a lamina propria that is thickened and heavily infiltrated with mononuclear and eosinophilic cells, the type of white blood cells that tend to accumulate when tissues are indolently inflamed or otherwise irritated." (52)

'Leukocytosis' is the name that medical pathology gives to an excessive number of white corpuscles in the blood. Doctors discovered this phenomena in 1846 and Wirchow classified "digestive leukocytosis" as "normal" since everyone seemed to suffer from it. This was upset over three decades ago by the findings of Paul Kouchakoff, MD, who showed that food in its natural, uncooked state did not produce leukocytosis, or actually the cooking of food was the cause of leukocytosis.

The white corpuscles are the defense organisms of the blood that prevent infection and intoxification of the blood. In any pathological condition, including the intoxification of the digestive system with cooked food or other toxic materials, these white cells increase from 5 or 6 thousand per

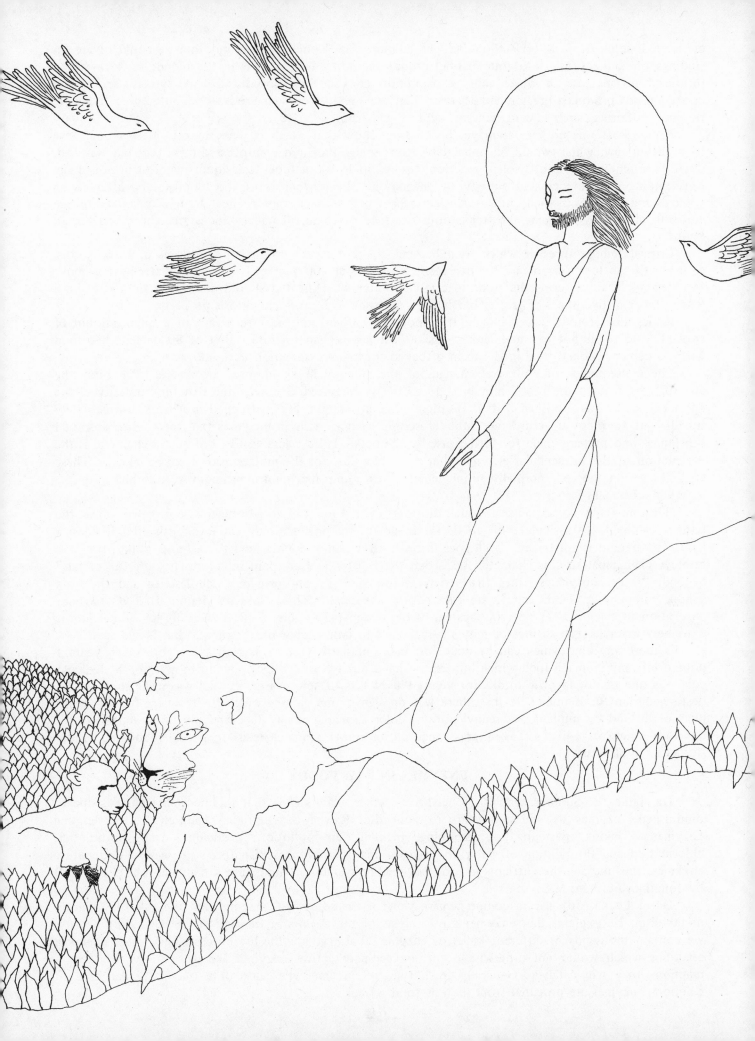

cubic millimeter to 7, 8 or 9 thousand per cu.m.m. Dr. Kouchakoff found that he could divide his findings on leukocytosis into four distinct groups according to reactions in the blood: 1. A raw food produced no increase in white cells. 2. Common cooked foods produced leukocytosis. 3. Pressure cooked foods produced greater leukocytosis than non-pressure cooked foods. 4. Manufactured foods are the most offensive, such as wine, vinegar, white sugar, ham.

Kouchakoff was no vegetarian yet his findings show that, to avoid leukocytosis, flesh would have to be eaten raw, which would be unpalatable to humans. Prepared or processed meat (cooked, smoked, salted) brought on the most violent reaction, equivalent to the leukocytosis count manifest in poisoning. This finding on the increased activity of phagocytes, the scavengers of the bloodstream, after eating cooked and processed food, makes it clear why raw foods so rapidly heal both acute and chronic ailments, simply by reducing the tremendous overload of toxic substances and germs the blood has to fight.

Critical temperatures at which food became "pathological" producing symptoms of leukocytosis, varied with the food: carrots at 206 degrees F., potatoes at 200 degrees F. and even water heated above 191 degrees F. Considering the toxic reaction of water when heated should discourage the use of herb teas in favor of live juices of greater biochemical potency and anti-leukocytosis properties.

Kouchakoff found that a largely raw food diet offsets the adverse effect of a small amount of cooked food so as not to cause leukocytosis. Most people can tolerate a diet of 80 percent live food with 20 percent cooked food in the form of baked tubers as a transition to an all raw diet.

The consequence of structural changes of the mucosal lining in sprue are several (52). First, the absorbing surface of the bowel may be reduced up to thirtyfold. Second, "the structural polarity of the epithelial cells has vanished . . . at their luminal margin are entrapped nutrients. Immediately subadjacent to these structures are submicroscopic particles rich in enzymes that metabolize absorbed substances and prepare them for further use by the body. Third, "less visible, but nonetheless real is the destruction of the intracellular enzymes that are responsible for the metabolism of epithelial cells. These enzymes within the cells normally supply energy to a pump mechanism and convert absorbed nutrients to other substances."

Here are a few consequences of such disorders (52): First, "in an advanced case of celiac sprue, the patient is unable to assimilate his food. He is slowly starving. He may eat ravenously, but it doesn't help. The patient is apt to say, 'It all goes through.' Bowel movements tend to be loose, bulky, foul and bubbly. Their most striking characteristic is that they glisten and are light in color. They are full of fat." Second, "fatty substances other than triglycerides, such as phospholipids, cholesterol and the lipid soluble vitamins A, D, E and K are also poorly absorbed." Third, loss of vitamin D leads to poor absorption of calcium. "The nervous system of the patient whose blood and tissues are low in calcium is extremely irritable. The slightest stimulus is sufficient to induce claw-like cramps of hands and feet."

Is there anything which can be done for such a patient? Yes! I was such a case. For many years, I poured into my stomach food which burned my hand but felt only slightly warm in my mouth. Ice cold cola was one of my favorite drinks for years. I used lots of spices. For a year I was using some of the best vegetarian foods but at 98 lbs., there was no sign of my gaining weight. After using indoor greens juice orally and by implant, for many months, color appeared in my face and my body started to fill out to a weight of 140 lbs. Taking grass juice on an empty stomach leads to partial rebuilding of the stomach cell structure.

ENZYMES IN RAW FOODS

Dr. James B. Sumner, a 1946 Nobel Prize winner, claims (58) that middle-aged feeling is due to diminished enzymes as you add years to your life. Raw foods contain health-giving, rejuvenating enzymes. Cooking, pasteurization, smoking, pickling, air pollution, pesticides, drugs, antibiotics, chlorination and fluoridation of water and many other interferences in nature's processes will denature enzymes, thus making the nutrients in food not readily available. These were the conclusions drawn (59) by Jonathan Forman, M.D.

David Locke (56) gives a comprehensive view of the source of enzymes and the role they play in metabolism. He explains that enzymes are catalysts of the chemistry of life. We are alive only because we contain thousands of different kinds of enzymes that regulate the life process. They cause chemical reactions which would not otherwise occur. Exceedingly active, enzymes are also choosy about what reactions they will catalyze. Generally, each type of enzyme will cause only one particular kind of reaction. Enzymes are procured from the raw food we eat.

The following is a summary from the works of Ralph Gerald (57) and Jean Bogert (54) on the role of enzymes in the human metabolism. Many enzymes consist of at least 2 parts, the apoenzyme and the coenzyme. This is especially true of the enzymes involved in cell metabolism; in digestion, coenzymes play a very minor role. It has been known for years that the apoenzymes are unable to act as catalysts except in the presence of their activating coenzymes. Many of the micro-constituents of food function as coenzymes, thus becoming essential nutrients. In this category are such materials as the ions of calcium chloride, copper, iron, magnesium, manganese, phosphate, potassium, plus the more structured micronutrients: the vitamins niacin, pyridoxine, riboflavin, thiamin.

Dr. Ingelfinger (52) entitled his article "For Want Of An Enzyme," because the digestive enzymes are just as heat sensitive as enzymes found in live foods. Jean Bogert, PhD (54) has said: "All enzymes are sensitive to heat and cold . . . The chemical cleavage which constitutes digestion is brought about through the action of enzymes . . the digestive enzymes all seem to work best at about the temperature of the body." To be more specific, the conversion of starch or glycogen into dextrins and maltose (sugars) requires pH 7 (same as water, neutral) and a temperature of 98.6 degrees F. (normal body temperature) in the saliva, pancreas and intestinal mucosa, where the reaction occurs. The breakdown of protein by chymotrypsin into polypeptides and amino acids requires a temperature of 99.7 degrees F., which means the body must generate some heat in order to make the conversion effectively.

How many cooked food addicts have their food served at body temperature? With respect to temperature, the rule is the higher the temperature the faster the reaction within limit. However, proteins are themselves sensitive to a rise in temperature, so that enzyme proteins are inactivated by a temperature only a few degrees above the normal range. A sustained fever of 106 to 107 degrees F. soon becomes incompatible with life, partly because the active enzyme proteins are damaged and thus the catalytic reaction terminates in death.

PROTEIN LOSS IN COOKING

Experiments on the destruction of protein by heating are many. More rare are experiments on meat protein. One such study (80) was sponsored by the United States Department of Agriculture which reported that cooking at 400 deg. F., average temperature in home cooking, "caused a very marked decrease (4 to 30 fold) in the soluble protein nitrogen of the steaks."

Non-soluble nutrients cannot be effectively utilized by the body. An editorial in Nutrition Review (79) reads: "It has been postulated that dry heat processing of protein produces a new lysine linkage which is either not digestible by enzymes or is slowly digested so that lysine enters the bloodstream too late to participate with the rest of the assimilated amino acids in tissue formation."

When protein is cooked with sugar in the form of glucose, destruction of amino acids has been repeatedly corroborated. This destruction may account for a 50% loss of lysine, argine, tryptophane and histidine content (79).

Evans and Butts (81) heated a mixture of 8 gm. of soybeans and 2 gm. of sucrose (sugar) for 4 hours at 120 deg C. On acid hydrolysis of the product, they found that 50% of the lysine content was lost. However, enzymatic hydrolysis showed a loss of 84%. This loss is significant, since lysine determines how well the other amino acids are utilized in protein building.

E.M. Olsen (82) in a study of heat treatment of wheatgerm meal observed that autoclaving for 45 and 90 minutes reduced the absorption of nitrogen to 77 and 63 percent respectively. The effect of 90 minute autoclaving was even greater on other specific amino acids. There was a reduction of absorption to 42% for lysine, and 54, 56 and 58 percent for isoleucine, valine and leucine, respectively.

Cooked food has lost more than 85% of its nutrient value. It acts as a poison in the body, especially if it is ingested hot, that is warmer than 100 degrees F. Most cooked foods are eaten at a temperature of 180 degrees F. Until the temperature is reduced to that of your body, the whole metabolism is in a state of emergency. A cup of hot soup or coffee increases body heat, causes perspiration and an increase in pulse rate.

Considering the small temperature range at which enzymes are active, you are doing similar harm by eating cold foods. Frozen protein in the form of ice cream is putrefactive in the digestive tract. Fruits and vegetables should never be eaten directly after refrigeration. It is best that fruit is left outside the unit for at least eight hours before eating. During sunny days, place it in the sun and let it absorb solar radiation.

"I do say to you: Kill neither men, nor beast, nor yet the food which goes into your mouth. For if you eat living food the same will quicken you, but if you kill your food, the dead food will kill you also. For life comes only from life and death always comes from death .   For everything which kills your food kills your bodies also.   And everything which kills your bodies kills your souls also. And your bodies become what your foods are,   even in your spirit ,   likewise, becomes what your thoughts are."
JESUS, ESSENE GOSPEL OF PEACE

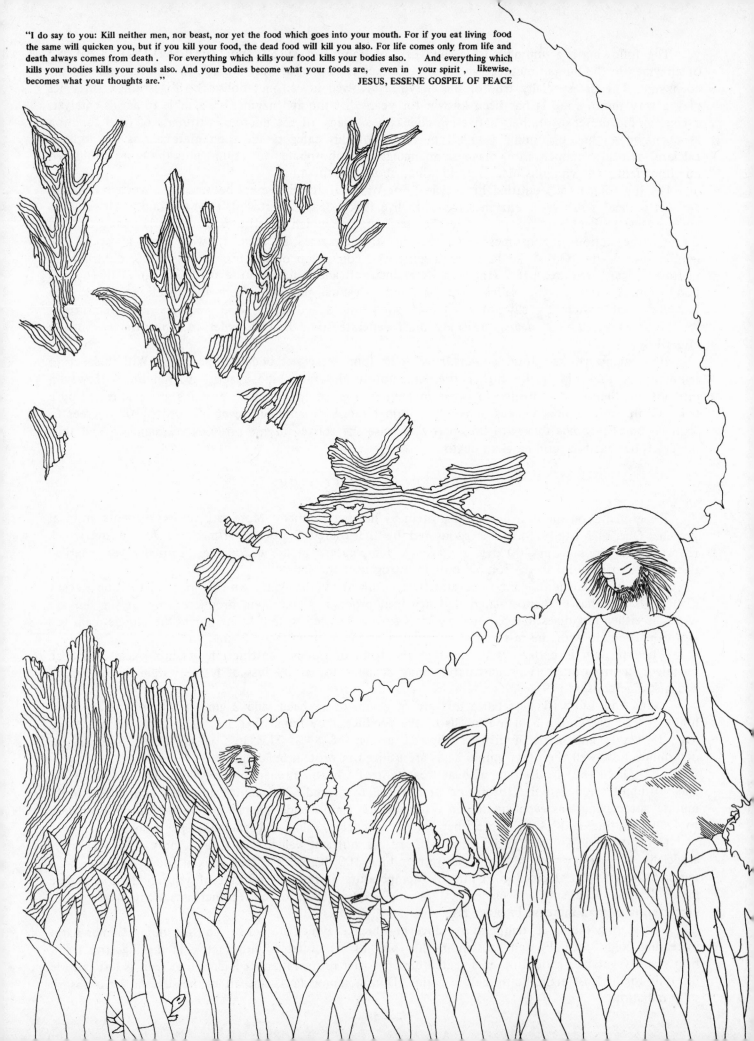

VITAMIN LOSS IN COOKING

Enzymes in food and enzymes in your body are not the only nutrients destroyed during cooking. Following is a list of the nutritional casualties: thiamin (64) loss in cooking is 25 - 45 percent, and can be as high as 96.4% at ph 7, 100 deg. C in 3 hours; can be 100% destroyed at ph 9, 100 degrees C. (62, 65); riboflavin, 40 -48% loss (63,64); biotin, not stable in alkaline solution, 0 to 72% loss (63); pantothenic acid, 0 - 44 loss (63); folic acid, 0 - 97% loss (63); inositol, 0 - 95% loss (63); ascorbic acid, 70 - 80% loss (64,68); vitamin A 10 -30% loss(64); Vitamin D-2 appreciable loss (66); Vitamin E, 50% loss (67) Deep fat frying and baking results in apprecianble destruction of all nutrients. Storage further destroys Vitamin E 47% of alpha tocopherol is lost from flour in 80 days of storage at 37 degrees C. (69). According to U.S .D.A. (70) preparation ansd cooking can effect as much as 45% to 55% loss of the B complex fraction or ascorbic acid in certain foods. Lecithin is destroyed in normal cooking.

LIVE FOOD VEGETARIAN DIET

Cooking does not improve the nutritional value of food. It destroys or makes unavailable 85% of the original nutrients. Cooked food is totally lacking in enzymes; most of the protein has been destroyed or converted to new forms which is either not digestible by body enzymes or digested with difficulty; many of the vitamins have lost their vitality. To purchase organic food and then to waste precious hours in destroying most of the nutrients is poor economy and unsound ecology.

Under a microscope the etheric body of a living cell scintillates with sunlight. Dead cells do not polarize light and the color display is extinguished. The minerals of live food act as magnets, holding the sun's energy, filling our bodies with sunlight. Technically, the electron orbit of a mineral takes a quantum orbit jump because of the absorption of sun energy. An inorganic mineral becomes an organic mineral through the action of sunlight on a plant. Live food elements make it possible to charge the body with an enormous amount of energy from natural breathing which provides optimal power for the mental and spiritual faculties. On a cooked food diet, to generate the same power requires forced breathing exercises.

Eating hot food deteriorates the taste buds, mucus membrane of the mouth and stomach, destroys on contact many of the enzymes and vitamins that are present in the digestive juices. The devastating effect of cooked food on animals has been well documented in laboratory experiments.

Francis Pottenger, M.D. carried out a 10 year experiment (73) using 900 cats which were placed on controlled diets. The cats on raw food produced healthy kittens from generation to generation. Those on cooked food developed our modern ailments: heart, kidney and thyroid disease, pneumonia, paralysis, loss of teeth, difficulty in labor, diminished or perverted sexual interest, diarrhea, irritability. Liver impairment on cooked protein was progressive, the bile in the stool becoming so toxic that even weeds refused to grow in soil fertilized by the cats' excrement. The first generation of kittens were sick and abnormal; the second generation were often born dead or diseased; by the third generation the mother was sterile.

Dr. Ann Wigmore states: "The most thrilling experience I can recall was to see cancer cells taken from a human body and thriving on cooked food, but unable to survive on the same food when it was uncooked." (Be Your Own Doctor)

Factors that are needed for building quality blood are lost from food in cooking. Dr. Koratsune, Japanese researcher, observed (83) in 1951, that as long as he ate uncooked whole rice and raw radishes, spinach, kale and grated raw potatoes, he found he had excellent quality blood, even though his diet was poor in protein and calories. However, as soon as he ate the same quantity of vegetarian food in a cooked form, he began to notice symptoms of edema and anemia.

Dr. Saxon Graham, State University of New York (Buffalo) with a group of researchers, observed (84) that "people who eat uncooked vegetables (lettuce, tomatoes, carrots, cole slaw, red cabbage) appear to have less stomach cancer than the general population." Their study was published in Cancer Journal.

Contrary to textbook dogma, some researchers believe (85) that raw food enzymes continue to work in conjunction with digestive enzymes in the stomach. In the intestine, the vegetable enzymes help to detoxify the intestinal flora as well as to normalize bacteria population of the colon. This reduces the number of decay-causing bacteria as well as stimulates the increase of the desirable lactic-acid-forming bacteria.

A heated seed does not germinate. Life has been destroyed. Ancient masters instruct us to soak the seed overnight and expose it to the sun before eating. The Bhagavad Gita, which is the common denominator for major Eastern philosophies, specifically says: "Pious men eat what the Gods leave over after the offering. But those ungodly cooking good food for the greed of their stomachs sin as they eat it."

Questions about the preferedness of a vegetarian diet to a diet that includes animal products have come up since the publication of THE SECRET LIFE OF PLANTS (232). If plants have feelings aren't vegetarians just plant butchers rather than plant and animal butchers?

Becoming acquainted with vegetarian literature means becoming acquainted with fruitarianism. Eating fruit that has ripened and fallen from a tree involves no harm of any living creature.

As Narcissis was preoccupied with his likeness and loved it most, it has taken we earthlings a little longer to see the green beings we've been sharing the planet with as "human" — "human" in the culinary realm meaning that which shall not be devoured.

Devouring animals means devouring 10 times as many plants as we would be by utilizing the plant food alone. It takes 10 pounds of plant products to produce one pound of "consumable" animal flesh.

The plant eater slaughters fewer green neighbors. When the plant eater turns to raw food, he or she needs about one quarter the food needed in cooked form. Most raw food eaters, eat greens because they need the power in the plants to keep them healthy in an unnatural environment. The aim of raw food eaters is to live in a natural environment on a diet of fruit alone.

To make the transition into a live food diet, gradually replace cooked vegetables, grains and legumes with raw foods: sprouts, vegetables, fruits and grasses. Decrease cooking time, follow the food combination chart carefully, and your body will come to choose an all raw food diet. Eventually eliminate all nuts, grains and seed, to achieve a low starch, low protein, low fat diet.

Suggestions

At least one day a week, fast on water or juices. For at least one day each week, eat only fruit meals. Cut down on the size of breakfast, eventually eliminate it, thus extending the length of the nightly fast. Eventually discontinue the use of electrical utensils. Cut down the use of all seasonings (vegetable powders, sea kelp, dulse, onion, garlic), herbs and spicy vegetables (green peppers, celery, mustard greens). The eventual elimination of spices and seasoning will diminish your craving for water. (In a polluted environment, additional fluids may be needed to flush the system.) In nature, all the needed fluids will come from fruit, sprouts and vegetables. Have, as your goal, the total elmination of all seasoning, and a mono diet (one food at a meal).

Before
Breakfast - Energize the mind and body with yoga. Follow with rejuvelac or the juice of a lemon in a glass of warm water.
Breakfast - Skip it, ideally. Otherwise, use juicy fruit, fruit salad, wheatgrass juice, greenjuice or vegetable juice.
Lunch - Fruit or sprouts. Try to eat a mono diet or combine food properly. Use perfect dressing, page 258 or dry seed cheese.
Supper - Sprouts, greens and vegetables. Use any of the sauces or salad dressings to enhance and increase the nutritional value of the meal. As your body becomes more and more conscious, the sauces will become undesirable and the simplest fare will be most suitable.
Daily - For at least one half hour, expose your body to the most perfect food - solar radiation.

Practice yoga asanas or exercise, deep breathing and meditation or prayer. Develop more and more awareness of the spiritual nature of the human being through the study of scriptures and works of ancient wise ones.

Continuously reduce the size of the meals. Jesus says: "Never eat unto fullness. Flee the temptation of Satan, and listen to the voice of God's angels. For Satan and his powers tempt you always to eat more and more. But live by the spirit and resist the desires of the body, and your fasting is always pleasing in the eyes of the angels of God. So give heed to how much you have eaten when you are sated, and eat always less by a third." (Essene Gospel of John)

When one changes one's diet from cooked to raw food, one may experience occasional cleansing reactions — fever, dizziness, tiredness, coated tongue, gas, diarrhea, open sores. These reactions may be a little more severe than those experienced when one gave up meat and started a vegetarian diet. For relief one should use zone therapy and space meals according to hunger. To slow the cleansing process, take daily a banana meal, or add a moderate amount of seed, or a baked tuber (potato, yam, carrot, beet, turnip) to the raw food (see: Crisis).

Some discomfort may have nothing to do with cleansing reactions, instead it is the result of breaking the health rules (see Appendix). For example, a meal should be completely passed from the stomach (with associated hunger pangs) before even considering taking sweet fruit, juice, melon or any other food. Otherwise fermentation, indigestion, tiredness, headache may result. This is especially true of individuals who like to have cereal for breakfast followed by a fruit lunch. The fruit catches up with the grains in the digestive tract, causing fermentation. Better to eat fruit first, and grains several hours later (or not at all).

There are some who have never emptied the stomach completely. Such people are never hungry, eat out of habit and feel stronger after a meal. The food dilutes temporarily the concentration of rot and ferment in the stomach. The new food is mixed with the remnants of previous meals. Within two hours, they are tired, sluggish. Thinking they are hungry, they eat some more. To get out of the vicious cycle, such individuals would benefit from a thorough stomach wash (see Fasting). When hunger returns, satisfy it with juices (beet, carrot, spinach, celery, indoor greens - see Appendix for proportion) and rejuvelac.

GRASS

"All flesh is grass and its beauty is like the flowers in the field."

ISAIAH 40:6

"One of the most popular current health fads is the use of wheat grass."

DONALD C. HEALTON, DEPARTMENT OF HEALTH
EDUCATION, WELFARE

The civilized human being has only to look in field and forest to learn from wild animals. They have no hospitals, no doctors, no medicines, yet they are ruled by the same laws of creation that govern people. If any animal feels sick, it nibbles on grass or fasts, depending on the instinctual commands of its body. There seems to be some sort of healing, protective property in grass which makes all animals — carnivorous as well as fruitarian — desire to nibble the green blade.

More than 60 percent of U.S. citizens are chronically ill, most are self-medicated. Can we learn from the animals how to rejuvenate a sick blubber — drowning America into a nation of healthy youth?

The human being has been eating fruit of the grass family since living outside of a natural environment. Wheat, rice, corn, bamboo, sugar cane are all members of the grass family. Liver, butter, wheat germ, grass powder and yeast contain all the vitamins science has been able to discover and isolate. Grass is a source of all five. Having used grass seed (grains) for food for thousands of years, the human being limits his and her health possibilities by failing to recognize the sustenance in the grass itself. Grass is a complete food. It should be included in the diet for both protective and healing value.

Dr. Wigmore, in one of her publications, reflects on the history of wheat, citing a prediction made many thousands of years ago on the continent of Atlantis, which later sank beneath the sea. It was then predicted that the real "health properties" of wheat would not be learned until some "far distant future generation" was given the key which would save a tottering "civilization from extinction". We are such a generation. Ann Wigmore advises wheatgrass as the tool for regaining health.

A few "experts" may discount the importance of the grass juice factor in the human being's nutrition, but those drinking the grass juice through these critical times will be better prepared to survive ecological crises. Scientific work will continue, and more specific facts about grass will appear. However, we can take advantage now of the "x factor" in grass juice and feel the difference in our sense of strength, health, spirituality, endurance and well being.

All animals obtain their basic nutrition, directly or indirectly, from grass. Through recorded history, the use of fresh green grass as a basic feed for livestock has revealed the vital need for year-round feeding of its life-giving juices. Dr. George D.A. Scarseth, director of research of the American Farm Research Association, West Lafayette, Indiana, says: "Somewhere in the food chain of all people something green was the starting point."

In the Journal of Nutrition (167) results were presented to show that various supplements rich in the known vitamins produced little or no growth response in rats on basal winter milk diet. This led to the conclusion that the growth-stimulating factor was distinct from all known vitamins.

In another experiment (37), rats were fed mineralized winter milk ad libitum plus two types of supplements, while their weight and general health was observed. Kohler found growth and health stimulated by 3 gm fresh grass, 3 cc grass juice and .6 gm of dried oat grass. Inferior growth response was produced by daily doses of 2 drops of cod liver oil, 1 cc orange juice, .5 gm brewer's yeast, .25 gm dried bran and 1.0 gm defatted wheat germ.

In a later experiment, (37) Kohler et al used herbivorous guinea pigs. He fed them mineralized winter milk plus supplements containing liberal quantities of all known vitamins. Brewer's yeast, orange

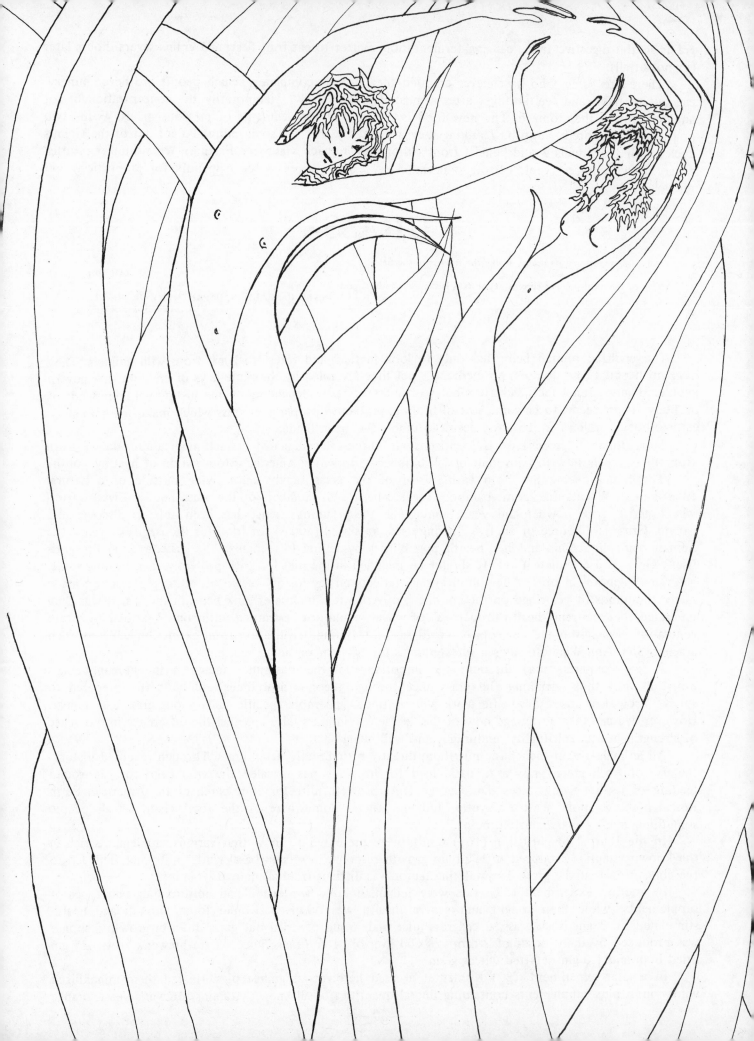

juice and liver extracts effected inferior growth. The remarkable growth produced by supplementing grasses, adds credence to the hypothesis that the "grass juice factor" described for rats is the same factor concerned in this later experiment.

Kohler showed that wheat and barley grass was most effective in producing an increased growth rate. It offset the abnormal weight loss (and eventual death) which was shown to set in on a milk diet. It was noted that extracted juice contains the active factor for both rats and guinea pigs. The activity of the grass juice disappeared upon storage at room temperature.

What was really conclusive, as Kohler stated: "The animals receiving mineralized milk, orange juice and grass juice grew at good rates and no abnormalities were observed. When the grass juice was omitted the animals died."

CHLOROPHYLL THE HEALER

"Chlorphyl will be the principal protein for the coming light bearing age. When freshly made in a drink, it contains synthesized sunshine, plus the electric current necessary for the revitalization of the body, and it will open areas of the brain that man yet known nothing about."

UNIVERSAL BROTHERHOOD TEACHINGS
'LET THERE BE LIGHT', ANN WIGMORE

For ages people puzzled over the question "What makes grass green?" About a century ago, chemists isolated the green pigment in growing plants and named it chlorophyl.

Certain beliefs evolved about this green fluid. The fact that herbivora build hemoglobin (blood cell pigment) on a diet composed of greens invites the hypothesis that derivatives of chlorophyl may be used in making hemoglobin. After years of research, Hans Fisher and his co-workers finally established the correct structure of hemin (a component of hemoglobin) by synthesis, and showed its true relationship to chlorophy (See Page 113).

They observed that the cholorophyl molecule closely resembles hemin, the pigment which combines with protein to form hemoglobin. The latter is present in the red corpuscles of the blood and by carrying oxygen to the tissues makes the production of energy and life possible.

One of the major differences between chlorophyl and hemin is that chlorophyl contains magnesium while the hemin molecule contains iron as its central atom.

Owing to the close molecular resemblance between chlorophyl and hemoglobin, scientist Hans Miller suspected that chlorophyl is nature's blood-building element for all plant eaters and humans. He writes: "Chlorophyl has the same fast blood-building effect as iron in animals made anemic."

What exactly is anemia? According to Webster's dictionary, anemia is a condition in which there is a reduction of the number of red blood corpuscles or the total amount of hemoglobin in the bloodstream or both. Thus anemia is an excellent vehicle for the study of the relationship between food and hemoglobin count.

J. Hughes and A.L. Latner from the Department of Physiology, University of Liverpool, in a highly discriminative experiment (86), finally resolved the question of the blood regenerating capacity of chlorophyl. Rabbits were made anemic by daily bleeding, reducing the hemoglobin level to two-fifths of the normal value. The rabbits were split into two groups. The experimental group received chlorophyl in oil in the diet, the control only oil. Both groups received a complete diet.

They performed five experiments, three with varying degrees of pure chlorophyl (synthetic), one with a large dose of crude (unrefined, as found in nature) chlorophyl and one with magnesium-free chlorophyl derivatives. The following is a summary:

1. Pure chlorophyl in large doses has no effect on the speed of hemoglobin regeneration after hemorrhage. It seems that large doses are toxic to the bone marrow.
2. Very small doses of the pure chlorophyl, markedly increase the speed of hemoglobin regeneration to approximately its previous level.
3. Crude chlorophyl is effective and non-toxic even in large doses.
4. Where effective, the anemic condition was overcome in 15 days.

Hughes concludes: "It seems therefore that the animal body is capable of converting chlorophyl to hemoglobin." This is in agreement with Zin (87), who, however, showed the effect of chlorophyl injection on the red blood cell count of animals not rendered anemic.

Other workers have reported curative effects from chlorophyl and its derivatives in a wide variety of anemias: protein deficiency, hemorrhagic, pernicious, hypochromic of unknown etiology and "experimental nutritional anemia" of unidentified character. Some reports are based on clinical studies, while others are the result of animal experimentation.

Patek and Minot (88) in a clinical study with rare type anemia caused by pigmenticity, observed a small positive increase in hemoglobin concentration on intravenous injection of chlorophyl derivative. Dr. Fisher in Germany announced that for some time he had been using chlorophyl in the treatment of anemia, with promising results (89).

In another clinical study Dr. Patek (90) used fifteen adult patients with chronic hypochromic anemia. They were given chlorophyl and allied substances and were placed on house diets free from meat and eggs, whereas the diet was adequate in all other respects. The crude chlorophyl was a tar-like substance extracted from alfalfa leaves. It was found pure chlorophyl alone was not effective. When chlorophyl and its derivatives were administered there was an increase in hemoglobin and an improvement in sense of well being.

Other workers have reported curative effects from chlorophyl and its derivatives in a wide variety of anemias: protein deficiency (91), hemorrhagic (86, 92), phenolhydrazine poisoning (93, 94), pernicious (91, 95), hypochromic of unknown etiology (90) and "experimental nutritional amemia" of unidentified character (96). Some of the reports are based on clinical studies, while others are the result of animal experimentation.

Thus we see chlorophyl can aid in rebuilding the bloodstream. Unless all causes of anemia are corrected, results from chlorophyl therapy are temporary in nature and not consistently workable with every individual. If, however, the individual is given organic live foods and one of the richest crude forms of chlorophyl, the results are always the same: the anemic condition disappears.

Chlorophyl has proven therapeutically effective in a wide range of disorders: external and deep internal infections, such as sinusitis, osteomyelitis, pyorrhea, peritonitis, gastric ulcers, chronic diseases such as anemia, arteriosclerosis, and mental depression.

In July 1940 (89) the first comprehensive report on the therapeutic use of chlorophyl was published in the American Journal of Surgery. Under these auspices, and with testimonials by many distinguished doctors, the green pigment was described as an important and effective drug.

Some 1,200 cases ranging from deep internal infections, such as brain ulcer and peritonitis to skin disorders and pyorrhea had been treated and documented; after treating with chlorophyl doctors were able to close their reports with: "Discharged as cured."

Ulcerated varicose veins, osteomyelitis (a serious bone infection), skin disorders and various types of infected wounds have been cured and healed. Applied locally in numerous cases of mouth infections, such as Vincent's angina and advanced pyorrhea, the results were immediate and positive. "The gums tightened entirely."

Other teams of specialists reported results just as favorable. Dr. Burgi (97) and his co-workers used chlorophyl in the treatment of anemia, tuberculosis, cardiac disease, arteriosclerosis and mental depression because of its "tonic" effect.

The efficiency of topical application of chlorophyl as a tissue stimulant and healing agent in cases of tropic ulcer, varicose ulcers, decubitus ulcers, pilonidal cyst, osteomyelitis and other conditions have been proven by Bowers (98), Morgan (99) and Boehme (100). Furthermore, doctors at Temple University in Philadelphia discovered (89) that the green solution seems to thicken and strengthen the cell walls of living animals.

Drs. Bertham and Weinstock (101) said: "Our evidence suggests that the method of treatment (chlorophyl, urea, benzocaine) described will materially reduce the period of disability (infected corns, ingrown nails, calluses and tape reactions) and avoid the possibility of reaction that might otherwise occur from the use of systemic antiobiotics."

Offenkrantz reported (102) the following study. A total of 79 patients with x-ray-proved duodenal and gastric ulcers were treated with powder incorporating water soluble chlorophyl 'coating' material and a recognized antacid. The treatment was not accompanied with the usual restriction on diet, smoking, alcoholic beverages or daily activity.

Of the group, 58 showed on roentgenological examination complete healing in two to seven weeks; 60 experienced complete symptomatic relief in one to three days.

The majority of the 27 patients who had a peptic ulcer of long duration previous to the chlorophyl treatment, had undergone treatment with accepted therapies incorporating strict diets, antacids, aluminum gels and mucin preparations.

In 20 out of the 27 cases, pain and other subjective symptoms disappeared with regularity in 24 to 72 hours after chlorophyl treatment started. No toxicity was encountered. Of 24 patients examined with x-rays after treatment, 20 showed complete healing after two to seven weeks of treatment. There was no recurrence of symptoms in cases showing complete healing, which were followed for a period of 4 to 11 months.

Boehme (100) reported over 50 cases of chronic leg ulcers with a high percentage of rapid healing. Many of these ulcers had persisted from one to eight years but chlorophyl therapy healed them completely in three to ten weeks. Carpenter (103), Carleson and Garsyen (104) and Juul-Moller and Mikkolsen (105) reported similar success with chronic ulcer and osteomyelitis.

Drs. Rafsky and Krieger reported (106) a case study of twenty patients with colon disorder several of whom had ulcerative colitis—"The method of treatment employed was as follows: Rectal installation of various dilutions of chlorophyl solution as retention enema once daily . . . patient instructed to retain fluid as long as possible. No evidence of irritation resulted from the treatment and the solution as a rule was retained for several hours. When the patients began to improve they were able to retain the chlorophyl solution overnight . . . Definite improvement was seen in the majority of cases."

Drs. F. Paloscia and G. Pollotten (107) used chlorophyl therapy with some success in the treatment of tuberculous empyema. Cancer (108, 109, 110) patients seem to have benefited to some degree from chlorophyl therapy, although results are inconclusive.

Dr. Edmond Fowler (111) in 1950 reported favorable side effects in the use of chlorophyl: "It should be noted that most of these patients in addition to an improvement in hearing and a lessening of tinnitus (ringing sound in ear) also improved in general health, gaining relief from a variety of other additional symptoms. There were no undesirable side effects. For what it may be worth, although most were older people, none have suffered from any coronary attack."

Can there be such a beneficial tonic, completely safe, without side reactions? Toxicity studies (112, 98, 106) have shown that chlorophyl is absolutely non-toxic when administered parenterally (intravenous or intramuscular) or by mouth to animals and humans.

Drs. Hughes and Latner (86) from their experiment using an oral dosage of pure and crude chlorophyl discovered that very small dosages of PURE chlorophyl exerted a favorable effect on blood regeneration, however, in large dosages it seems to be toxic to the bone marrow. In the case of crude chlorophyl, large doses exerted a favorable effect on hemoglobin regeneration. It seems, therefore, that there is some factor in the crude chlorophyl which counteracts the toxic effects of the pure chlorophyl.

Wheatgrass juice is a crude chlorophyl and can be taken orally or as an implant without risk of toxic side effects. Nature always provides what is safe for the body.

Dr. Lawrence Smith (112) professor of pathology, reports in his study on the effect of water-soluble chlorophyl preparations on cultures of various of the more common pathogenic bacteria. The results tend to support the premise that chlorophyl acts to reproduce an environment unfavorable to bacterial growth rather than to act directly upon the bacteria themselves.

Rapp and Gurney, as quoted by Offenkrantz (102), at Loyola University established that water-soluble chlorophyl inhibits the action of proteolitic (breaking down of protein into simpler substances) bacteria and enzymes. Hence when taken internally, via mouth or rectum, it inhibits the putrefaction of protein by some of the bacteria commonly found in the digestive tract of meat eaters.

It was observed by Drs. E. Ammann and V. Lynch (169) that chlorophyl-sensitized photochemical degradation of uric acid was found to occur in vitro. It is not known at this time whether uric acid reacts with chlorophyl in vito in same manner as in vitro.

Dr. Miller and co-workers (113) established that water soluble derivatives of chlorophyl had the ability to inhibit the formation of fibrin clots when thrombin was added to fibrinogen.

Rapp and Gurney, as quoted by Offenkrantz (102), demonstrated that water-soluble chlorophyl had the ability to raise the pH in human saliva, thus making it more alkaline, which is very favorable to carbohydrate digestion.

Considerable evidence is being accumulated which indicates that a chlorophyl-rich diet can effect the survival of experimental animals undergoing lethal doses of radiation. In 1950, Lovrou and Lartigue (114) reported that green cabbage supplement increased the resistance of guinea pigs to radiation. Further studies by Duplan (115) with green cabbage, Spector and Colloway (116) with broccoli, and Colloway et al (117) with broccoli and alfalfa indicated that certain plants may reduce the effect of radiation on guinea pigs.

In the experiment, every animal which received no greens died within 10-15 days, while mortality among the greens eaters was only about half as great during the same period. Daily, we are exposed to radiation from many sources. Chlorophyl-rich foods should be included as part of protective living.

In a private communication on December 6, 1961 to Dr. Ann Wigmore from Bloomfield Laboratories, High Bridge, New Jersey, Dr. Earp-Thomas confirmed the efficacy of chlorophyl-rich wheatgrass in neutralizing the toxicity of sodium fluoride, which is a rat poison and is used in the fluoridation of drinking water. He said: "Fluorine rapidly combines with calcium phosphate and other kinetic elements to lose its toxic properties, and harden teeth and bones. That is why fresh grass would act like a catalyst to speedily change the acid fluorine into a beneficial component with a positive reaction. By using wheatgrass which is comparatively rich in calcium phosphate, it would remove any free fluoric acid and change it and its negative charge to an alkaline calcium phosphate fluoride combination with a positive reaction."

It is evident that chlorophyl used without any additional dietary changes has a great effect on a wide range of disorders. Total, consistent healing would be observed by medical doctors if, in their approach, they eliminated the cause of disease: toxicity. Treatment with drugs tends to suppress symptoms which are actually the attempts of a toxic body to cleanse itself. In the majority of cases the problem is dietary in nature, and unless some drastic changes are made in diet, the same or different symptoms will appear at a later date.

The human being dies from more than 250 diseases, whereas powerful grass-eating animals such as the elephant, steer or horse are prone to only five or ten diseases. Scientists have no explanation other than the fact that these animals live on a diet, produced by Mother Nature, not factories.

We see that people could benefit in health by adopting a chlorophyl-rich diet, which includes plenty of juice from wheatgrass and other greens and foods rich in all the known nutrients, such as sprouts and fruit.

GREEN JUICE FOR REJUVENATION

The blood of all life is one. The juice in the cells of plants is very much like the juice of animal cells. Drinking the juice of early immature greens and sprouts is drinking the nectar of the rejuvenation of youth. Old cells are made youthful cells. The elements that are missing in your body cells — especially enzymes, vitamins, hormones — can be obtained through this daily green sunlight tranfusion.

Brown Landone, in an article "Make Cells Grow Younger" wrote: "More than twenty years ago experiments were made on old decrepit rats. They were so old that, proportionately, they were about as old as a man of ninety years. These decrepit old rats were fed with what were called immature foods, that is, foods which had not finished their growth, sprouting new stems and very young leaves. The results were amazing. The decrepit old rats were transformed, and their bodies began to grow younger.

"At about the same time other scientists discovered a root-auxin in plant roots. When they extracted this auxin from the tips of young growing roots, and pasted it on the edge of a leaf, roots grew even on the edge of a leaf. This is the miracle of auxinon foods — they induce growth after their own kind of activity. A root auxin will grow roots and a youth auxinon will grow youthful cells.

"Youth-growing substances from new growing sprouts will induce cells to grow younger. There is 'something' in the chemical substance of a young growing auxinon which, when you eat it as food, makes the cells of your body reproduce younger cells instead of older cells.

"The best auxinon foods I know of are found in Mung Bean sprouts. Mung beans are Chinese beans."(170)

Similarly, Dr. Weston Price, isolated a substance from tips of young spring grasses which promoted healing and regeneration. (171)

Dr. C.F. Schnabel writes: (168) "It is well known that grazing animals can live on grass alone, and pretty poor grass at that. It has been assumed that herbivorous animals could live on any of the common green crops, but this is not the case. A guinea pig is herbivorous, and yet it will die in 8 to 12 weeks on a diet of head lettuce, cabbage or carrot, and will grow at only half its normal rate on a sole diet of spinach. But a guinea pig thrives on a sole diet of grass. A superior race of guinea pigs was developed on a sole diet of 20% dehydrated grass . . . Grass seems to be unique in that it can serve as a source of energy without injuring the liver or kidney."

V.E. Irons & Co., manufacturers of Green Life, have experimented extensively with animals to show that grass is a "complete food." Fifteen years ago, the company offered a $10,000 reward to any laboratory which could isolate a vitamin or any other nutrient (with the possible exception of Vitamin D and B-12, which are synthesized within the body of a vegetarian animal) essential to health, which is not found in fresh organic grass. The reward is still available.

CHLOROPHYL JUICE may be extracted from many plants. The choices possible are: barley (bitter), rye (dry), alfalfa (takes a long time to grow and has very long roots), rice (little juice), weeds (don't grow easily indoors), comfrey (difficult to juice, although as a healing herb it is as effective as wheatgrass), spinach (low in enzymes, high in oxalic acid), celery (high in minerals, lower in enzymes and chlorophyl).

Wheatgrass has been chosen over other greens because it has all the characteristics desirable for health: it is a high chlorophyl, high vitamin, high enzyme, low protein, low mineral, no starch food.

"Dr. Earp-Thomas, scientist and soil expert from Bloomfield Laboratories, has isolated over one hundred elements, including all the known minerals, from fresh wheatgrass. He concludes that it is a complete food. Fifteen pounds of fresh wheatgrass is equivalent in nutritional value to 350 pounds of the choicest vegetables." (Ann Wigmore; Be Your Own Doctor).

Wheatgrass juice contains crude chlorophyl (70 percent of the juice solute) and can be taken orally or as a rectal implant without risk of toxic side effects.

Peak nutritional value of grass is reached on the day the first joint begins to form. Dr. Schnabel states: "Unjointed grass has no stem. What appears to be a stem is several leaves rolled together, Grass has a stem only after the first joint forms and the sole purpose of the stem is to bear the reproductive parts. That is, the first joint in the grass culm separates the vegetative from the reproductive stage of growth. A grass culm will grow up again and again if it is not cut before the first joint forms, but it will die if it is cut or grazed even one day after that time. The first joint in a grass culm can be detected as a swelling in the culm within an inch or two of the ground; it feels like a head in a rubber tube." (168)

It is interesting, that according to agricultural researcher, Pfeiffer (172), if one dehydrates the grass, the protein composition can be as high as 47.4 percent. Farmers have noted that hay, dried grass, fed in too liberal a quantity, can make animals sick. It contains too much protein. Dried wheatgrass has 3 times as high a protein concentration of beef. Hence, wheatgrass juice is suitable for people, but dehydrated grass preparations are not, unless in very dilute form. Dr. Pfeiffer proved that on the 8th day of growth, all the essential amino acids are present in grass.

Harvey Lisle, (173) a biochemist, says "The things that count in your wheatgrass is the quality which cannot be named. To give an example; vitamins cannot be measured in terms of mathematical units because they are in fact quality factors derived from the sun and planets and impressed into the plants. Vitamin A is a factor derived from the sun's infra red or warmth rays. Vitamin D is the chemical form factor derived from the sun's ultraviolet rays. Vitamin C is the order factor derived from the influence of the planets. Vitamins are not something which can be measured or weighed any more than love can be measured or weighed. The only practical way of measuring vitamins is by feeding tests on small animals."

WHEATGRASS FOR HEALTH

"Wheatgrass is not a 'cure.' However, through scientific investigation and experimentation, we have discovered that it furnishes the body with vital nourishment, which, when missing, yields sickness . . . . Many physicians here in Boston have tested the miraculous effectiveness of the wheatgrass therapy."

"All things whatsoever we shall ask in prayer, believing, we shall receive" Mathew 21,22   BE YOUR OWN DOCTOR, ANN WIGMORE

At times I jokingly inform new acquaintances that our institute is the only group permitted by the American establishment to grow "grass" for human consumption. While many are taking drugs and being jailed, we at the Institute use grass freely with the blessing of the establishment. If only they knew, the use of grass is the most revolutionary concept introduced into the diet of society. Our grass is a body "high." Drugs of all sorts become completely unnecessary. Mind and body no longer follow the orchestration of foreign chemistry but become one's own domain. As the use of grass becomes widespread it will reshape the health of society. Taverns will be replaced by juice bars, pharmacists will take up farming, the war industry will make peace buttons, drug manufacturers will study the mystics, our politicians will become astrologers, doctors will push grass, hospitals will be converted into museums, and the lion and the lamb will rest side by side.

Use the grass therapeutically, or as a supplement to your diet. It is a must if you do not obtain food directly from a garden. Food loses much value if it is not eaten immediately after harvesting. Wheatgrass chewed several times a day, closes the harvest gap supplying the missing nutrients. "You can take the grass out of the country, but not the country out of the grass." When tender and less than 4 days old, grass shoots can be cut fine and added to salads and all cooked or blended preparations as a nutritional booster. One teaspoon of grass juice mixed into any of the blended green sauces before serving gives an unusually exotic sweet taste. When preparing any non-acid vegetable drink, add a teaspoonful of grass juice.

Many of our digestive enzymes have been destroyed by the antigens created by pollution and cooked foods. Grass juice will help to build them. When combined with fasting and live foods it will lead to rebuilding of the bloodstream and return of youth.

As a neutralizing agent, it corrects the acid-alkaline balance of the body. As a general healing herb, it may be applied internally or externally wherever sores or bleeding occur. Cuts, skin irritation and burns heal quickly with application of the pulp soaked in grass juice. Pain from these afflictions, from blows or insect stings is relieved by immersing the area in wheatgrass juice for 15 minutes.

To soothe the eyes and improve vision, use the grass juice as an eye wash. Purchase an eye cup from a pharmacy. To eliminate sediment from the juice, strain it through a clean cheesecloth. Wash the eye for at least one minute. You may experience a brief burning sensation.

Applied to cotton and inserted into the ear, wheatgrass juice has been reported to relieve pain from ear inflammation. Similarly, it has relieved toothache. To speed recovery, fast for a few days and do some therapy on the feet.

It is an excellent gargle for sore throat, and has a cleansing, clearing effect on the nasal passages when sniffed up the nose and expelled from the mouth.

A poultice of wheatgrass pulp will, in time, make moles, skin growths and blemishes vanish by making possible the elimination of stored toxins in the skin.

Taken as a douche, the juice relieves vaginitis.

A tablespoon of juice helps to relieve indigestion. For a detoxifying stomach wash, drink four ounces of wheatgrass juice. Let it remain in the stomach for at least half an hour. Drink one quart of warm water while doing abdominal breathing, then regurgitate.

The stomach wash may be used as an antidote to some ingested poisons. After drinking the grass juice and water solution, regurgitate immediately. Follow this with two ounces of wheatgrass juice every two hours. Retain each dose at least 20 minutes.

A mother shared this story about her son and his friend. The boys had inadvertently used water hemlock in their weed salad. After eating, both boys became ill and were hospitalized. The mother took grass juice to her boy, giving it to him every couple of hours. He recovered. The other boy died.

Pure air is most important for vitality but the right diet can somewhat compensate for the lack of it. Living food and chlorophyl-rich greens can insure survival. If you insist on living in a city, indoor greens can create a natural atmosphere in your home. It will provide an adequate oxygen supply. Keep your windows closed. Live in top floor apartments.

GRASS JUICE REJUVENATION REGIME

"The sorrow on this planet is due to men's inability to control their bodies. Healing is the first essential knowledge.

Healing is not in faith; it is in the raising of vibrations; it is in the quickening of the body.

Our new children will discover in radioactivity powers of which man has not dreamed. He will control the health of himself, and he will see the source of himself.

Man seeks for the energy of the sun. The energy of the sun is in the fleetness of the deer and the strength of the elephant. Grass is the flesh and the flesh is grass. Chlorophyl is the blood and the blood is chlorophyl.

Food fashioned by the sun and eaten in the wholeness of the cell is the manna from heaven. Food murdered by the cook is the corpse of the manna and generation of the dissolution of the body.

All food has its own rate. Dead meat is lower than the infra-red rate. The blood of living fruits and plants is in the ultra-violet rate. Here is the energy of the sun; here is the life-blood of divine beings. Crush the living sap from the spinach and the tomato. Drink this living light and cleanse the veins and wake the psychic nerve-center. Get back your heritage.

The various chemicals in your body are only different because their vibrations are different; so one chemical can be turned into another by accepting a certain vibration."

TEACHINGS OF THE UNIVERSAL BROTHERHOOD
(YOGA FOR YOU, BRAGDON, LANCER BOOKS, NYC)

The cause of fatigue, disease, old age and death, according to W. Hay, M.D. (174) is threefold: (1) failure (or inability) to remove waste matter, which acts as poison in the body; (2) failure to replenish the body with living food and (3) failure to think creative thoughts and eliminate destructive emotions.

During healing, waste elimination can be more important than nutrition, although many micronutrients can play their role in neutralizing the released poisons.

The lungs eliminate not only carbon dioxide, but also expel air pollutants plus gases generated in the body by putrefaction. The skin primarily expels excessive salt and other irritants, plus some waste originating from protein, fried foods, dairy products and starches. Skin breathing if stopped even for a few hours can result in fatal poisoning. The kidneys expel protein waste products primarily. Their malfunctioning can result in death within 5 days. The bowels take the major burden of elimination. Over 75% of food waste is bacteria.

In therapeutic amounts, wheatgrass internalizes a maximum of green chlorophyl and enzyme-rich, liquid food, to detoxify the body by increasing the elimination of hardened mucus, crystallized acids and solidified, decaying fecal matter. Its high enzyme content helps to dissolve tumors. It is the fastest, surest way to eliminate internal waste and provide an optimum nutritional environment, so that the cosmic cell consciousness can rebuild your body.

The wheatgrass regime is economical, efficient, and easy to carry out. All needed equipment may be ordered by mail. In your home you can produce an organic live food diet at a cost of 50 cents per day. Generally, you may maintain your usual activities while detoxifying and rebuilding your body.

To improve health most rapidly, you may switch immediately from a regular diet to one of cooked and raw vegetables for at least one week. Next, adopt the rejuvenation regime. At all times combine foods properly. After two weeks of this regime, you may go on a fast one day each week. If relatively healthy, you may replace grass juice with fresh organic fruit or vegetable juices.

You may speed the process of detoxification by using some of the other aids to elimination. Massage and zone therapy will help to dissolve debris in the body. Enemas, colonic irrigations, herbal laxatives, sauna baths may be used in tolerable amounts.

During the day, the skin normally excretes two or more pints of fluid. A daily warm shower and loose clothing permit elimination of offensive odors. While bathing, vigorously scrub the soles of the feet with a stiff brush to activate all internal organs. A soft, natural bristle brush may be used on the whole body with great benefit to circulation and vitality.

A salt bath can aid elimination by osmosis; toxins are drawn through the skin by a salt solution of greater concentration than that of the bloodstream. To a tub of luke warm water, add two to three pounds of pickling salt (or Kosher, sea salt or the recommended amount of Batherapy)—the water should taste briny. Immerse yourself for twenty to forty minutes. On an empty stomach, drink about three cups of warm linden flower tea to induce sweating. After the bath, rest for an hour under linen or cotton covers while continuing to sweat. You can take this salt bath at least three times a week. When available, the best results are obtained from swimming, on sunny days, in warm ocean water.

If salt bath causes any discomfort, soreness or dizziness one should discontinue the bath. If you feel weak, have someone with you while bathing. The water should have a salty taste, not as strong as brine.

Daily sunbaths, increased gradually from five minutes to half an hour, will provide missing nutrients and increase elimination via the skin.

Conserve your energy with silence. Stay away from emotion draining discussions of politics, religion or gossip. Rest as much as you need, even if it be twenty hours per day. Fill your heart with love. In the silence of your thoughts, tell each person you meet how much you love him or her. Empty your heart of resentment, fear, despair, jealousy, anger.

Practice yoga breathing exercises each morning upon rising and during the day when you have a few moments (at least three times a day). Most of us take twelve to twenty shallow breaths per minute. With practice you can reduce this to only four deep breaths a minute. If you are like the average breather, you are using only one-sixth of your lung capacity. With practice, you will be able to utilize at least three-quarters of your lung capacity. Correct breathing rids the lungs of accumulated impurities, makes breathing easier, improves thinking and strength and gets rid of many physical disorders.

Start each breathing routine with a few minutes of exercise. First, draw your shoulders forward as close together as you can. This induces exhalation of stale air, and creates a vacuum, which, when released, causes the lungs to fill with air. Set up a count, four beats for inhaling, twelve beats for holding the breath and eight beats for exhaling. Holding the breath is very important, for it increases many fold the amount of oxygen absorbed. .

HOW TO DRINK YOUR GRASS

When first using wheatgrass, a good practice is to take very small quantities, one or two tablespoons at a time. Take enough to make you uncomfortable, but not so much as to make you feel sick. Wheatgrass juice is a powerful cleanser. Because of its high enzyme content, it starts an immediate reaction with toxins and mucus in the stomach, often causing distress. Nausea after taking the juice shows that it is needed and should be taken regularly.

At least 30 minutes prior to taking grass juice, it is good to drink rejuvelac or the juice of one-fourth lemon in a glass of water. If you have a sour stomach, mint-papaya tea is preferable. This rinses mucus from the stomach, minimizing discomfort. If there are ulcers or a growth in the stomach, it is best to skip the lemon, or use it in small, tolerable amounts.

Very sick people find even the smell of grass juice nauseating: my suggestion is to have someone else juice it for you, mix it with rejuvelac, and sip it through a straw. This way you don't have to smell it while juicing, building up a lot of apprehension about drinking it.

In an empty stomach, the wheatgrass juice is immediately absorbed through the mucous membrane. Soon after I started using the juice I noticed that within five minutes after drinking it, protruding veins in my hands became scarcely visible; a sign that it was already at work in my tissues.

After drinking 3 or more ounces of grass juice do not take any solid food for at least one hour. However, to relieve nausea, some find rejuvelac or the juice from celery leaves or carrots an excellent mixer or chaser for this chlorophyl cocktail.

Grass juice in one or two ounce doses can be taken immediately before a vegetable sprout meal. It will not cause any problems, for it is quickly absorbed.

For those with a delicate digestion, I recommend resting at least five minutes before taking the drink and at least 20 minutes of lying down after drinking it.

Place left hand on stomach and right hand on heart. This will set up powerful energy currents, giving you the right polarity for digestion.

If nausea or dry heaves occur, retain the juice for twenty minutes. Drink some water. Then vomit to remove toxins contained in the stomach.

Those who have any disorders of the mouth cavity, gums or teeth should retain the grass juice in the mouth for at least five minutes. Those who find it difficult to drink the juice may absorb much of it directly through the mucous membranes of the mouth. After holding the juice in the mouth for at least five minutes, spit it out. In addition, take two grass juice implants daily. The first few days, take four ounces in each implant, increasing it to eight or more ounces.

Many individuals, especially anemic people, have obtained satisfactory results when they used the grass juice in homeopathic proportions, i.e. 1 part grass juice to 10 parts distilled water (or even higher dilutions).

Those who have difficulty drinking the grass juice may try an alternative approach. Drink 1 ounce of grass juice at breakfast. At noon and evening drink 4 ounces of a mixture of buckwheat, sunflower green and/or alfalfa sprout juice. Take at least two grass juice implants daily. You may, if you prefer, take your entire dose of wheatgrass juice by rectal implant. Other green juices mixed with less potent ones, such as carrot or celery may be taken until the desired ingestion of grass juice is reached.

Daily Regime

On awakening ask God to guide you and to encourage you to persevere. Feel certain that you will receive   all that you need for this day. Read some inspirational messages. Feel free and secure in God's hands. Decide to be loving in all your encounters. God will give you today many new lessons about the mysteries of the universe. Love will enable you to hear and see the Divine. Never give up your God-given birthright of a healthy body.

On rising, drink two cups of rejuvelac or warm water containing the juice of one lemon or lime. Take an enema, followed by an implant of four to eight ounces of grass juice.

Follow this regime for at least 21 days before you start the city Sproutarian diet. Therapeutically, it is beneficial to fast for two to four days on grass juice, lemonade, juicy fruit and/or vegetable juices (see Fasting), then resume sprouts for one day to slow the cleansing reactions. Follow with another 3 days of the grass juice fast. Continue this regime for at least four weeks.

Breakfast:

Onarising, one or more cups of warm water, peppermint or herbal tonic tea. Exercise, yoga & breathing, prayers, thirty minutes. Later, one cup of lemon in water or rejuvelac or one fresh, organic, ripe citrus or apple juice. Use tsp. of lemon per cup. Thirty or more minutes later have a grass juice drink (1 to 4 ounces). One hour later, favorite sweet juicy fruit (no banana or avocado) or vegetable juices (see Appendix).

Lunch:

Herbal tea, vegetable broth or water. In thirty minutes, follow with grass juice. Wait for at least thirty minutes, or until hungry. Then, if available, have juice from carrot, celery and spinach, alfalfa, parsley and indoor greens, and wait another thirty to sixty minutes, before you have the sprout salad. Make one to three cups. Alfalfa and sunflower greens, plus buckwheat lettuce should predominate. Add washed dulce leaves and a few fenugreek sprouts (may add one or two favorite vegetables). Occasionally, if you want to slow the cleansing reactions, include with the meal ¼ cup of seed cheese or perfect dressing (See Page 258). On other occasions, you may use the green sauce with sprouts.

Supper:

As at lunch, grass juice, sprout salad - no seed. To achieve best digestion, chew each bite at least 50 times and eat little. If you have trouble chewing, blend or juice your food. Space meals according to hunger. Even when hungry, postpone the meal by drinking juice or water. If hungry at bedtime, take tea, grass juice or celery juice.

For the recovery of health by natural means you need a strong desire for health and willingness to go through the agony of a healing crises, sound knowledge of health and the basic physiology of the human body and the determination to pursue health steadfastly.

Once the cleansing reactions diminish in frequency and severity, perhaps after several months, you may reduce the intake of wheatgrass juice to one or two ounces per day. Eventually, take it only when you desire the juice. If you don't have a juicer, you may chew the grass, swallow the juice and spit out the pulp. Two ounces of grass is equivalent to one ounce of juice.

ENEMAS

"One who practices basti or yoga enema never suffers from constipation and other abdominal disorders. It further increases appetite and insures remedy for flatulance."

Gherandasamhita I, 49

"Seek, therfore, a large trailing gourd, having a stalk the length of man; take out its inwards and fill it with water from the river which the sun has warmed... enter your hinder parts, that the water may flow through all your bowels... then let the water run out your body... and you shall see with your eyes and smell with your nose all the abominations and uncleanesses which defiled the temple of your body... I tell you truly, baptism with water frees you from all these. Renew your baptism with water on every day of your fast, till the day when you see that the water which flows out of you is as pure as the river's foam."

Jesus, THE ESSENE GOSPEL OF JOHN

Of the 22,000 operations I personally performed I never found a single normal colon; and of the 100,000 performed under my jurisdiction, not over 6% were normal.

Harvey Kellogg M.D. Battle Creek, Mich.

"The fact that chronic constipation might exist in certain individuals as an almost permanent condition without apparently causing ill health is due solely to the power and protective action of the liver. It is only an evidence that some individuals possess the caecum and colon of an ox, with the liver of a pig capable of doing any amount of detoxification."

William Hunter, M. D. London

Accumulated, putrefied, hardened waste in the colon, quite often of many years' duration, places a great strain on the eliminative organs, disturbing especially liver and kidney function. A chain reaction develops: fats, proteins and carbohydrates are not properly metabolized; electrolyte balance is upset; the entire body is placed under stress.

"The colon is a sewage system, but by neglect and abuse it becomes a cesspool. When it is clean and normal, we are well and happy; let it stagnate, and it will distill the poisons of decay, fermentation and putrefaction into the blood. It will poison the brain and nervous sytem so that we become mentally depressed and irritable; it will poison the heart so that we are weak and listless, poison the lungs so that the breath is foul, poison the digestive organs so that we are distressed and bloated and poison the blood so that the skin is sallow and unhealthy. In short, every organ of the body is poisoned, and we age prematurely, look and feel old, our joints are stiff and painful; neuritis, dull eyes and a sluggish brain overtake us; the pleasure of living is gone."

V.E. IRONS, INC.

Studies (174) done by W.H. Hay, M.D., show that most normal individuals who have one daily evacuation, do not completely expel one meal for three days. Partial retention of meals, for up to three days means that the bowel is continuously filled with putrefying and fermenting material. He says that the number of bowel movements should be the same as the number of meals during the day.

Dr. W.F. Koch (228) strongly advocates the use of enema, in conjunction with liquid diet, during the cleansing regime. He states: "At least a liter should be held by the colon and it should be so manipulated that the fluid passes over into the caecum where most of the putrid material is held, often in diverticulae. But in old chronic cases of constipation, the crypts of Lieberkuhn are jammed full of fine sandlike deposits that hold the germs that develop the poisons. The bowel should be expanded by the enema to open these crypts and let their contents out. It may take from 4 days to 2 weeks to get the colon clean when one is taking no solid food whatsoever but only liquids as watermelon juice, apple or pear juices. Grape juice is not used and citrus fruits are not either for reasons explained earlier. Vegetable juices are easy to prepare now with the modern kitchen appliances. Cabbage juice, carrot and beet juices are very desirable."

The digestive tract lining is the hidden portion of the human skin. Most people bathe the outer skin, but never think of bathing the inner membrane. In most humans it is filthy, in need of a good washing. When we eat natural foods – raw fruits and vegetables, such cleansing is unnecessary. But if one is filthy inside, one must take an internal bath – putrefaction will cease, gas will be eliminated, permeability of the membrane lining the digestive tract will be re-established and it will become once again the home of friendly bacteria.

Purchase from a pharmacy a No. 16 catheter (20 French Size, Code No. 3720X) and glass connecting tube. (Davol Inc., Box D, Providence, R.I., or Metropolitan Supply Co., 1458 Cambridge St., Cambridge, Mass.) Attach them to the rubber tubing on the enema bag. Use a glass pipet. Fill the enema bag with one quart of water at body temperature. Hang it three feet above the floor. Lubricate the rectal tube and anus with oil or water-soluble jelly, such as HR or KY. Kneel with the head touching the floor and trunk raised, or lie on a slant board, feet higher than the chest. Insert the tube about fifteen inches. Open the clamp to let the water flow in. When you have taken as much as you comfortably can, lie on your back and massage the abdomen for at least two minutes. To increase elimination from the ascending colon, lie flat on the back, extend the legs into the air and ride an imaginary bicycle upside down. Retain the water for 2 to 10 minutes. Sit or squat on the toilet seat for at least five minutes to insure expulsion of all the water. For those who are having difficulty retaining the implant, two to three warm water enemas prior to the implant will generally insure retention of the juice.

WHEATGRASS JUICE IMPLANT

Wheatgrass juice can be inserted into all body cavities for rejuvenation of localized areas as well as absorbtion into the blood works for feeding the whole body.

Wheatgrass juice will reside in the mouth, stomach, intestines, colon, rectum, genitals, nasals, eyes, skin and ears. Chewed wheatgrass (juice, spit out the pulp) will remove most discomforts of the lung and heart in a matter of five minutes. It is desirable to apply wheatgrass to all body parts for long term rejuvenation effect and for quick reduction or removal of pain and discomfort.

At initial stages, in order to gain extra healing power, without the discomforts, besides drinking a small quantity (start with 1 tablespoon to one ounce or muscle test for best dosage), one may also take a significant quantity through the colon. The bulb implant is quick and requires no water enemas and will help greatly in healing hemeroiods as well as being absorbed into the blood. One can go back to normal activity immediately after the implant. For an implant going into the transverse colon using a catheter, one or more enemas of water are required to clean out thoroughly along with a slant board treatment for 20 - 30 minutes. The catheter implant of 3 - 6 oz. (with extra water as needed) will dissolve old debris, heal ulcerations, shrink the colon down to normal size, overcome diverculations and get rid of worms and gas. On a healing program, it can be administered 1 - 2 times daily for a period of at least 2 months.

Bulb Rectum Implants

Two to three ounce bulb enemas (infant size) may be purchased from a drugstore. Fill the bulb with grass juice (no water is required, the rectum has solid waste and it will not be absorbed). Put the bulb in a cup of hot tap water for a few minutes to warm up the juice. Lubricate the tip of bulb and anus. Bend down, slowly insert the tip, press out the full contents and pull out the squeezed bulb. Go back to normal activities.

The bulb retention enemas are ideal for folks who are looking for a quick energy increase, for the totally exhausted, where there's poor digestion and a very acid body or extreme cases of enervation or prediction of short life by physicians. In extreme cases, one does best by having the bulb implant administered every 2 – 3 hours, and, as much as possible, the person should take walks when there is some energy. Folks who were super toxic, acidic, with unclean stomachs and bedridden, after having implants administered 4 – 6 times per day, after 3 – 7 days, felt strong enough to pursue the program on their own. For best results, the person should be encouraged daily to do some walking or trampoline exercise.

Wheatgrass juice implants alkalinize the system, giving an increase of red blood cells and hemoglobin. The primary function is to feed the body, resulting in strengthening the blood and increasing enzymes and chelated minerals, all helping one to recover quickly.

The transverse colon has a liquidy waste and should be flushed out first. Most transverse colons are sagging and divirticulated. The implant will feed colon cells leading to the return of normal structure and osmotically entering into the blood system. Examination of the iris will give you a good idea of the state of your colon.

Enema Colon Implant

A grass juice enema (implant) helps to cleanse and rebuild the colon, destroy putrefactive bacteria, and is absorbed into the bloodstream. It is valuable for those persons who feel nausea when drinking the juice. An implant should be taken by the chronically ill for at least two weeks during the cleansing period. It is beneficial to the chronically constipated and to heavy meat-eaters. After one week of daily implantation, you may discover a fantastic release of worms and/or mucus in your bowel movement.

For the implant fill the enema bag with 4 to 8 ounces of grass juice. Lie on the slant board, trunk raised, so that the grass juice flows into the transverse colon. Retain it for at least 20 minutes. Spend this time doing Yoga postures, zone therapy, face massage, or meditate, pray or sing. Allow gas to be expelled. Check the initial urge to expel juice by applying pressure with finger between anus and sexual organs. Expel the juice within 30 minutes. If you're active, take implants only in the evening. According to Dr. Wigmore, these chlorophyl implants can actually sustain life when oral nourishment is impossible.

Before the implant, wet your face, scalp, chest, sores, congested areas, varicose veins with grass juice. It will speed healing and beautification. You can rub as much as 1 cup of wheat grass into your bod (better than drinking or implants) in 20 minutes. It is al absorbed. Rub self with wet cloth and you will notice no wheat grass green juice left on your skin. It is all absorbed. You can taste it in your mouth.

If implants cause gas pains it is best to expel the grass juice after the twenty minute period. Follow the implant with a warm shower. Rest, if you feel tired. Do not eat for at least one hour.

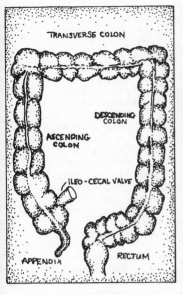
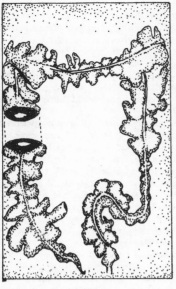
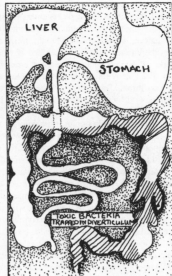
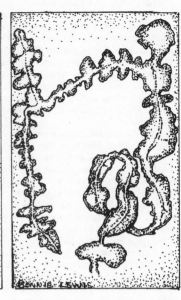
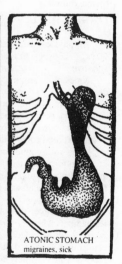

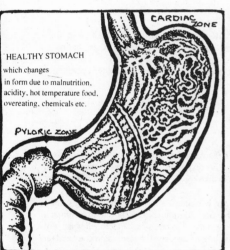

HEALTHY STOMACH

which changes

in form due to malnutrition, acidity, hot temperature food, overeating, chemicals etc.

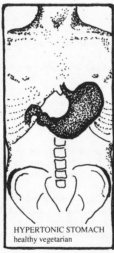

HYPERTONIC STOMACH
healthy vegetarian

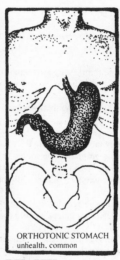

ORTHOTONIC STOMACH
unhealth, common

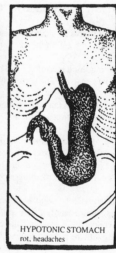

HYPOTONIC STOMACH
rot, headaches

ATONIC STOMACH
migraines, sick

VAMANA DHAUTI
Emesis-Stomach Wash

"Emesis clears heaviness of the head; clears the vision; removes nauseative dyspepsia. It benefits persons in whom bile is apt to pass into the stomach and decompose the food. For, if vomiting precedes the meal, the latter will always enter the stomach without being contaminated, and so the sense of loathing is removed which proceeds from oiliness of food, as also the depraved appetite — namely, the longing for sharp, sour, or pungent things. Emesis is also beneficial for flabbiness of the body, and for ulcers of the kidneys and bladder. It has a powerful effect in anesthetic leprosy; in persons with an unhealthy color of skin; in gastric epilepsy, jaundice, asthma, tremor, hemoplegia. It is also an effective treatment in cases of impetiginous skin diseases in which there are ulcers covered with scabs. Emesis is a great help for persons whose temperment is primarily bilious, and who are lean of habit. Hippocrates advised vomiting to be induced monthly and for two consecutive days. On the second day the difficulty of the first is obviated and that which has enterd the stomach is fully emptied. Hippocrates claimed that health was conserved thereby. To exceed this may be harmful. Emesis carried out in this way gets rid of mucous and bile, and cleanses the stomach. For in the case of the stomach there is no cleansing secretion like that for the small intestine — where the bile cleanses the mucous membrine as it passes down the bowel."

Translator O.C. Gruner, M.D. of Canon of Medicine, book one, section 1010, written by Avicena, an eleventh century physician.

"The following rules are to be observed in the administration of emetics and enamata. Vomiting may be induced during the six winter months, as this is the phlegmatic time of year and diseases are centered about the head and in the chest. During the warm weather enemata may be used, as this is the hot season when the body is more bilious and heaviness occurs in the loins and knees, when there are fevers and colic in the belly."

A REGIMEN FOR HEALTH, Hippocrates, father of western medicine.

"Purity has four stages: The first stage is the purification of the body from excrements, impurities, and bodily growths and discharges. The second stage is the purification of the bodily senses from crimes and sins. The third stage is the purification of the heart from blameworthy traits and reprehensible vices. The fourth stage is the purification of the inmost self (Sirr) from everything except God. This last stage is that of the Prophets and Saints." Al—Ghazzali

"One is considered to have gone thru emesis sucessfully who expels the mucous, bile, and air in succession and who feels that one's stomach, sides of the body, sense organs and body—channels have been cleansed and that one's body has become light. If the emesis goes wrong, then there occur eruptions, welts and itching on the body, imperfect cleansing of the stomach and body channels and heaviness of the limbs. Thirst, stupor, fainting, provocation of vata, loss of sleep, and loss of strength, etc., occur in cases of over—action of emesis."

CHARAKA SAMHITA: SIDDHISTHANA, chapter 1, by Chakara, highest authority for over 2000 years in traditional Indian Ayruvedic Medicine.

"An important part of the Egyptian concept was the beliefin a close relationship between the anal region and the cardiovascular system. A number of prescriptions noted that retention enemas were valuable because they refreshed the anus and the heart...

For the public health, the people were exhorted to frequent fasting and the regular use of emetics and enemas. The daily life of the people were strictly regulated by hygienic laws governing the buriel of the dead, diet, sexual intercourse, care of infants, and cleanliness of the body and in the home..."

EPIC OF MEDICINE, Dr. Felix Marti—Ibanez, M.D., former professor and chairman of Department of Medicine, New York Medical College (C.N. Potter, NY 1959).

The stomach is the major area of digestion within the intestinal tract. If it is not kept clean and totally emptied periodically, the tissue becomes poisoned by the stagnation, with weakening of muscles, resulting in failure to hold the stomach in proper place. This produces gastroptosis, or dropping of the stomach, which is very common among cooked food eaters, with its physical existence showing up in the iris, and is indicated in swollen, thick lips. The condition leads to the dilation of the small intestine and the reabsorption of its contents, which, when combined with the cesspool of the distended part of the stomach, can result in migraine headaches, pressure on the eyes, nausea, nightmares, bad breath, fatigue, and hypoglycemia.

The cleansing and purification process of the intestines should be handled as a sacred ritual, knowing it will lead to health, joy and spiritual growth. I have done as many as 40 emesis within a 20 hour period using one half to one quart liquid for each washing. It was a way of getting rid of severe headaches. First, the indigested, fermented, spoiled food came up. Then many forms of mucus, with the major part of vomit as dissolved acids — mostly lactic — with a ph of 3 — 4 (very acid), which on a few occasions burned my throat. The last stage is the release of bitter, colorful bile, which might require at the most 2 washes. And then the joy; headache all gone and the removal of the toxic acids led to such energy that I would stay up another 24 hours. No food is to be eaten until one becomes very hungry.

The Vamana Dhauti has a strengthening effect on all body organs, especially the lungs, nerves and brain. It may be practiced safely once a week, and under proper guidance, even more than 3 times a week. During fasting, use it as often as needed, that is when there is headaches or nausea.

To execute the Vamana: In the morning upon awakening, drink a large quantity of warm water (some use salt, but I find it unnecessary since it can lead to absorption if the proportions are not just right, 1 tablespoon to 1 quart). I have found that for most folks ½ to a full quart is enough. Shake the abdominal regions either by jumping up and down or rolling the stomach with nauli kriya. This should make you feel nauseous. Contract the stomach and vomit the entire content. Some folks need to tickle the roof of the mouth with 2 — 4 finger rapid movements and pressure, and others suck in air. The performing of Mool Bandha and Vddiyana Bandha, with mastery, can turn the act into gentle movement, creating an upward, flowing, wavelike body contraction. Continue the vomit until only belches of air come up. Repeat with more water until only clean water comes up and all discomforts are gone. If water doesn't come up after 10 minutes, discontinue and try again the next day, unless dealing with headache. Then try it later in the day. Drink only water and do not eat. Do reflexology.

If digestion is good and you have no late meals, the stomach should be empty in the morning with very little mucus and possibly some acid. This is a good check on one's eating habits and strength of the digestive fire. The wash can take 3 — 15 minutes in such cases.

Severe acidity, associated with migrain headaches, lower body aches and sciatica pain, are all helped, and, if practiced long enough, are usually relieved within a short time, but it can take as long as 24 hours. Because the practice can be exhaustive, after the initial emptying of the stomach content, one does well to spend as many hours as possible in a warm tub of water with 3 pounds of table salt or epsom salt. During the soak, if feeling nauseous, do stomach wash, then go back to the tub. The skin acts as a second kidney and drains the acid into the water. Drinking hot tea helps and if dizzy spells develop, have someone help you out to rest in bed if feeling nauseous. I have gotten rid of the mentioned discomforts in my body, which come up because of abusive eating habits, by soaking 4 — 10 hours with continuous additions of warm water. (For additional information, read Life In The 21'st Century, V. Kulvinskas, pgs. 273 — 297 by Mat Rosmarynowski)

FOOD AND STUFF TESTING FOR ALLERGIC RESPONSE

All physical manifestations have an electomagnetic field associated with them, and are either in harmony, indifferent or in conflict. We wish to establish ways of choosing our food, clothing, affirmations, thoughts, feelings, colors, space, etc., to enhance our life and grow in strength, beauty, joy, peace, harmony and love.

Kinesiology, muscle testing, biolcinesiology and pendulum testing are scientific outgrowths of folk's intuitive observations of life's phenomena poetically described as turn ons, bummers or jives. The tests will give you simple indications of:
1) Which foods weaken or strengthen you.
2) Which herbs or food concentrates (and which brands) to use and their dosages.
3) Exact size of meal for best digestion and strength.
4) Good food combinations.
5) How to structure your program so that there is a daily increase in strength.

Emotions play a major role in the success of a healing program. One should re—examine attitude and secret negative affirmations about self—jealousies, anger, vengence and lack of forgiveness for self and others. If good food, no matter what the dosage, gives a negative response, check out your thoughts and feelings, forgive all and go out and do something nice for someone — especially one for whom you may have a dislike for. Use positive affirmations before eating.

For example, there are some folks who have an allergic reaction to wheatgrass, but when the emotions are corrected, show a strengthening effect. Remember, when the test is administered, if your stomach is not empty it could cause a nauseous feeling. Usually, after 20 minutes you should do a stomach wash, resulting in feeling wonderful. Even when there is no food, wheatgrass and other greens pull in toxins and can make you feel sick. A stomach wash will bring relief. Smaller dosages with the right attitude will not give any problem. Muscle test and be safe. All sour foods — rejuvilac, seed cheeses, saurkraut and fat foods should definitely be tested for therapeutic value and dosage.

Three different testing methods may be used:
Method 1
Both persons are standing. The person to be tested (Pat) has both hands at her side. The person testing (Doc) faces the person's side. Doc puts left hand on top part of Pat's arm and right hand under region between wrist and elbow. During testing, Doc will pull Pat's arm towards self with palm to establish strength and resistance.

Method 2
Pat stands erect with arm extended from shoulder with palm facing down and other arm relaxed at side. Although either arm may be used, most practitioners have the right arm extended. Doc faces Pat and places one hand on Pat's wrist palm down and the other on Pat's shoulder, palm down for balance. Doc will test Pat's ability to resist downward pressure.
Method 3
Pat presses with all strength the thumb tip to form a circuit. Doc grabs ends of the two fingers and tries to pull them apart.

The basic procedure is as follows: establish a standard level of strength of Pat by Doc saying, "Resist me." Doc pushes down or pulls. Both parties should use the same amount of strength when testing for the effect of "stuff" in body. If a full jar or large quantity of testing material is available, just a touch of the finger will be enough to contact. If no weakness is discovered, determine dosage by starting with a small quantity and increase until there is a weakening effect, then test positive with herb or supplement. Recheck the smaller quantity which should be your optimal dosage.

Many other nutritionally minded folks are shopping in health food stores, grocery markets and co—ops with the help from the pendulum. One can be purchased or made with a 4 — 7 inch long crystal, fish sinker, ring, small glass or mahagony weight on the end of a string. Allow the pendulum to swing horizontally and ask it to indicate by either clockwise or counter—clockwise which direction is "yes". Now ask, for example, "Is the celery in this quantity good for me?" and watch the direction of rotation.

I have found the muscle test and pendulum in aggreement and have helped me and many others in knowing what to eat. For additional information, read "Which Vitamin, Which Herb", by John and Margaret Barton, P.O. Box 64, Talent, Oregon 97540. They operate a school. Or Life in 21st Century, pgs. 219 — 222.

One of the greatest secrets of the military training in survival is the fact that a person can use ones own urine for nourishment. The 3 — 5% toxins within urine are quickly filtered out within the intestinal tract and act as laxatives. With 4 days of urine drinking, the taste becomes almost like water. It is rich in enzymes, minerals, vitamins and some amino acids. One can live for a minimum of a month on solely urine. This has been tested by miners trapped in a cave, where it took 35 days to excavate. Their health actually improved. With this knowledge you never have to panic, as you can always travel on your own liquid and any grasses available in fields to an area of safety. Much has been written in the books of the oldest natural healing practices of the Ajervedic system and the body liquid was called the "divine nectar". For more information on this subject and it's therapeutic and survival usage, read "Water of Life", Armstrong, Nutribooks, Provo, Utah and Shivambu Kalpa, Pauls D.O., Orthobionomy, 5502 MacDonald Avenue, El Cerrito, California 94530.

SOME SESAME SECRETS

My research shows that you don't have to go to a miller to dehull your sesame seeds in order to remove the oxalic acid content. Everyone can try the following experiments:

Soak 1 cup sesame seeds overnight, blend with 2 cups of water to a cream. Very likely you will muscle test a weakening effect at this stage. Pour the milk through a strainer then test the husk left in the strainer and notice the weakening effect caused by the calcium oxalate found here. Then, muscle test the strained milk without the hulls. Most folks will find 4 - 8 ounces strengthening, but beyond that quantity will cause weakening. Again, pour this milk through the strainer and the substance will increase in strengthening the person. Next, muscle test for seasonings, like banana, pear, apple juice, honey, seaweed, etc., to determine whether it should be taken plain or flavored. Likewise, test all frequently eaten foods at least once for allergic reactions through muscle testing. If it tests alright when fingers are in contact with the food, then try varying dosages held in a glass with the palm wrapped around the glass. When a weakening dosage is reached, reduce the amount. If it strengthens, this is the dosage for optimal strength and health.

GROW YOUR OWN GRASS

"And God said, let the earth bring forth grass."

GENESIS I,II

"There is no unbelief. Whoever plants a seed beneath the sod and waits to see it push away the clod. He trusts in God."

ELIZABETH YORK CASE

It is easy to become a grass farmer in your own home. If you intend to use wheatgrass, read the instructions, then start planting. Drop by to see the indoor gardens at Hippocrates Health Institute.

Dr. Ann Wigmore, over a period of years, has developed and perfected this method to meet the needs of her growing community. It is organized to produce up to twenty trays daily. After the grass is harvested, the sod is stored in deep piles covered with plastic sheets in our basement. The earthworms and micro-organisms convert the seed husks, stubs and earth of the sod into the best compost obtainable in a period of three to six weeks. Then the soil is recycled into the planting trays. You may have to add lime or kelp.

The best earth is dark, porous, and pleasant smelling. Black humus found in the woods is excellent. It is springy and alive with helpful organisms which are present to feed the rootlets of the wheatgrass. Without them the plants cannot be properly nourished. With each harvest, they continue to improve the soil. If you use commercially prepared soil, be sure it has not been sterilized. Dead earth cannot foster the growth of high quality live plants. Chemical fertilizer kills the life of the earth and should not be used. Use the best soil you can find.

Earthworms should be kept in a can with some compost. They can be found on top of any soil after a good rain.

Obtain the best wheat available. To get started, purchase it from a health food store. It should have a germination rate of at least 90%. Purchase the wheat berries in hundred pound sacks. Find other people to order with you. An order of at least 300 pounds will mean a tremendous saving on freight costs. Store the grain in a cool, dry place.

The hard spring wheat seed is soaked in tepid (about 70 degree) water for 12 hours in summer, 24 hours in winter. Use two parts water to each part wheat.

PLANTING

We use the large 18 x 26 x 2 inch baker's sheet "trays" which can be obtained from a commercial restaurant supply house for 50 cents to $2.50 apiece, depending on condition. Use one to two inches of soil. Or you can use wooden fruit boxes lined with plastic to keep them from leaking. Use five to seven inches of soil. Any container or baking pan is suitable for growing.

To produce better quality grass by continuous improvement of soil, add about a dozen earthworms to each container. They will regenerate the soil and leave their castings, one of the best fertilizers.

The soil should be thoroughly moistened, but free from puddles which would drown the seed.

Spread the soaked wheat seed evenly over the surface of the soil, seed touching seed, but only one seed deep. Do not press the seed into the soil. Soil should be scarcely visible through the layer of seed.

To conserve moisture and increase temperature, the tray is covered with a sheet of plastic, placed over it loosely, to permit a supply of air. The trays are left in the basement for three days. Any semi-dark spot with a temperature of about 70 degrees will do. A very rapid rate of growth can be obtained by keeping pans inside an almost closed large plastic garbage bag, in indirect sunlight. Be sure to water adequately. Plants initially grow faster in dark places because they are reaching out for light.

When the grass is about one and a half inches tall, the covering is removed and the grass is brought up from the basement to shelves located in the sunniest part of the house, near a window where it will receive some sunlight.

The soil should be watered as needed, but not drowned. In seven to fourteen days, depending upon temperature, soil and light, your grass will be around seven inches high and ready to harvest.

HARVEST

Using a sharp knife, or scissors, cut the grass at the roots. If you are using the whole plant — root, berry and stem — pull the grass from the soil in small sections. Harvest only the amount needed, since refrigeration of cut grass entails some nutritional loss. You can delay maturation time by keeping the grass tray in a cool place.

JUICING

The simplest, most natural way is to chew small amounts of grass, swallowing only the juice. At the Hippocrates Health Center, Dr. Wigmore has been using a manual juicer designed especially for grass because its slow rotation prevents oxidation of the juice (see Appendix, Food by Mail). The use of a blender, centrifugal juice extractor or any other high speed machine oxidizes the juice. This greatly reduces its nutritional value.

Feed the grass into the receptacle. The juice flows out the spout. The machine ejects the dry pulp. The juicer should be disassembled and washed every evening after the last use. Clean the strainer thoroughly and dry the whole unit carefully.

Following are suggestions for the best use of the manual juicer:

1. A new unit should be thoroughly cleaned with biodegradable soap.

2. Don't tighten the clamp screw with wrenches or exert a great deal of force; it can cause the clamp to break.

3. Adjust the pulp outlet screw and lock ring for easy turning and maximum juice flow.

4. To prevent rusting, occasionally oil with cold pressed seed oil.

5. Let the juice sit for a couple of minutes after juicing so that sediment will settle in the bottom of the glass. Do not drink the sediment.

6. Filter the juice when using it in an eye cup.

7. Mixing indoor greens (sprouts, celery, parsley, spinach or weeds) with grass, makes the juice more palatable. Use a small quantity of grass during each feeding of machine. You might have to run the pulp through several times to get all the juice.

8. Although inefficient for this purpose, one can use the machine to juice carrots and other tubers, plus the squashes. First, slice or grate them. Run through several times. It is not good for juicing fruit as the acid reacts chemically with iron.

9. The machine is ideal for use in time of power failure and famine.

I have found that a conventional grain mill can be converted into a grass juicer (good for all greens) with minimal effort. Adjust the screw for fine ground flour. Run the grass through. It will come out as finely ground pulp. Place the pulp in a strainer. With spoon press on the pulp. Collect the juice in a bowl. It is fast and efficient.

One box of wheatgrass, if properly planted and cared for, should produce up to two and a half pounds of grass. Generally, one pound of seed will produce four pounds of grass. With the grass juicer you can extract at least ten ounces of juice from one pound of grass. Hence, you can anticipate, on an average, at least 24 ounces of juice per box planted. This amount of juice will provide a husband and wife with three daily drinks of at least two ounces each. To obtain this quantity, you will have to plant two trays every second day. After you start the operation, your first harvest will be between the seventh and the fourteenth day.

COMPOSTING

After harvesting the grass, dump all the soil from the "planting box" onto a large, plastic sheet on the floor. Separate out the worms and the plant material. Return the worms to your earthworm farm. Place the stubs and roots along with your organic vegetable garbage in the bottom of the planting box. Cover the waste with the soil you have separated out. You may compost the whole stubble mats by stacking them in a large wooden box, galvanized garbage can, or directly on the basement floor. Add a few earthworms. If compost develops a strong smell, a 'starter' can be used which would prevent the odor and speed decomposition.

Every eight plantings, mix a handful of sea kelp fertilizer and a light sprinkle of lime onto the topsoil of each box. Moisten the earth thoroughly and you are ready for your second planting, which should be a replica of the first.

INSTANT GRASS

You may purchase all the material you need from the health food dealer and department store. This method is ideal for teaching children about gardening. Let them do their thing in soil. This is the quickest, least expensive method, good for those who want small amounts of grass. Ideal for students, nurses, communes, politicians, truckdrivers and up-tight individuals. The next gift you give to your loved ones should be a tray of grass. Share the grass with strangers.

From a grocery or department store purchase non-aluminum baking trays. I found the Ekcoloy brand, size 9¼ x 5 x 2 inches at a cost of 79 cents each to be the best. Look around in your neighborhood garbage cans for the best deals on containers for growing.

Obtain two large, heavy duty plastic bags. Fill one with the best available soil. Add soil to baking tray. From your salt shaker, sprinkle some sea kelp onto the soil. Mix it into the soil. After planting the wheat, insert the tray into an 18 x 14 inch plastic bag. This will create a greenhouse effect. Keep the tray in a window. In three days remove the covering. In seven to fourteen days the grass will be at least seven inches high and ready to harvest.

There is no reason to wait until the grass is 6.3451 inches long before you start enjoying its luscious foliage. Taste it daily at different stages of growth. You will notice that after you remove the cover, the stems are crisp and sweet, very much like sugar cane. Cut off just the amount you intend to use, perhaps a handful, chew it before breakfast and before every non-fruit meal.

After the first harvest, the second growth of wheatgrass is not worthless. It may be harvested and used, but the third growth is of little value.

After harvesting the grass, store the sod in the plastic composting bag. The first mat should be placed with the roots downward. All the others should be placed root side up. Drop a few earthworms into your compost pile. It will not emit any offensive odors and will insure plenty of soil for planting. Make certain this bag is not closed tightly, the worms need air to breathe. In three to six weeks, the sod will break down into soil to be used in planting. In the meantime, you will be using the soil which you have stored in the other plastic bag.

HOW TO GROW WHEATGRASS WITHOUT SOIL

This is the hydroponic way to grow wheatgrass, alfalfa or aquarian greens. Everyone can have this grass juice. Takes only few minutes day. Requires no soil. No heavy earth pans to lift. If you have high quality seed, and enough light, you can expect dark green 6 inch sprouts in 8 to 14 days. Juice from the grass is sweet.

Obtain baking pans. Easy to handle is 12" x 18" x 2" size. Soak the seed as described previously. Place 1 to 2 layers of   cotton or paper towels, cheese cloth   or equivalent   (wash them out thoroughly between plantings) on bottom of pan.

Soak the towel with water. Avoid puddles which might drown the seed. Sprinkle the soaked seed densely on towel, one next to another, one layer thick. Bless the seed. Ask the Lord for a harvest.

Cover the pan completely with one layer of plastic. Keep it in a warm place, 70 to 80 deg. F. (Room temperature). Check once a day, add water to keep the towel wet. The first 3 days provision of adequate heat is critical.

Remove the plastic on the 4th day. Let vegetation grow from 8 to 15 days, to a height of 5 to 7 inches. When harvesting, pull the greens out, or clip with knife or scissor. Remove the seed husk. If buckwheat, sunflower or alfalfa and the roots look healthy, not brown, you may eat the whole plant. Otherwise, compost the roots.

Consider: To reduce the care of plants, place a half inch of untreated sand or tiny pebbles, on bottom of pan. Flood it with water to the level of sand. Cover it with layer of wet towels. This will provide continuous humidity and water for growth. You may make a hole in bottom of pan and plug it. You may drain the water every 4 days if it should become smelly and refill it with clean water. For faster growth and sweeter taste, you may add a few pinches of kelp or liquid seaweed to the water solution.

Another simple, efficient method of growing wheatgrass or other indoor greens: thoroughly soak peat moss in very warm water. Mix crude sea kelp into it, one teaspoon to each ounce dry peat moss; fill the tray with the mixture and plant in the usual manner.

PIE CRUST Method. This method is best for city, apartment dwellers. It is very economical, takes up a small amount of space and has no odors. Material needed: 25 pounds (or 60 pounds) peatmoss, liquid (or powder) kelp fertilizer and a dozen baking pans. One 12 by 20 inch baking pan can require about 3 tbs of liquid fertilizer and one pound peatmoss.

Mix water with liquid fertilizer (3 tbs per quart) or kelp powder (2 tbs per quart). In a large bucket mix peatmoss and fertilizer solution to the consistency of mud. Use the wet soil to make a pie crust (about ¼ inch thick) on the planting tray.

The seeds should have been soaked in the usual manner. Spread them densely. Cover them thoroughly with a plastic sheet, or place the tray inside of a plastic bag. Check daily to be sure that the peatmoss is moist. Sprinkle gently with water as needed. After 3 days remove the plastic.

Throughout the 7 to 10 days of growth, to increase heat and humidity, you may cover the tray at night with plastic. Every couple of days mist the greens with a dilluted solution of fertilizer. As the greens develop roots into the soil, you can flood the tray with water, let the tray sit for couple minutes, then drain the water.

After the growth is complete, you can place the whole mat, with the greens, inside of a plastic bag and refrigerate it. Harvest as needed. After all the greens are cut, place the mat in your outdoor compost heap.

The quality of this grass is no different from grass grown in soil. When I omitted kelp, it grew half as fast, developed little color, was dry and had a flat taste. In place of peat moss you may use untreated sand and water.

Another method is to sprout one-half cup of wheat in a wide mouth quart jar. After four days of sprouting, tip the jar on its side. Rinse as needed, draining thoroughly. Grow grass to desired height.

REASONS FOR FAILURE AND CORRECTIONS

Many people who use good quality seed, discover that their grass crop is very sparse. The fault lies in soaking the seed too long or having the soil too wet or too dry. If the seed has germinated too long before planting, the sprouts will not take root and will die.

Mildew may start to form on the stems and in the soil. Soaking seed in dilution of liquid sea kelp, fertilizer, as well as choosing hard winter wheat might correct it. It can also be caused by too much dampness or too densely planted grass. To correct this condition, permit the air to circulate. The moving air will reduce the possibility of bacterial growth. A fan directed at the grass can keep the air circulating. Mildew does not destroy the quality of grass, but wash the mildew off the grass before juicing.

You may find small insects on the soil. They are quite harmless. Often they are associated with inferior quality seed or incompletely decomposed soil.

The grass juice may taste flat, or even bitter, due to poor quality soil. Correct this by searching out better soil. Introduction of sea kelp into the soil will make the juice sweeter.

Infrequent watering will produce dry grass with little juice.

Insufficient light will cause the grass to be dry and pale in color. If you live in the north, you can supplement natural light with a 40 watt combination of incandescent and flourescent light or Vita-lite.

The grass may be growing poorly due to clay-like soil. Correct this by adding peat moss and sand. During the first few plantings mix one part soil to one part peat moss. Additional worms will aerate the soil, making it more porous.

SPROUTS FOR HEALTH AND ECONOMY

"Moisten your wheat, that the Angel of water may enter it. Then set it in the air, that the Angel of air may embrace it. And leave it from morning to evening beneath the sun, that the Angel of sunshine may descend upon it."
Jesus, Essene Gospel of John

"WANTED: Alive, a vegetable that will grow in any climate, rival meat in nutritional value, mature in three to five days, may be planted any day of the year, requires neither soil nor sunshine, rivals tomatoes in Vitamin C, has no waste, can be eaten raw ."

Dr. Clive McCay of Cornell University composed this ad, which would perplex all of us if it were carried in the daily papers. The Chinese, centuries ago, captured the "good guy soybean" and have been fletcherizing it ever since.

A ban of Robin Hood type outlaws, headed by the soybeans, now includes such big-timers as garbanzas, untamed peanuts, ho chia mung beans, as well as wheat, alfie, and the radical radish. The only qualification for joining this underground band of revolutionaries is to be an organic, sproutable seed.

If the sprouts ever join forces, on a large scale, with the creeping weeds and biblical grasses and start infiltrating the supermarkets and sneaking into the salad bowls of outstanding members of our society, they will cause the most radical revolution in our diet and destroy many of our highly respected utensils, as well as our institutions.

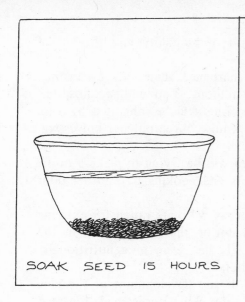

SOAK SEED 15 HOURS

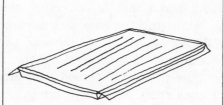

WET SOIL, PEATMOSS, TOWEL, OR PAPERTOWEL ~ SPREAD AN EVEN LAYER OF SEED ~ COVER WITH A PIECE OF SHEET PLASTIC

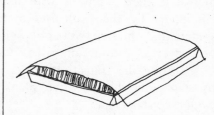

LET SIT THREE DAYS OR UNTIL YOU CAN SEE THE SPROUTS PUSHING UP THE PLASTIC

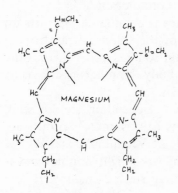

MAGNESIUM

CHLOROPHYL MOLECULE

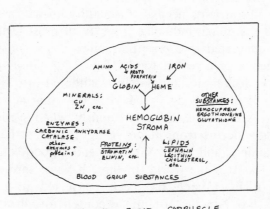

THE RED BLOOD CORPUSCLE

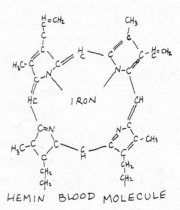

IRON

HEMIN BLOOD MOLECULE

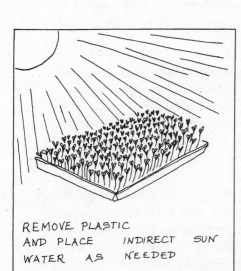

REMOVE PLASTIC AND PLACE INDIRECT SUN WATER AS NEEDED

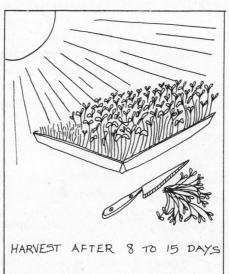

HARVEST AFTER 8 TO 15 DAYS

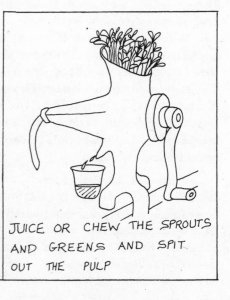

JUICE OR CHEW THE SPROUTS AND GREENS AND SPIT OUT THE PULP

These lowly little warriors will lead civilization into a new world of humanity and the era of fruitarianism.

The sproutarians have been preparing for decades. They have sharpened their wits by fasting, increased their strength with live food, and gained followers in the millions. You will see hospitals eliminated by the explosives of live food. Drug factories and research firms will be inhabited by wise spiders and their networks of webs. Old age homes will be replaced by tennis courts; butcher knives will be converted to museum pieces; vivisection will be considered sadism.

During the transition, those who have not yet discarded their greed will be trying to make a profit by selling, to the receptive, plans for converting stoves into refrigerators and cooking pots into indoor garden containers.

Sprouts are one of the essential ingredients in the diet of the Hunzas, who are noted for extreme long life and unsurpassed health. Such foods provide them nutrients during the cold winters in the Himalayan Mountains. All peoples of Asia are familiar with sprouts. Today, even in a nutritionally backward country like America, sprouts are becoming daily fare for millions.

The seed is a storehouse of food energy intended for early growth and development of the new plant. The dry seed is characterized by a remarkably low metabolic rate. When moistened, the seed starts transforming the stable nutrients into life components.

The chemical changes which occur in the sprouting seed activate a powerful enzyme factory which is never surpassed at any later stage of growth. This rich enzyme concentration induces a heightened enzyme activity in your metabolism leading to regeneration of the bloodstream and digestive processes.

Dr. Francis Pottenger, Jr., found that sprouted legumes and grain contain a complete protein. In tests on rats, sprouts sustained life through the reproductive cycle for many generations, thus proving that they can adequately supply all nutrients needed for healthy growth and reproduction.

Once the seed has sprouted the mucus-inducing property of most legumes is eliminated. Sprouts do not cause gas. Crude protein is converted into essential amino acids; much of the starch is transformed into simple sugars, making sprouts a predigested foods. The seed may contain some starch, whereas the shoot contains only sugar. Hence, it is more completely assimilated into the body. You eat less. Ease of digestion means you will have more of the body's vital force for other activities.

The vitamin content of the seed increases tremendously when sprouted. Depending on the seed, optimum vitamin content generally occurs from 50 to 96 hours after it begins to germinate. Sprouts are an especially good source of Vitamin C and the B Vitamins and a good source of Vitamins A and E.

Wheat is one of the staple foods of the world. In three days of sprouting, its weight doubles and it becomes sweet. Much of the original starch has been converted to natural sugars, making it less mucus-forming. In four days of sprouting the Vitamin E content of wheat increases 300%. Some of the Vitamin B-complex components increase from 20% to 600%.

Drs. Graves and Miller of the Agricultural Experimental Station at Beltsville, Md. showed the power of sprouts in restoring fertility to sterile cattle. 11 cows were involved. They had been bred recently many times without success. 7 of the 11 had been bred for 6 to 14 months. 3 of them were over 8 years old, however they had reproduced successfully in the past. 4 were heifers. Each animal was fed 5 pounds sprouted dry weight. The rest of diet was equal weight of silage. At the end of 60 days, when bred, all cows were made pregnant.

In "A Review of Literature Pertaining to the Value of Sprouting Cereal Grains For Livestock Feed": "The value of sprouted oats for improving fertility in cattle was studied at several stations. Moore reported results with 4 shy breeders whose rations were supplemented with oat sprouts. Two of the four conceived after receiving the supplement. No controls without the supplement were reported. Winters discussed results in which 8 of 10 hard-to-breed cows conceived after being fed 2½ to 5 pounds of sprouted oats for a period of 21 to 90 days. Mosley et al reported five cases in which all conceived at service after initiation of oat sprout supplement. Again no controls were reported. Cunningham reported conception as the result of supplementing 7 shy breeders with oat sprouts for 70 to 150 days. Miller and Graves reported that 57 of 88 cows conceived within 4 services after oat sprout feeding was started.

In a bulletin, Dr. J.J. Fayne states: "Tests were made many years ago by the Department of Animal Husbandry of the United States of Agriculture in Beltsville, Md., to determine the importance of sprouted oat in restoring fertility. The success was no less than amazing. In every case tested the cows that had lost, or outgrown, their ability to reproduce became mothers again, giving birth to fine, normal, healthy calves. The same sprouted grain diet was given to another group of cows that were so completely sterile they had never reproduced although they had been bred many times. With the addition of nourishment found in these grain sprouts they all became mothers with every evidence of healthy reproductive ability. Bulls that had became sterile were also restored to normal fertility again in every case tested." (The Miracle of Alfalfa).

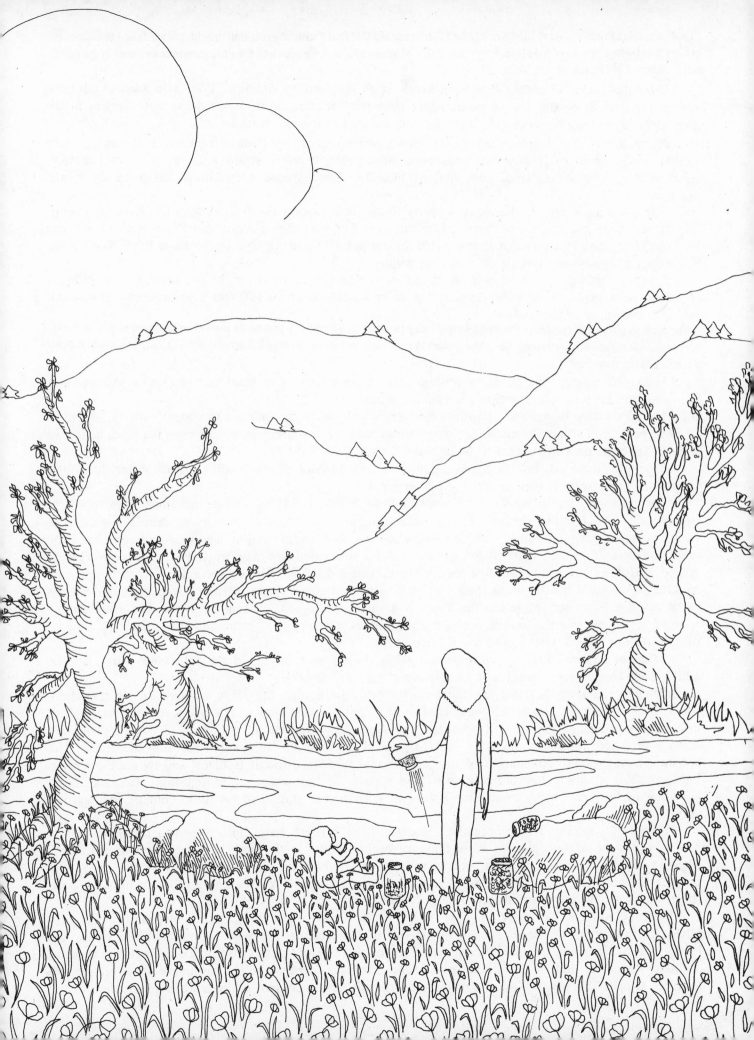

Dr. Ehrenfried Pfeiffer, told at Bio-Dynamic Soil Conference in 1951 that "without exception they had never failed to restore to fertility a bull when they have fed him a very limited diet of green alfalfa for a time and then fed generous amounts of sprouted oats." (Three Fold Farm, Spring Valley, N.Y.)

Over the years, Vitamin E has been heralded as the fertility vitamin. Those who want to continue sexual activity, especially for purposes other than reproduction, should include sprouted grains in the diet. Otherwise, they may experience exhaustion and earlier loss of youth.

Rutin if rare, it is found in few foods. This bioflavonoid is very high in buckwheat. It has an action similar to Vitamin P. It increases endurance of capillaries under strain and exposure to radiation, shortens any kind of external and internal bleeding time., speeds coagulation and increases mental acuity.

The soybean is one of the most versatile foods. It is among the few seeds which have an alkaline ash. It will sour just like milk. Sprouted, it makes a delicious cheese and yogurt. It keeps well and can be bought organically grown for as low as 16 dollars per 100 pounds. Sprout for three days. Refrigerate. The best use of soybean sprouts is in making yogurt.

Alfalfa, although the smallest seed of the legume family, turns out to be the favorite. Nutritionally it should be superior to all other sprouts for its roots extend up to 100 feet into the earth to seek out minerals and other nutrients.

The sprouts differ from proteins like meat, seeds, dairy products and grain by having its protein in the form of amino acids, enzymes, chlorophyll and hormones. Thus, the protein is either in predigested form or in a form which the body can easily utilize. No uric acid is generated.

The total amount of available protein after germination of a seed increases by a few percent. However, the protein concentration per seed decreases.

The percentage of protein in sprouts is inversely related to the increase in weight. Alfalfa seed is 1.5 to 30% protein. The alfalfa sprout increases approximately sevenfold in weight over the seed, hence we would expect its protein content to be between 2 and 5%.

If people are to eat food that is best suited to their physiology, they will eat fruit. After three days of growing some sprouts become like fruit in many ways.

For example, according to Composition Of Foods, U.S.D.A., we can make the following observation about mung beans: The germination process converts starch to simple sugars. The carbohydrate content of mung bean sprouts is the same as in casaba melon. The moisture content of the seed increases from 10.7% to 88.8% in the sprout, comparable to any fruit. Protein is converted to amino acids, and its concentration is reduced to that of a dried fig. The caloric value is slightly less than that in papaya and a little more than that in honeydew melon. One cup (one fourth pound) contains forty calories. Sprouted mung has the Vitamin A value of a lemon, thiamin of an avocado, riboflavin of a dried apple, niacin of a banana, and ascorbic acid of a pineapple. For a complete nutritional analysis of sprouts and grasses write to Omangod Press (176).

Years of experimentation with sprouting has led me to recommend the following: mung, alfalfa, aduki, buckwheat lettuce, sunflower greens, wheatgrass, fenugreek.

Other seeds I do not feel are the best for health, although they may be used during transition. Chick peas continue to be starchy and gas-forming; lentil, unless sprouted 3 or more days, are high in uric acid producing properties; if sprouted too long, they become very fibrous. Sprouted grains are slightly acid and mucus-forming; it is best to grow them for 4 to 8 days and use only the shoots. The alkaline, high protein combination of soy sprouts makes them difficult to digest and they are often gas inducing. If you desire soy beans, convert the sprouts to cheese for easier digestion. Rice and millet continue to be very starchy even after 7 days of growth; the grass is of low fluid content and it grows very slowly.

Ernest T. Krebs, Jr., biochemist, believes that sprouts have anti-cancer factors. He states: "Nitrolosides are anti-neoplastic. When they are broken down in the body they release two chemicals. These two chemicals are cyanide and benzaldehyde. Body cells, the normal cells of the body, can protect themselves from such released chemicals; but cancer cells are incapable of doing this. . . both these chemicals kill unprotected cancer cells." (219)

Krebs continues: "Consider quickly, just the nitriloside content of the diet of primitive man. He relied heavily upon the fresh succulent sprouts of the grasses, the wild legumes, millet, vetch, the lupines, wild beans and the like. Vitamin contents of these plants at the sprouting stage often exceed by 20 times or more, that of the mature plant. The nitriloside content in the sprouts of some grasses and legumes is often 50 times or more greater than the nitriloside content of the mature plant. Indeed, the nitrilosides and other accessory food factors that occur in prodigious quantities in the sprouting stage of the plant may be completely absent in the mature plant."

After I moved into the Institute, my first observation of the regenerative powers of this highly nutritional food was in the body of one of Ann Wigmore's guests.

Joe was an architect, past 50 years of age. For the last ten years he had not been able to carry on his practice because his right arm was paralyzed. He was very emaciated.

Daily, for a duration of four months, he ate two meals of sprouts, raw vegetables, little seasoning, and no other food. At the end of three months he was reduced to skin and bones. In the fourth month, I witnessed gradual regression of the pallor in his arm, as the blood and nerves regenerated. He left the Institute a month later. We shook hands. He proudly extended the right one. Proof of the regenerative power of sprouts.

Because I observed that sprouted grain caused me to experience mucus discharge, tiredness and sexual stimulation, I stopped using it in my diet. For a spiritual path, sprouted grains should be used in small quantity, if at all.

When organic produce was not available in Boston four years ago, I lived totally on sprouts, kelp, dulse, wheatgrass, buckwheat lettuce, sunflower greens and sesame-sunflower seed yogurt all winter and experienced, at every meal, the joy of eating this tasty food. I continue to use grass juice and a mixture of sunflower and buckwheat greens in conjunction with my fruit diet.

This simple diet has greatly improved my health, and keeps my energy level high. I have become more conscious of my body's needs. Although I work hard both physically and mentally, I need very little sleep, and seldom feel tired. Meditation is easier, and I am more flexible for yoga.

HOW TO USE SEEDS AND SPROUTS

Sprouts provide the most nutritious and varied menu available. They are an excellent supplement to any diet and should be included in every meal.

Sprouts can be grown in any utensil without thought to soil conditions, climate, composting techniques, blight or bugs. They are simple to harvest and to store for future use. They are not contaminated by insecticides or pesticides or made defective by heat, cold, preservatives, irradiation or aging.

A sprout diet can be very inexpensive — as little as 15 cents a day or 69 cents if you include seeds, fruits and vegetables. Sprouts are extremely versatile. They can be used as a salad, as a base for soups and casseroles, snacks, cereals, or as drinks made with the help of a blender.

The soak water from most seeds is rich in water-soluble nutrients and enzymes which improve digestion. It can be blended with sauces and seed milk. Some of the soaked seeds can be used immediately. After three days of growth sprouts are ready for eating. In another four days, you can pick greens from mason jar gardens. If soil is used, you can grow greens that will surpass store-bought lettuce in taste and nutrition. Juice may be extracted from seven-day grasses to be served as health-giving food. Juices eliminate hunger and enable one to reduce healthfully. Following is a list of some of the uses of seeds:

1. Soak Water: in sauces, soups, seed milk. Recommended: fenugreek, wheat, buckwheat, oat, sweet rice, alfalfa. Wash seed, soak one part seed with two parts water. Let soak water of grains ferment for at least 24 hours.
2. Soaked Seed: in bread and casseroles, use grains and chick peas; in salad dressings, cereal and blended drinks, use sesame, sunflower, almond, and pumpkin.
3. Sprouts: raw as snacks, substitute for nuts: soy; mixture of wheat and chickpea; mixture of sesame, pumpkin and sunflower. Use only natural seasoning.
4. Greens: On soil — buckwheat, sunflower, wheatgrass, in jars — raddish, fenugreek, alfalfa, sunflower.
5. Blended Beverages: almond, sesame, sunflower. Yogurt: soy, sesame, sunflower, almond. Sandwich spreads from all sprouts. Add to breads, soups, casseroles, and salads.
6. Juices: as a supplement to the diet or as tools for rebuilding health through live foods and grass juice fasting. Use wheatgrass (sweet), barleygrass (bitter), alfalfa (strong), oatgrass (mild). Sprouts and indoor greens may be juiced. The juice from alfalfa, feungreek, sunflower greens and buckwheat greens may be mixed into carrot or celery juice.

Each of the dishes can be enriched with seasonal green herbs, dried sea vegetables and weeds. A sprout diet is ideal for students, city dwellers, and those up north. It is an inexpensive way to live organically.

Let the young ones do the sprouting; they will learn a lot about the fundamentals of life. It takes at most eight minutes a day to produce all the sprouts a group of five can eat. You will discover the adventure of instant farming, as you watch life unfold. Serve sprouts as conversation pieces at your next party.

Considering the uncertainty of our times, it is good to know that you will be able to provide food for your family and be assured good health. There is no survival food better than sprouts. Sprouts generally increase many times in weight over dry seed. The seed can be stored for a long time at the lowest possible cost. Several hundred pounds of seed can provide complete tasty meals through famine, war, strikes.

SEEDS FOR SPROUTING

Any live seed will sprout. Don't germinate any seed which are known to produce poisonous greens such as members of the nightshade family, which include potatoes, tomatoes, and petunia.

Grains such as wheat, rice, barley, oat, and rye should be sprouted for more than three days. By then they will have swelled to twice their original size with a stem about one-fourth inch long. Aduki when sprouted 3 to 5 days tastes like fresh garden peas. Mung, soy, lentil, peas, and radish are most palatable in three or four days when they are still sweet and tender. When grown for six or more days, and exposed to light the last three days, they are beautifully green, but become fibrous like a plant and somewhat tough unless cooked.

Garbanzas (chickpeas) are at their best in two days. When combined with sprouted wheat and sea kelp, they make a most delicious snack. Most nuts, if fresh and alive in their shells, can be brought to their former tree-ripened vintage by several days of sprouting. Before sprouting remove the shells without damaging the nut. Peanuts, after four days of sprouting, lose much of their legume flavor, and develop an enticing sweetness.

Sesame, flax, and chia are best after 24 hours of germination. Sesame develops a bitter taste if sprouted much longer. Use it, instead of strong condiments, to give tang to your salads.

Alfalfa, clover, and fenugreek are at their best after at least one week of sprouting. Sprouted sweet corn becomes like candy. Sunflower and pumpkin sprouts are ready in two to four days; they are tastier than the dry seed.

Some garden vegetable seed may be sprouted for two to six days. Experiment with spinach, swiss chard, celery, garlic, lettuce, okra, parsley, rutabaga, turnip and anything else you can find.

The seed you collect from weeds can be another source of sprouts. Amaranth, burdock, wild carrot, clover, dandelion, lambsquarter, peppergrass, plantain, sorrel, wild dock, wild onion and garlic can be added to your sproutable seed vocabulary.

For the highest nutritional value, buy organically grown seed. At least make certain that the seeds intended for sprouting are viable and have not been treated with chemicals. If purchasing seed in small quantities, which is the expensive way to shop, buy them from health food stores or mail order houses. A good quality seed should have a minimum of 90% germination rate.

For sprouting, choose any container, but avoid soluble toxic metals such as aluminum, copper, iron. I have used a variety of glass containers, unglazed flower pots, mason jars, sprouting kits, strainers, perforated fruit cans, towels, perforated galvanized 20 gallon cans. Mason canning jars are adequate for small quantities; for larger quantities, use 25 pound capacity enamel roasting pans. For banquets, I have used large   buckets, the bottoms of which are perforated with one-fourth inch holes.

GENERAL SPROUTING METHOD

This method works well for all seed. You may buy the large mouth mason jar from hardware stores or grocery markets. This inexpensive sprouter can be made by removing the inner disc from the lid. Using the disc as a pattern, cut an exact replica from copper screen, plastic window mesh or stainless steel screen. Use the screen to replace the disc on the lid.

A more clumsy looking, but just as effective sieve for the jar can be made by placing nylon or cheesecloth mesh on top of the jar and then tightening the lid (or using a rubber band). Wash the seed thoroughly and soak them overnight in a container of tepid distilled or untreated water, at least two parts water to one of seed. The smaller the seed, the shorter the soaking period. Alfalfa seed does well with three hours, but will not be harmed by 15 hours, soaking. The larger seed (chickpea, mung) may be soaked up to twenty hours.

After the initial soaking, drain off the water. Wash the seed; pour off the water. Place the container in a dark warm spot at 60 to 70 degrees temperature to hasten growth.

Twice daily the seed should be rinsed with tepid water. Pour the water directly into the container, then let it drain off. If not using a mason jar with screen, use a fine-mesh strainer to aid in pouring off the water without losing any seed. Seed hulls float or sink, and can easily be removed. They can cause the sprouts to spoil prematurely.

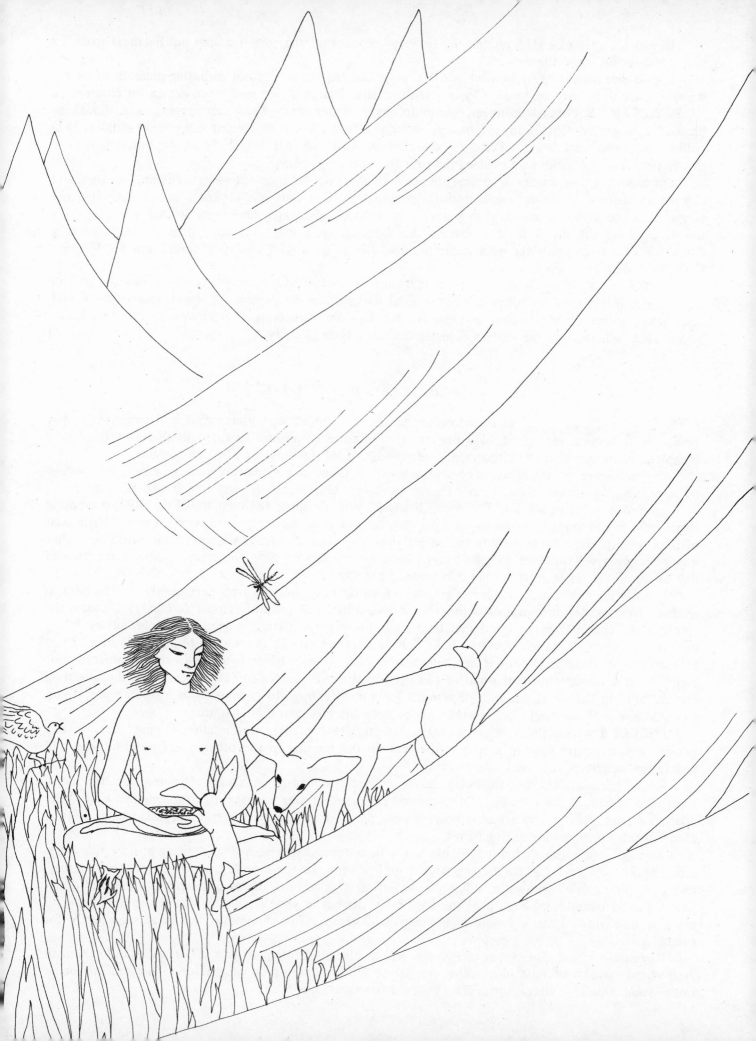

If you use metal or glass containers, be very careful that the sprouter does not overheat from the sun, which would roast the sprouts.

If you desire chlorophyl in your sprouts, after the first three days of sprouting place them on the window ledge until they are green. Clover, radish, alfalfa, fenugreek, do well when grown for chlorophyl.

SOY BEAN. Soybean, sunflower, pumpkin, have tender easily breakable sprouts, and should be handled very gently. Obtain any 32 ounce, or larger, fruit juice or shortening can, crock, stainless steel coffee pot, or enamel bucket. Perforate the bottom with one-fourth inch holes. Or purchase a large flower pot, and add some clean pebbles to cover the bottom opening.

Purchase the best quality sprouting soybeans (if they are old they rot easily). Peking, Otootan, and Cayuga are known for their quick, uniform germination. Eliminate the broken, dark or shrivelled old beans. Soak the soybeans overnight in warm water. Pour off the water. One more soaking is required for the beans. Pour off the water and remove the damaged seed. Place the good ones in your sprouting container. Flood the container with water three to five times a day, letting it drain from the bottom. Keep the container covered.

MUNG BEAN. If you want a sweet, tender mung sprout of high moisture content, soak the seek in warm water for at least 15 hours. Sprout in total darkness, at 80 degrees or higher, and wash at least three times a day. They are ready in three to five days. Before serving or storing, wash away the green husks. They will float to the surface. This is the mung bean at its best.

SPROUT SALAD IN ONE JAR

May vary the flavor of salads according to the mixture of seed you sprout in a single jar. A few radish or fenugreek seeds add piquency to any mixture of mung, lentil, and alfalfa seeds. For a complete, really hearty meal, sprout sunflower, alfalfa, lentil, fenugreek and mung together.

If you happen to get alfalfa seed with a low percentage of germination you can lessen the spoilage by sprouting them with mung beans. I have used one tablespoon of alfalfa with two tablespoons of mung per one quart mason jar. The mung beans provide air space between the little aflies, preventing them from smothering. In three to six days, the jar will be completely filled with sprouts. Alfalfa seed of poor quality cause the sprouts to rot on the third day. The seed from Wittmer, Deaf Smith and other quality sources will produce excellent crops with a minimum of care. Generally, alfalfa, after the 4th day of sprouting, needs at most only one washing per day.

Sprouts may be stored in the refrigerator, where they continue to grow very slowly. If you have to be away from home for several days and have started a batch of sprouts, refrigerate them; on return, the sprouting process may be be continued to completion. If sprouts start to spoil, it is the result of drying out. After washing away most of the hulls, I have kept sprouts in damp cloth bags, plastic bags or jars for one month without loss in vitality, crispness or taste. If your home is below freezing temperature at night, build a wooden box for sprouting and insulate with hay, leaves or newspaper. When the sprouting jars are kept in this chest, the heat of germination will be enough to prevent them from freezing. If still too cold, use a 25 watt light bulb in the box, or keep the box near a heat source.

POCKET GARDENING. When taking a car trip, back-packing, mountain climbing, carry in one pocket several plastic bags of seed mixture and do the farming in the other one. Sprouting seed will reduce the weight of your pack considerably.

While backpacking the following seeds are recommended: mixture of mung, alfalfa, lentil, sunflower, fenugreek for sprouting; finely ground sesame-sunflower seed for making ferments; kelp, dulse and dried fruit. Heavy duty reusable polyethelyne plastic bags can be the sprouter, salad bowl, bag for cheese making and soaking of dried fruit.

At night, wash the seed, fill a plastic bag with water and the washed seed, using at least two times more liquid than seed. Fasten the bag with a rubber band. In the morning, squeeze a neck on the bag, and pour off or drink the water. After the water has drained, give the seed another washing and drain. Leave a small opening in the top of the bag. Place the bag in your pocket and let the sprouts grow till evening, then rinse. If it is a cold night, sleep with them. After three days the sprouts are ready for eating.

If you are in the country, generally you will be able to identify at least a few weeds. Add them to your sprout salad and dine like a king or queen. Or carry a supply of sea vegetables and oil for an exotic salad. Don't be stingy, invite the birds and beasts to your feast.

SPROUTING ERRORS

1. Soaking the seed more than one time. Soaking the seed for too long or too short a time. Larger seeds tolerate up to 20 hours of soaking; four is best for small ones. Be sure to use plenty of water for soaking. In summer, soak a shorter period of time than in winter.

2. Choice of poor quality seed with a low percentage of germination. This is especially true of alfalfa and soy.

3. Damaging some of the sprouts by mishandling, causing them to rot.

4. Because of poor drainage, some sprouts or seed become waterlogged.

5. Failure to wash the seed at least once a day, leading to dehydration of some sprouts, killing them. The same condition may result from not keeping the container covered. You don't need to bother with covers when using mason jars; the screen seems to retard evaporation.

6. Keeping sprouting containers in the hot sun.

7. If your alfalfa crop spoils within five days, it usually indicates too hot a temperature or poor quality seed. Move the sprouts, if this happens, to a cool place or an air-conditioned room. Overheating, caused by infrequent washing, overcrowding, or lack of air, can also cause spoilage.

8. Mildew may start to form on many of the larger seeds because of improper ventilation and infrequent washings.

9. The sprouting container or the plastic cover may have started to mildew because it was not rinsed.

10. Quality of water used in seed soaking. Alfalfa can be killed with tap water. Seed will grow if blades of fresh grass are allowed to soak with the seed. Distilled or spring water is best for sprouting.

11. If you work with distaste, the seed will not grow. A 1969 Time magazine article on science, disclosed that good vibrations (love, joy, music) will cause the plants to grow up to twice as fast as normal. Bad vibrations were shown to stifle growth, causing death.

Thoughts of love and well-being are states of consciousness. They affect everything — other people, animals, plants and minerals. One should strive for harmony instead of negating the life force of other beings. When you sprout, if you discover that the seed grows slowly it might not be a problem of technique, it may be your state of consciousness. So love and be joyful, for the sprouties are watching you.

VIKTORY GARDENS FOR SURVIVAL

Instant Aquarian Salad Greens are a delightful collection of vegetation which can be grown in eight days to replace the expensive, unnutritional store variety. You don't have to rely on lettuce, spinach or celery which might have been harvested several weeks ago. Aquarian greens are grown in exactly the same manner as wheatgrass. Obtain unhulled seed which is suitable for sprouting (or planting). If you cannot obtain them organically grown, they may be available at feed stores or as bird seed (which, however, are quite often inactivated by heating) at the grocery store. Look in the Yellow Pages under Seed.

BUCKWHEAT LETTUCE is a succulent, tender, clover like green. Soak seed 3 hours before planting. During the first three days it is important to keep the trays in a very warm area (65 - 80 deg. F.). It is best to remove the cover when the plant is about ¼ inches tall, which is usually within 3 days of planting. Otherwise, the stems will be very long, the greens will be poor in color and the husks will not drop off. It is ready to harvest within one week when the husks have fallen off. If you plan to juice the buckwheat, plant the seeds more sparsely; allow them to grow for three to four weeks or even up to the flowering stage. Since the seeds have an uneven rate of sprouting, after the first harvest, you can expect a second crop from the slow starters. Buckwheat may easily be grown on wet towels, in place of soil, in a baking tray (see wheatgrass).

SUNFLOWER GREENS have a taste very much like watercress. Unhulled sunflower seed will give you a much larger harvest than the hulled, with minimal loss. Soak the seed 8 hours. Generally within 8 days most of the husks fall off. Harvest the crop before the greens become bitter to taste. If overproduced, you can refrigerate for up to 4 days or transfer your indoor garden to a cooler place to slow down the growth. I have had good success in sprouting, up to 8 days, unhulled and hulled sunflower seeds in jars, without soil. Before eating, be sure to remove the hulls. Sunflower greens are easy to juice and make a nutritious booster to carrot or any green juice.

FENUGREEK. These greens provide a piquant salad seasoning. You can start eating them after five days and continue till about the fourteenth day. They can be grown on soil or sprouted in jars. You can grow a mixture of buckwheat, sunflower and radish on a single tray to provide all the desirable greens. By combining this vegetation with a sprout mixture of alfalfa, mung, lentil, a few sunflower and fenugreek, you can provide yourself all the needed nutrients directly from your own indoor garden. The indoor green salad tastes delicious plain, or may be served with olive oil and kelp.

In addition, the following plants provide variety in the family indoor garden: 15 plants of comfrey, 5 plants of zucchini, 5 plants of kale, 15 plants of cherry tomatoes, 5 pots of alfalfa plants. Have them at different stages of maturation. They will give you a continuous variety of salad greens (See Appendix: Miniature Indoor Vegetable Gardens).

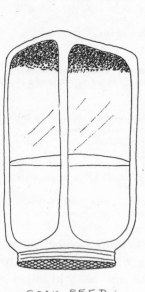
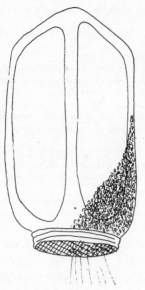
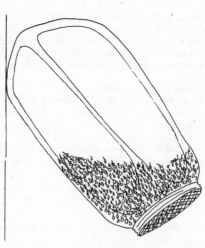
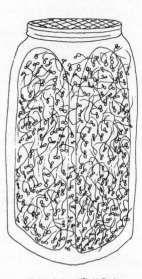

SOAK SEED:
alfalfa 4 hours
beans and grains
15 hours

POUR OFF

SOAK WATER

LET JAR SIT

AT A SLANT

RINSE TWICE
A DAY~
READY IN
4 TO 8 DAYS

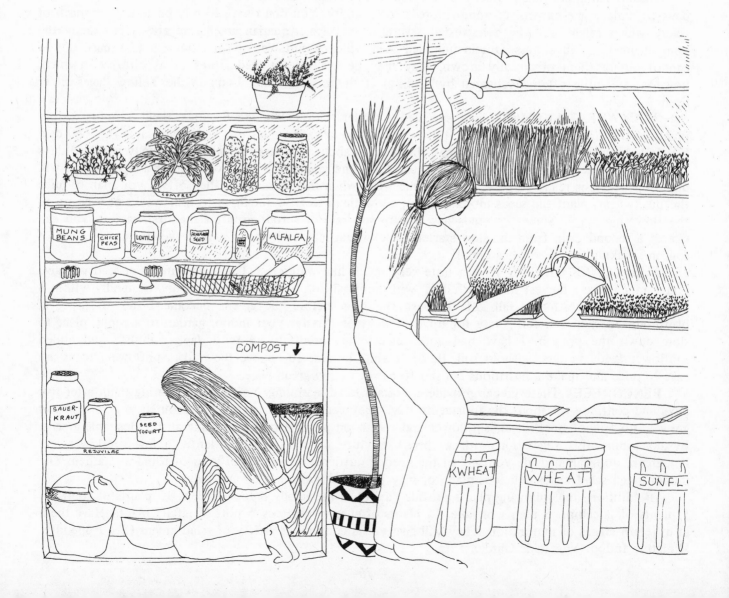

MINIATURE INDOOR GREENHOUSE. Once you have collected and dried a good quantity of seed from the field or purchased them from a nursery, you are ready to enter the green world of indoor farming. At the start, it is inadvisable to employ extensive planting, either in quantity or species. You can familiarize yourself with the growing of wheatgrass, buckwheat, sunflower vegetation and sprouting. These mastered, try a few favorite greens. Expansion, which most likely will be encouraged by other members of the family or commune, can be stopped only by usurping all the window space.

Start with a sunny location, a southern exposure if possible. East-West planting can be satisfactory, but, in winter, a northern exposure cannot supply enough light for most plants.

An indoor garden may be a very wide shelf built into a bay window on which you can put a prefitted waterproof tray, about three inches deep, filled with a layer of sand or pebbles no more than two inches deep. The pebbles must be kept continuously moist for good humidity. Set potted plants on this tray. Or use an outdoor window box simply mounted from an inside window ledge. This has advantages, for you may plant outside in summer and if you selected plants that can survive all winter indoors, you can simply detach the box and switch it to the indoor hooks.

An unused bedroom or properly insulated garage can also serve as your indoor farm. You can built a 12 x 16 foot greenhouse for as little as ten dollars by using two by three studs and heavy duty plastic. Send for plans. A prefabricated fiberglass greenhouse size 6 x 12 x 6 feet, for less than $100.00, can be obtained through several mail order houses advertised in Organic Gardening and Farming magazine. The greenhouse can be set up on the ground or on a flat roof, making it suitable for city dwellers.

Many homes have sunporches, unused during winter, where temperatures rarely drop below freezing. An open porch can be enclosed, with the aid of heavy duty plastic, into an effective greenhouse.

You must prepare for heavy winter winds. To insure that the plastic will not be torn by wind, reinforce it on both sides of the sheet with wires running crisscross, anchored to ceiling and floor, and to the two bordering vertical structures. The wires should be strung into one to two foot squares. First, string the outer mesh, then fit in the plastic, follow by installation of the inner mesh.

For extra warmth, you might consider two layers of plastic with a four to six inch air space separating them. The addition of a rubber-insulated window would provide temperature control, eliminating the need to tear down the structure for summer ventilation. The floors of most porches are not windproof. They should be insulated to reduce heat loss. Lay heavy duty plastic on the floor, then top it with an old rug.

Such an instant greenhouse should be finished by the middle of autumn. It is inexpensive, perfect for growing most vegetation. During the day, especially if it is facing south, the temperature can reach up to one hundred degrees. At night it will seldom go below freezing. For more heat on cold nights, leave a window or door ajar between the greenhouse and the living quarters.

HERB GARDEN IN YOUR KITCHEN

Pick a sunny day for planting. Soak the seed for two to three hours

The soil should be slightly acid and not too rich, except as qualified in this text. The choice of a planting container will vary with the plant's root length and spread. Use appropriate pots, perforated cans, window boxes, shallow baker's trays. Hanging baskets can increase space and provide decorative effect with a herb like oregano or nasturtium. An inexpensive method for planting is to fill heavy duty plastic bags with soil. Placing another bag over them creates a warm, moist, miniature greenhouse. Large or tall plants can be placed in pots on a pebble and water tray. In your unique household, use your imagination to create a work of green art.

Plant the seed in soil appropriate to them. Don't bury them too deep. The soil should be porous, without puddles. The seed will germinate faster if you lay a plastic sheet loosely over them. This will provide moisture and warmth. It should be removed soon after the shoots penetrate the earth.

Plant roots should not stand in water; place pebbles in the bottom of containers to provide drainage. Water the plants according to performance, as the soil demands. Misting can give additional moisture, especially for rosemary and other water-loving weeds or herbs. When the weather is above freezing, nearby windows should be opened, but avoid draft. Most herbs will do best at a temperature no lower than 55 degrees Farenheit and will tolerate up to 75 degrees if there is abundant humidity.

During the transition to good nutrition, cooking herbs can supply enticing flavors as any veteran cook knows. A sage having a wild thyme is a familiar activity in the stewing pot. Herbs like tarragon, chervil, mint, and basil may be used both in salads and in cooking.

Because of the volatile oils which give herbs their characteristic aroma, they should be harvested immediately before they are to be cut up or ground into the salad dressing. It is best to prepare the dressing at the dining table to let others enjoy the fragrance.

Pot the following plants late in August, unless otherwise stated, and allow them to remain outdoors in the container until frost threatens before taking them inside. When they are placed in the window garden, prune.

LEMON BALM is a 24 inch perennial. The crushed leaves release a lemon fragrance. Use it in drinks, salads, and cooked vegetables.

CHIVES, an attractive perennial, is known for its delicate onion flavoring in salads and cooking.

SWEET FENNEL is a biennial herb, 12 inches to 4 feet with many yellow flowers and feathery leaves. Use it for flavoring or as a vegetable.

MINT gives a pleasant aroma to any salad, dessert or drink. It enjoys a heavy soil, plenty of water and good drainage.

NASTURTIUM can be grown indoors in a sandy soil, from seed or 4 inch cuttings. The leaf stalk will climb a guide stick up to 10 feet tall. Its greens and beautiful flowers taste much like watercress. If more foliage and fewer flowers are desired, increase the richness of the soil.

PARSLEY is a small biennial with dark curly leaves. It can be grown from seed. Use rich, well-drained soil, and continuous watering, without waterlogging. When leaves coarsen, cut back to encourage new shoots. Use it fresh or dried in salad or in cooking.

SORREL can be grown from seed. Remove flower stems as soon as they appear and gather leaves frequently for salad. It has a strong lemon taste and can replace the use of citrus in your salad bowl. You may gather sorrel plants from outdoors in late autumn, obtaining at least two dozen of the young ones. Avoid any additional transplants, for it tends to weaken the plant.

THYME may be grown from seed or bought as a plant. Obtain the lemon scented. Use the leaves and flowers for seasoning and in salads. Likes plenty of sun and fresh air.

ROSEMARY and sweet marjoram were favorites of castle casements. There are no sweeter plants, except wheatgrass, for the window of an indoor garden. This nearly ever green perennial shrub should be pruned and its pot lowered each spring next to a warmth-giving, sheltering wall or hedge. It must be brought in before the onset of cold September nights. It loves lime. Work finely ground plaster into fresh, rich soil to keep the fresh green tips growing all winter. Use it in salads and dried for seasoning.

LETTUCE: Oakleaf, Salad Bowl, Early Curles Simpson, Grand Rapids, Early Prizehead — grows indoors with little care, faster than other varieties. For continuous supply, sow new seed every two weeks. They will grow as leaves rather than heads, if several plants are placed in one pot or if planted close in a box. A good practice is to start at least sixty plants in a flat baker's tray. Keep in a cool place. Once the seedlings develop some height, transfer some of them into 4 inch pots in a warm location.

SALAD CRESS will grow from seed into lush salad greens in ten to twenty days.

SPRING KALE is a hardy, fast growing (thirty days) salad green. As the outer leaves are picked, new ones continue to grow from the center.

SQUASH — summer yellow, zucchini (also cucumber) can be grown in 5-gallon cans. Very productive. To insure continuous crop, don't let any of the squashes mature on vine and go to seed. Water frequently, add compost and kelp periodically.

COMFREY THE MIRACLE HERB

COMFREY leaves, when young, make a good salad green or blender preparation. The plant is a perennial which prefers rich soil, plenty of moisture, and full sunlight. It multiplies rapidly by root division. It has a deep tap-root and it is hard to eradicate once it has taken a liking to your soil. Well-drained, porous soil will prevent rotting of this fleshy root. Every ten days you can expect an abundant crop of twelve inch leaves with long, liquid-loaded stems. For continuous growth, the plants should be cut once a month to prevent blossom formation, though the flowers are tasty in salads. To start them, obtain the roots from mail order house or nursery. Plant at least ten roots, placing each one in a gallon can.

Dr. Walter J. Bray, at the World Confrey Conference meeting, reported that the amino acid balance in leaf protein is generally superior to that of soybean or beef, with deficiency in comfrey leaf extraction of only methionine, which is probably due to processing. Furthermore, vitamin B12 is found in comfrey. (Let's Live, Aug. 1974, p. 106)

Comfrey has been called the MIRACLE HERB. Because of its astringent and demulcent property, comfrey has been successfully used in all forms of respiratory disorders such as asthma, TB, emphysema, cold and flu. Comfrey tea or juice has resolved intestinal scars and necrosis of tissue and healed duodenal, gastric and kidney ulcers. It has been reported to stop internal bleeding within thirty minutes of ingestion when all other methods had failed. Apply it to all external sores, wounds, or lacerations. It is great for ulcers, insect bites, growths, broken bones, burns, gangrene. The active healing agent is allantoin which is found in the leaves and roots.

When my heel bone was scraped one fall, swelling doubled the size of my heel and ankle. The doctor who examined me predicted I would be limping and in pain for at least six weeks. However, after application for one week of a poultice of crushed comfrey, the swelling and pain disappeared.

Another use of comfrey is for chest ailments. To induce sweating, apply a poultice to the chest at bedtime and drink a tea from the dried leaves, using two ounces of comfrey to one quart water. It is a laxative and can be used cooked, raw, juiced, or in tea.

Comfrey may be juiced in any centrifugal juicer. First, juice a cup of carrots. Blend comfrey leaves with the carrot juice in blender. Pour the mixture, slowly, into the juicer. A delicious comfrey sauce can be made by blending equal portions of comfrey and buckwheat greens (or zucchini) with a little avocado or olive oil. For seasoning add garlic, and/or tomatoes.

LIGHTING. While using such lights, you are in no way duplicating the sun's rays. Use the lights in moderation. For maximum sunlight, you can remove the shades from all windows in the room and open the curtains during the day.

Fluorescent tubes emit the rays at the blue end of the spectrum and the incandescent tungsten filament bulb supplies the needed rays from the red end of the spectrum. Vita-lite approximates sunlight spectra.

All house plants and greens, with the exception of grasses and sprouts, may require extra light during the short winter days. It is good practice to combine an incandescent and a fluorescent light unit to prevent the plants from developing light spectrum deficiency.

Herb gardens can be maintained indefinitely with proper feeding, annual soil changing, re-potting, seasonal shift to the outdoors, renewal of annuals and the necessary pruning. Once your love of indoor gardening has progressed beyond the embryo stage, you can find in most public libraries an extensive range of literature to familiarize yourself with details about herbs, weeds and organic gardening.

For additional information write to Department of Agriculture.

If you have access to a garden, plant a large crop of berries and fruit trees. Until they start producing fruit, the following crops are especially suitable for obtaining delicious cleansing juices: zucchini and yellow squash; cucumbers are tastiest when matured yellow; large and cherry tomatoes; celery, spinach, kale, beets, carrots. Be sure to prepare the soil properly if you want tasty vegetables.

By discovering the type of music the plants love, you can increase the growth rate. If the leaves start turning yellow and look wilted, apply a small amount of organic fertilizer to the soil. You can purchase it at most health stores. Or apply a compost broth made by soaking some compost in water and using the fluid for watering. In emergency, place one ounce of wheatgrass juice or one tablespoon or sea kelp in one quart of water, mix and serve it to the plant.

TOPS FOR WINTER SALAD

During the summer, beet, carrot and parsley greens are passed over for more conventional vegetables, but during the winter when the common greens are scarce, their tops will add sunlight nourishment to your salad.

Dig the roots in November, at least a dozen of each, according to family need and taste preference. If you don't have a garden, purchase the tubers from organic distributors or a local organic farmer.

For the indoor garden, choose undamaged roots with stems of at least one inch. Obtain any large size container: wooden box, bathtub, galvanized ash barrel, bushel basket, window box, or grape box lined with plastic. Tip the container on its side at a 45 degree angle. On the lower side, place six or more inches of sand, then a close-spaced layer of roots. Cover this layer with sand about one inch thick. Repeat this layering until your box is full. The roots should not be in direct contact with one another; some sand should separate them. Cover the tops with a one inch layer of sand. The inclined position of the tubers enables you to use shallow boxes for the planting; they are easier to handle.

Keep the soil moist; the tubers will produce new growth from the nourishment stored in the roots. As they grow, cut the shoots to use in your salads.

Beets, turnips and carrots may also be grown for greens in water. Take a one inch section from the stem end of the tuber, place it in water in a shallow tray. You may sprinkle in kelp as fertilizer. Keep it in a sunny window.

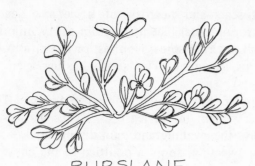

PURSLANE

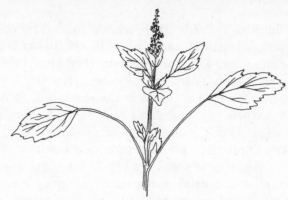

LAMB'S QUARTER

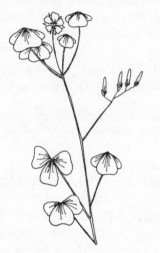

SOURGRASS

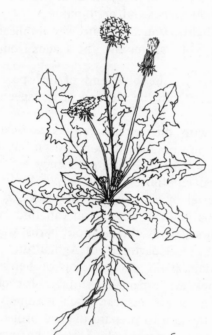

DANDELION

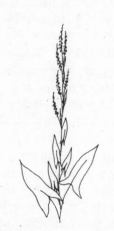

SHEEP SORREL

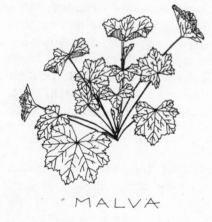

MALVA

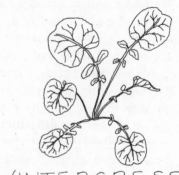

WINTERCRESS

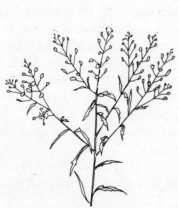

PEPPERGRASS

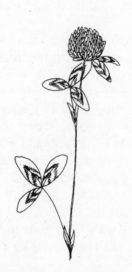

RED CLOVER

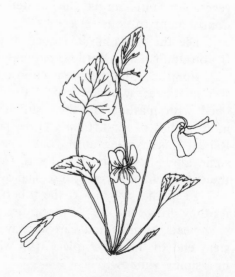

VIOLET

You will be considered a beneficiary of uninformed gardeners or lawn addicts if you pick the dandelions off their conventional lots. Use them freely in all your salads: the bitter taste reduces the need for other seasoning and the high Vitamin A content will insure of eyesight to find them again. When picking, be sure that they have not been sprayed with a weed killer.

During late autumn, before the ground freezes, dig up a bushel of dandelion roots, the bigger the better. Pack them in sand, as you do the tubers. In a few weeks tender dandelion shoots will be ready for your salad.

You can plant chicory roots in exactly the same manner as dandelion.

Celery, onion, chives, swiss chard and cabbage roots may be replanted after the first hard frost into pots or any other containers. Set them in an area of strong light. With proper care they will produce shoots all winter long.

WEEDS FOR HEALTH AND SURVIVAL

There is great evidence that weeds are nursing themselves back into the human diet, much to the benefit of our health. Grandma's remedies are being carefully examined as 'possible temporary cures' by the lab-oriented scientist and commercial producer. Many evening adult-education classes and day colleges have courses on weeds, herbs and mushrooms. Presently, even pharmacies carry books on herbal medicine and the complete works of Edgar Cayce, who writes about herbs, weeds, sprouts and live food in his "Diet and Health."

Pictures of common wild greens may be found in books on edible weeds (see Appendix). No matter where you find them, weeds can be exotic companions in any salad, blended with avocado to make delicious sauces, juiced for health-giving drinks, included in your cooking, or fed to your pets. When dried and ground to fine powder, they make excellent spicing for soups and salads.

If you have an outdoor garden during the summer include at every meal many of the weeds so bountifully available between the cultivated vegetables.

You will readily find in any garden chickweed, ground cherry, lambsquarters, purslane, wild mustard, sorrel and violet. Red clover, peppergrass, sheep sorrel, shepherd's purse can be located in the vicinity of a garden. They generally prefer a soil of poorer quality. Then there are those that do very well in a more moist, damp locale, such as chicory, watercress, peppermint, and "live forever."

Generally, when preparing salads from the "wild", eliminate the heavy stems; use the tender parts and possibly the fruits and flowers. Include no more than three types of greens per salad. Since each weed has a very unique taste and aroma, anything more is bound to lead to disharmony in the sensory orchestration. Use the more tasty, non-poisonous flowers to complement the greens. For a delightful drink, you may juice all the weeds in the manual grass juicer. If they taste too strong, mix them with carrot juice.

Do not delay acquaintance with weeds and grasses; someday there may be nothing else to eat. The once-fertile land is being destroyed at a fast pace by "advanced" forms of agriculture.

Dr. Wernher von Braux states: "If we continue as we are, the starvation and high infant mortality now limited to local pockets of mankind will become widespread." In order to grow, seeds need a good environment. They certainly cannot thrive in soil saturated with insecticides and synthetic fertilizers. The time is near, and unless the agricultural community makes a 180 degree turn back to the natural way, which doesn't seem likely, the mass famines predicted for our generation will become a reality.

If your body is highly toxic, a rapid transition to a simple diet of weeds and grasses might induce uncomfortable cleansing reactions (you will think you are starving). This will be true especially if heavy debris of medication, nicotine, and chemical reside in the fat of the body. Make the switch slowly, while there is still time available. Learn to live simply.

Spend your weekends in the fields and forests gathering wild fruits, nuts and weeds. They are more tasty and diversified than store-bought produce.

Scientists are discovering how nutritious nature's vegetables and weeds are in comparison with commercial vegetables.

Lambsquarters exceeds its overrated close cousin, spinach, in Vitamin A and C, matches it closely in iron and potassium and exceeds all common greens in calcium content. The surprising fact is that it contains 4.5% protein, which is higher than any other green or fruit. Hence, it's excellent material from which to build healthy muscles and bones. The ripened fruit can be dried and ground in your Moulinex coffee grinder. It is one of the most common edible weeds in any garden or neighboring field.

The Vitamin A content of dandelion exceeds all the store-bought greens by at least four times. Purslane tops all the greens, except parsley, in organic iron content. Sorrel nearly matches dandelion in Vitamin A and potassium, and contains three times more Vitamin C than lemon. Grass exceeds even the common weeds in nutritional value.

You can see why nature's supermarket, which is free, can be a better bargain for health, taste and nutrition than the cities' stale, embalmed foods. A weekly trip to field and forest can supply you with all the greens you need for the week. Those which are unsuitable for food are bitter, sometimes contain milky juice, or have many thorns. To the list of edibles, add wild fruits such as strawberries, blueberries, raspberries, blackberries, apples, grapes, cranberries, gooseberries, plus an array of mushrooms and nuts. Eat mushrooms only when identification by an expert proves their safety.

When it gets too cold for food-hunting ventures outdoors, start duplicating the summer season indoors. No project is more useful than growing your own greens and herbs indoors. Using a window box, or kitchen window, you can easily grow a variety of vegetation to use fresh or dried in salads or in cooking.

While weeds are ruling the garden, let some of them go to seed for planting indoors. The use of weed seed came to mind when I was searching for seed to plant indoors to produce tasty greens.

FOOD STORAGE

If you have planted a garden, you will want to save quantities of beautiful tubers, sturdy greens and fruits for the colder, sterile part of the year. You will have many foods to store if you made weeds, garden greens and fruit the main fare of your summer diet. Storing will extend the season and increase the value of the home garden by making much of the produce available all year round. In Boston, we have kept apples, tomatoes, carrots, beets, cabbage, Jerusalem artichokes in good condition, some of them as late as May.

If you are not a gardener, organic vegetable crops should be purchased in the fall when there is a surplus and the prices are low. This is especially true of apples and carrots, which become unavailable as the season progresses. As you travel, purchase them from organic dealers by the carload and store them for winter.

The storage facility may be a closed garage, a cold room in the cellar, a specially built room in the apartment or an outdoor pit. In every case, screening is necessary to prevent entry of vermin and flies. Storage in darkness is most effective. Ventilation reduces the possibility of molds. The nutritional and taste value of stored produce depends upon its quality, its stage of maturity, correct temperature, and appropriate moisture.

A closed garage, especially when insulated, can provide storage space for fruits and vegetables well into spring. Be sure there are none of the noxious odors often associated with tools or engines for food tends to absorb some of this toxic material.

If space is available, one of the best ways to keep fruits and vegetables is to build a special room in the basement. A 6 x 8 foot enclosure provides adequate storage to supply a family of six.

Choose the north, or cold side of the house, away from the furnace. Use a corner of the house for two of the walls. There should be a window in at least one of the walls to provide needed ventilation. Build the frame for the other sides with two by three studs.

For paneling, use the cheapest available lumber or heavy duty plastic. For effective insulation, build double walls. Presently, the market carries many inexpensive, insulating sheets. They may be used for paneling. To find them, look in the yellow pages under plastics and insulators.

Keep the room dark with heavy black curtains over the window. Keep the room clean to prevent growth of bacteria. Be sure not to use any toxic products or sprays in cleaning the room.

When storing, temperature and humidity play a major role in determining the useful life of the produce. Sprinkle the concrete floor with water or keep it covered with a layer of earth; moisten as needed. Dampness can be reduced by ventilation during days when the temperature is just above freezing. Never ventilate on warm days for this will result in moisture deposits on the produce.

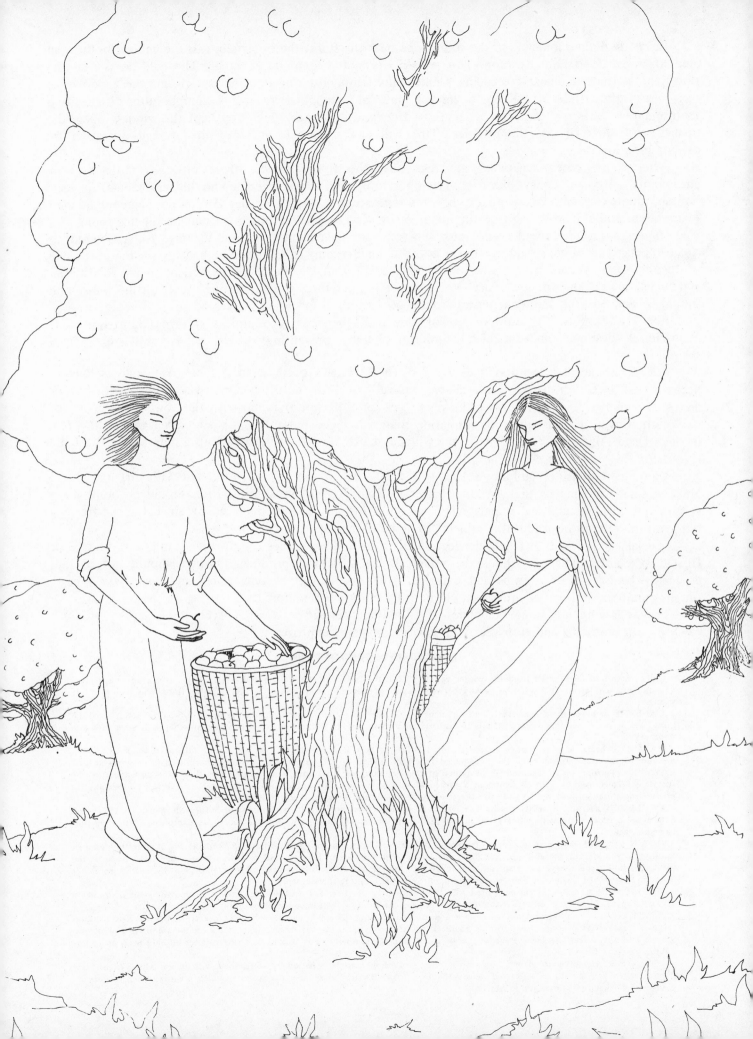

Install two thermometers in the room: one near the floor, the other close to the ceiling, both in an area of major food concentration. This will give you the temperature range. The cold air is near the floor; the warmest air near the ceiling. Control the temperature by opening and closing the windows on days just above freezing. Keep a log of date and time of recording temperature of the two thermometers, outdoor temperature, length of time and degree to which you kept the window open, the quality and shelf life of the produce. This will enable you to improve the storage operation by experimentation.

Arrange the green vegetables in racks near the floor. Enclose them in moist cloth bags or cheesecloth containers; they like a cold temperature, just above freezing, no higher than 40 degrees. Squash, pumpkin, and sweet potato have better keeping quality in dry 55 to 65 degree Farenheit temperature and should be kept on the upper racks. You may keep unripened bananas in this room.

If you are a city dweller and must rely on your apartment for homesteading, you can build, at small expense, an effective storage bin. Choose a small room, large closet or hallway on the north side of the house. It should have a window opening to the outside. Purchase a small, used air conditioner and install it into the window space. For a lower temperature, glue insulating sheets on the walls. You should be able to keep the temperature around 40 degrees. Build some shelves.

For hardy souls, the outdoor pit or trench is the most economical storage compartment. It maintains a desirable uniform high humidity, thereby preventing tubers, celery and apples from shriveling.

Select an elevated location and dig a ditch 12 inches deep, 2 to 3 feet wide, and as long as necessary. If boxes or barrels are available, insert them into the ditch. Otherwise, line it with hay or leaves to a depth of 6 inches. Place the vegetables carefully in a pyramid with tips toward the center of the ditch. Cover it with layers of insulating material. Place burlap on top and cover this with a few inches of sod. Mark the area so that you will be able to find it easily. Draw up a map of the vegetable layout for easy, exact access to the pit.

You might consider building a large pit partly below the ground, insulated with dirt and straw. Make a small opening so that you may enter it. Some sort of cross ventilation should be built. Keep vermin out with screen. Seal it only when all the warm air has been replaced by air just above freezing temperature. Obtain books on this subject from the library and use common sense.

Special care should be taken in selection of fruits and vegetables for storage. Don't store bruised or frosted vegetables. The skin should be intact. Don't store wet produce. Produce should not be old, especially beets, carrots, turnips and parsnips, otherwise it will become tough and tasteless. Cabbage, onion, pumpkin, and winter squash should be fully mature when stored.

The following are some guidelines for the most effective storage of common garden produce. Record your methods, and each year you will find ways to improve.

●●●●●●●●●●●●●●●●●●●

APPLES should be selected from the winter variety. Store the fully colored, undamaged ones. They like a cold temperature and medium dampness. They may be packed between layers of leaves or straw. Place the box near the floor. Will keep into late spring.

CABBAGE can withstand light frost. Pull up plants in the middle of November and sink the roots in boxes of sand. Place the boxes on a shelf near the window. Plants like plenty of circulating air. If there is no early warm-up, they will keep into late February.

CARROTS, beets, winter radishes, rutabagas and turnips are best stored in moist, not wet, sand. Pull the roots, keep an inch or more of the stem and store all the undamaged tubers in labeled boxes. Carrots are sweetest if permitted to grow for at least six months. Turnips and rutabagas may be pulled at the beginning of November, but other tubers should be pulled before the first frost. They may be kept all winter in a garden if heavily mulched. In storage, keep them near the floor; periodically, to provide moisture, sprinkle a little water on the sand. At the Institute, we keep them until late March.

CAULIFLOWER and brussels sprouts can withstand a light frost but should be brought in before the heavy winter freeze. Otherwise, protect them with a heavy mulch and pick them as needed. In storage, sink the roots into damp sand. Will keep four to eight weeks.

GRAIN and seed keep best in a cool, dry room. An air conditioner in your storage bin will keep the temperature low enough during the summer to prevent spoilage. Keep the room well ventilated. They should not be stored the same place as the vegetables unless the area is dry. You can keep them near the ceiling, which is drier than near the floor. Use the storage room for fruits and vegetables during the winter; store grain and seed there during the summer.

ONIONS must be gathered before a hard freeze; be sure they are firm and will not dent easily around the stem. They like a dry, cold space. Place them on higher shelves in boxes near the window. Will keep well into spring.

PUMPKIN, squash, and sweet potato require a warm temperature. They should be picked before frost. Dry the sweet potato for two weeks after picking. Don't sort or handle them after storage. Leave at least 2 inch stems on the pumpkin and squash. Store all of them near the furnace where the air is dry and the temperature is around 55 to 65 degrees. Should keep up to late February.

POTATOES keep best stored in a cool, moist place in covered barrels or wooden boxes lined with heavy paper. Light turns them green. They should be harvested before the first frost. Be sure to remove the sprouts, which are toxic, before you use potatoes. Will keep all winter and longer.

TOMATOES should be kept on the vine as long as possible. Cover them at night to protect from frost. Pick the well developed, green ones and lay them in boxes, carefully, no more than three layers thick. It is the middle of January, and I'm still eating tomatoes from our garden. I took no special precautions except to keep them in unheated room. To ripen the stored tomatoes, place them in a 60 to 70 degree temperature, preferably in a window space. Once you have tried it, you will do it every year. There is no comparison in taste between the tomatoes you have grown in organic soil and tomatoes of questionable quality shipped from far away places.

Indoor gardening and proper storage will assure you of a fresh vegetable diet the year round.

SEED STORAGE

DRY ICE METHOD: Will keep seed from molding and will kill larvae that may already be in the seed. Will preserve seed indefinitely: friends have reported the method has worked well for seeds stored five years. HOW: From Deli, Pizza parlor or Specialty Food store, obtain free 1 gallon plastic or glass jars which they use for spices or pickles. Scrub jar and lid. To prevent rusting, varnish the lid. Cover a lump of dry ice (about ¼ the size of your fist) with enough thickness of cotton cloth to prevent freezing the seeds. Place the package of ice in bottom of jar and fill it to the top with seeds. Replace lid but don't screw on, just lay it down on top. When the ice melts, seal the lid real tight. You will have the seeds surrounded with an inert gas (nitrogen) thus preventing mold, decay or bugs.

DEHYDRATION SALT METHOD: The best temperature for seed storage is 45-50 deg. F. If dry conditions are maintained at this temperature, the seeds or grains can be kept in a viable state for many years. The following method has worked well for many friends.

Obtain cans from Sears & Roebuck Co. (permarex trash cans) or from some other source with tight fitting lids. Large heavy duty plastic bags may be purchased at most coin laundries or hardware stores.

There are two salts — calcium chloride (CaCl) and silica gel — which have the property of absorbing moisture from the air. Look in Yellow Pages under chemicals. Don't purchase from wholesalers, retailers or scientific supply companies. Instead buy directly from plant or industrial supplier. Difference in price is tremendous. For example: CaCl from Fisher Scientific Chemicals was $26 for 5 lbs. whereas from Maxi Chemical Plant it was $6.80 for 100 lbs. CaCl is much easier to obtain and works as well as silica gel. Purchase large quantity then share it with friends.

Choose a dry day. Place seeds into plastic bags. Close them loosely. Place the bags into can. Obtain a shallow round pan, fill to ¼ in. depth with CaCl and place it on top of the bags. Be sure it is secure. Tightly seal can lid. Keep the can in the coolest place available.

Calcium Chloride becomes wet and shiny after some time due to its reaction with the moisture present in the air and should be replaced when the solid powder or lumps have been transformed into the liquid stage. Depending on the moisture content of the area the powder will be changed every 1 to 6 months.

Silica Gel is blue in the dry state and turns pink after it has absorbed water. It does not change to another form as does calcium chloride and can be renewed over a low flame or stove until the blue color returns.

For every day sprouting keep a small jar of seed with large enough quantity to take care of your needs for at least a month. Thus, the can will be opened only a few times which will minimize the likelihood of spoilage of seeds by molds, bugs or flies.

Plastic buckets are fine for short term storage, but eventually the contents will begin to smell like the plastic. Also water will condense on the inside, making it damp and the seeds will mold. Animals can also eat through plastic. Gallon jars, as well as gallon jugs, are great for smaller amounts as long as they are kept out of the sun or else water will condense inside.

THE SPROUTARIAN

"When the leaves and blossoms wither, the fruit remains."   Sri Rama Krishna

"The Fruitarian who perserveres will attune himself to wondrous health, beauty and life secrets."
— FRUIT THE FOOD and MEDICINE OF MAN, M. Krok

GREENS ARE YOUR MEDICINE

Until civilized human beings recognize that greens are for healing and fruit is for meat (Ezekiel), they will not have achieved their natural diet. Trees once provided coverage for the land and supplied the most natural food of human beings. Civilized humans had to destroy segments of the tree population before they could plant grains and vegetables.

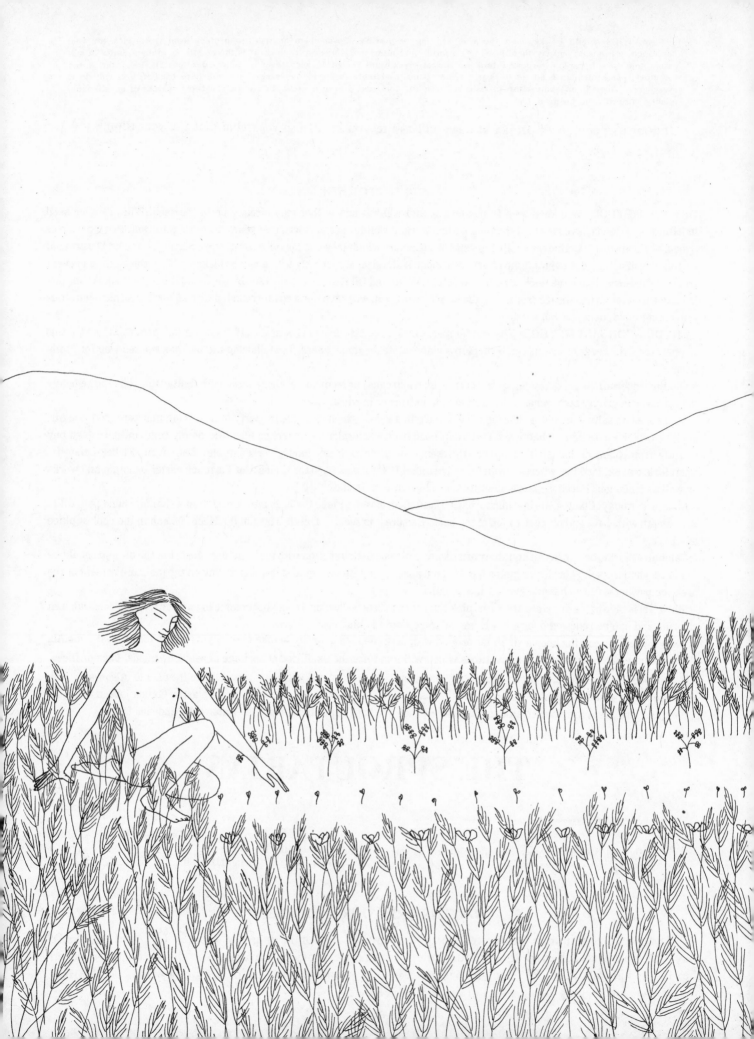

Why should one eat a fruit diet, is it not enough to eat raw foods? No. Greens are therapeutic and as a result medicative. Most medicine has its origin in seed or greens. If you live in the unhealthful environment of polluted cities, you will continue to need greens. However, once you move to the higher altitudes of subtropical mountains, or, at least, take residence in a warmer climate away from polluted areas, you no longer need greens.

Scientists have observed some toxic side effects from a vegetable diet. Most of the vegetables that people eat are not grown in their original state. They are difficult to produce and contain many natural poisons (See Appendix Natural Toxins in Food and Man's Higher Consciousness). People were never intended to eat vegetables as food. They adopted this habit because they migrated from their natural home in tropical and subtropical regions. The human being discovered the therapeutic value of vegetables after becoming sick from unnatural foods in an unnatural environment (166, 245).

A raw vegetable diet is high in rough fibre which may act as an irritant to the delicate stomach lining. Dr. A. Thomas states: "The fibre of vegetables provides no nourishment and must be eliminated at great expense of energy."

Although fruit is the food best adapted to human digestion, a diet limited to fruit would make the city dweller's organism too sensitive to the damaging effects of air pollution. By including protective foods, such as sprouts, weeds and grasses, we minimize the destructive effect of pollution and ingest the most concentrated sources of life nutrients.

Grass juice heals and dissolves the scars that are formed in the lungs from breathing acid gases. The effect of carbon monoxide is minimized since chlorophyl increases hemoglobin production. The sproutarian needs very little food; hence, the bloodstream will not be congested with incompletely metabolised food, toxins or the waste products of metabolism. As a result the eliminative organs can more efficiently deal with inhaled air pollutants.

Some sprouts are much like fruit in composition and are preferable to grains and seeds. The earthy mineral matter has been reduced to about one fifth of its previous value. They are low in protein, low in fiber and high in vitamins and enzymes.

Grass, like all plants or sprouts, reaches its highest nutrient content at the earliest, most rapid stage of growth. It is especially rich in enzymes and chlorophyl, the sun factor which regenerates the bloodstream. It is low in protein and high in natural sugars.

Dietary Regime

BREAKFAST - Best to skip it altogether. Thus you will be fasting at least 16 hours a day. If you must eat, have a juicy, sweet fruit, seed milk or fresh juices. Don't do it out of habit, only if you feel very hungry.

LUNCH - Sprouts, with or without dressing (such as perfect dressing page 258). Use more or less a quarter of a pound of mixed alfalfa sprouts, sunflower and buckwheat greens, sea vegetables (washed dulce is best, soft, not fibrous), zucchini, beets and other favorite in season vegetables and non-starchy sprouts.

SUPPER - Sweet or sub acid fruit salad or one fruit only or indoor greens or vegetable juice.

To be a gluttonous raw foodist is probably worse than to be a frugal meat-eater. To cut sleeping time, go to bed slightly hungry.

You may reverse lunch and supper. For ease of digestion, it is better to have one day of sprouts and vegetable juices and the following day only fruit. Eat moderately.

Fast on water or juice at least once a week. Practice deep breathing, yoga asanas and meditation.

Do not overstrain yourself. Whatever you do, get into it gradually because your body has a difficult time adjusting to rapid changes, whether for good or bad.

Whenever possible, take drives outside the city limits. Spend your weekends, vacations and holidays in the isolated countryside, and, if possible, in nudist camps. Expose your body to the healing sunshine, in moderation, and, if possible, in nudist camps. Expose your body to the healing sunshine, in moderation, between the hours of 10 and 3 p.m. Purchase a home outside the city; become a commuter. Best, move away from the city altogether.

There are many ways and means to maintain yourself in a rural area. You will discover that clothing, rent and food costs will be much lower. If you have skills — carpenter, plumber, mechanic, handyman, gardener, masseur, healer, teacher — you will have no difficulty. Otherwise, you can go to the city to work for a couple of weeks. This will usually provide enough revenue to support yourself for at least four months. Organize communes which are self-supporting through crafts or growing organic foods to be sold or exchanged with communes or city dwellers. Age is no hindrance to change in life-style.

FRUIT IN THE SYNTHETIC JUNGLE

"My fruit is better than gold, yea, than fine gold." Pro. 8:19

"And the land shall yield her fruit, and ye shall eat your fill." —Leviticus 25:19

For the fruitarian, tropical fruits are preferred to northern ones. The idea that people should eat only food grown in their own locale originates in a basic, well-founded mistrust of other people and the high cost of transportation. If you do not grow the food yourself, you do not know if the food was grown organically and with love. Shipment introduces unknown dangers of contamination. However, locally grown fruit may be as contaminated as that grown far away. Try to know your food producer to determine the quality of the food you eat.

Tropical fruit will always have enjoyed longer and more concentrated sun exposure than northern fruit. As a result, it will supply you with more trapped sun radiation when you eat it.

The cellulose in some fruit may be an irritant to delicate stomachs. If so, chew the fruit, swallow the juice and spit out the pulp. This way you can stay on a liquid fruit diet without any juice extractor and still enjoy the act of chewing. For minimal internal fermentation and optimal assimilation, grapes and apples are best juiced.

BANANA should be bought green and ripened at home. If green bananas turn evenly yellow in less than 24 hours, the ripening of the banana has been forced with the use of ethylene gas. Request ungassed bananas from your dealer. If he or she is not willing to provide them, get them from a wholesale fruit dealer (look in the Yellow Pages). Almost every city has such an outlet. You will probably have to purchase a 40 pound box. This can be divided among other health seakers. Generally, during the summer months many grocers carry naturally ripened bananas because gassed bananas spoil quickly in hot weather.

Bananas take 4 to 12 days to ripen. A temperature between 65 and 70 degrees is adequate but do not let the temperature drop below 60. Variation in temperature will prevent the bananas from reaching their full sweetness and bright yellow color. Don't buy unripened bananas, unless they are green in color, from an air-conditioned market, for they will never ripen properly.

When properly ripened, the banana is at its prime taste when its color has turned deep golden yellow speckled with brown.

If the ripening temperature is too high, the banana might ripen to softness and excellent taste but continue to be green with dark spots on the ends. There is no comparison in flavor or fragrance between naturally and forced-ripened bananas.

After the banana has ripened to the stage you like, refrigerate. Once the ripening process has been stopped by cold, it never starts again. If the skin turns brown under refrigeration, don't be alarmed as the inside will remain tasty. Before serving, remove the skin. Such bananas do well in blender preparations.

COCONUT may be purchased either in the fibrous green husk or as a brown nut with three exposed eyes. It should feel heavy with liquid — shake all coconuts, pick the heaviest one. Be sure the coconut is not losing water or shows mildew or rot in the area of the "eyes" as these signs indicate that it is old and probably rancid. Under semi-tropical conditions, one can obtain coconuts free. Unripened ones (water coconuts) are best. With a screwdriver, remove the stem. Force a hole. Drink up with a straw. Don't spill the water on your clothing — it will leave a permanent stain. Split the green husk coconut open with an axe or machete. The brown nut can be cracked with a hammer. Scoop out the delicious jelly with a spoon. Jelly coconut is quite low in fat; it is sweet and easily digested. Mature coconuts are high in fat and fibre content and are difficult to digest. This saturated fat can be cholesterol-forming.

AVOCADO — On the weekend or on Monday, fully ripened avocado, mango and papaya can generally be purchased at reduced cost from large markets because of fear of spoilage. The avocado should give when pressed with the thumb, otherwise it is not ripe. If it is very dark and soft you can be sure that the avocado is spoiled.

The alligator skinned avocadoes from California are tastiest. Even when overripe, with flesh color turning from green to slightly brown, can be eaten. Avocado should never be eaten directly from refrigerator. Let is warm up to room temperature so that the body has an easy time digesting the fats. Avocado should be soft, fully ripe, when eaten. Some skins turn black or brown when fully ripe, others only soft. Never over eat on avocadoes. It can give bad indigestion. Limit yourself to one per day.

The individuals, which have liver or gall bladder disorders, or suffering from cancer and other serious ailments, should exclude avocado, as well as coconut, sprouted grain, nuts and other heavy food from their diet.

MANGO has been called the "apple of the tropics," when it is fully ripened, it tastes like a juicy peach with a light tart tang. No other fruit compares in taste with the possible exception of the cherimoya. When eaten the fruit should be yellow in color. When fully ripened, the skin can be peeled off with the fingers.

PAPAYA takes on a bright yellow color when ripe. Do not eat it green, for you will be disappointed in the taste, although underripe papaya are a valuable digestive aid. It can be allowed to ripen from green to its juicy state in a period of a week. Cut the fruit in half, scoop out the seed, and eat the meat from the shell with a spoon.

CITRUS at its sweetest and juiciest comes from the Rio Grande Valley in Texas and the Indian River Valley in Eastern Florida. When purchasing oranges, examine the stem. If it is orange in color, you may be sure the fruit has been colored. Since citrus stops ripening after it has been picked, be sure you are obtaining fully ripened fruit. Unripe green-speckled fruit tends to be acid and may withdraw alkaline minerals, in particular calcium, from your teeth causing them to crumble prematurely. Use such fruit in moderation unless obtainable in a fully ripened state. The acid PH of such fruit makes it excellent for dissolving hardening deposits in tissues, arteries and joints.

Under ripe or over ripe oranges can create overacid condition in stomach which can give sour taste in mouth and headache. This is true of all citrus fruits plus tomatoes and pineapples.

Buy citrus in crates. They are less likely to have strong preservative content. Buy the citrus in season. Tangelo, tangerine and ugli are generally less sprayed. Before eating the fruit, aerate them in sunshine or wash them in water which has some wheatgrass juice added.

When purchasing inorganic citrus, lime is preferable to lemon because it is less acid, has a delightful tang and is not as heavily enbalmed with chemicals. If you should be going to the wholesaler, purchase citrus with the other produce. It will keep a long time, even without refrigeration. Lime is cheapest during the summer months.

PINEAPPLE should not be purchased unless they are ground-ripened and heavy with juice. When unripe, they tend to be very acid and can damage your teeth and create sores in your mouth. Picked green, they will never ripen fully. When ready to eat, the pineapple is yellow, very sweet in taste, highly juicy and non-acid. In the ripened state, the leaves can be pulled out without resistance. The section close to the stem should be discarded or blended as a seasoning for salad. Dried or fresh pineapple blends delightfully with avocado.

MELON are available in a wide variety. Each one has a season and some overlap. They contain the most perfect, inexpensive, sweet, alkaline, nature-distilled water, far superior to polluted, chemical-filtered tap water. Melon your fruit vocabulary by familiarizing your taste buds with Persian melon, honeydew, cantaloupe, Spanish crenshaw or watermelon. At the Institute, we use them all year round. If you cannot purchase them from a food store, contact a fruit wholesaler.

Always purchase whole melon, for, when cut open, they tend to absorb toxic material. Most stores are filled with poisons.

WATERMELON comes with or without stripes, green is the common color, weighing from 5 to 60 pounds. The juice has a flushing action on the kidneys, gall bladder and bladder. The seed can be blended to make delicious drinks (strain out the pulp) or when dried can make a fine tea. The seed contains cucubocitrin which is used to dilate the capillaries, and reduce high blood pressure.

CANTALOUPE is the melon first in season. Vine-ripened ones are best. You can recognize them by a shallow depression at the end of the melon, formed when the canteloupe separates from the vine. Less mature melon retains a portion of the stem. The surface nettings of a ripe melon are well raised, coarse, and stand out in distinct relief over the entire surface. It is yellow all the way to the thin skin. Melon in general should be heavy with juice. Press with your thumb, it should give slightly. When blended, it makes a most delicious drink.

Do your melon shopping intelligently by increasing observation of what constitutes a tasty fruit. Eat them alone, never with other foods.

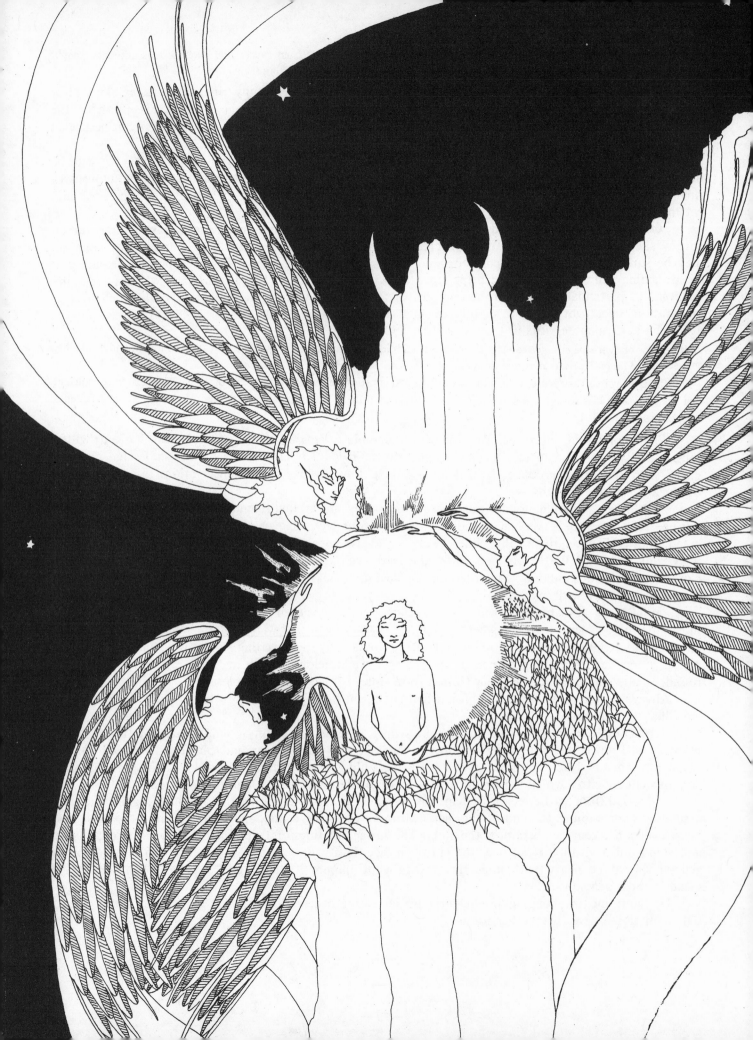

FASTING NOT STARVING

"And he said unto them, this kind can come forth by nothing, but by prayer and fasting."   MARK 9:29

". . . If we fast two days a week, then eat only fruit and obey the other laws of life, we can approximate the longevity of the Biblical patriarchs."
                                                    PROFESSOR EDMOND SZEKELY, COSMOTHERAPY

Fasting is the most powerful of all tools for cleansing the body. Most people ingest, as part of their diet, preservatives, insecticides, lead, arsenic, medication, and nicotine. Their bodies accumulate toxic waste products from wrong and/or badly combined food and from excessive eating.

The body has a limited capacity to eliminate this toxic load. When the accumulation starts to interfere with proper function, the body sends out warnings: aches, pains, visible signs of disorder. It is time for housecleaning.

Here are some of the most obvious signs of toxicity:

1. Unclear head, frequent upset stomach, aches and pains, and menstrual cramps.

2. Chronic constipation and associated tightness in the region of the shoulder blades; dizziness, inability to concentrate, uncontrolled temper; black, offensive-smelling fecal matter: healthy color is light brown or color of food eaten ; offensive body odors.

3. Continuous tiredness. The requirement of many hours of sleep. The more toxic one is the more sleep one needs. The more one eats, the more sleep one needs. In a natural environment a healthy person needs one to three hours; in a city environment, two to six hours. It is best to sleep when you feel like it. There are times when you can substitute meditation or relaxation for sleep. Meditation produces relaxation which gives you good digestion with resulting low toxemia.

4. Sallow, aging skin; dull or bloodshot eyes, insomnia and that "I'm getting old" feeling. Lines on the face.

5. Addiction to sweets, coffee, cigarettes and starches. Overeating. No appetite. Eating from habit or "to keep up strength." Headache upon waking, or after missing a meal which is relieved by eating.

6. Waking in the morning with a stuffy nose; mucus in the throat; acid, bitter or salty taste in the mouth; encrustation on the eyes; wax in the ears.

7. Coated tongue from years of mucus-forming foods. Natural mucus is a clear, slimy fluid which is secreted in the respiratory system, the genito-urinary and the intestinal tracts. It moistens the organs and protects them from irritating chemicals. A diet that includes albuminous foods — dairy products, grains, nuts, meats, fish, eggs — impart to the various mucus secretions their colored, sticky, viscous consistency. The blood, lymph and cells become saturated with the abnormal mucus. The body tries to discharge it through the organs of elimination. Doctors call this cleansing process an acute disease. Colds are not the result of virus or germs. A cold acts as a safety valve for relieving the bloodstream and the lymphatic system of congestion which can otherwise lead to catarrhal infections, tuberculosis and tumors. Fighting colds with Vitamin C results in acidification of mucus, which prevents its elimination via the respiratory system. It must instead be expelled by the kidney. The overall effect is strain on the kidney.

Many individuals are congested with as much as fifteen pounds of extraneous mucus. As the mucus is eliminated, there is an increase of the permeability of digestive and respiratory tracts and the cell walls. Thus, more nutrients will reach the inner cells and waste elimination will improve. You will naturally eat less, because more of the nutrients are made available.

The aim of fasting is to rest the body so that the vital force which normally would be used for physical activity and for digestion and assimilation of food is freed for cleansing and healing. Drugs only hinder.

Fasting is one of the most effective natural methods of rebuilding the body's own dynamic healing powers and overcoming many major ailments. Doctors recommend it for patients afflicted with colds, sinusitis, tonsillitis, laryngitis, pharyngitis, bronchitis, pneumonia, bursitis, neuritis, colitis, dysentery, carditis, arteriosclerosis, hepatitis, nephritis, arthritis. The disease is named according to the area of congestion or inflammation in the body.

It is best to start fasting before any such disorders develop. A fast of one or two days a week should be part of the health regime. What you miss in the pleasures of eating, you will make up manyfold in the joy of living. It will improve your health, increase the activity of the spiritual life, sharpen your wits, increase youthfulness and beauty.

Anyone planning a water fast should first improve his or her diet by eating organically grown vegetables, fruit, seed, sprouts and grasses for several months. There is a good reason for this. The body stores various natural and civilization made toxins because it has a limited capacity for excretion and neutralization of poisons. This task is made especially difficult because the body has also to eliminate the waste products of daily metabolism. During fasting, much of the body fat is rapidly used up, suddenly liberating stored poisons. If inorganic foods have predominated in one's diet, during fasting a urine analysis will reveal a high level of DDT and other pesticides. A gradual cleansing releases the poisons slowly, never overtaxing the capacity of the eliminative organs.

"And many unclean and sick followed Jesus' words and sought the banks of the murmuring streams. They put off their shoes and their clothing , they fasted , and they gave up their bodies to the angels of air, of water , and of sunshine. And the Earthly Mother's angels embraced them, possessing their bodies both inwards and outwards. And all of them saw all evils, sins and uncleansinesses depart in haste from them.

And the breath of some became as stinking as that which is loosed from the bowels, and some had an as issue of spittle , and evil smelling and unclean vomit rose from their inward parts . All these uncleannesses flowed by their mouths. In some , by the nose, in others by the eyes and ears. And many did have a noisome and abonimable sweat come from all their body, over all their skin. And on many limbs great hot boils broke forth, from which came out uncleannesses with an evil smell, and urine flowed abundantly from their body; and in many their urine was all but dried up and became thick as the honey of bees; that of others was almost red or black, and as hard almost as the sand of rivers. And many belched stinking gases from their bowels, like the breath of devils. And their stench became so great that none could bear it. "
THE ESSENE GOSPEL OF PEACE

Reactions during the fast or cleansing diet will vary with the individual, depending on how badly the body has been abused. Possible symptoms: nausea, irritability, headache, fatigue, aching muscles, sleeplessness, and in rare instances, rash, vomiting and open' sores.

Some reactions common to all are heavily coated tongue, foul breath, loss of weight, periodic irritability and a sense of weakness. These are all signs that nature is performing surgery.

Gas dissolved from cells and excreted into the digestive tract can cause symptoms of toxicity and can be a source of pain and discomfort due to pressure. An enema or zone therapy on areas related to the digestive tract, pituitary gland and neck can help to trigger the expulsion of the gas. Aniseed, caraway seed, cloves, sweet fennel, ginger, peppermint or parsley will help to expel gas. Mix ½ teaspoon of the ground herb in one cup of hot water. Steep for five minutes. Drink it hot.

The area of congestion in your body will determine the type of eliminative crises you will experience. For example, a congested lymphatic system may be cleansed via boils and open sores. If the reactions become too severe, after the crisis is past, break the fast and repeat it several weeks later.

The first two to five days are usually the most difficult. It takes perserverance, will power and self control to overcome habitual eating. Many signs of discomfort will appear on the first day when the body starts its cleansing. Headaches and muscular pains are the result of released toxins which irritate muscles, nerves and tissues.

Generally, painful reactions are of short duration, no more than a few hours. Lie down and wait for them to pass. Zone therapy often helps.

Periods of great discomfort could be a sign that the concentration of toxins in the colon is higher than in the bloodstream and the poisons are being reabsorbed. During the first three days of the fast, an enema should be used every evening to cleanse filth from the colon; afterward as frequently as needed. As the body becomes more and more purified through improved diet and fasting, the use of enemas while fasting will become unnecessary. Baths should be of short duration, in lukewarm water.

Every day, about 10 in the morning, or in the afternoon, take a short sunbath. If you are in a natural setting, discard all clothing to improve elimination and absorption of oxygen and solar radiation through the skin. Daily exercise of short duration, will prevent flabby tissues.

Generally the cleansing symptoms during fasting are mild. You are more likely to experience the joys of fasting: a sense of lightness, clearheadness, wit, spiritual joy, love and the absence of digestive strain. No matter how well you feel you should spend most of the time resting.

WHEATGRASS FAST

The very aged, those who are just starting a cleansing rejuvenation regime, those with a seriously weakened constitution, the underweight, those suffering from chronic disorders such as cancer, diabetes, advanced osteoarthritis, and diseased liver should not consider an extended water fast. They respond best to plenty of rest, a cleansing diet, a vegetable juice fast, a very short water fast or a partial fast. For them, the wheatgrass fast is ideal.

Advantages of a wheatgrass juice fast over the water fast are many. Generally the energy level remains high, permitting activity. Released acetone, uric and other acids are neutralized by the alkaline organic salts of wheatgrass juice, preventing acidosis, producing calm and permitting sleep.

Abnormally high blood pressure drops rapidly toward normal soon after beginning a fast. It remains at a safe level, enabling very sick people to fast without danger of exhaustion. The chlorophyl-rich juice acts as a natural builder of hemoglobin and the red blood cell count. One is able to begin to digest food without difficulty should it become necessary to break the fast before the time planned.

A wheatgrass juice fast with watermelon, taken at a separate meal, is helpful in overcoming rheumatism, cancer, leukemia (diseases which result from eating animal protein) as well as diabetes, alcoholism and obesity (diseases which result from starches and processed carbohydrates). The high enzyme content of wheatgrass juice helps to dissolve tumors. The high alkaline fluid content of watermelon neutralizes acids and flushes the toxins out of the body.

Ann Wigmore and I have guided many "incurables" through the wheatgrass juice fast. It is very cleansing; at the same time it provides one of the most effective nourishments for the body. We have seen good results in all chronic disorders, "provided the essential organs have not been irreversibly damaged by the disease or by medical treatment."

For those who have taken a lot of drugs — LSD, marijuana, hashish, heroin, or conventional medicine — grass juice is to be preferred over all other fasts. Improving the diet and following it with a grass juice fast gradually rids the body of stored drugs. Those who have used a lot of hallucinogenic drugs can anticipate a duplication of their effects as the stored drugs re-enter the bloodstream.

PREPARATION FOR THE WHEATGRASS FAST

It takes about seven days for wheatgrass to grow to optimum nutritional value. If you plant a tray daily, the first tray will be ready in a week. If you have been eating a regular diet, start eating raw and cooked vegetables for four days, followed by three days of sprouts and organic juices & fruit.

The night before starting the fast, skip the evening meal. In morning, if you are able, do a stomach wash (unless you have known lesions or pain in the stomach). Fill one quart of warm water and drink as much of it as you can. Inhale. Pump your abdomen in and out about seven times. Exhale. Tickle your throat with two to four fingers. Repeat this process until able to regurgitate. A stomach wash is not a requirement for the fast.

Before going to sleep, take a thorough enema. To insure restful sleep, do zone therapy. Keep a glass of water at your bedside. If you waken in the night with cleansing reactions, such as headache, take a few sips. You will fall asleep.

First Day Fast - A colonic irrigation (look under Physiotherapist or Wholistic Clinic or Naturopath in the Yellow Pages, or check with Health Food Store) to cleanse the colon is a good preparation for the first wheatgrass fast. From many years of wrong diet, most people's colons are contorted and convoluted with accumulated wastes, sometimes up to thirty pounds of fecal matter. If you can't have a colonic, take at least three enemas.

Length of Fast - At least seven days are recommended, but duration varies with the capacity of the individual, usually three to forty days.

Amount of Wheatgrass Juice - We recommend drinking wheatgrass juice three or four times each day(see:Food Testin for Allergic Response to determine the exact amount that is right for you) and taking two wheatgrass implants. If it is very uncomfortable to drink it, you may instead take three rectal implants. If you like, you may take only indoor green and sprout juice, instead of grass juice and implants.

Fluids: It is best to choose one type of drink for the day during the wheatgrass juice fast in addition to the wheatgrass juice itself. Herb teas, distilled water, the juice of watermelon (chewing the fruit, spitting out the pulp), a mineral drink (add to one quart of distilled water, two cups of a mixture of chopped buckwheat greens, wheatgrass, grated carrots, crushed weeds, chopped alfalfa sprouts, let it set for 24 hours, strain and drink), fresh apple, grape, carrot, celery, rejuvilac (see pg. 257), or watermelon rind juice are good.

Daily Regime: Sleep as long as you wish. On waking, massage the face, neck, hands and feet. With an open window, practice deep breathing (avoid drafts). Drink warm liquid such as deluted rejuvilac, lemonade or herbal tea. Soak your feet in hot water (may add 1 cup of salt) and scrub the soles with a stiff brush to aid elimination. The feet have a high concentration of sweat glands. Keep a box of small pebbles to walk on or apply firm pressure to the soles of the feet. Do at least five minutes of zone therapy on the feet.

Thirty minutes later drink the grass juice. Most of it will be absorbed in twenty minutes. If you feel uncomfortable, follow it with half a glass of rejuvelac. If you feel nauseated, you may do a stomach wash to remove poisons pulled into stomach by the grass juice.

Take a warm water enema; expel all water and follow with an implant of wheatgrass juice.

About two hours after the grass juice, take a glass of juice, tea, water or a mineral drink. Two hours later, take 4 - 12 oz. fluids (see pg. 95 for choice) followed in thirty mnutes by grass juice. Follow this pattern until you have taken three or four drinks of the grass juice. You may omit one or more glasses of fluid if you feel it is too great a strain on the kidneys or if it interferes with sleep.

Thirty minutes later drink the grass juice. Most of it will be absorbed in twenty minutes. If you feel uncomfortable, follow it with half a glass of rejuvelac. If you feel nauseated, you may regurgitate after twenty minutes.

Take a warm water enema; expel all water and follow with an implant of wheatgrass juice.

About two hours after the grass juice, take a glass of juice, rejuvelac or a mineral drink. Two hours later, take some juice, rejuvelac or a mineral drink followed in thirty minutes by grass juice. Follow this pattern until you have taken three or four drinks of the grass juice. You may omit one or more glasses of fluid if you feel it is too great a strain on the kidneys or if it interferes with sleep.

WATER FAST

The water fast is best for healthy people who have lived naturally and want to improve their spiritual and physical wellbeing. However, anyone, even exceptionally sick people, after months of improved diet and juices, can consider a water fast of short duration — one to three days.

There are no age limits for a fast. A child should never be encouraged to eat if he or she feels no hunger, even for days. Children know more about their body needs than the adult. One should go on a fast voluntarily and with desire. Otherwise there will be less benefit. Fast with joy.

For best results, three days prior to the fast begin a diet of higher vibrations than the one you are now eating. If you eat   cooked food, switch to all raw food; if you are using raw food, eat only fruit; if you are using fruit, take only liquid fruit, such as citrus or melon. All could benefit from a three day fast on wheatgrass juice prior to the water fast.

Whenever feasible, fast in a natural environment. Seashore, forest, or countryside are ideal places. During the first fast, it is helpful to have a companion for the joy of sharing.

Since you are likely to chill easily, it's preferable to pick a warm season, but don't let that prevent you from fasting in winter. You can hibernate and keep warm as the animals do.

You may start with a fast of a day or two, about two weeks apart, after which longer fasts may be undertaken. Choose a weekend. For a three day fast, you may start on Thursday by skipping supper. The first day, Friday, will be tolerable and you should have no difficulty in going to work. Do not drive, your reaction time is slowed, making you accident-prone.

A fast of three to fifteen days may be taken with safety by those who enjoy moderate health.

Fasting in serious illness for extended periods of time should not be undertaken except under the direction of a doctor versed in fasting and food therapy. Once you become familiar with fasting through many short fasts you can progressively increase the duration. A fast of thirty or more days should not be undertaken unless you can live comfortably on a diet of fruit for at least three months. Do not try long fasts in a polluted environment. Read books on fasting. Consult others.

For those who fast in a non-polluted environment, especially in mountain regions, there is a cleansing bonus. Many report experiencing one to four days of diarrhea and regurgitation of black soot. People in the city accumulate, during the first year of residence, up to one pound of soot in the lungs. During a clean air fast the pollutants from lungs and cells are osmotically moved into the digestive tract by the action of the clean air.

Usually each individual can determine the duration of the fast on the basis of age, physical condition and strength, nature of any ailment, level of toxicity, previous diet, mental attitude, weather conditions, level of air pollution, the demands of the daily work and activities.

Rest is extremely important to avoid overtaxing the body while it is engaged in the eliminative process. Sleeplessness and nervousness are signs of severe toxicity. For temporary relief, take an enema and do zone therapy. You will generally achieve sound sleep within five minutes. However, as the fast progresses, you will experience vitality with only a few hours of sleep.

Avoid television and radio. If you must read, read on fasting, meditation or sacred writings. Practice breathing exercises and meditate on the teachings of the ancient wise ones. Reading should not be of such an intense nature that it leads to overexcitement and exhaustion. Keep your emotions on a calm plane.

Conversation should be kept to a minimum. Commune with the angels of life so that they will rebuild you. Be happy. Nature is so forgiving. You will soon have a healthy body.

Use distilled water during the fast. It is a better solvent for toxic material than regular water. Drink enough water to satisfy thirst. There is no benefit gained by excessive water intake. It puts a strain on the kidneys. If there is a burning upon urination, or if the urine contains sediment, increase the intake of water. Dilute it with 1 part grass (or fruit juice) to 5 parts of water to neutralize poisons.

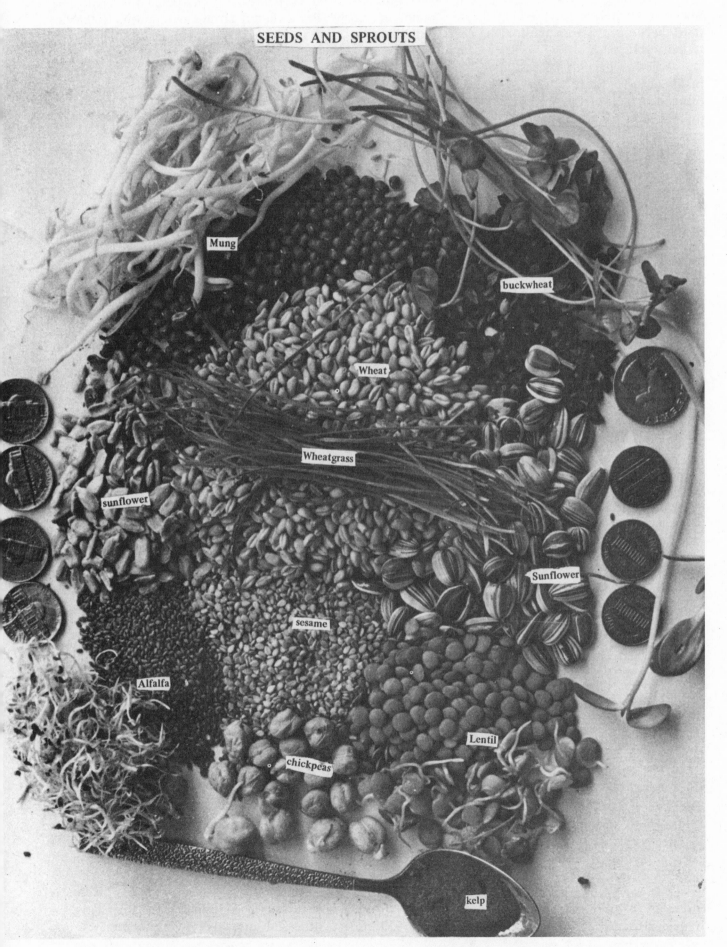

Mung

buckwheat

Wheat

Wheatgrass

sunflower

Sunflower

sesame

Alfalfa

Lentil

chickpeas

kelp

BREAKING THE WATER FAST

Depending on the severity of the toxic condition, the tongue may remain coated for some time; hence the criterion for breaking the fast when the tongue clears cannot always be applied. If the fast must be broken before the tongue clears and hunger returns, repeat it at a later date until all signs of toxicity disappear.

Whether the fast be only a few days or up to fifteen days, it should be broken gradually. Take as many days to break a fast as the number of days fasted. Never end a fast during a period of acute discomfort (crisis). Wait until you feel better. End the fast at midday with four ounces of citrus juice diluted with water and drink it every two hours. Sip it slowly, take at least half an hour to drink the cup.

This will start the flow of digestive juices. Continue taking citrus juice until you feel ready to take more concentrated juices. When ready, drink wheatgrass or vegetable juice, or start eating juicy fruit such as the mango, orange, peach, melon or cherry. Later, you may have heavier fruit such as apple and papaya. Soon you will be eating simple salads without dressing.

During the first night after breaking the fast, generally, you may anticipate spending more time on the toilet than in bed. Some individuals may have as many as ten bowel movements within a 24 hour period.

AFTER THE FAST

Food should be at room temperature. Your stomach has contracted; eat small meals. Many people, after breaking the fast, have a tendency to stuff themselves. This is a mistake. Not only does it lessen the effect of the fast but it can do serious damage.

One should practice water fasting at least one day a week and twice a year go on longer fasts of at least one week in duration.

Fasting was part of the required discipline for initiation into the Mystery Schools. The Essenes and Pythagoreans had the student go through many years of trial, study and purification to familiarize his or her self with eternal truths. For the final initiation, to develop the highest degree of purity, the student had to go through 40 days of fasting as a preparation of the intellect for understanding the cosmic mystery. Fasting and little eating is the key to high intellect and the spiritual path.

The Holy Bible is filled with references to fasting ranging in duration from one to forty or more days. Jesus fasted often; he advised seven day's fast on water, air and sun.

AQUARIAN LIQUID DIET

"The fruit of the vine that I shall drink new (fresh) with you in the kingdom of heaven." 　　　　MATT. 26:29; MARK 14:25

"Where there is no vision, the people perish, but he that keepeth the law, happy is he." 　　　　PROVERB 29:18

"Jesus says, 'Drink ye all of this, for this is my blood of the new testament which shall be shed for many unto remission of sins. And I say unto you, I will not drink henceforth of this fruit of the vine, until that day when I shall drink it NEW WITH YOU in the kingdom of my Father.' The 'new' or fresh juice of fruits is to be shed and taken for remission of sins instead of the animal sacrifices of ancient and modern customs. Get your blood transfusion from the omnipresent Christ life in the juice of fruits and vegetables for that will give you life besides everlasting."

JOHNNY LOVEWISDOM

In a study on the 'grass juice factor' in diet, Dr. Kohler et al discovered that an animal can be raised on a total liquid diet for the entire life span. He states: "An interesting fact brought out by this work is that guinea pigs can be raised on a liquid diet in spite of the fact that their digestive tract is equipped to handle large amounts of roughage."

Dick Gregory, the famous pacifist comedian, vowed not to touch solid food till the end of war on this planet. He has been on a liquid diet for over 30 months. He runs at least three miles daily. To celebrate the 100th day of the fruit juice diet, he ran 15 miles. During his visit at the Institute, he informed us that he drinks one gallon of fresh fruit juice one day; the following day one gallon of distilled water. It took about three years of purification and fruitarian diet before he achieved optimum energy on this liquid diet. In 1972, he ran for 20 miles in the Boston marathon race. He tells you in his book (see Appendix) just exactly how anyone can become a fruitarian and why.

For therapeutic reasons and ease of digestion, one should juice all vegetables. Dr. Walker, who was given up to die, regained his health completely by using raw juices. He continues to be very active in naturopathy and in writing well past the age of 100. He eats little and juices most of the vegetables.

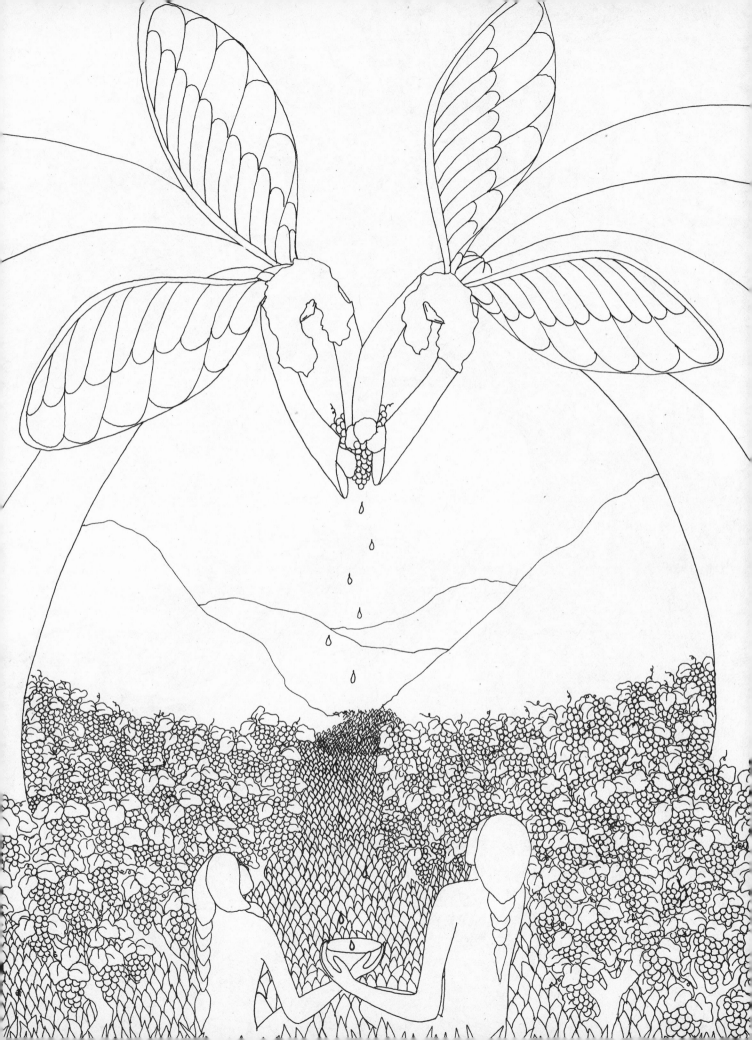

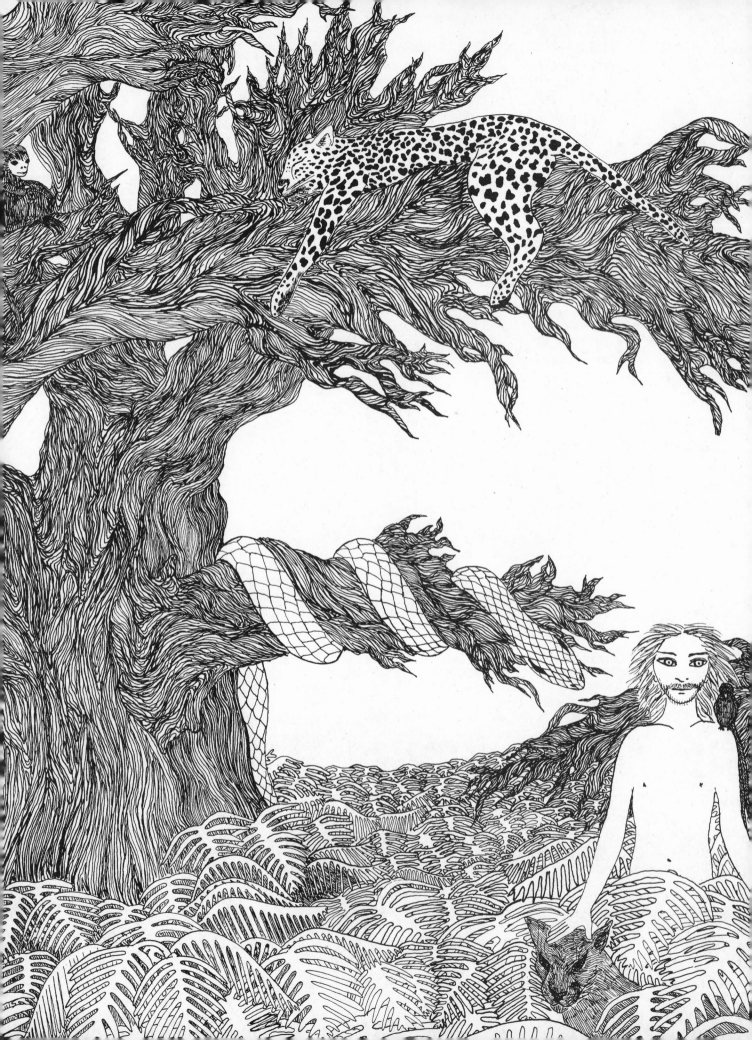

Newspaper clippings, London Times, 1959, reported: "Britain's most talked about woman today is Dr. Barbara Moore, a 57-year-old Russian born physician-scientist who walked 110 miles on two successive weekends on a diet of fruit and vegetable juices. The slim woman doctor has come within minutes of beating soldiers and civilians of all ages by marching 110 miles in 26 hours and 29 minutes. The record 26 hours and 24 minutes is held by 3 British soldiers. She says, 'Indian Yogis taught me the art of deep breathing and cures without surgery. When I was 30, I began experimenting on myself. First I lived on a vegetarian diet, then on raw fruit and vegetable juices. My daily diet is a simple four small glasses of mixed juices, ranging from orange to cucumber or pumpkin juice, plus pure water and honey. I eat no starch, no protein, no fibre, no milk. Meat and protein foods fill the body with toxins which cloud the brain. I sleep only 2 hours a day. I have cut down my breathing rate to six times a minute, half the normal speed, which also reduces my heart beat all adding to my long life process.' Her husband is the sculptor, Henry Moore. 'He knows that I have the body of a woman of 32, the vigor, stamina, and endurance of a man of 24. My last illness was leukemia, which crippled me for three years, until I cured myself.'

A child starts the days as a liquidarian. Mothers' breast milk can be fed for up to three years or more as the sole nourishment and yet the child's body will manifest health and show no signs of degeneration.

Every study in longevity shows that frugal eating, predominantly of liquids promotes health and prolongs life.

When one is a liquidarian, the occult apparatus will function at the level intended by creation. Waste products from the digestion of solid food will not interfere with the nerve linkages. Oxygen will circulate more freely because of the absence of pressure on the arteries and veins by gas generated from fermentation of undigested food. Vital energy will be centralized in the upper chakras instead of in the stomach to carry out digestion. Sleep will be practically eliminated. One will have time for meditation and experience all the esoteric privileges at one time restricted to a select few. One will be on the path of transcending time and space.

With a liquid diet, one has to redesign his/her life. It must be spent in the service of Humanity, Perfection and Love. The less a person uses and indulges, the more perfect he or she becomes. Humans gain in perfection as they conquer their appetites and desires and they devote their lives to the discovery of the "heaven within." This is not an easy road, but "If any man will come after me, let one deny himself and follow me."

RETURN OF THE FRUITARIAN

"Love and all things shall be added unto thee."

CHRIST

"The plant-eaters form still at the present time, as they have always done, the great majority of animals on earth. The highest developed plant-eaters are the fruit-eaters. The highest fruit-eater is the human being."

DR. ABRAMOWSKI (FRUITARIAN DIET AND PHYSICAL REJUVENATION)

"The oldest inhabitants of Greece, the Pelasgians, who came before the Dorian, Ionian and Eolian migrations, inhabited Arcadia and Thessaly, possessing the island of Lesbos and Lokemantos, which were full of orange groves. The people with their diet of dates and oranges, lived on an average of more than 200 years."

HERODOTUS As quoted by Hotema in MAN'S HIGHER CONSCIOUSNESS

"Preliminary studies of fossil teeth have led an anthropologist to the startling suggestion that the early human ancestors were not predominantly meat eaters, or even of seeds, shoots, leaves or grasses. Nor were they omnivorous, Instead, they appear to have subsisted chiefly on a diet of fruit"...Every tooth examined from the hominids of the 12 million-year period leading up to Homo erectus appear to be that of a fruit eater. Every Homo erectus tooth was that of an omnivorous. Homo erectus was the first form of human being known to have migrated out of Africa.

N.Y. Times
Sunday 5/15/79

"The fruitage of the tree of life is all too fine to feed the carnal mind."

AQUARIAN GOSPEL OF JESUS THE CHRIST Levi

"My fruit is better than gold, yea, than fine gold."

PRO. 8:19

They will actually sit, . . . under vine and under fig tree, and there will be no one making them tremble.

MICAH 4:4

Fruit is the only cuisine that is karmaless. All other food involves killing, whether it be of animals, plants or seed. Fruit is offered from the tree by God. When ripened to perfection by the sun, it is plucked from the tree by the wind and laid as an offering to humans or animals. In taste it is perfect. Human beings aid in the beautification of the planet by eating the fruit flesh and depositing the seed in fertile soil. The children of these men and women shall eat from that tree.

Fruit is the most perfect food for human kind and also helps human beings to advance much further in esoteric studies and the spiritual life. It is the easiest food to digest. The vital force of the body can be centered most of the time in the head instead of expending its energy in digestion. It is the least mucus-inducing of all foods, thus it opens the sinuses where the breath of life is centered. Through yogic breathing exercises they are charged with prana (vital force). The electromagnetic nature of air makes the circuits of the brain start functioning at a new level of awareness during meditation and daily life.

The most advanced form of communication with the cosmic consciousness takes place when all food is removed in a state of fasting. If the human temple has been cleansed previously, then there will be perfect reception and heightened awareness.

On starting a fruit diet, a good practice is to go on at least 24 hours, but no more than 48 hours, of dry fasting (no water). Follow with three or more days of acid, sub-acid fruit juices diluted with distilled water. Take up to one gallon per day. Such juices are easily obtainable by sucking on the fruit and spitting out the pulp.

Afterward, choose fruit that agrees with you. Eat one type of fruit at a meal, no more than two pounds. Fruit from trees, vines and shrubs, are all suitable foods. If mixing fruits, follow the food combining chart. Eat the juicy, acid, quickly assimilable, cleansing fruit first; twenty minutes later, you can eat the more concentrated fruit such as banana or avocado.

"Genesis I:29 describes juicy fruit and succulent herbs which bear their seed for propagation as the only food designed for humans. If the seed of fruit and herbs is used as food of humans, such seed cannot bear of yield. This is the only distinction the Creator used to divide the tree of life from the tree that gave mortality to human beings. Genesis I:II, 12 states that seeds are to yield each for its kind; propagation is their sole purpose. We eat apples, peaches, oranges, and cast away the seeds or we eat grapes, tomatoes, berries, and, even if swallowed, the seeds are cast off in fertile fecal matter to grow afterwards. But if we eat almond, walnut, peanut, grain, legumes or seed food, the seed is destroyed forever.

"There is another proof that the forbidden food was seed: the result of eating it produced a disturbance in the reproductive sex function causing shame to the first couple. Seed was the fruit from the 'tree of knowledge of good and evil.'

"In no way is it ever indicated that any sexual act or anything else was the cause of defilement in paradise originally but it plainly accuses eating forbidden food as the sin. When Adam explained that he hid and was afraid because he was naked, God replied correcting him, "And who hath told thee that thou wast naked but that thou has eaten of the tree whereof I commanded thee thou shouldst not eat?

"Modern attempts at fruitarianism acknowledge the need of a stimulating sex element, justifying their use of nuts, without realizing that an undefiled love relationship on juicy fruit could lift one's body and mental powers above defilement.

"It was only by using external stimulants or our intoxication through acid forming seed and animal protein decomposition, alcoholic beverages and drugs that humans acquired short-lived strength to do evil things."

(Johnny Lovewisdom)

CHEMISTRY OF FRUIT

All fruit have an alkaline ash. Whether food is alkaline or acid is determined by comparing the residue ash. If it contains more alkaline than acid mineral (i.e. if the minerals calcium, magnesium, potassium and sodium predominate over chlorine, nitrogen, sulphur and phosphorus), it will be classed alkaline. All grains, with the exception of millet, have an acid ash. Wheat and oats are the most acid.

Because fruit and vegetables contain citric, milic, and other acids, they will have an acid pH reaction in digestion, but because of the high content of alkaline-forming minerals, their reaction is always alkaline in the bloodstream. This helps to neutralize the waste products of metabolism which are always acid.

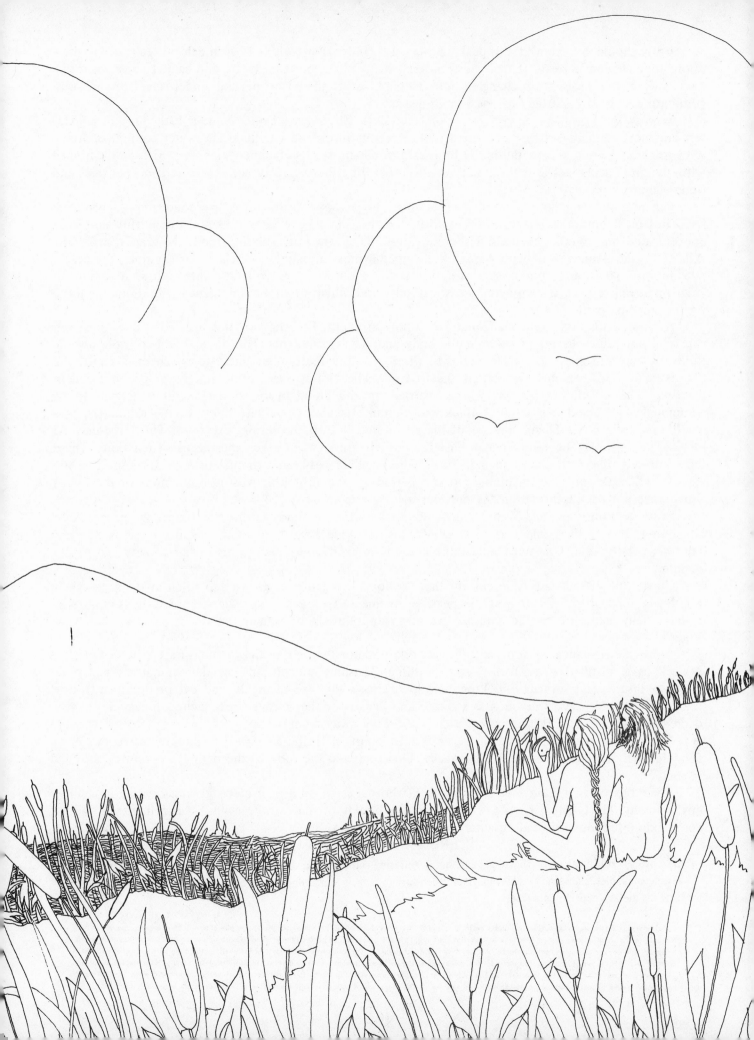

Fruit should be eaten at the peak of ripeness. Under-ripe fruit is high in acid juices and will draw upon your alkaline reserve. It can cause blisters, loss of calcium from teeth, and canker sores. Over-ripe fruit are in the process of changing into alcohol. Both the over-ripe and under-ripe fruit are very stimulating and are disturbing to one's inner peace.

William H. Diefenbach, M.D.   of New York City, says "Fruits contain little protein and fat but are most valuable sources of mineral salts, carbohydrates and vitamins. The water content of fruits, with mineral content, keeps the blood in a state of alkalinity. Its alkaline elements, which are combined with the fruit acids, act as natural laxatives by promoting the secretory action of the liver, pancreas and other secretory glands."

Persons suffering from acid dyspepsia must avoid sour fruits until the condition is corrected. Diabetics must limit the intake of sweet fruit. Bananas, dates, avocados, figs and dried fruit are highly concentrated and should be used with reservation. They are not cleansing foods. In grapes, avoid the skin and seed. Stoned fruit with tender flesh are the most digestible as a class: for example, the peach, persimmon, mango and apricot. An exception is the avocado — its high fat content slows digestion. In yoga philosophy, fruit is considered sattwic food, food which promotes the highest vibrations for those on the spiritual path.

At first, fruit may seem inadequate to supply strength. Digestion of this light food does not form uric acid and other toxins to saturate the body and act as stimulants. Too, in a toxic body, the organic fluid of fruit dissolves old waste deposits, products of a faulty diet, and stored chemicals into the bloodstream. This can make one tired and irritable. The bloodstream, urine and sweat become acid in reaction. The circulating poisons will be carried by the bloodstream to the excretory organs to be eliminated. The blood may become thick and viscous. It cannot circulate freely in the capillaries; as a result one feels cold. There may be discharge of mucus into the respiratory tract. The feces may be loose. The lips may be swollen and blistered, which are signs of fever and cleansing reactions. These signs are very likely to persist in individuals who vacillate between extreme diets, such as macrobiotic and fruitarian. A fruit diet maintained over a period of several months will flush out most of the toxins which have not been removed on the previous dietary regime.

Fruit is both food and drink. Adequate intake of pure fluids during the transition insures daily evacuation. If one lives under tropical conditions, working in hot sun, one can lose a gallon of fluid daily via perspiration. One must adjust the amount of fruit consumed to his or her activity and to the climate.

On a fruit diet, it is very important that the food is organically grown and eaten at the stage when it is ready to drop off the tree at the peak of ripemess. To make such a diet complete, it is important to have daily exposure to the sun, to live in an unpolluted atmosphere and to conserve one's sexual fluids.

Have the first meal at noon and the last one no later than six in the evening. Fast at least two days a week using distilled water, fruit juice or nothing. Consume enough bulk or take enough sub-acid sweet juice to insure daily evacuation. Progressively decrease the size of meals, and eat predominantly ripe, juicy fruit. Avoid heavy fruit such as avocado and banana or the fibrous fruits such as pineapple. Yearly, decrease the number of meals you eat each week. Stay away from nuts.

Peter Max, the well-known artist, is fast becoming a fruitarian. "God is the greatest cook. When food falls off the tree that means it is ready. God prepared the food to the right temperature, taste and energy."

Over the years, I have met a few women who persisted on a fruit diet and frugal eating in a sunny environment. Thirty-five year old women had the bodies of fourteen-year-olds — sparkling eyes, radiant complexion, lustrous hair and an aura of God-consciousness.

FRUITARIAN DILEMA

To be a healthy fruitarian up north without eventually suffering some undesirable consequences is difficult, if not impossible. A total mucusless diet, unless rich in chlorophyll or green sprout juice, is just as dangerous. Consider the following story of Dr. S. Bass and his dietary experiments (234):

"After trying many food programs I came under the influence of the writings of Arnold Ehret whose simple philosophy of health and disease appealed to me. He claimed that fruit was the perfect food of man, and that one could live on it alone and be perfectly nourished. He allowed some green leafy vegetables, 'if desired,' and on rare occasions [only during the winter] nuts in limited quantity. The very persuasive style of his writings fired me with so much zeal that I decided to try his system of living on fruit alone for two weeks. After the two weeks I went on a fruit diet that included proteins such as nuts and followed this with longer periods of an exclusive whole fruit and juice regimen. I experienced states of euphoria, buoyancy and the ability to do more work, mentally and physically. These apparent improvements propelled me to search for more knowledge concerning nutrition in order to attain physical perfection.

"In my fervor I finally decided, in 1941, to live on an exclusive fruit and fruit juice diet and at the same time continue to work. The diet consisted of MANY FRESH ORANGES AND ABOUT ONE PINT OF PINEAPPLE JUICE DAILY. I lost at the average of one-half pound per day for about ten days. Thereafter, I lost about four ounces daily. After the third week my weight remained almost stationary and I lost only three additional pounds from the third week to the tenth week. I felt better and stronger for the first three weeks but after the third week on my fruitarian program, I observed a drop in energy which was accompanied by an intense DESIRE FOR PROTEIN FOODS. Though it was difficult to keep away from protein foods I managed to do so. While on this program I noticed symptoms such as mild BLEEDING OF THE GUMS, with some RECESSION, and some pitting of the TEETH. Also present was a general EMOTIONAL SENSITIVITY and irritability. At the conclusion of this regimen I returned to protein foods [nuts, cheese, etc.] for two months. I followed this with fourteen days EXCLUSIVELY ON A GRAPEFRUIT JUICE DIET. After this period followed a mixed fruit and vegetable diet for several weeks. I then went for seventeen days on a grapefruit juice diet. At this time I noticed greater recession and bleeding of the gums along with toothaches and the loss of two tooth fillings.

"It was at this point that I began to have serious doubts about the efficacy of living on fruit alone. I was forced to reconsider Ehret's theory as a result of the new physical and mental disturbances that I experienced. I became disillusioned and disheartened and did not know which way to turn.

"A few years later, after four years of college work, I became a practitioner and was then in a position to observe clinically the ill effects of EXCESSIVE FRUIT EATING, or an exclusive fruit diet, on a large number of people. Overindulgence in fruit [alone with other carbohydrate foods] is the most common violation among vegetarians, natural hygienists and other followers of radical food regimens.

"The harm which results from EXCESSIVE FRUIT EATING is not quickly discernible. It sometimes takes many years before the ill effects manifest themselves. In some cases negative results occur within six months; in others it may take one to three years and even longer. Fruit contains the simplest sugars, such as glucose and fructose, which are monosaccharides and enter the blood stream rapidly. The immediate effect, WHEN FRUIT IS EXCESSIVE, is stimulation; that in many creates a feeling of exhilaration. But the later effects of OVER CONSUMPTION are great restlessness, nervousness, argumentativeness, inability to concentrate, hypersensitivity, loss of weight, lassitude, fatigue and loss of appetite that alternates with food binges that are extremely abnormal.

"AN EXCESSIVE FRUIT SUGAR intake leads to what can be called carbohydrate intoxication which will interfere with normal protein metabolism even though the protein intake is sufficient. Signs of protein deficiency that have been noted following carbohydrate-protein imbalance are ridging and splitting of fingernails, anemia, loss of hair, general loss of energy, venule and capillary breakage [rupture of the small hair-like blood vessels close to the skin surface], swelling of the ankles and feet, varicose veins and hidden fluid retention, slow clotting of the blood and delayed healing of wounds. Hemorrhoids frequently swell a few hours after a binge on dates or dried figs. Emotional outbursts after the slightest provocation may follow with long-term violators. Some may become insomniacs, while others want to rest and sleep almost constantly. Many more abnormalities could be mentioned to illustrate that one cannot be indiscriminate in eating even natural foods.

"THE OVERCONSUMPTION OF FRUIT SUGARS AND MORE COMPLEX CARBOHYDRATES leads to oversecretion of insulin by the pancreas [hyperinsulinism] which is followed by a rapid "burning-up" of sugar in the blood. This results in low blood sugar and a lack of energy; that in turn creates an irresistible desire to indulge in sweets again. Thus a vicious cycle is established which can be controlled only by proper regulation of sugar intake. In some individuals long continued overactivity of the pancreas caused by high sugar intake can lead to a form of diabetes."

The following lessons can be learned from the experience of Dr. Bass. Professor Ehret developed his practice in the days of relatively low pollution when the fruit was grown organically and was generally picked tree ripened right from one's locale. They were grown with love by happy farmers. Today, under city conditions, fruit is not fruit.

Under city conditions, the carbon monoxide (CO) content in the air is two to four hundred times higher than in the pollution free countryside. The CO gas inactivates the hemoglobin oxygen carrying capacity and will bring on anemic condition. Over 75% of city dwellers are anemic. Likewise, many essential dietary factors are used up by the body to neutralize the corrosive effects of the many airborne gases and chemicals. A diet rich in chlorophyll (or sprout juices) can effectively and quickly correct anemic conditions (see: chlorophyll). A diet of fruit is inadequate to compensate for these dietary losses. I have witnessed several cases of young persons on a mucusless diet in Washington, D.C., N.Y.C. and Boston who were anemic. The condition was not corrected until they included fermented seed preparations (which created some mucus) or increased the intake of sprouted green juice to several glasses daily.

A diet with emphasis on citrus and pineapple can dissolve any fruitarian. One purchases in the city inorganic fruit in an unripened state which is embalmed with chemicals. Even when organic, the fruit is generally picked unripe and has gone through nutritional losses due to the timelapse between the harvest and the time of eating. These highly acid fruit will inactivate some of the hemoglobin, produce gum bleeding and dissolve teeth. I have seen in my practice several such cases where in a single summer in Boston on a diet of grapefruit and oranges the front teeth were reduced to half of the original size.

Vegetarians often overindulge in carbohydrates (in the form of grains, bakery products, potatoes, dried fruit and in some cases fruit) or proteins (nuts, seeds and legumes) which is their stimulating substitute for the flesh foods they have given up. The same is true for fruitarians; they are prone to excess in sweet or acidy fruit.

Overindulgence in fruit (as well as any food) will magnify overacidity, since the condition will come not only from unripe acid fruit but also from fermentation. Fruit in excess quantity stays in the digestive tract for a long time because of bulk and does not allow the stomach to empty from one meal to the next. It goes through the same process as a grape in the manufacture of wine. The overindulgence and associated fermentation leaves marks on the face in the form of a swollen lower lip (see physiology). Furthermore, through overeating of fruit, the high sugar content can bring on carbohydrate metabolic disorders. This is very infrequent and will appear only in individuals who have associated complications already. The gorilla, which consumes up to 40 pounds of fruit in a single day, is not noted for sugar disorders; however, the overindulgence is the responsible factor for the short lifespan of this animal.

Even in an ideal environment many experimenting fruitarians, because of a long past history of dietary processed foods, must go through the suffering of rebirth which takes much longer than two months. It can take up to a year, and longer, to become totally detoxified and feel the strength that can be experienced on a totally frugal fasterian fruit diet.

If one does a rapid diet change, the internal body acids which are dissolved by fruit juices can make one feel very weak, lead to the discharge of large quantities of mucus through the mechanics of a cold or flu or bring on open sores and blisters as the toxins are being discharged through the eliminative function of the skin.

If the cleansing process is too speedy, one should go back to vegetable juices, mucus lean sprouts, avocado, banana and some fermented seed sauces. Do occasional fasts. Wait for a time when you can afford to have unlimited rest in a favorable environment to do a complete detoxification program.

The fruitarian program when diligently pursued in an ideal environment can result in the most dramatic rejuvenation. I would like to share the experience of a few such individuals.

Several years ago, I picked up two hitchhikers, a man and, what I thought, his teenage daughter. She had the physical features of a woman, but everything about her gave the impression of a little girl. She was 18. Her iris was completely clear and glistened in blue colors. Her hair radiated with life and her skin was without blemishes, luster clear. She spoke with wisdom, frolic, wit and zest. To my surprise, she had been a fruitarian for ten months.

She became a fruitarian in an unusual way. She was obese. The doctor told her she needed to lose 60 pounds. He gave her a calorie chart and a conventional diet. After experimenting on a variety of foods, she saw that she had no desire for most foods unless they are processed or highly seasoned — two dietary no-no's. So she decided to do the weight loss in the quickest possible manner. She decided to eat only fruit because it tasted good and was low in calories. She also decided to eat very little. The cleansing activities of her body caused her to pass out several times; there were also occasional vomit fits and some other symptoms of detoxification. Her parents tried to force her to eat other foods, especially meat. The family doctor wrote up medical prescriptions. She cooperated with neither her parents or the doctor. Instead, she ran away from home. During a period of 6 months she lost 70 pounds. By continuing the fruit diet, she gained 15 pounds. Her current food intake is one orange a day. She takes in sun rays and plenty of outdoor physical activity. There are days when she eats nothing.

The second case is a man of 38. I have been acquainted with him during the last two years. He, during a period of 3 months while living in the nude in a Florida orchard, regenerated his features to that of a young man. His face lost all of its lines and wrinkles and much of his receding hair line grew back. His diet consisted primarily of treeripened organic oranges, tomatoes from a local garden and occasional avocado from the neighboring trees.

FUTURE FRUITARIAN FARMS

Dear Victoras, As we are preparing to depart for Central America where we are interested in setting up our first community, I would like to share a few thoughts & feelings & suggestions with you. Since mail is so expensive we will not carry on much correspondence with fff folks, instead we will send you reports of our experiences and answer any questions you or others may have. While you will probably continue the communication flow — by person as well as newsletter or any other convenient media

If there is room to accommodate more than the 8 - 12 of us who are going now we will let you know so that whoever is interested can join us. Many fff folk have idealized conceptions about what it would be like living in such a community — this leads to confusion when confronted by the bare facts of real life situations with ordinary, less than perfect human beings who fall far short of such high-minded ideals.

However it is helpful to spell out in detail such practices and goals that outline the differences between the typical usual spiritual community & our group. The things we have already excluded from our lifestyle can best be expressed in the negative: NO FIRE — which implies no cooking, or heat, or smoking (tobacco or marijuana), 75 - 100% fruit diet, little or no clothing, shelter or other material things. Of course retain legal papers, i.e. passport etc & clothing to appear in civilization.

The question of whether Western material civilization will survive does not concern us because we do not feel that it is possible to evolve while we are experiencing such pollution as we have to endure in the cities.

We wish to lead lives guided by the principle of Ahimsa — harmlessness — which we expect will lead us to experience greater harmony with nature — awareness of other beings (no longer considered as objects of exploitation). All of us already have completed the transition away from using animal beings for food and are becoming more sensitive to our fellow insect and plant beings though it is hard to anticipate how we will be able to avoid stepping on them even after every other level of oppressing other beings has ceased. But our experience has shown us that we receive guidance at every step of the way and at the appropriate time I'm sure that the answers will be provided.

We do not use the label fruitarian because we have found that practicing glutarianism even with fruit is nearly as much of a hindrance to elimination as with a conventional diet. Besides, there are many who identify themselves as psychadelic fruitarians who use substances other than fruit to achieve their "high", "heavenly", "paradisical" state of consciousness. Then we also find other juicearians (liquitarians) who use "dry" supplemental "vitamins" & "minerals" as stimulants to keep their energy level up; in addition some fruitarians use "cooked juices" packed in some non-biodegradable bottles and cans. Others even use honey which they might label bee fruit. Then there is the well known use of herbs which Johnny Lovewisdom labels Vitarianism when combined with fruit. We need not discuss the use of seeds & nuts.

The usual explanation of fruit diet is similar to the rationale of the vegetarian diet, health & ethics (compassion). Healthwise it provides the least poisons or stimulants to the body of any food, when fully ripe, and aids in the elimination of previously stored toxins. According to fruitarianism it is the only way of eating that does not destroy the plant or its potential for growth (seed), rather it is often considered an aid in propagating the plant/tree by placing the unbroken seed in a location which might be more conducive to its growth away from the bearing plant while using the liquid flesh part of the fruit as a source of nourishment.

Love, Just   4/1/74

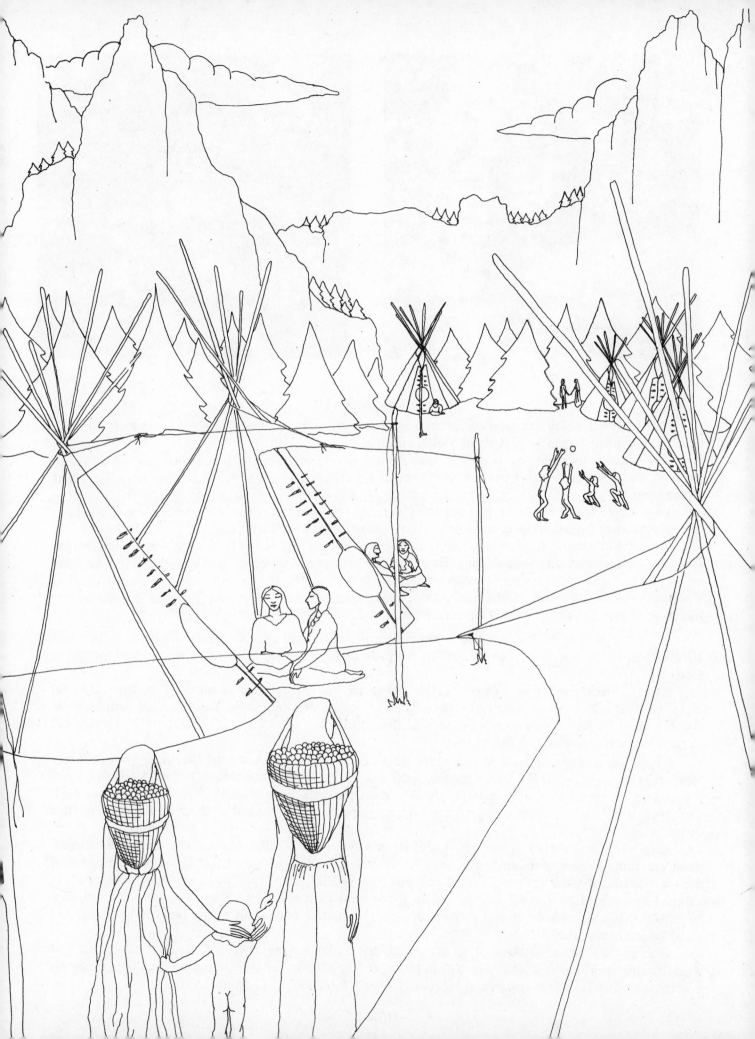

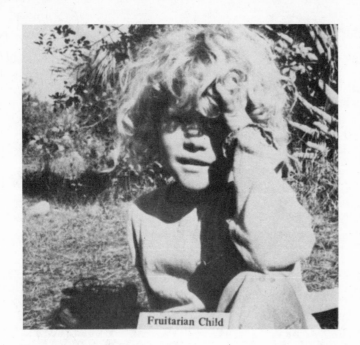
Fruitarian Child

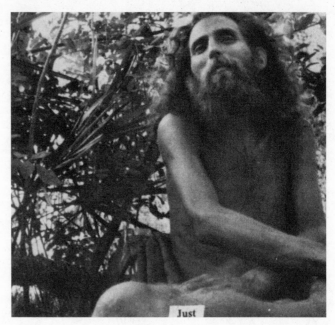
Just

FRUITARIAN PATH

Pollutants are much heavier than air; as a result they sink to the lower levels. Live at least 50 miles from centers of pollution, preferably at a high altitude.

High altitude is where you find more sun, cleaner air and increased solar radiation. Grown at higher altitudes and near the equator with more ultraviolet rays, fruit have up to ten times the vitamin content of the same fruit in the U.S.A.

Your lungs will increase in size and your stomach will become more and more of an appendage. The stomach was originally to be used only under unnatural conditions for survival.

One should choose tropical mountains to live in. Avoid locations with a wide temperature range. They are not conducive to simple living. However, the highest known concentration of centurians occurs in high mountains with extremely cold winters, such as the Himalayan Mountains (Hunzas) or Ural Mountains (White Russians), as well as subtropical Andes mountains. One can survive the cold as long as one has pure air and knows the secret of correct breathing.

After complete detoxification, not only will urine, saliva and skin secretions be alkaline, but also, they will have the taste and fragrance of the fruit eaten. Such a body is a delight to companions and to God.

As you adopt this simple diet your craving for food will keep getting smaller and smaller (also your digestive tract will contract to one-fourth, or smaller, of its previous size). Your strength will increase. On a fruit diet, less energy is wasted in digestion. Fruit has no starch, little fiber. Hence, you will experience increased vitality in all activities.

I lived for months on fruit and for three weeks on orange juice. After the fourth day of juices, the cleansing reaction ceased. My breathing was such as I had never experienced it before. I felt like I was doing deep breathing exercises continuously. My nasal passages felt expanded manyfold. This mucusless diet opened my sinuses completely and my breathing apparatus functioned at the level intended for this divine organ.

After the juice diet, I tested my body. I ate a few nuts. Within minutes, my head was clogged; nasal breathing became difficult; my lungs felt congested. Within an hour I had the most painful bowel movement. Initially, the fruit-feces came out soft and slightly firm. Then came the nuts, undigested, in round balls as hard as a rock. I tried a similar experiment with cooked food one day later, a small meal of brown rice and cooked vegetables. Same result — the matter passed out of my body in an undigested state several hours later.

One of the big advantages of an improved diet is higher sensitivity of taste, smell, touch and digestive organs. They will tell you which foods are non-foods for you. As your body increases its vitality on a diet closer to its needs, it vigorously rejects food which is harmful.

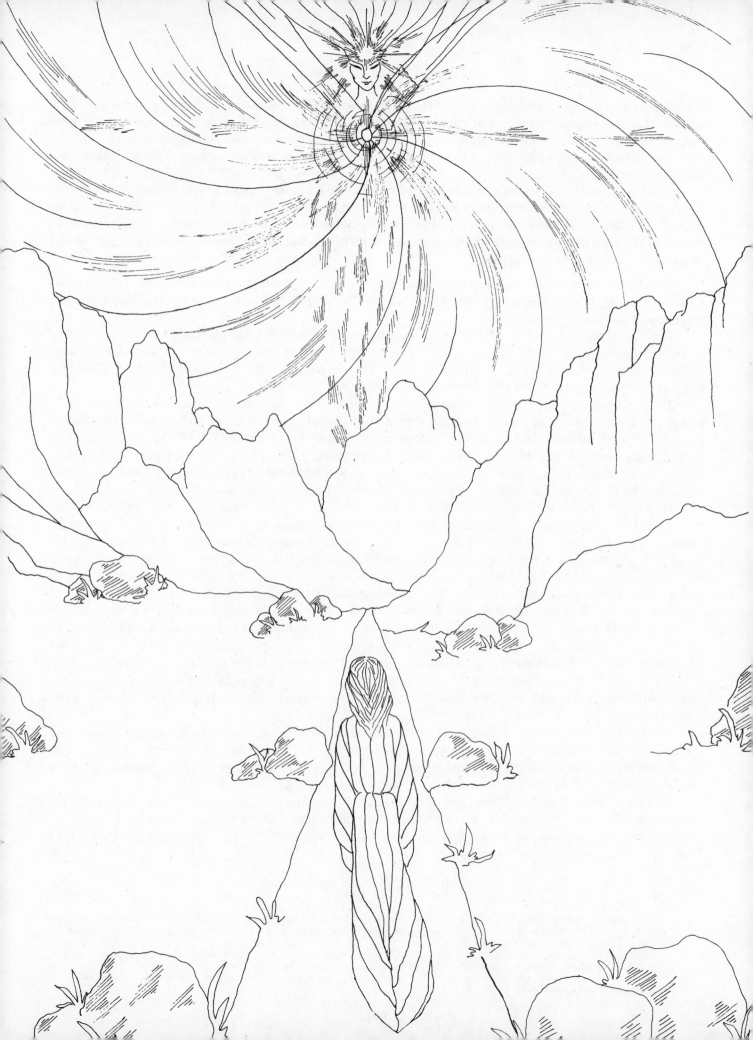

WHERE TO LIVE LONG

In choosing a country for a warm climate settlement, it is advisable to take into consideration the politics of the land. If the country is heavily dependent upon the import of food and essential commodities, the people would be in a desperate situation in times of food scarcity experienced by the exporters. The natives would take their vengeance out on foreigners.

It is good to choose a country which has a good size population of English speaking people or one in which English is the official language of the country.

Countries, such as Australia, New Zealand; islands off the coast of Africa; British Columbia, or even American States such as Texas, New Mexico and Arizona, although they might not be ideal, can provide survival accommodations during the oncoming ecological disaster. Before finally settling in your desired location, experiment with 3 month gatherings (see Grapewine in Appendix) to see how it feels to live under a new environment. Much information can be shared at a gathering so that you can make a better decision on a choice of land.

The temperature in subtropical mountains can be varied by moving up or down the mountain. If you want snow, climb a thousand feet and you have your own Alps. If you want to experience the tropics, just descend a few thousand feet.

The tropics at sea level are not an ideal place to live. Continuous humidity and decay of vegetation is not conducive to good health and long life. The high content of water vapor, carbon dioxide and sulpher derivatives makes the air unfit for humans. The air at high altitudes is quite different. The ideal temperature ranges from 60 to 90 degrees, with low humidity.

To avoid nuclear fallout, settle in the morning shadow of the high Andes mountains. Fallout travels east to west while the earth rotates 17 miles a minute so fallout cannot descent fast enough to reach the morning shadow of the Andes. A.E.C. measurements show the least fallout in the world in cities immediately west of the high Andes such as Antofogasta, Chile and Quito, Ecuador. The higher strontium 90 count in East South America is highest in Rio de Janiero. The northern part of the globe, including the U.S.A. has the bulk of fallout now. (Order of Paradise, Johnny Lovewisdom)

If possible, move to the higher altitudes of the tropical or subtropical regions of Mexico, Texas, South America, Australia. Avoid all areas where non-organic gardening is practiced. Use the readings of Edgar Cayce and other prophets as an aid to the choice of area. Much of our land mass will be revamped by geological turmoil, especially the coastal areas like California, New York, Boston. As your diet improves, away from pollution you will develop the uncanny power of prophets, primitive people and animals. It will guide you to avoid natural catastrophes which will ravage the land.

Nobel Prize Winner, Alexis Carrel, spoke of the availability of infinite access to all universal information. This takes place as soon as human beings become more like the divine beings they were created to be. Carrel said: "Each part of the body seems to know the present and the future needs of the whole and acts accordingly. The significance of Time and Space is not the same for our Cells as for our Mind. The body perceives the remote as well as the near, the future as well as the present" (Man, the Unknown). You need only to train the mind to have access to this information through daily meditation.

Take tools and books — ancient scriptures, human physiology, astrology, geography, yoga and esoteric studies. A shortwave radio will keep you in touch with civilization. A sailboat can aid you to reach uninhabited islands, free from the plagues of civilization. It will provide transportation for your brothers and sisters, plus supplies.

Having chosen a locale, unless you are capable of keeping your own and God's company, take along at least one other person. It is always wise to think in terms of starting a community for spiritual development and the new life styles that will follow the collapse of the present earthlings' attempts at living. You are forerunners of a new future.

THE FRUITARIAN HEADS

"The ancient wise ones taught that there is a spiritual realm within the human being. "The kingdom of God is within you," (Luke 17:21). That includes everything and all. The spiritual realm of the human being is located in the spiritual chambers of the skull, called the "Golden Bowl" (Eccl. 12:6).

"These Chambers, the functions of which are unknown to modern science, are five in number . . . and they are symbolized in the ancient scriptures by certain five as: 'The Five Golden Emeralds' (Is. 6:4), the 'Five Loaves' (Matt. 14:17).

"The Sankhys doctrine states that the Five Physical Senses . . . are the exteriorized products of the five corresponding spiritual centers which are as follows:

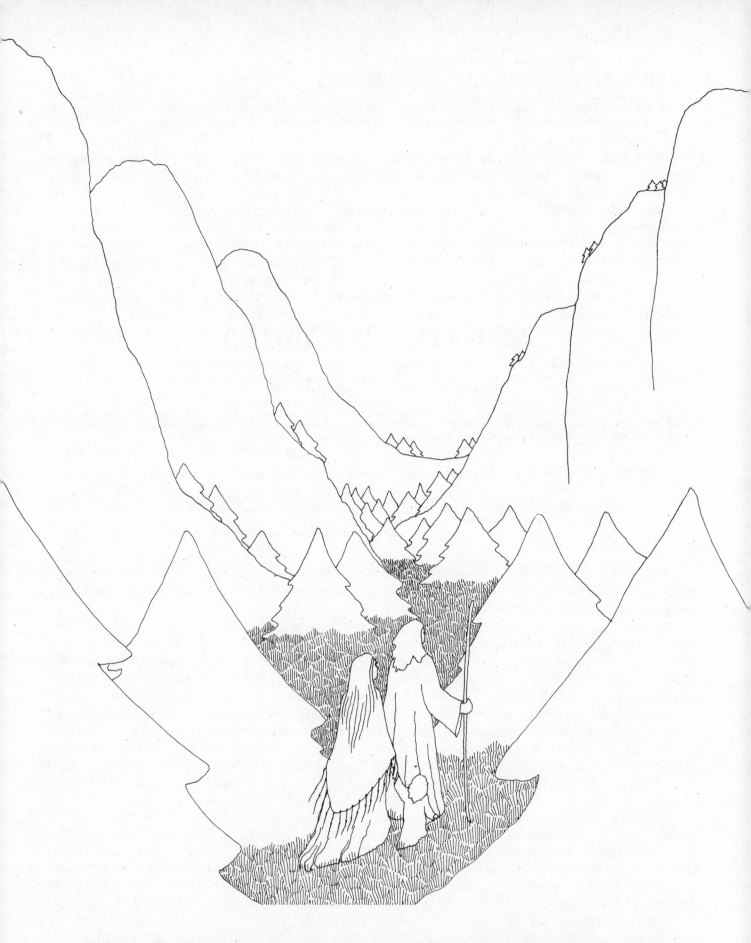

"Seth and children dwelt on top of the mountain below the garden. They sowed not, neither did they reap. They sought no food for the body, not even wheat; but only offerings. They ate the delicious fruit of the trees that grew on the mountain . . . Then Seth often fasted as did his oldest children. Each forty days. For the family of Seth smelled (like) the smell of trees of the garden when the wind blew from that way. They were happy, innocent, without fear; there was no jealousy, no evil action, no hatred among them; there was no animal passion. From no mouth came either foul words or curse, neither evil counsel or fraud."

THE FORGOTTEN BOOKS OF EDEN, SETH BOOK I, XI:10

1. Frontal Sinus — a cavity in the sphenoid bone of the skull.
2. Sphenoidal Sinus — a cavity in the sphenoid bone of the skull.
3. Maxillary Sinus — largest of the five, and resembling a pyramid in shape.
4. Palatine Sinus — a cavity in the orbital process of the palatine bone and opening into either sphenoidal or posterior sinus.
5. Ethmoidal Sinus — this chamber consists of numerous small cavities occupying the labyrinth of the ethmoidal bone, and in these cavities are situated the small, mysterious glands known in occult science as the Intellectual organs." (166)

The Sinuses communicate directly or indirectly with the nasal cavity. They are lined with mucous membrane extending into them from the nose. For protection, nature has placed the sinuses in a bony enclosure. To prevent their destruction by polluted air or wrong food, they become filled with mucus.

On a frugal, liquid-fruit diet or water fast, eventually these sinuses are opened. Therefore I do not recommend such practices in the city as the polluted air will destroy their spiritual function. With proper diet, proper environment and proper meditation, the sinuses become a receiver-transmitter which enables one to reach other individuals and to be in touch with the cosmic consciousness. In my mathematic studies, I have found that there is a one to one correspondence between circuit theory and nerve network theory. The brain can duplicate all the functions of a radio except on a much higher frequency. If you are tuned in to the universal spirit, you will be able to follow its guidance.

AQUARIAN FAMILY

"The Mother explained the future body to the children of the Ashram: Transformation implies that all this purely material arrangement will be replaced by concentration of force, each having a different mode of vibration; instead of organs there will be centres of conscious energy moved by the conscious will. No stomach, no heart any longer, no circulation, no lungs; all this disappears and gives place to a play of vibrations representing what these organs are symbolically. For the organs are only the material symbols of centres of energy; they are not the essential reality: simply, they give it a form or a support in certain given circumstances. The transformed body will then function through its real centres of energy and not any longer through their symbolic representatives such as were developed in the animal body."

SRI AUROBINDO, ADVENTURES OF CONSCIOUSNESS

"Beloved, let us love one another, for love is for God, and everyone that loveth is born of God and knoweth God."

1 John 10.7

"Fruit diet will once more enable mothers to suckle their young by producing an abundance of milk, rich in all necessary constituents but free from any dangerous matter."

FRUIT DIET AND PHYSICAL REGENERATION, DR. ABRAMOWSKI

You will find that on a diet of fruit in tropical mountains, all your needs will be provided for as are the needs of the beasts and birds of the forest. It will be easy to redirect sexual energy to the more creative life of physical and spiritual unfoldment.

Survival into the 21st Century is possible only with spiritual unfoldment. Our material needs are minimal. Today you are not doing a child a favor by bringing it into the world. If you want children, adopt them. If you choose to have a child, loving thoughts, a great desire for a child, celibacy after conception and happiness are the most important ingredients to develop in him or her a superior intellect, spirituality and vitality.

Chastity should not be drudgery. If it is, then the sexual experience has much to teach you and this incarnation demands it. Approach it with loving heart and best nutrition. Spend days of abstinence to rebuild your reserves. Follow the natural rhythm of the female. A light fruit diet prevents pressure of intestinal gas and waste on the seminal vesicles so that a man is not plagued with sexual tensions. A light diet also prevents irritation of the sexual organs in both female and male. The practice of Karezza (intercourse without loss of sexual fluids) is an alternative to those who are into this pastime.

In nature the function of sex is to insure the continuation and perfection of the species. If anything such as toxicity from eating meat, high protein seeds or stimulants threatens the existence of a human individual, instinctually the sex drive becomes more intense. Nature attempts to create descendants in whom she can attain the perfection she failed to achieve in this generation. In nature the unhealthy organism, provided it still has enough energy and internal nutrients, participates more intensely in sexual activity than the healthy one. In a healthy organism, the sexual energy is channeled to cell regeneration and the continuous joyous perfection of life.

Human Godliness, with consciousness of everlasting life and ascension to the bliss of perfect attunement with the universal rhythm, will be ours when we return to a sunny land and a fruit diet. By altering the electromagnetic sex currents, Ida and Pingala — male and female elements — through mind and body chemistry, the Kundalini force will rise to the thousand petalled lotus.

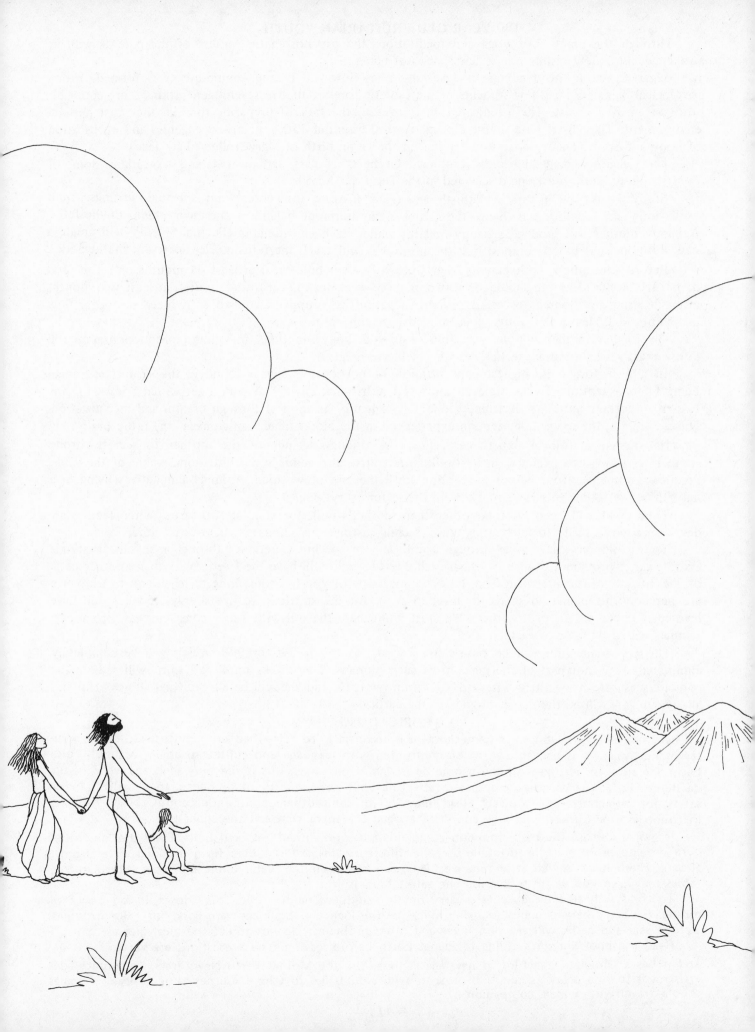

100 YEAR OLD FRUITARIAN YOUTH

Through the practice of yoga and meditation, the psychosomatic centers of the parents will be awakened, ultimately resulting in a new species of being.

Edgar Cayce in his readings of Jesus describes how the Essene community was formed. From astrological calculations, a few students of the esoteric foresaw that in several generations there could be born on earth a Christ. They dedicated their lives to the task of preparing for him the most perfect environment. They lived on a simple diet, performed essential duties, practiced eugenics and purification of body and spirit. Their preparation resulted in the virgin birth of Mary, followed by Jesus.

The Essenes were great healers, prophets, teachers, scholars, agriculturists and vegetarians. Some of their scholarly works are being discovered in the Dead Sea Scrolls.

Study books on natural childbirth and your favorite intellectual and spiritual writings. Your aspirations and activities will change the nature of the hormone balance — the environment of the fetus. A happy mother will produce a happy, healthy child. Each emotional-intellectual activity will create a new hormone and blood composition; the hormones will teach the fetus music, poetry or mathematics.

Before conception, both parents **should** detoxify their bodies for at least six months on a live food diet. Part of the cleansing should be a two or more week fast. On a fruitarian diet, at least two months after cleansing reactions have ceased and menstruation has stopped or has been reduced to a clear flow lasting no more than a few hours, you are ready for conception.

On this natural diet, you are conscious of all your body functions, including reproduction. You will know exactly when you are fertile and when you are pregnant.

In all life forms the highest concentration of nutrients is always found in the seed. The human being is no exception. To maintain an improved nutritional environment in a detoxified body, stop the loss of important nutrients (lecithin, Vitamin E, calcium, hormones) through orgasm and menstruation. During orgasm, the oxygen deprivation experienced in the bloodstream can damage the fetus brain .

Heightened emotional experience causes the ductless glands of the mother to secrete strong stimulants, which are excreted in her milk. Intercourse also reduces the nutritional value of the milk. Practice continence from before conception until the end of weaning. Animals and natives living in a natural setting follow this pattern. There is a time for everything.

Your child will need no food other than mother's milk for at least two years. When teeth start developing one is ready to start eating fruit. A child instinctively chooses fruit over all other food.

Your child may have gone through a million years of life experience through many incarnations. Provide an environment of love in which each day the child will have the freedom to open another petal of the infinite lotus centered in God. Be open; each one of you has something to teach and to learn. We are here on this planet to share, to love, to strive for the spiritual, to live simply. If what you have learned is good, pass it on to others. We must impregnate the soil with a new consciousness. From such families will grow the new earth.

The fruitarian child will be physically a youth at 80 or 240 or 978. Aging will be completely eliminated. It is not part of the makeup of such humans. The child's mind and spirit will radiate the consciousness of an infinitely wise and joyous universe. He and she will be all-knowing, all-powerful and all-loving. This will be the return of gods to the earth.

TROPICAL TRIP

Before heading for the tropics or warm climate it is important to be detoxified on a mucusless diet(see:Frutarian Festivals). It is bad enough to be confronted with language and cultural problem without also becoming sick. In dealing with the people be loving at all times, this is the only language everyone understands. If famine becomes widespread, affecting your new country of residence, there will be no safety for foreigners like yourself. Head home or for some other country. Be careful about settling in countries where there is a large contrast between the super rich and the super poor.

In warm climate the most common complains are sores, infections and boils. Even the "detoxified pure"develop problems from drinking bacteria infested water. A friend died from drinking water from a stream. Fresh juices served at commercial stands can have polluted water, milk and sugar mixed in. Vegtables may give you worm problems. The safest food is fruit.

To cope with ameobic dysentery carry tincture of Ipecacuanha. Take small doses, it can cause vomiting. Bayberry bark is good for many ailments. Burdock and Echinacea are good for skin troubles. Golden seal and garlic will aid skin, liver and other problems. Do not forget the local grasses.

Read the book Pilgrim's Guide to Planet Earth before leaving. The suggestions are verv and it has a complete directory of new age centers. Use the Mother Earth News free contact advertisement to find other sisters and brothers who would like to take a journey. For safety, females should travel with a male companion.

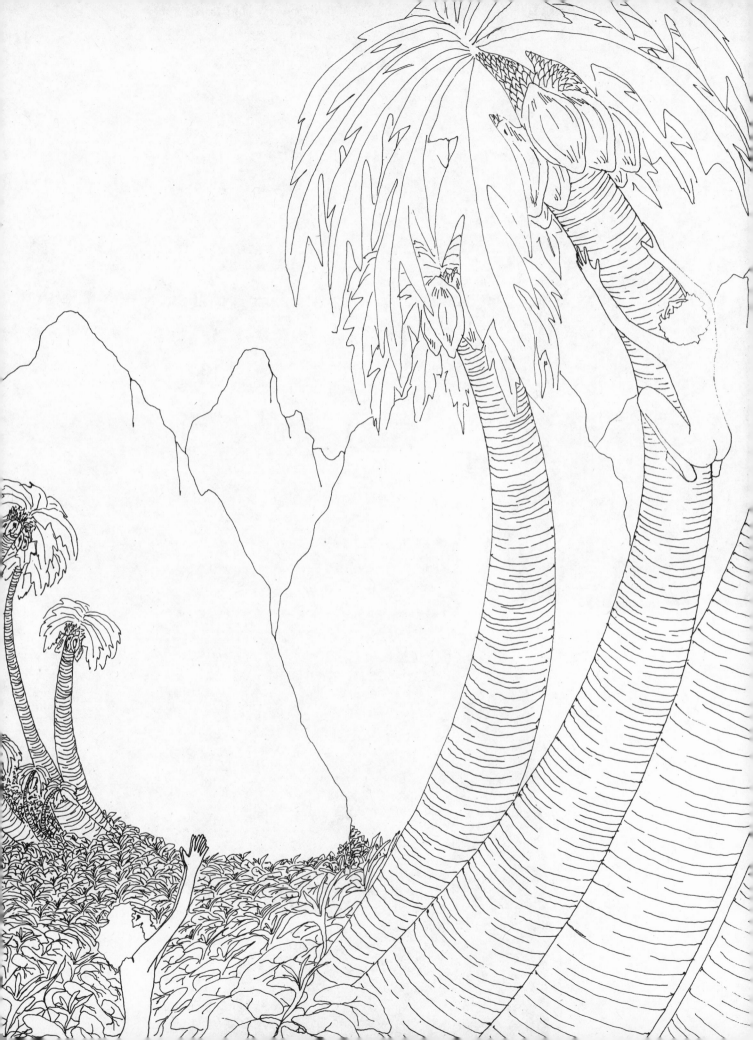

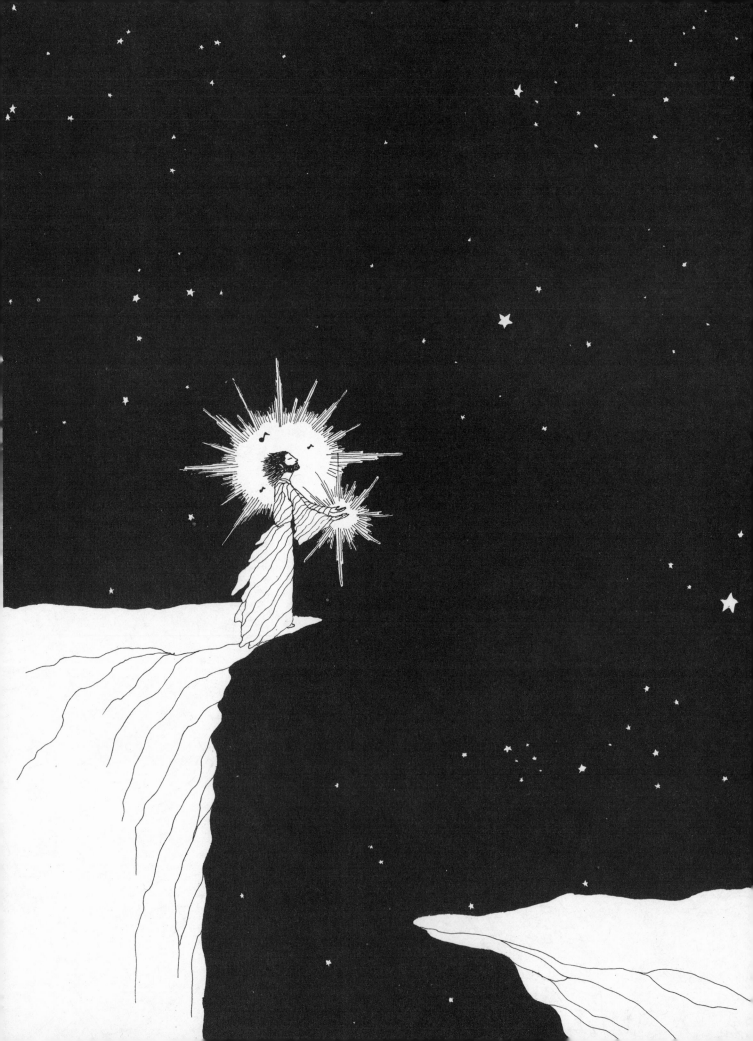

BREATHARIANISM
SUNSHINE FOR LUNCH

"NOT FOR EVERYBODY"   HESSEIAN WALL

"I can't believe that," said Alice.

"Can't you?" said the Queen in a pitying tone. "Try again. Draw a long breath and shut your eyes."

Alice laughed. "There's no use trying," she said. "One can't believe impossible things."

"Idaresay you haven't had much practice," said the Queen. "When I was your age, I always did it for half an hour a day. Why, smetimes I've believed as many as six impossible things before breakfast."

"In Christ we shall neither hunger nor thirst."   JOHN 6:35

"It is written that it is not by bread alone that one can live, but by every word which proceeds from the mouth of God '
                                                                                       Mathew 4:4

"The human being was created perfect, and placed in a garden of fruits and streams. He and she were free of all bodily appetites and had no desire to taste the fruit or quaff the water. Moreover, they had been commanded by Divine Providence not to eat or drink as that would inject foreign substances into their perfect bodies, causing them to deteriorate, decay, and die. People were mere children when a hundred years old, and none of the infirmities of age. When ready to pass on to the region of the superior life, it was a gentle slumber."

                                                                    FABLES OF ANCIENT MAGI

"Let they who seek, not cease seeking until they find, and when they find, they will not be troubled, they will marvel and will reign over the All."

                                                        THE GOSPEL ACCORDING TO THOMAS

"If you do not take food, that already frees you from this unconsciousness that you have no longer to assimilate and transform within you: that liberates energy in you. Then, as there is an instance in the being to make up for energy spent, if you do not gather it from food, i.e., from below, you make automatically an effort to draw it from the universal vital energy which is free around you. And if you can assimilate that energy, assimlate it directly, then there is no limit to your energy."
                                                                                       SRI AUROBINDO

Breatharianism was the most perfect state of the human being. He and she lived on solar radiation. The food and drug addicted masses through habitual gluttony have closed the entry of the spirit. When the stomach works, the vital force is centered in the digestive organs instead of the five sinus chambers in the head. Few search out the cosmic truths of life and put them into practice. "O how narrow is the door and how difficult is the road which carries to life, and few are those who are found on it." (Mat. 7:14)

Every life process is reversible. It might take from a few weeks to many years to make the transition back to the most fitting diet for the human being — paradisiacal fruit. Those who have the soul of Methuselah and a body fit to climb the peaks may well transcend even this height to attain breatharianism. Professor Hilton Hotema discussed the subject in   Man's Higher Consciousness. The lungs, not the stomach, are the life organs. The life line is the spinal cord, not the alimentary canal. The most vital function is breathing. "If human beings consumed only radiation through his and her respiratory organs as they did in an early Golden Age, when they lived a thousand years according to tradition, if the radiaiton were never polluted, if the procreative function remained dormant, sickness would be unknown." Professor Hotema emphasized that the return must be slow and carefully thought out: "The return or transformation to breatharianism, where food is no longer essential for body stimulation, must be slow and gradual. People must slowly reduce the amount of food ingested daily in order to give the body time to meet the new conditions and adjust to the perfect physical state of long ago, when the air people inhaled supplied all the stimulation the body needed." (166)

As one decreases food intake and evolves into a breatharian life-style, physiological changes may be anticipated. The textbook,   The Human Body (183), describes the early stages of growth of the alimentary canal: "The human digestive tract . . . in the embryo is relatively straight and uncomplicated but as development proceeds, the tubes become coiled in the abdominal region as a result of its rapid increase in length in contrast to the development of other parts of the body."

It is possible that in one or more generations, the abnormal length of the alimentary canal could be eliminated, starting with the diet and life-style of the mother. At an early fetal stage the alimentary canal is the length of the spine. By the time one reaches adulthood the canal is thirteen times the length of the spine.

There is an exchange of material between mother and fetus. If the mother is toxic and full of mucus this enters the fetal digestive tract, causing it to distend. Some newborns from extremely toxic mothers immediately vomit mucus or have a bloody stool of mucoid material. Due to faulty diet, distention of the digestive tract increases through childhood and adulthood.

A similar convolution can be observed in the development of varicose veins. At birth, the blood-carrying tubes are straight, unconvoluted and without blockages. But after many years of misuse of the body, toxic deposits cause them to stretch and bulge into varicosities. A similar phenomena, perhaps, occurs in the development of the intestine. A dietary change can reduce varicose veins to their original structure. Is it possible that, similarly, the digestive tract can be reduced in length?

When people lived on solar radiation and air, they received the exact energy needs of the body. Lungs and skin collected the needed energy and eliminated waste. When you try to balance food intake you are apt to get too much of one nutrient and not enough of others.

Depending upon the climate in which people live, in order to compensate for the intensity of sunlight, the skin pigment gets darker or lighter to insure that the right amount and quality of rays will enter the cells of the body. Pigment acts as a filter which reduces both the intensity and the quality of the light spectrum that penetrates the skin.

Dr. Alexis Carrel states that "the body seems to mold itself on events. Instead of wearing out, it changes. Our organs always improvise in meeting every situation; and these means are always such that they tend to give us maximum duration."

In our time there are enough examples of individuals who have transcended the nutritional myth to give us the feeling that "what was, can be."

One heroic figure is Barbara Moore, M.D. of London. A news release (185) reads:

"A woman of 50, who looks like she was only 30, claimed yesterday that she hates food, has beaten old age, and expects to live at least 150 years. She has set out to do it by giving up food.

"Twenty years ago she ate three normal meals a day. Slowly for 12 years she reduced her eating until she was keeping fit on one meal a day of grass, chickweed, clover, dandelion and an occasional glass of fruit juice.

"Five years ago she switched entirely to juices and raw tomatoes, oranges, grasses and herbs. Now she drinks nothing but a glass of water flavored with a few drops of lemon juice.

"She says, "There is much more in sunlight and air than can be seen with the naked eye or with scientific instruments. The secret is to find the way to absorb that extra — that cosmic radiation — and turn it into food.

"Each year she goes to Switzerland for the better air and climbs mountains on a diet of water from the streams. 'You see', she explains, 'my body cells and blood have changed considerably in composition. I'm impervious to heat and hunger or fatigue.' She continued:

" 'Winter or Summer, even in Switzerland, I wear only a short sleeved jumper and skirt. In cold weather people stare at me. While they shiver in furs, I am warm. I'm as strong as a man, and need only 3 hours sleep for mental relaxation. As my body is free of toxins, I'm never ill.

" 'I had to advance slowly from vegetarianism to uncooked fruit and then to liquid. Now I'm working towards Cosmic Food (Air). I've passed the eating stage and could not eat if I desired as my alimentary canal has changed considerably. It is no longer a filthy tube and is unable to handle any fiber.

" 'Instead of thinking my life will end in ten years, I'm growing younger. Anyone can do the same if they try. The tragedy is that eating is one of the great pleasures of life. To stop eating is to experience discomfort only when the body is adjusting itself to the new course, which was the original course. I now find even the odor of food nauseating.' "

In 1961, Dr. Morris Krok of Durban, S. Africa, published "Conquest of Disease," where he reproduced a part of a speech by Dr. Moore, (186). This is an extract:

"By experimenting on myself, I've found that neither energy nor body heat comes from food. It's a fact, paradoxical, yet true, that I spent three months in the mountains of Switzerland and Italy eating nothing but snow and drinking only snow water.

"I was climbing mountains daily, not just fasting and sitting down and reading a book or gazing at the sky. No, I was hiking daily from my hotel to the mountains, often 15 miles, climbing up to seven or eight thousand feet, then coming down and walking another 15 to 20 miles to my hotel.

"During my fasting I climbed mountains daily; and if I could not on account of bad weather, I'd walk 30 to 40 miles. That proved it to me. Year after year I've done the same thing to find out whether it's true of not. For one year it may work and the next it may not work with the same body. So I've done it year after year and find that neither energy nor heat of the body comes from physical food.

"When I discovered this I went a step further, I wanted to see whether I could live without food at all, not for two or three months, but for a longer period. I found this also possible, but not quite on an ordinary level, as it were. I can do that in the mountains, but it is more difficult when I come down to an ordinary level. I find the air is different.

"I hope in time to live entirely on air. . . . I'm a very busy person and have little time to sleep. I'm never tired or hungry."

In the press and occult magazines, there are reports of many examples of breatharians:

Balayogini Sarasvati (Amma, India) for 3 years lived on water only (187).

Marie Frutner, a Bavarian girl who lived on water without food for 40 years, was under observation for a time in Munich in 1835 (188).

Judah Mehler, Grand Rabbi, 1660-1751, ate and drank sparingly one day a week, broke his fast about twelve times a year on Jewish holidays, led a busy life as Rabbi of 3 communities, lived to be 91 (Ripley's Believe It Or Not).

Dr. T.Y. Gan (197) gave the following report on Yand Mel, age 20, who hasn't eaten for the last 9 years: She shows no signs of starvation, leads a perfectly normal life except for having lost desire for food. Her alimentary tract has become dormant and rudimentary; she takes no water.

Caribala Dassi, sister of Babulamboxer, pleader of Purilia, has been living for the past 40 years without taking food or water and has done her regular household duties with no apparent injury to her health (189).

Dhanalak Shumi of Marcara, India, age 18, for over a year took no food or water; she leads a normal healthy life. At age 14 her appetite diminished until she could not assimilate anything. The Indian government sent her to be examined at the Bangalore General Hospital, Bombay (190).

Teresa Avila, Bavarian Peasant, born 1898, has taken no food, no water and no sleep since 1926; she is not thin or sickly, works in her garden, and is described as one of the happiest persons (191).

Giri Bala, Bahar, West Bengal, now over 70 years, as a child had an insatiable appetite but has taken no food nor fluid since she was 12. She has never been sick, is an expert in pranayama and yoga, is always gay, looks like a child, does normal housework, has no bodily excretions. Her case was investigated by the late Sri Bijaly Chand Mahtab, Maharajah of Burdwan (192).

There is a beautiful simplicity in this approach. It enables one to get away from the gross and intoxicating nature of food which leads the average person to spend at least one third of his and her lifetime in the unconscious state of sleep and the rest of it in a stupor of unproductive, demoralizing labor.

The ancient ones taught in their texts that people were and are breatharian — living on solar radiation and air. Could it be possible that they were right?

LIGHT IS LIFE

"Truly the light is sweet, and a pleasant thing it is for the eyes to behold the sun."

ECCLESIASTES 11:7

Light has a physiological effect on all living things. Summer sunlight provides its worshippers with a great deal of vigor and vitamin D. Research teams are discovering that dependence on the sun is even more extensive, possibly making the difference between health and premature death. It might be stated, even more strongly, that the long term effect of air and sunlight is much more important than the diet itself. Dr. John Ott, Chairman and Executive director of the Environmental Health and Light Research Institute, states (193):

We are just beginning to find out that light entering the eyes, in addition to vision, stimulates the activity in both the pituitary and pineal glands and possibly other areas of the midbrain region that control the endocrine system and the production of hormones.

Dr. Ott became interested in light research because of a personal experience. He retired to Florida hoping the sun could improve his arthritic leg. Sun soaking failed to help. When he broke his sunglasses, sunbathing without them improved his condition in a few days, even enabling him to throw away his cane. He reported in the Optometric Weekly:

"Life on this earth since the beginning has evolved under the full spectrum of natural sunlight. Recent experimental studies have indicated that abnormal growth responses developed when any part of this natural sunlight spectral energy was blocked from entering the eyes. As people have become more civilized, living under an environment of artificial light, behind window glass, eye glasses, and particularly sun glasses of different colors, the balance of the wavelength energy entering the eye has become greatly distorted from that of natural sunlight."

Dr. Richard Wurtman, associated professor of endocrinology and metabolism in the Department of Nutrition and Food Science (M.I.T., Camb., Mass.), states, "The role of pineal cells appears to convert a neural input controlled by an exogenous factor (light) to endogenous glandular input (its hormones)." Dr. Wurtman recapitulates another study where the function of the spiritual "third eye" is discussed: "That pineal might have some photoreceptive capacity, at least in vertebrates, was postulated about 60 years ago by a Swedish anatomist. Noting that frog pineal cells are surprisingly similar in appearance to the cone cells of the retina, they speculated that the function of the frog pineal was to act as photoreceptor, or 'third eye'."

People spend over 90 percent of their lives in buildings and vehicles; they have declared themselves independent of the ocean of light in which they are immersed. Dr. Wurtman forsees a new concern in the near future "if, in fact, excess exposure to artificial light, or inadequate exposure to natural light has a harmful biological effect, we may soon find ourselves worrying about 'light pollution'".

Glass windows shut out the greatest part of the ultraviolet end of the light spectrum. Artificial lights are no substitute for the rays of the sun. A few years ago, the Russian scientists Dantsig, Lazarev and Sokolov states: "If the human skin is not exposed to solar radiation (direct or scattered) for long periods of time, disturbances will occur in the physiological equilibrium of the human system. The result will be functional disorders of the nervous system and vitamin D deficiency, a weakening of the body's defense and an aggravation of chronic disease." (193)

Dr. Ott reported in studies of insects that when you block out any part of the natural sunlight spectral energy from entering their eyes, abnormal growth of the body may result.

In a paper published by the Building Research Institute, Dr. J. Hardy says the penalty for shutting out even a small degree of natural light may be acceleration of the aging process.

Dr. Ott reports (193) that cell cultures exhibit a wider range of behavior patterns when subject to distortion of natural light:

"A blue filter that transmits only the shorter wavelengths produced an undulating of boiling motion not noticeable at normal speed but only apparent when the action is speeded up many times through time lapse photography. This abnormal activity closely resembles that of cells being attacked by viruses. When a red filter is used in the light source, restricting all but the longer wavelengths at the other end of the visible spectrum, the final death of the cell results from a rupture of the cell wall and hemorrhaging out of the cytoplasm."

Considering that pollutants in the air act as filters changing the quality of light from the sun which made life possible, there may be a compelling reason for leaving the city: "People are made of billions of universes called cells" which research shows to be light dependent. Therefore, so are people." Dr. Ott says: distortion or deficiency of natural light can cause "a biochemical or hormonal deficiency in both plant and animal cells."

Dr. Ott foresees (193): ". . . perhaps sometime in the near future the relationship between the full spectrum of the sun's natural rays and health will be better understood. Then to keep well and happy, we may find ourselves being put on 'light diets' in the same way we go on food diets today."

Research and direct observation show there may possibly be a great error on the part of the orthodox nutritionist who emphasizes the myth of a well balanced diet. Dr. Ott finds it very difficult to explain why some individuals develop nutritional deficiency symptoms while others do not on exactly the same diets.

We already know that vitamin D, which is essential to health, need not be introduced into the diet because it is created through the action of light on skin cells. This may be true for other vitamins as well. Vitamin B deficiency does not seem to affect all individuals living on identical diets.

"Residence in the tropics make it clear that a typical nutritional deficiency disease, such as beri-beri, may only affect a small percentage of the individuals living on the same diet in any particular village. Its incidence among the Philippine Scouts, for example, serving under American Officers varied between 100 and 600 from year to year out of a total of 5,000 men living on identical diets" (194).

George Ohsawa often says, "generally speaking, avoid consuming anything that contains vitamin C." The macrobiotic diet doesn't produce an obvious vitamin C deficiency. According to nutritionists, vitamin C cannot be stored in the body. You need a daily dosage. The temperature, alkaline environment and oxidation in the blood stream destroy it. Yet, macrobiotic followers do not develop scurvy. The same observation can be made about sailors who lived on board ship on identical diets. Many developed no scurvy symptoms long after some had died from the disease. It is possible that some individuals were actually manufacturing the vitamin in their bodies?

Dr. J. Lovewisdom, after several years on a largely fruitarian diet, performed an experiment which demonstrates the adequacy of air, sun and water to sustain health. He lived in the high Andes. He says: "My first long fast was endured 7 months and 7 days and 4 months later I again fasted 6 months and 17 days taking nothing but 99% pure water. Most everyone who fasts, fasts on 99% pure water since ordinary tap water contains considerable mineral matter, but I did not want the inorganic earth minerals so I used pure distilled water with a compensatory 1% from acid fruit juice of 'organic water.' The 'organic water' doesn't have a toxic waste of even 1%. Altho this 99% pure water had hardly any taste of color noticeable to others, adding the fruit juice did make it possible to drink great quantities of water, a gallon a day, that washed the whole alimentary tract. So diluted, it could not start digestive functions which brings back hunger that makes a fast practically impossible to continue. This way the digestive tract benefits from a complete rest without any unbalanced 'feeding while fasting,' so the water goes thru fast, sometimes 15 minutes after taking, serving as a natural enema. Thus my secret of such long fasts is simply in keeping the whole length of the intestines well washed, rather than letting the food residue, and even aged deposits from before one's fast, poison the blood and thus paralyze the body's muscles, cause toxic headaches, coat the tongue and even kill one." (Vitarianism, Spiritualizing Dietetics)

A yogi cataract surgeon from India said that "the peasant in India who works all day in the fields under the sun, in the evening will have a frugal meal of rice. They have been eating the same thing for ages and yet no nutritional deficiency. They get the food from the sun the way God intended."

Drs. Omen and Hipsley when studying the interior native population of New Guinea found that they showed excellent health and muscular body build. By orthodox standards, protein intake was insufficient — 15 to 20 grams daily. However studies disclosed that an additional 25 to 45% of protein was provided by internal bacteris "Clostridium refringes B," which fixed nitrogen from the air to form amino acids.

George Lakhovsky, a Russian-born scientist and medical doctor, who lived and worked in America in "The Secret Life" (195) discusses an experiment where he relates cosmic radiation to nutrition. The experiment is as significant as the demonstration of Einstein's Theory of Relativity which showed that matter can be converted into pure energy and vice versa.

"Lakhovsky's thesis is that 'body growth and maintenance depends not on food, but on cosmic rays; the body itself being a condensation of these rays' which are said to be 'streams of substance of ultra-sonic form which condense into minerals' as they contact the earth's atmosphere.

"This datum he deducted by measuring the amount of iron in unicellular organisms kept in sealed tubes. After a period of time, he found that, as the cells multiplied, the iron content of the organism increased" (195).

Several years ago, the Soviet Academy of Science publication "Transactions" (Vol. 128, No. 4) published the findings of Dr. Mikhail Valsky. Dr. Valsky incubated hen eggs in an incubator containing special air in which harmless argon gas replaced the ordinary air content. The egg-embryo died in 4 hours.

He then put other eggs in air containing the normal amount of oxygen; however, he replaced nitrogen with argon — this time the eggs lived 12 hours. Finally, the eggs were put in air containing normal components except that the nitrogen atoms were tagged. It was observed that the eggs definitely absorbed nitrogen-tagged atoms and grew chickens. Dr. Victor Kavalsky commented on Valsky's findings: "What used to be regarded as an inert gas (nitrogen) has been proven to be a gas assimilated from the air to become a part of the proteins which form animal organisms" (198).

Scientific advances show that the entire material universe is only a visible manifestation of varying condensed wave forms. Dr. H.H. Shelton, New York University wrote:

"We live in a world of waves. The further we delve into the ultimate structure of matter, the more obvious it is that nothing exists except in wave form. Electrons, long thought to be the ultimate particles of which all matter is formed, have now been shown to have a reality only as a wave form, while the atom consists of a bundle of such waves." (166)

Today it is common scientific knowledge that for most known particles, there is an anti-particle; when they come together, both are annihilated, leaving no trace. Similarly, in sound when two identical waves are out of phase they will cancel one another under proper geometrical arrangement.

Two wave forms can be added and new ones formed. Through selected filters, a complex wave form can be filtered into simpler components. In the field of nuclear physics, this could be equivalent to transmuting one atom into other atoms, not compounds. This alchemist's dream has been fulfilled in nuclear labs through the use of enormous amounts of energy and the particle accelerator. In the human body such reactions are carried out through the use of low intensity biological energy and the most precise bio-nuclear forces.

L. Kervran (196) presents overwhelming evidence that the alchemist's dream is active in the biological laboratories. L. Kervran describes the following experiment which showed transmutation of nitrogen into carbon and oxygen:

"In 1961, a rat was confined to a sealed tube for two months (along with chlorella and oxygen). The animal survived the experiment. When the sealed tube was opened it was found that the percentage of nitrogen in the air inside the tube had decreased by two thirds while the oxygen simultaneously increased."

Kervran shows that to produce potassium from the fusion of sodium and calcium about four electron volts (4ev) of energy is required. This could be furnished from the sun by a short ultra-violet ray, wave length 3,000 angstroms. Other experiments show that matter is being created from solar radiation through the condensing effect of cell geometry. As an example "the nitrogen diet is lowered below the level of normal excretion by the intestine. The excreted quantity remains higher than the total ingested quantity. Since nutrition could not supply nitrogen, endogenic production must be responsible" (196).

Emma Dietz of Harvard University in the Journal of Chemical Education wrote that chlorophyll "absorbs energy from the sun and in some unknown way uses it for the manufacture of sugar, starch and protein."

Dr. Dietz finds it difficult to comprehend that chlorophyll and hemoglobin should be so similar in structure yet play such different roles. "In the slow development of the chemistry of these two pigments, it has been an increasing source of wonder to chemists to find that two substances of such widely differing origin and function are yet so remarkably alike in structure."

Is such discrepancy between structure and function possible? I believe it is not. My belief is that hemoglobin, which constitutes a major portion of the blood solids, when unobstructed by food, in a high altitude tropical environment, will maintain the body in good nutritional balance indefinitely by converting solar radiation into essential nutrient vibrations. Nutrients are trapped solar vibrations which constitute the basis for diet. The bulk that is associated with food has to be expelled once the energy has been stripped from it. The thousands of individuals who have lived without food give weight to this argument.

The plant kingdom is made up of "light eaters." There are also some highly evolved spiritual beings who likewise are "sunlight and air eaters." The hemoglobin rich blood is changed by its encounter with light as it journeys from sun illumined skin on its journey to bring light to the dark interior of the body. The skin is the organ of "light" nutrition assimilation, just as the lung is the organ for the ingestion of "air" nutrition.

LOVE LIGHT

All matter is light waves in motion, and within light and its spectrum lies the secret of all life. The very air we breathe is permeated with the forces of light and color and the vital energy or prana that imparts and sustains life. We extract this living force from the food we eat, the water we drink, and the air we breathe.

As a wave of light is projected through space, it creates a certain rhythm — a harmonious vibration of etheric matter. The trinity of colors red, yellow and blue have a definite correspondence with the three basic elements hydrogen, carbon and oxygen. The chemicals and minerals are there because of the action of the color of the sun's rays. When we breathe we absorb prana, cosmic and solar radiation and not just oxygen and other chemical ingredients.

The source of all terrestrial life — the Sun — contains within it everything of which the earth is composed and the human body as well, if it is not too depleted. That is, if we are getting the proper quantities of necessary air and food elements, the body has the ability to choose the specific color it needs from the sun. When we sunbathe or airbathe our skin breathes and our aura picks up the color it needs and rejects the others. When we eat any kind of food we are actually eating color from the sun.

COLOR CHAKRAS

Color is the great cosmic healing force which works directly on the etheric cells, replenishing and revitalizing them. Light and color have a direct action on the protoplasm of the body. They penetrate and influence the body activity by arousing sympathetic vibrations within the organism. Let us suppose that we are eating the right kind of food and yet we are not able to assimilate the elements we need. The scientific application of one or more of the visible colors will aid our bodies in making use of these elements. When light and color enter the body, the homogeneous particles are thrown into sympathetic vibration and the organism is vitalized and recharged. Health is the condition of perfect equilibrium, perfect rhythm and harmony throughout the organism.

It is important that we live in harmony with the colors of our own aura. A great deal of discord and antagonism between members of families and groups of people closely associated arises from cross-vibrations due to inharmonious color combinations within the personal aura and environment. When the auric emanations of any two individuals in close proximity to each other are not in harmony, there is no possible chance for peace and mutual understanding to exist between these persons unless they can neutralize the inharmonious vibrations by manifesting some other color vibration which will blend with the former. If these persons can through meditation, love or through the use of the Color Rays (colored lights) open a channel for the regenerating White Light to change and raise the unstable vibrations and establish its own equilibrium, then disharmony will no longer be active.

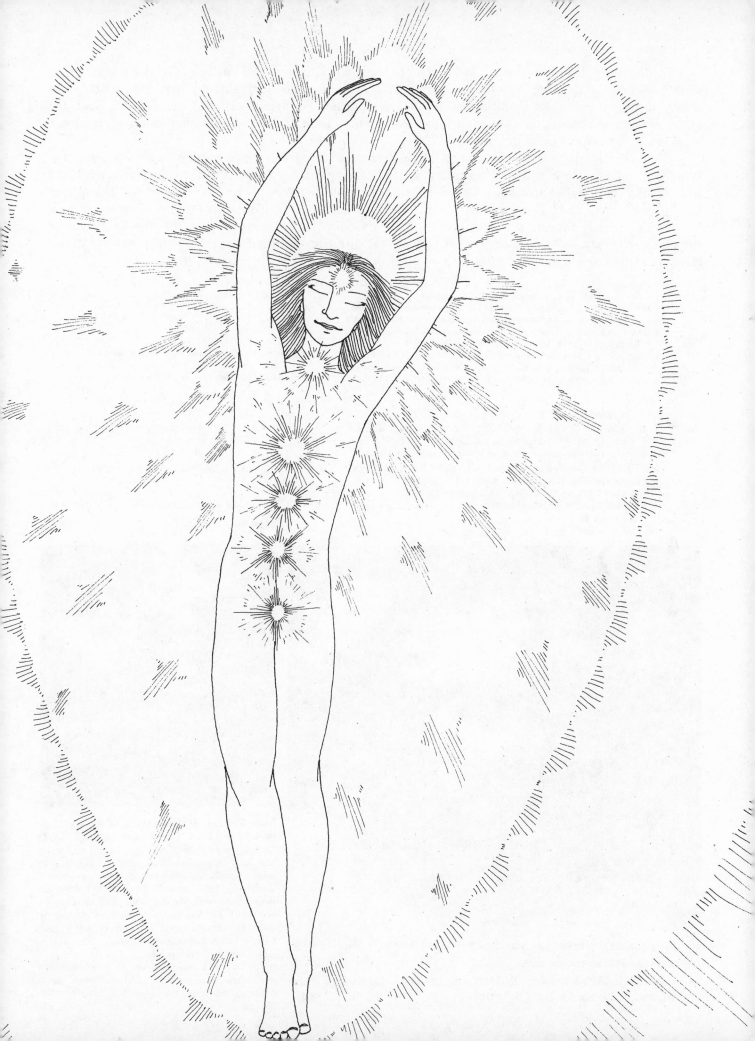

In the near future we will all be able to experience visibly and audibly the color and sound vibrations emanating from the human form. "We as individuals undoubtedly have no existence in reality other than waves, multitudinous and complicated centers, perhaps, in what we call the ether. We are analogous, in a sense, to the sounds that issue from a piano when a chord is struck or when a symphony orchestra sounds" (200).

The chemistry of the fruitarian bloodstream contains the seed which will compose the symphony of the new body. Many mortals are working hard to give birth to the new from the soil of the old. Sri Aurobindo says, "The body could become a revealing vessel of a supreme beauty and bliss, casting the beauty of the light of the spirit suffusing and radiating from it as a lamp reflects and diffuses the luminosity of its dwelling flame, carrying in itself the beatitude of the spirit, its joy of the seeing mind, its joy of life and spiritual happiness, the joy of Matter released into a spiritual consciousness and thrilled with a constant ecstasy" (201).

SUGGESTED READING MATERIAL

1. Search Magazine July, 1957, Article "Their Food Is Thin Air" K.M. Talgari.
2. SPIRITUALIZING DIETETICS, VITARIANISM, Prof. Johnny Lovewisdom.
3. LIVE 1400 YEARS, THE EMPYREAL SEA, Prof. Hotema [Health Research].
4. MAN'S HIGHER CONSCIOUSNESS, Prof. Hotema [Health Research].
5. THE SECRET OF LIFE, Dr. Lokovsky, M.D. [Health Research].
6. FOOD SCIENCE FOR ALL AND A NEW SCIENCE OF SUNLIGHT THEORY OF NUTRITION, Dr. Bircher — Benner, M.D. [Health Research].
7. MAN, THE UNKNOWN, Alexis Carrel, Nobel Prize Winner [DeVorss Books].
8. A REVALUATION OF ULTRAVIOLET AS A VITAL PART OF THE TOTAL SPECTRUM by John Ott Sc. D [Obrig Labs Inc., P.O. Box 1899, Sarasota, Fla.].

1. IEEE Trans. Biomed. Engin. 15:4 Tan 68.
2. J. Anim. Sci. 27:684, May 68; Light, Nutrition & Reproduction.
3. J. Dairy Sci. 50:4475 Sep. 67; Sex & Light.
4. Science, 161:489, 2 Aug. 68; Xtra retinal response to light.
5. VOP PITAN 25:82, Sep/Oct 68; The Effect of Natural Ultraviolet Radiation on the Blood Ascorbic Acid level in Animals.
6. ERGONOMICS 11:23, Jan. 68. Light Effect on Man.
7. Clin Pediat (Phila) 8:499, Sep. 69. Light on Light.
8. ARCH BIOCHEM 123:468, 11 MR 68, Free Radicals in Skin.
9. J. Vitamins 13:173 & 130, Jan., 67.
10. New England J. Med.. 280:1075. 8 May 69.

"And seek not what you shall eat and what you shall drink."   LUKE 12:29

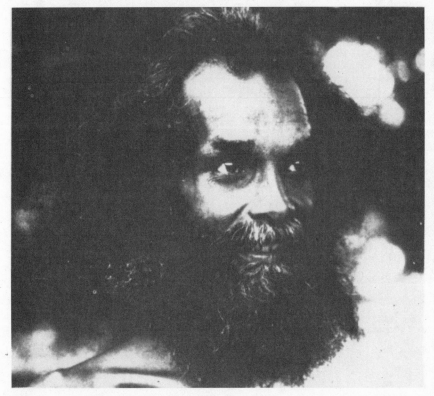

Shivapuri Baba, 112 years of age, who died recently at the age of 135. He was a fruitarian for at least two decades.

LONG PILGRIMAGE, J. Bennett. (Hodder Group Sales Div., Saint Paul's House 8/12 Warwick Lane, London E.C.4 Britain)

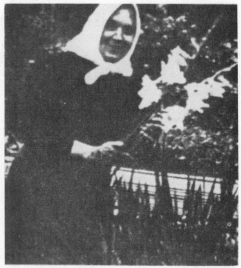

From TERESE NEUMANAITE, J. Burkus (Suduvos Press 4434 S Fairfield Ave, Chicago, 1953). Teresa , since 1926 , has daily 1 tsp of water and holy communion. Her sleep is a 20 minute meditation . Her favorite work is growing flowers for the church. In physical activity she never seems tired. She is psychic and has done astral travel. Her foodless living has been attested by scientific committees (dr. Fr. Gerlich , Die Stigmatisierte Teresa Newman von Konnersreuth, I 128-136; Also J. Teodorowicz, in the Life of Teresa Newman, p. 326 - 343). She is stigmatic, during which period she losses up to 6 pounds. She gains the weight back after an evening rest.

LONGEVITY

LOST WISDOM OF THE ANCIENTS as shared in publications of Health Research:

Why the unprepared mind cannot separate truth from falsehood. Physical instruments show the inner or solar being exists in a vibratory plane far above that of the body. The body is physical, the occupant of it is 4th dimensional. Mind power is infinite and limitless; it crosses the time-space barrier; it penetrates steel as easily as space.

The individual controls his or her destiny, works out salvation and completion by knowing the following: the divine processes of the body, the dormant organs and lost powers, the mysterious chambers in the skull (the sinuses), the workings of the glands, the positive and negative solar organs in the body, the seven seals or chakras, how the kundalini gives liberation to the yogi and bondage to the fool, purpose and development of pineal gland and pituitary body, the laws of rhythm, polarity and correspondence; cosmic polarity, cosmic trinity; how to transmute sex force into brain power, the five kinds of cosmic prana, breathing, law of birth, death degeneration, regeneration, immortality.

The meaning of immortality. The symbology of the sacred beetle which is self-begotten. When the creative fires have passed up through the spine and activated the pituitary and pineal glands opening the single eye that fills the body with light, the human being is then raised up, not from an earthly grave but in a state of consciousness where the glory of God can be realized.

The human being was placed in a garden. This home was not a hostile region of ice and snow, but a place perfect for habitation and equal in state to the perfection of the being created to occupy it, thus perfect correspondence prevailed.

And then, according to the Bible, it required only eight generations for the human being to disrupt that harmony. And in eight generations more the degenerative effect of the disruption caused the human life span to hit the low mark of 148 years, in the case of Nahor (Gen. 11:26). And it has hovered around that point ever since.

People were free of all bodily appetites and desires. Perfection lacks nothing and needs nothing. It is completion. But civilization is opposed to perfection.

Better living for longer life will never be taught in public institutions. Better living for longer life brings reproach down upon all who favor it publicly and was the basic cause of the crucifixion of the gospel Jesus.

Authors of natural history assert the wild hog in its native state lives to the age of 300 years; the eagle lives 500 years; some parrots live 600 and 700 years and some turtles live 500 years.

The human being, the climax of Creation, the most perfect organization produced in billions of years, should logically outlive all other animals. No scientist has ever been bold enough to place a limit on human duration. All data on that point is based on past experience, and experience is what has been but is not what should be.

If one animal can live 500 years, why can't the human being? It's possible to learn the reason for a turtle's longevity. By applying those principles to our way, we too would live, to say the least, as long as a turtle. Some day it will be done when medical art has vanished and passed into history.

Flora Thomson of North Carolina died in 1808 at the age of 152. Zora Agha died in Turkey in 1935 at the age of 162. Jose Calverto of Mexico died in 1921 at the age of 186. Thomas Garn of England died in 1795 at the age of 207. Le Chung-Yun of China died in 1933 at the age of 256. Numas De Cugna of India died in 1565 at the age of 370. According to Homer, Dando the Illyrian, lived over 500 years. (MAN'S HIGHER CONSCIOUSNESS, Hotema)

Wm. F. Warren, in his book, PARADISE FOUND OR THE CRADLE OF THE HUMAN RACE presents the opinion that humankind originated on a tropical continent, now at the bottom of the ocean, the famed Hyperborea of the ancient Greeks, a land of fruits and flowers whose inhabitants, a race of gods, lived more than a thousand years without the infirmities of aging.

The consensus of writers on the subject from the time of the ancient Greeks to the present day unite in contending that the human being is a tropical inhabitant and lived for centuries in health and vigor.

No feature of the Adamic period in the Bible is more strongly painted and emphasized than the warm climate of the Edenic World. The human dwelling naked in Eden's clime says in plain language that there was no alternation of summer and winter. This eternal summer, it must be seen, is necessary to make complete the harmony of the ancient historian's account.

The interminable struggle of the body to live under hostile conditions of the environment and abusive treatment provides material for the silly stories that fill medical books, in which the numerous phases of that life-and-death struggle are given names in Greek and remedies in Latin and never a hint as to the basic cause of that life-and-death struggle.

Probably no one has investigated more thoroughly the topic of longevity than Professor Hilton Hotema, who, past the age of ninety, continued to publish his results. He felt that a frugal fruitarian diet with fasting, pollution free air, high altitude of mountains — preferably tropical — loving friends and infrequent sex activity were essential prerequisites for a long life. Here are a few historic notes, where he traces fruitarian diet and longevity as found in Man's Higher Consciousness (166):

Herodotus wrote:

"The oldest inhabitants of Greece, the Pelasgians, who came before the Dorian, Ionian and Eolian migrations, inhabited Arcadia and Thessaly, possessing the Islands of Lesbos and Lokemanos, which were full of orange groves. The people, with their diet of dates and oranges, lived on the average of more than 200 years."

LI-CHING YUN GAVE HIS AGE 197 INQUIRY PUT AGE AT 256

"Your body may seem much the same to you as it was a year ago, plus or minus a few pounds or inches, but . . . in a single year 98% of the old atoms will be replaced by the new atoms which we take into our bodies from the air we breathe. the food we eat, and the water we drink."   DR. PAUL G. AEBERSOLD, Atomic Energy Comm. (140)

"Li Ching-Yun, resident of Kaihslen, in the province of Szechwan, who contended that he was one of the world's oldest men and said he was born in 1783 — which would make him 197 years old — died today.

"Compared with estimates of Li Ching-Yun's age in previous reports from China the above dispatch is conservative. In 1930 it was said Professor Wu Chung-chien, dean of the department of Education in Minkuo University, had found records showing Li was born in 1677 and that the Imperial Chinese Government congratulated him on his 150-th and 200-th birthday.

"For the first hundred years he continued at his occupation (gathering herbs). According to one version of Li's married life he had buried twenty-three wives and was living with his twenty-fourth, a woman of 60 . . . Many who have seen him recently declared that his facial appearance is no different from that of person two centuries his junior." (S. Fred Strong, New York Times, May 6, 1933. p. 13)

William Goodell learned while he was in Canton in 1833 that Li "was a vegetarian who ate only herbs that grew above the ground and fruit of high alkaline content." Richard Lucas believes "Li's longevity was due to his strictly vegetarian diet, his calm and serene attitude toward life and the fact that he used two powerful rejuvenating herbs prepared as teas. One of the herbs was Fo-ti-Tieng and the other was ginsing." (Nature's Medicines, Wilshire Book Co., N. Hollywood, Calif.)

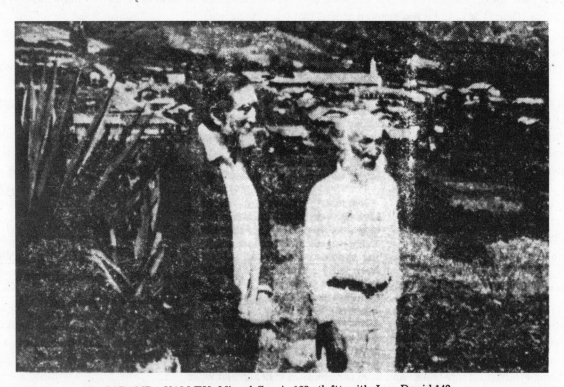

VILCABAMBA VALLEY. Miquel Carpio 123, (left) with Jose David 142.

Dr. David Davies, a professor at London University, 1973. on a field trip discovered Vilcabamba Valley, Ecuador, Dr. Davies stated: "Their diet is mainly vegetarian — oranges, bananas, apples and lots of vegetables. They eat only an ounce of meat a week and virtually no animal fat."

Pride of the clan was an energetic farmer Jose David. "I could hardly believe this man was 142 years old," Dr. Davies said. "He was grumpy because we were interrupting his work. He could not wait to get back to hoeing his vegetable garden."

(National Tattler, June 24, 1973)

"Dr. Guillermo Vela of Quito found a strikingly low caloric consumption also among the elderly of Vilcabamba. The average daily diet provided 1,200 calories. The daily protein intake was 35 to 38 grams, and of fat only 12 to 19 grams; 200 to 260 grams of carbohydrate completed the diet. Protein and fat again were largely of vegetable origin, with only few grams of protein daily from animal sources. Needless to say, one sees no obesity among the elderly in either Vilcabamba or Hunza; neither were there signs of undernutrition."

(National Geographic, Jan. 1973)

Again:

"'The pelasgians and the people who came after them in Greece, ate fruit of the virgin forests and blackberries from the fields."

Putarch observed:

"The ancient Greeks, before the time of Lycurgus, ate nothing but fruit."

Onomacritus of Athens, a contemporary of Peisitratus, said:

"In the days before Lycurgus, each generation reached the age of 200 years."

Philochorus said of the Pelesgians:

"Their heroic spirit and their strong arms to destroy their foe were formed of shiny red apples from the forest. Apples were their favorite foods, and the speed of their feet never lessened. They raced against stags and won. They lived for hundreds of years in the world of Cronus: but their vast stature never diminished as they grew old, even by thumb's breadth. The dark lustre of their hair was never tainted by a single silver thread."

"The human being is potentially immortal . . . a self-repairing machine; yet the individual becomes decrepit and dies, and the reason is a mystery."
                                                              DR. LINUS PAULING, Press, Feb. 19, 1960

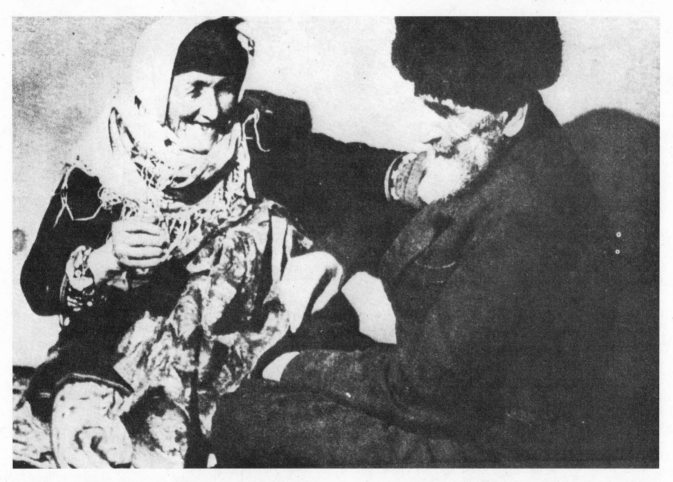

Shirali Mislimov with his wife, a mere teenager of 120. According to Soviet records he was born in 1805 in Azerbaijan, a constituent republic of the USSR noted for the longevity of its people. He wed at 65.

The Soviets claim that Shirali Mislimov is 167 years old, that he was born in the high mountain settlement of Lerik in Azerbaijan, a constituent republic of the Soviet Union, west of the Caspian Sea, on May 19, 1805, one year after Napoleon I became Emperor of France.

Like other centenarians of his region, Mislimov attributes his longevity to long-lived parents, his delayed sex life — he was not married until he was 65 — and to an active and serene life both as farmer and carpenter.

Never obese, competitive, or ambitious, never gluttonous for the delights of food and flesh, convinced that a thin horse is necessary to run a long race, Mislimov tells researchers that he has always been satisfied with his role in life, and that he has always practiced self-control.

In the town of Barzava, he works daily in the fruit orchard he planted more than 100 years ago; he takes long walks always with his grand or great-grand children. He eats sparingly, mostly vegetables and fruit, drinks wine, abstains from tobacco, rarely worries.
                                                                    PARADE, SEPTEMBER 24, 1972

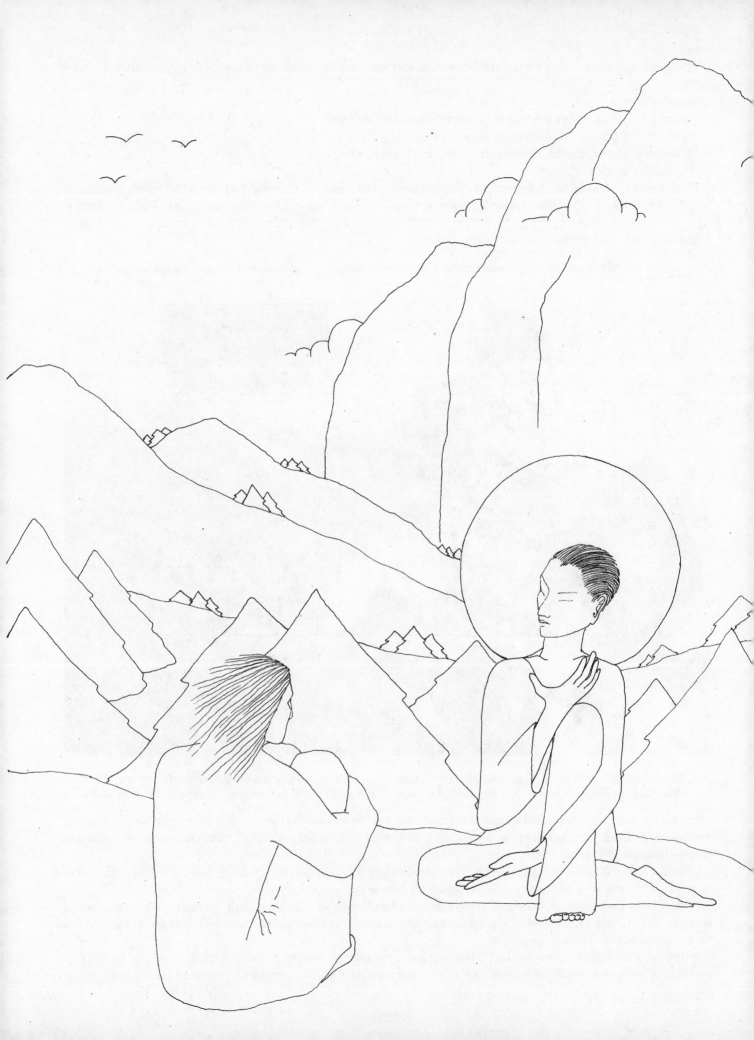

YOGA

INTRODUCTION TO GOD

You don't have to be living on a mountaintop in a detoxified body to pursue a spiritual discipline, though it might help. Yoga is a discipline compatible with whatever life-style you choose. It is the most complete, most basic system I know for developing a healthy body, mental alertness, emotional stability and spiritual growth.

Yoga means union. There are many paths in Yoga for it is all life inclusive. There is no mystery in yoga — it is not difficult to find teachers and books. It is available and useful to anyone at any stage of his or her development.

Although yoga may be learned from a book, it is wise to study with an experienced teacher. Such a teacher can teach you, from the beginning, correct technique, help you to choose the exercises which will most benefit you, and restrain you from doing those which are too strenuous for you.

A yoga class can give you the support of group energy. The group consciousness will encourage you to persevere in mastering this discipline. Group yoga will open to you the joyous experience of chanting and dancing, making and listening to inspiring music with your brothers and sisters.

Serious practice of yoga can take you as far as you want to go. Whether you develop slowly or quickly does not matter. Do not be anxious; just do what feels best to you. You may not wish to go beyond the practice of hatha yoga.

If you commit yourself to yoga and practice it regularly, it will serve you in this world. It will make you healthier, stronger, a better worker, more clear-thinking, more relaxed and loving.

Meditation will open the door to God Who is within you. You will gain access to eternal knowledge and experience the universal truths in whatever religion or philosophy you pursue.

Eventually you can know all, become perfectly humble, desireless, happy to serve, to become the eyes, ears, hands, feet of God. You will be prepared to survive the purificatory cataclysms of earth or die without fear.

WHO IS GOD?

The entire universe, material and spiritual, is manifested out of, sustained by and eventually dissolved back into an eternal, changeless, supreme reality which is pure consciousness called God.

The entire range of manifested things in the universe are various complex patterings of this basic essence and thence they ultimately return. The appearance of the various distinct manifestations in the universe are the product of constantly changing time-space relationships. These outward appearances have no permanent reality and are an illusion in the sense that they hide the real inner essence of God.

Science progressively approaches this central concept of yoga philosophy. It has been discovered and proven that matter is merely a concentrated form of energy. In its effort to discover the smallest and most basic material constituents of the universe, modern science first discovered the atom and then the components of the atom: protons, electrons and neutrons. More recently a host of new basic atomic particles, such as positrons, mesons, neutrenos and photons have been discovered and there is no end in sight. The further science goes, the more subtle, the more energy-like and the less material are the particles it finds and the less limited by time and space they seem to be. The ultimate end of this investigation will undoubtedly be pure consciousness.

All change is due to motion or the rearrangement of energy patterns relative to each other. Time as measured on any level of manifestation is merely the comparison of changes. Space is merely the comparison or the measurement of the interrelationship between sustained or standing cyclical vibrating energy patterns which are familiar to us as the various shapes and forms found within the universe.

The appearance of matter or any energy pattern in the universe is like a stationary eddy over a stone in the bed of a stream. The same water never flows over the stone and yet the eddy above the stone remains permanently the same, as a conditioning of the flow of the water. Absolute being or pure consciousness moves with infinite speed through every manifestation in the universe. The energy patterns in the universe, material or otherwise, are only visible details of the otherwise homogeneous flow of pure consciousness.

God as pure consciousness, sum of all existence, cause of all creation, the eternal changeless principle within every manifestation in the universe, registers and experiences every vibration pattern and hence the form, motion and condition of every manifestation. Since it is moving through every manifestation at infinite speed, these patterns are transmitted throughout the entire universe instantaneously. At the level of pure consciousness the entire universe can be seen from any point in space. All the energy in the universe is present in its entirety within every infinitely small point in space simultaneously and passes through all of these points in an infinitely short period of time. Infinity passes in a split second of the eternal now. Past, present and future exist in the present instant and that instant is eternity. Every point within God or pure existence receives and gives love, radiates and absorbs the radiations of all other points.

The more subtle and rapid in vibration any level of existence, the more permanent and less subject to change it is. Pure consciousness is omnipresent, motionless, with an absolute, transcendent quiescence which nothing can perturb or influence in any way. This is the anvil against which the souls of people are forged. Great mystics, who have experienced states of ecstasy and illumination, speak of a presence, a stillness, an absolute peace.

Pure consciousness within us is enlightenment in all the processes of living. In God-consciousness, full enlightenment can be experienced in any point of space in any manifestation in creation. God, or pure consciousness, the ultimate conscious energy, is the cosmic supply of all the substance of which everything is created.

MANY BODIES ONE SOUL

We are well aware that we are more than just our physical body. We are equipped with a series of subtle energy bodies called vehicles or sheaths of the soul. The subtle bodies interpenetrate each other and occupy the same space. These organized vibration patterns are used by the highest aspects of our consciousness as instruments of action and expression. The physical body is but the densest and least permanent of this series of bodies.

There are four bodies which compose our personality nature. These are the physical body, the etheric body, the astral or desire body, and the mental body. The physical and etheric bodies actually form one unit since the etheric body is composed of the matter of the higher subplanes of the physical planes.

The etheric body has the same shape or form as the physical body and interpenetrates the physical body in the same way that air interpenetrates the porous body of a sponge. For every physical organ there is a corresponding etheric organ which interpenetrates it. The etheric body is the energy matrix; around its substance the physical body is organized. Defects in the etheric body are often reflected in the physical body as disease. The condition of the etheric body is in turn determined by the nature of our emotional and mental activity. The condition of the etheric body determines the amount of physical vitality which we feel or possess. A healthy etheric body gives a person a quality of radiance and magnetism.

Memory is dependent upon the etheric body; memory pattern impulses must be transmitted through it in order to register in physical brain awareness. Emotional feelings and mood dispositions exist in the desire body. The etheric body reflects the patterns existing in the desire and mental bodies and impresses them on the physical nervous system and endocrine glands, causing the physical body to respond.

Mistreatment of or accidents to the physical body also affect the etheric body since it must employ its energy to repair the physical body. If, due to mistreatment of the physical body, the etheric body is overworked, the etheric vitality is drained and the etheric body is unable to properly transmit the impressions made by the mental and emotional bodies. The person in this condition seems to be mentally and emotionally unresponsive.

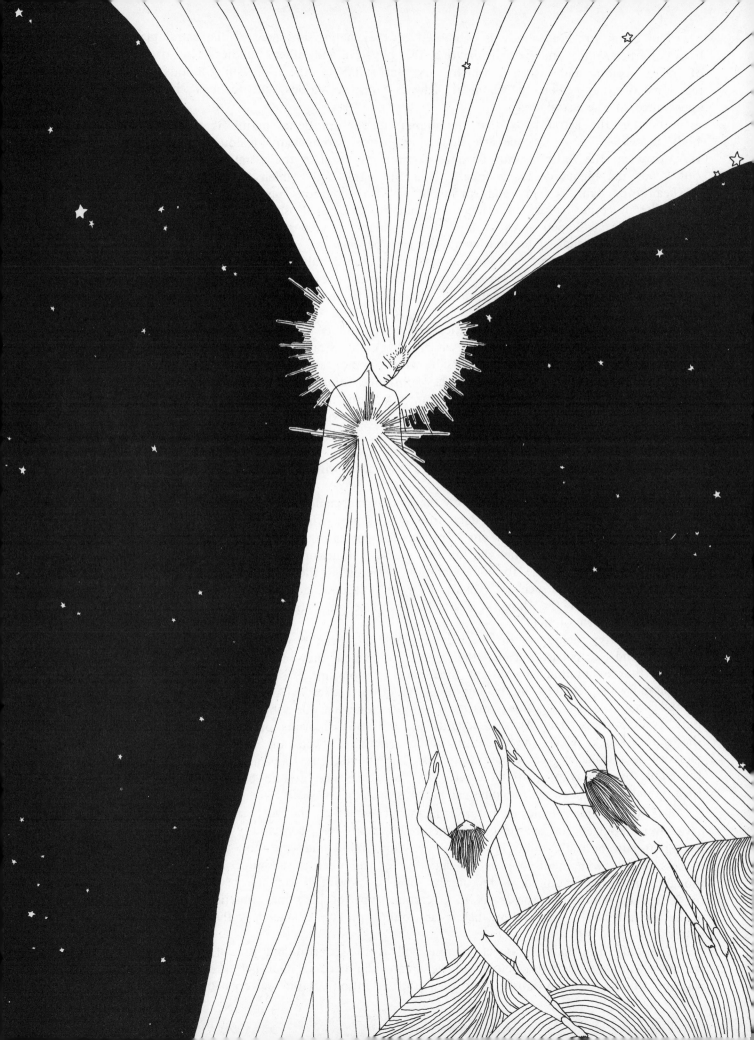

The astral or desire body is composed of the energy substance of the astral plane. The astral body interpenetrates and extends beyond the physical and etheric bodies. This ovoid is composed of many colors and textures which vary according to the prevailing moods and emotional reactions of the person to whom it belongs. As the moods and feelings change, so does the appearance of the astral body.

It is in the astral body that the drama of our emotional nature is played out. This is the body in which we experience love, hate, joy, sorrow, compassion, jealousy, humor, awe, reverence, fear, courage; the entire gamut of human emotions. It is in the astral body that the war between our lower and higher desires is fought. It is the astral body which reveals our emotional habits by its beauty or ugliness. Pure and spiritually uplifting emotions reveal themselves in the astral body as areas of pure color, of pure spectromatic or pastel shades. Destructive emotions reveal themselves as misshapen areas of grey, brown, black, muddy red, slimy green or other dull colors. A person's emotional state and character can be read by a clairvoyant who is able to see and interpret the color, shape, contour and texture of the astral body.

Any long-held emotion leaves a sort of permanent imprint or preconditioning in the astral body which makes it easier and more automatic to indulge in the same emotion in the future. The astral body attracts and incorporates into its field of activities the substance and energy of the astral plane around it. It automatically attracts and is influenced by those astral thought forms and environmental astral influences which our own astral body vibrates in resonance with. We cannot attract anything from the outside which is not already present to some degree within our own being. We select and qualify the substance which we incorporate into the astral body according to the emotions we allow our attention to dwell upon. The higher and purer the quality of our emotions, the higher will be the vibratory rate of the astral substance we incorporate into our astral bodies.

Most thought forms are not merely mental patterns but also have astral matter incorporated into them according to the emotions we associate with the idea or thought form pattern in question.

The mental body is composed of the energy substance of the mental plane. It is the central clearing house of all input of data from the senses, the emotions and the higher faculty of intuition. It is responsible for our capacity for logical thinking, planning and purposeful action. The mental body is also the seat of the memory function where our thoughts, experiences and concepts are stored in the form of vibration patterns. If the thought pattern relates to a concrete situation or an object such as a chair, it is an exact scale model of that object or remembered scene of activity. If the thought is an abstract concept, it takes the form of a beautiful, intricate geometrical pattern of light.

Once energy belonging to the mental plane has been organized into a vibration pattern, the patterns tend to persist because the energy of which they are composed vibrates in a cyclical manner, thus maintaining a constant time-space relationship.

Memory is achieved by reading these vibration patterns (Akashic Records) within one's own mental body. Akasha, meaning space, is simply homogeneous vibration of energy on any plane of pure consciousness. The Akashic records are vibration imprints on the homogeneous vibration of the pure Akasha. When the attention or consciousness dwells on any such vibration imprint, the memory is recalled to conscious awareness. The memory is transmitted from the mental body to the brain by means of patterns created in the desire and etheric bodies which, in turn, transmit their vibration patterns to the physical nervous system.

The unconscious mind is nature's memory; whatever thought, emotions and perceptions we have ever indulged in are recorded there. Whenever we consciously finish with a thought or feeling, it automatically drops into the unconscious mind and continues to operate as an automatic process which will predispose us to act, think, and feel in a similar way in the future. Any thought or feeling indulged in repeatedly forms a powerful complex of vibration patterns in the subtle bodies which predisposes us to a certain type of behavior, sometimes even against our will or better judgment. This is how habits are built up. Our character is the composite of our habit patterns.

The most fundamental aspect of free will is the control and use of our attention. Whatever we allow our attention to dwell upon, we create and become. Our habits develop according to the way in which we have most often used the attention. Habit patterns obey Newton's first law which states that any object in a state of rest or uniform motion relative to its surroundings will remain in that condition unless acted upon by an outside force. Therefore, to change habits, we must apply will in the form of concentration to direct the flow of attention to new modes of behavior until the old habit vibration pattern is deflected into a new one. Once this transference has taken place, the new habit is just as easy, or easier, to maintain if it is in harmony with cosmic law and the vibration of the universe which constitutes the total environment. Good habits are self-maintaining energy patterns.

There are certain constructive mental habits which we need to develop. It is important to finish a thought, and, when speaking, to finish a sentence with its line of reasoning. We should never attempt to finish another person's expression or idea or to interrupt until he or she has finished the idea which he or she wishes to express. Breaking off in the middle of a thought or a sentence creates an incomplete thought form and litters the psychic atmosphere with useless matter.

Mantras, sounds, music all create their characteristic vibration patterns in mental energy and on the other subtle planes. The spoken word is particularly powerful in creating thought forms. Much harm can be done by idle chitchat. Unless we have something worthwhile to say, we should say nothing. It is the spiritual duty of everyone to think and concentrate before speaking.

The mind moves in cycles of concentration and relaxation. We should observe the mind in all its modes of activity from the level of consciousness; only then can we control it and master it. We must master the mind or it will master us.

Yoga practice is based on learning how to gain control over the attention. The individual who can master his or her attention can master anything. Concentration is sustained attention on one subject or process.

The more microscopic attention becomes, the more macrocosmic its experience. The more one concentrates within a point, the more that point becomes inclusive of the whole universe. Concentration produces intelligence and not vice versa. One who truly learns to concentrate will never lack intelligence.

Meditation is concentration on that pure existence out of which the entire universe is manifested. The place where that universal essence of consciousness must first be found is within the individual. To accomplish anything in life we must always start with ourselves. If the attention is kept constantly on the essence of pure being which is pure consciousness within ourselves, we realize our identity with that pure consciousness which is God.

The mental body is the great communicator between the various aspects and vehicles which compose our nature. Pure consciousness has direct perception of truth, but the mind must be the transmitter and communicator of that truth. The mental body is the link through which the purpose of the soul is translated into action on the mental, astral, etheric and physical levels.

Chaos on any level can only be overcome by reordering that chaos from the next highest plane. Each body may be controlled by the body which is next highest in vibration, and all bodies may be controlled by pure consciousness. The disorder of the physical body can be overcome by the directive imprint of the etheric body. The disorder of the etheric body can be healed by the soothing vibrations of the astral body. The emotional turmoil of the astral body can be balanced and properly directed by the purposeful, rational guidance of the mental body. The mental confusion, inaccurate concepts, and ignorance of the mental body can be overcome by the direct knowing of pure consciousness.

It becomes clear that the physical body and the subtle bodies must all work together as a team. This can be accomplished when their vibratory rates are in proper attunement with each other, just as the strings of a piano must be tuned so that the notes are in harmony with each other. The soul, the supreme musican, cannot play a beautiful melody of harmonious living until our instrument is perfectly tuned and the vibrations of all the notes are in proper mathematical relationship to each other.

The mineral kingdom has only an organized physical body. The vegetable kingdom has an organized physical body and an etheric body; thus it is capable of growth and reproduction. Animals have an organized physical, etheric and astral body. Animals are capable of emotional feeling, but not of logical feeling and thinking. We have an organized mental body as well, which makes us thinkers capable of independent judgment, planned action and free choice. For this reason, we are individually responsible for our actions. We can logically choose between good and evil, harmony and chaos. We have an all-knowing body of intuition on which we can learn to rely for direct guidance. On the intuitional level, the knower and the object known become one through the omnipresent, instantaneous circulation of the energy of consciousness.

The next step in our evolution is to go beyond the mental level to the Buddhic plane. When this is accomplished, we will leave the human, or fourth kingdom in nature, and enter the fifth kingdom of souls. Mental human will become superconscious human. A few spiritual pioneers of the human race have already done this or are in the process of doing it. The safety and peace of the human race depends on whether enough of its members reach this stage of development. Mental consciousness is no longer adequate to deal with the problems confronting our civilization. Only by developing the intuitional body can we go further.

HOW TO BE A GOD

"If you keep my commandments you shall abide in my love . . . these things I have spoken to you that my joy may be in you and your joy may be fulfilled."
(John 15:11)

Yoga may be thought of as a spiritual technology or system of techniques whereby one can directly experience ultimate reality within. In yoga intellectual knowledge alone is at best like a blueprint of a house; it may be a fairly accurate representation of the house but it is no substitute for actually being in the house and having the direct experience of the house itself. Its value is merely to make it easier to enter and find one's way around the house. In yoga all knowledge must be based on direct personal experience of consciousness. Therefore, in yoga the Guru or spiritual teacher does not impart knowledge but only the means by which the knowledge may be directly experienced by the student. That is, he or she teaches the practice of the yoga discipline or technique whereby the student may gain direct experience. There is no place for belief or blind acceptance of doctrine in yoga. One either knows and has experienced or does not know and has not experienced.

The omnipresent consciousness which is God is also present in humans. Through the process of meditation it is possible for us to purify our minds and to attune our own consciousness to the consciousness of God and therefore participate in the direct knowledge which God-consciousness affords. Our mind, body and senses are instruments organized in such a way that consciousness can express itself through them. When a certain stage in evolution is reached, we recognize our origin in God and seek consciously and deliberately to cooperate with the evolutionary purpose of supreme consciousness. At this point we consciously enters upon the spiritual path.

In meditation the attention is made to dwell upon the attention itself and is thus directed back to its source in God or pure consciousness. When this happens, pure consciousness begins to manifest itself through the human mind and makes the mind aware of its direct knowledge of anything in the universe, and thus the intuitive process begins to operate. Only through the perfected intuitive process can absolutely reliable knowledge be obtained because only God has complete knowledge of all the infinite, indirect causes that have brought any state of affairs into being and which will determine its future outcome. Only pure consciousness can exist in the center of every manifestation and have complete knowledge of all things by being all things.

Therefore, the chief aim of yoga is to awaken and perfect the intuitive process within human beings. It is not sufficient merely to intellectualize about God; one must experience God directly within oneself.

One of the unique aspects of the Eastern methods of teaching which applies to yoga in particular is the Guru-student relationship. This relationship is considerably different and more all-inclusive than the teacher-pupil relationship as it is usually conceived of in the West. The Guru must serve in the role of spiritual awakener and must exemplify and demonstrate the total spiritual way of life. He or she is more than just a person who imparts information. He or she is a master psychologist who understands the innermost phsychological workings of his or her pupils and acts as a spiritual catalyst to set in motion the spiritual and intuitive processes within the student. The Guru-student relationship is in many ways more intense and intimate than that of parents, minister, and psychiatrist rolled into one.

In reality, because there is only one consciousness and one mind in the universe, there is only one teacher. Regardless of who is teaching, if he or she tells the truth, it is the same

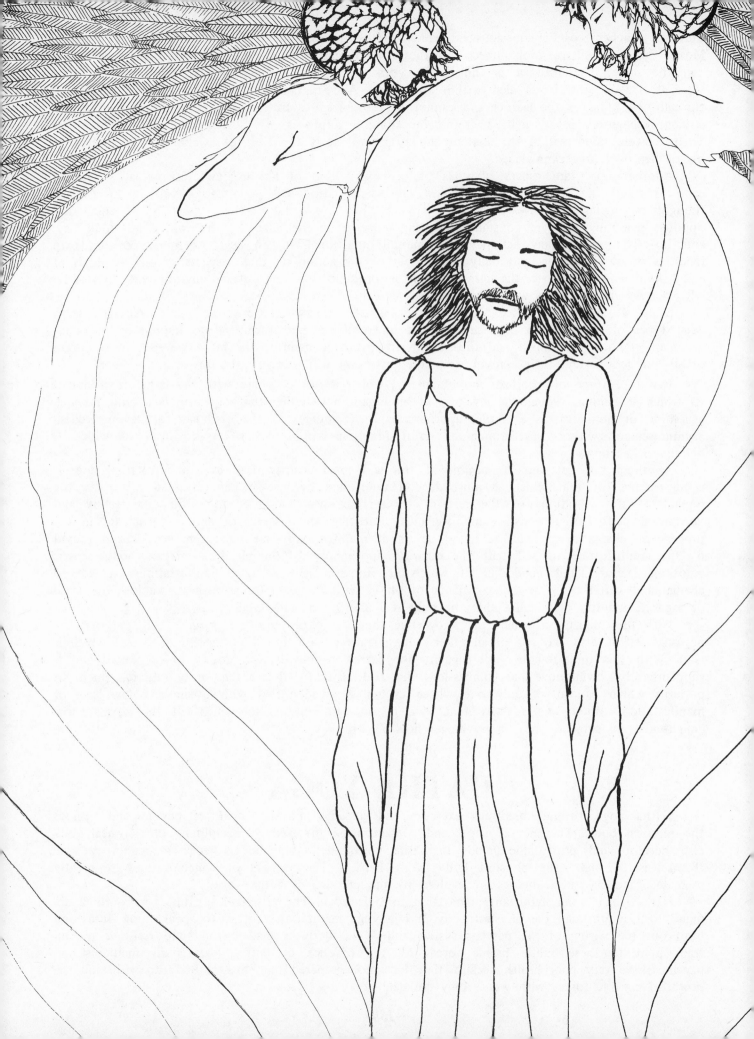

universal teacher, cosmic consciousness which speaks through them. The prophet may be Buddha, Moses, Jesus, Shankara, Mohammed, but the consciousness which reveals itself through each is one and the same. Therefore, it is said in the yoga tradition that God and the Guru are the same since it is God who is revealed within the Guru. All experience and knowledge must be filtered through the mind of the learner and cannot be recognized as truth unless consciousness within the student recognizes it as such. Therefore, teaching is a process of reminding the student of what cosmic mind within the student already knows. It is a process of awakening the student to his or her own inner knowledge.

Another important aspect of yoga philosophy is that of Karmic law. Karmic law is simply cause and effect. "That which you sow, the same also shall you reap." Karma can also be thought of in terms of Newton's third law — "For every action there must be an equal and opposed reaction." We are constantly creating ourselves in the image of that which we think, say, and do. To perform any action, be it mental, emotional, or physical, we must use our own faculties of mind, feeling, and body. The effect of the action on these aspects of our nature is of equal kind and degree to the effect which is produced on the outside environment. Inevitably, whatever we do to others we do to ourselves equally.

Since we must experience the consequences of our own actions, we must eventually learn what types of conduct are in harmony with universal law and thus lead to happiness, and what types of conduct are selfish and thus self-destructive and painful. The more we seek to be aware of all our actions and their consequences, the faster we will learn by this process.

Evil is a force of manifestation of energy, which is out of phase with the larger environment to which it belongs. Whenever any part of an organism (whether that organism is a human being, a nation, or humanity as a whole) appropriates the resources of the organism for its own selfish aggrandisement without performing a useful function within the larger organism to which it belongs, it becomes evil.

Anything that gets out of harmony in this way must destroy itself as a manifestation since it is destructive of that which it must depend upon and because it cannot stand up under the impact of the vibrations of the rest of its surroundings. In order to fulfill our destiny and become a perfect divine instrument, we must both be an observer of and a participant in the process of change and evolution on all levels of manifestation. We must remove delusion caused by the identification of Self with the outward appearances of the physical universe, body, senses, emotional nature, and mind; all of which are impermanent relative manifestations, subject to change and suffering. With the experience of union with Supreme Consciousness, we lose the sense of separate identity and realize that the only real identity is with God.

With this realization comes the knowledge that the entire universe is one's Self and that the personal self is also the self of all other beings, since all are united in the Supreme Self which is God. With this understanding, all capacity for hatred or ill-will toward any object ceases and is supplanted by divine love and compassion. One realizes that evil is a temporary misarrangement of patterns which can affect only one whose awareness is identified with a similarly low level of manifestation. When one realizes that evil is due to illusion to which all the permanently enlightened are subject, one can no longer hold ill will.

HATHA YOGA

Hatha Yoga, through breathing exercises and sustained physical postures, purifies and cleanses the physical body. The mental effort and concentration involved in disciplining the physical body also develop and purify the mind. In hatha yoga, the subtle bodies work harder in exerting themselves to make the physical body work harder. The powers of concentration are greatly increased, and the subtle bodies are evolved by the practice of hatha yoga.

Hatha yoga is an important preparation for raja yoga. The powerful spiritual forces which are made to flow through the physical body in raja yoga meditation can, so to speak, blow fuses and burn out the wiring of the nervous system unless the body is made strong and resistant to and transparent to these subtle pranic forces by the practice of hatha yoga. Many mediums and psychics have very poor health because they have not prepared the physical body to withstand the powerful psychic forces with which they are dealing.

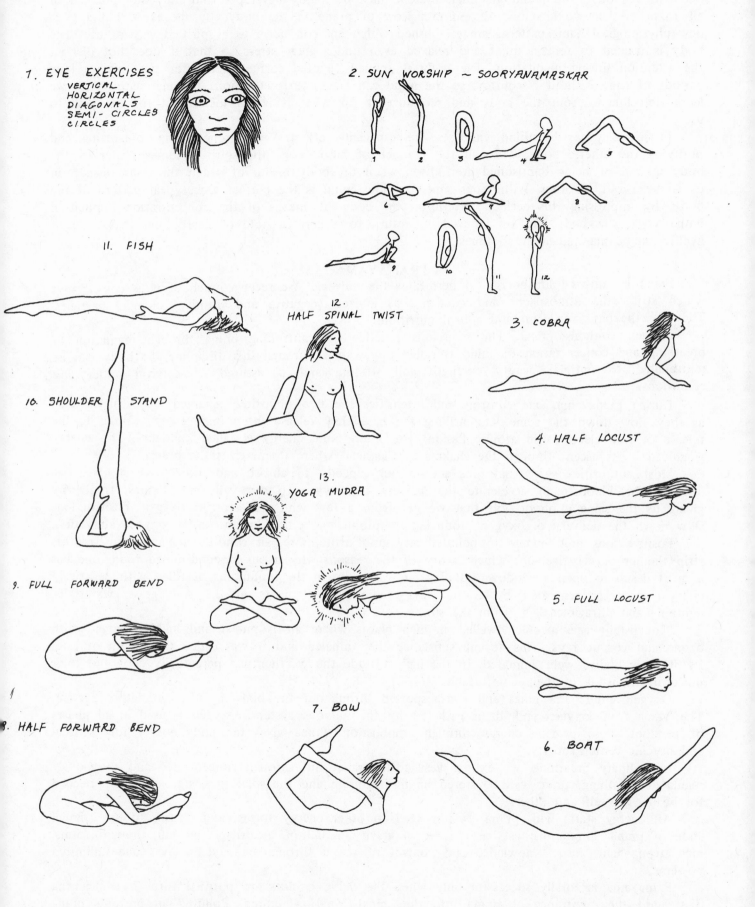

1. EYE EXERCISES
   VERTICAL
   HORIZONTAL
   DIAGONALS
   SEMI- CIRCLES
   CIRCLES

2. SUN WORSHIP ~ SOORYANAMASKAR

11. FISH

12. HALF SPINAL TWIST

3. COBRA

10. SHOULDER STAND

13. YOGA MUDRA

4. HALF LOCUST

9. FULL FORWARD BEND

5. FULL LOCUST

8. HALF FORWARD BEND

7. BOW

6. BOAT

The nervous system and glandular system must be highly developed and the body purified of all toxins which would block the smooth flow of prana in the body. By means of hatha yoga new physiological habit patterns are established which are conducive to a spiritual way of life. The body is trained to remain quiet and relaxed even under great stress so that it does not distract the attention during meditation. The body is trained to hold correct meditation postures for long periods of time without discomfort so the mind can engage in meditation. Through hatha yoga we learn detachment from the body and recognize it for what it is, an instrument for the soul to use.

In hatha yoga, breathing exercises are especially effective in strengthening, organizing and purifying the etheric body. Through the practice of hatha yoga the spirit becomes leader of the body instead of being imprisoned in it. Even when the body is out of order, the consciousness in us is never out of order. Within our superconscious mind is the perfect archetypeal pattern of the body. By impressing this perfect pattern on the body by means of the concentration implicit in hatha yoga, the body can be induced to return to a perfect state of health and that state of health can be maintained at all times.

PRANAYAMA

Prana is universal life energy. It permeates the universe. We receive much of it as cosmic rays which strike the atmosphere and condense as ionized (negative and positive) charged particles. They are the basis for plant and animal nutrition.

Oxygen contains prana. The conscious practice of controlling prana through regulation of breathing and concentration of mind is called pranayama. Through this discipline the body can be rejuvenated to optimal beauty, strength and wisdom and is assured of survival under any conditions.

During pranayama, one controls and intensifies the two oppositely charged electrical currents as they flow down the spine. On striking the base they release interatomic energy similar to the release of free electrons in atomic fission. The interatomic energy is called kundalini. This energy is guided in its ascent through the chakras to the head where it energizes the brain.

Most authorities agree that ions act on our capacity to absorb and utilize oxygen. Negative ions in the bloodstream accelerate the delivery of oxygen to our cells and tissues, frequently giving us the same euphoric jolt that we get from a few whiffs of straight oxygen. Positive ions slow down the delivery of oxygen producing symptoms markedly like anoxia, or oxygen starvation.

Positive ions predominate in polluted city air. Furthermore, air conditioners and many motors strip the air of negative ions which is one of the reasons why in an air-conditioned room one has a great desire to open a window. Country air, especially in the mountains, is filled with negatively charged particles generated by cosmic rays & radioactive elements in the soil, grass, waterfalls, lightning and ultraviolet light from the sun.

"In distant ages people dwelled in high places where air is purest and highly charged with ozone and cosmic rays. This cosmic substance they inhaled and it was called the Breath of Life. By it their bodies were animated. In the high altitude the weather was perpetually cool, but their powerful vitality kept them comfortable." (166)

Oxygen enters the lungs and is transported throughout the body by the circulatory system. The prana from oxygen and air is gathered by the nervous system. Oxygen is used in all phases of metabolism to provide energy through combustion. Prana gives the body energy for spiritual and psychic center activity.

In ordinary breathing, we extract very little prana. But through concentrated and consciously regulated breathing, prana can be stored up in the brain and the solar plexus to use when needed for healing oneself and others.

All energy starts with prana, is converted to other energy forms, and returns to the original state of prana. Prana manifests as a force of gravity, radiation, electricity, motion, thought forms, magnetism, light, heat. Knowledge and control of prana through pranayama gives one unlimited powers.

Pranayama is totally successful only when the nerve circuits are purified through a cleansing diet; until then, entrance of prana into the spinal canal is limited. Polluted air prevents prana from entering the divine chambers (sinuses). However, some individuals are able to circumvent these limitations because of inherent high vitality.

The practice of pranayama aids in cleaning out mucus and recharging the cells with high electropotential because of the alkalizing effect from increased breathing.

Retention of breath builds a strong body and mind, producing the vitality and increased concentration. When the breath becomes steady, the mind becomes calm and steady filling one with bliss. Through energy centralization combined with calm, the endocrine glands are rejuvenated producing clairvoyance and enlightenment; longevity is insured.

Your lungs will strengthen as they begin to process more oxygen with less effort; the heartbeat will grow stronger pumping an increased volume of blood to the muscles. Sagging tissues will regain youthful firmness. Your face will have better color; the hands, feet and ears will feel warm due to improved circulation; your lips will become redder. Because of increased mental and physical powers, you will develop a better self-image and tolerate more easily the stress of modern living.

Body temperature is controlled through automatic change of breath between the right and left nostril. The right represents the sun power, heat and energy. The left nostril represents the moon, the cooling power, and the expansion of the mind. Tibetan yogis, through breath control, are able to generate such intense heat that they can dwell naked in arctic-like mountain weather, even melting the snow surrounding them.

With the coming famine, oxygen shortage, and fuel shortage, we will all be forced to become ascetic yogis in order to survive. We may have to live on fewer breaths, be exposed to extreme heat and cold without the aid of air-conditioner or stove, tolerate many days without benefit of a meal and then possibly only a handful of blades of grass or weeds, have the strength to walk for days without sleep; be quiet and at peace in a world afflicted with violence, famine, insanity and disease.

Points To Remember In Pranayama

1. For beginners, the practice of breathing exercises twice a day, or even once, is sufficient.
2. Assume your favorite posture: lying, standing, kneeling, or sitting in a comfortable cross-legged position with spine straight for the duration of the exercise. Face north.
3. Advancement may be slow, but you will see weekly improvement.
4. Practice on an empty stomach and after bowel evacuation, if possible.
5. Breathe through the nostrils.
6. Never practice to the point of exhaustion. Go only to the limits of comfortable tolerance. Never strain, especially if you have health problems or when physically tired.
7. Do not retain breath longer than feels comfortable. If you develop chest pain, stop until pain is relieved.
8. Practice in a well-ventilated room free from disturbance and noise. Dress in loose clothing.
9. In the city, exercise in the early morning hours before city traffic builds up. Keep wheatgrass and other plants in the room. Use a dust free room containing minimal furniture. Choose a color for the room which feels harmonious to you. In spite of the appealing fragrance, incense burning is not desirable since it contaminates the air.
10. Get the assistance of a qualified teacher for perfecting the beginning exercises, as well as for instruction in the study of the more advanced pranayama.

Every cell in your body is performing respiration, but the lungs and skin are the main systems of breathing which consists of these processes:

1. Puraka — state of inhalation, lungs are filled with air.
2. Kumbhaka — state of retention. Toxic gas from cells enters the lungs. Prana and oxygen from the lungs enter the bloodstream to be delivered to all body cells.
3. Recaka — state of exhalation of toxic substances from body.

In pranayama, rounds and cycles describe the pattern of the breathing exercise. A cycle consists of one inhalation and one exhalation or one inhalation, one retention and one exhalation. Pranayama is done in proportioned ratios. The most common ratios are 1:2:1 and 1:4:2. In the ratio 1:4:2, we mentally count 1 'Om' during inhalation, 4 'Om's' during retention and 2 'Om's' during exhalation. Multiples of these ratios are used as one's powers increase. For example, if you start with the ratio 1:4:2, you might be able by the second week to increase the ratio to 2:8:4, by the fourth week, to 3:12:6. If you find difficulty in retaining the breath, continue the same ratio a few more weeks. Some teachers do not recommend retention of breath for beginners because they sometimes tend to overstrain.

Cleansing Breath

One should practice the cleansing breath at least several times a day, especially before a meal, and whenever opportunity presents itself in a natural pollution-free setting. It should be performed especially when one starts feeling drowsy from inactivity. (Oxygen is the only stimulant without side effects.) Other breathing exercises should always be preceded by the cleansing breath.

Assume a comfortable posture, relax the body, make the mind calm. Concentrate on the normal breathing for a few minutes.

First exhale as deeply and vigorously as possible and then take a deep breath. Exhale immediately through the nose strongly contracting the abdomen. Repeat rhythmically five to ten times. Then take a deep breath, retain for a comfortable period and expel. Continue the exercise for five to twenty rounds or until you perspire and feel fatigue, but do not overstrain. Stop if you feel giddiness or pain in the chest or abdomen. Take a few normal breaths and rest. After finishing the exercise, assume a relaxation pose for about five minutes.

This exercise clears the entire sinus and respiratory system enabling you to benefit more from the other exercises.

One Nostril Breathing

Close the right nostril with the right thumb. Slowly inhale deeply through the left nostril. Then exhale through the same nostril. This is one cycle. Six cycles make up one round. Daily, increase the number of rounds from one to as many as twelve.

Next, inhale through the right nostril by closing the left with the little and ring finger of the right hand. Then exhale through the same nostril. Repeat as with the left nostril breathing.

Alternate Breathing

Close the right nostril with the right thumb and inhale through the left nostril. Close the left nostril with the little and ring finger of the right hand, remove the thumb and exhale through the right nostril. Then inhale through the right nostril, and close it with the thumb, and exhale through the left nostril. Do this half a dozen times. This is one round. According to your capacity, increase to twelve rounds.

Alternate Retention Breathing (1:2:1)

Place the right thumb on the right nostril and inhale deeply through the left nostril, as if flooding the forehead with air. Then close the left nostril with ring and little finger. Retain the breath twice the time required to inhale. Remove thumb and exhale through right nostril allowing the same length of time as for inhalation. Repeat the process. Draw the air through the right nostril. Retain it as before. Exhale through the left nostril by removing the ring and little finger. This is one cycle. Six cycles constitute one round. Start with three rounds and gradually increase it to fifty. It is here that the 1:4:2 ratio and its increments may be used.

Complete Yoga Breath

To increase lung capacity, do deep breathing for at least ten minutes. The exercise expands the chest cavity in all directions; all parts of the lungs are brought into activity, including the most remote air cells.

Practice occasionally before a large mirror, hands over abdomen to feel the movement. You may stand or sit or lie on your back, hands at sides with palms upward, heels together, toes pointing upward. Breath steadily and continuously through both nostrils.

1. Fill the lower lungs by lowering the diaphragm as the abdomen gently expands.
2. Then fill the middle part of lungs, pushing out the lower chest.
3. Then fill the upper portion of lungs, expanding the upper chest, thus lifting the chest.
4. Then to fill the uppermost part of the lungs, slightly draw in the lower abdomen.
5. At the end of inhalation, occasionally raise the shoulders slightly thus permitting air to enter the extreme upper lobe of the right lung.
6. Retain the breath at least fifteen seconds.
7. Exhale slowly, slightly contracting the abdomen. When the air is completely exhaled, relax the chest and abdomen.

Practice this exercise; eventually it will become your normal way of breathing. The healthy primitive and any healthy infant breathe in this manner, but civilized adults have adopted unnatural breathing.

Even when we inhale an average amount of air, this exercise can distribute the oxygen to all parts of the lungs. However, to facilitate optimal health, one should do deep breathing several times a day at least.

Breath Of Fire increases oxidation in the cells, purifies the blood and stores up pranic energy. Keep the spine straight. Place great emphasis on the exhalation; don't strain, begin slowly. Initially do no more than three minutes continuously. Increase the time weekly up to twenty minutes. Exhale forcefully and rapidly through both nostrils. The diaphragm should expand like bellows down and out on the exhale, and contract in and up with the inhale. Do for 30 seconds, then inhale deeply and hold for 15 seconds.

Concentrate on the solar plexus to store up the pranic energy. Exhale forcefully and deeply. Take a few slow deep relaxing breaths, then repeat.

Advanced pranayama practitioners, especially when doing the breath of fire, should be in a pollution-free environment and should abstain from all solid food, obtaining their nourishment in liquid form. Success in pranayama is measured by the duration of breath retention. By a slow and steady process some yogis are able to retain breath for as much as five minutes at a time.

For the study and application of the science of pranayama and kundalini one should consult additional books. The initial exercises of pranayama can be performed without being concerned with the kundalini energy, but those wishing to pursue advanced study should be under guidance of an experienced teacher or reside in an ashram.

RELAXATION

Relaxation is essential to constant purification and strengthening of the body. It is as important an aspect of hatha yoga as the exercises. After each exercise, there should be a period of relaxation. The relaxation posture is done by simply lying on the back, legs out straight, hands by the sides, eyes looking directly upward with the back of the head on the floor.

All the muscles of the body should be completely limp. In order to achieve a sense of limpness and abandon, it may be helpful to raise each leg separately about two inches off the floor and then let it drop as though it were an inanimate object. In the same way raise the right arm slightly and let it drop. Then raise the left arm slightly and let it drop. Raise the hips slightly and let them drop. Raise the chest slightly and let it drop. Finally roll the head slightly from side to side. By this time you should feel limp as a rag doll. Let your entire body lie absolutely still and motionless and observe the internal results of the exercise you have just done. Notice how the breathing, heartbeat, muscles, tendons, joints, spine, and nervous system are readjusting themselves. In the beginning of the relaxation it may be helpful to do deep diaphragmatic breathing while lying on your back. As you inhale deeply the stomach should expand outward and as you exhale the stomach contracts. It is easier to achieve correct diaphragmatic breathing when reclining because in sleep diaphragmatic breathing occurs automatically.

As the body relaxes let the breathing become more slow and shallow until it seems to be suspended. Feel more and more that you are breathing (pranic) energy currents until you experience a feeling of weightlessness or floating in space. Feel as though the body has been transformed into a field of energy or magnetic force. Feel this energy revitalizing and regenerating every tissue and every cell of your body. The practice of this type of relaxation is an excellent preparation for meditation and the practice of raja yoga. Until one is able to relax it is impossible to meditate. After two or three minutes of this relaxation you will be refreshed and ready for the next asana or exercise.

By relaxing in this way after each exercise, the body is able to expel all the waste products which have been created and mobilized in the tissues during the physical exertion. Elimination of these fatigue toxins prevents fatigue and there is less strain on the heart and other internal organs. At the end of a yoga session you should feel less tired than when you began.

How To Become Completele relaxed

Any hatha yoga session should terminate in a relaxation period lasting ten or fifteen minutes. When the body is slightly tired but the mind is alert and conscious and the emotions are at rest you are very susceptible to constructive suggestions which will sink deep into the unconscious mind and take root there. For this reason the final relaxation is combined with suggestion. Begin by following the relaxation procedure outlined above. When the whole body is still and limp, focus your entire undivided attention on your toes. Feel everything that is happening in the toes. Be aware of the coolness of the air next to the skin, the feeling of density in the bones. Feel the toes pervaded and tingling with subtle vital energy and let the toes become completely relaxed. Feel as though you are communicating with the actual cells in them. Now purposefully and with full consciousness relax your feet and the ankles in the same way. Successively relax each part of the body from the feet to the top of the head, limb by limb, joint by joint, organ by organ. You may name successively each part of the body you are relaxing to yourself: "I am relaxing my feet; I am relaxing my thighs; I am relaxing. . ." Next, relax the calves and shins, then the knees and knee joints, then the pelvis. As you relax each part of the body do so with full undivided concentration. Concentration is not antithetical to relaxation. Concentration means to bring all your psychological forces to one focus of awareness. It is a process of unifying all the activities of the mind. When the mind is unified there can be no warring dualities, and, hence, no tension. Tension arises out of opposing psychological drives. It becomes evident that concentration is the real secret of relaxation. The activities of the body always mirror the activities of the mind. Whatever the mind envisions the body creates on the physical plane. When the mental and emotional activity is brought to a state of balanced equilibrium the body relaxes automatically. Bringing the mind to a state of balanced equilibrium by concentration on any part of the body automatically relaxes that part.

Next, relax the spinal column; feel each separate vertebra settle into place. Feel the spinal nerves tingling with pranic energy. Remember that your attention is consciousness and that wherever consciousness is focused vital force automatically manifests as the lower overtones of that consciousness. Consciousness creates the healing regenerating energies in the body.

Within your Superconscious mind is a perfect archetypal image of your body complete and beautiful in every detail. Quiet the mind in focused concentration and let this image of perfection precipitate on the physical octave of vibration and rebuild and regenerate the body as a perfect temple for your soul to manifest through.

Next relax all the back muscles, then the side muscles and stomach muscles. Allow at least 30 seconds for relaxing each part of the body. Next, relax each of the internal organs. Feel as though you are communicating with the individual cells in them. Relax the kidneys, bladder, liver, large intestines, small intestines and stomach; let your breathing slow down until it becomes imperceptible. The breathing should reach a point of relaxation where it seems suspended. You will seem to breathe by a pulsating flow of pranic energy throughout the body. Breathe energy through every pore and every cell. Now feel the heart relaxing deeply after each slow beat. Feel pulsations of vital energy flowing through the body with each heartbeat.

Now relax the chest and shoulders; sink back against the floor as all tension goes out of the muscles. Now while keeping them absolutely still and motionless, relax your fingers and thumbs. Feel them tingling and vibrating with energy. Now in the same way successively relax the hands, wrists, forearms, elbows and upper arms. Next relax around the base of the neck and the collar bone.

Next relax the neck, the link between the head and the body. Relax each part of the neck: the throat, larynx, vertebrae, muscles, tendons, veins, arteries, the thyroid and parathyroid glands. Now, while the mouth remains closed, let the jaw hang loose. Let your face become serene, impassive and expressionless. Now carefully relax your eyes. Let them sink deeply back into their sockets. Feel the eyes and eye sockets being enveloped by a warm soothing tingling sensation which is dissolving away all eye strain and fatigue. Next, relax the ears and all the delicate organs in the inner ears. Now feel the entire scalp tingling with cool soothing sensations right down through the roots of the hair. Let this tingling energy penetrate the skull and envelop the entire brain in the cool, soothing, clarifying sensation of pranic vibration. Feel all the brain cells being healed, regenerated and vivified.

Now that you have relaxed every part of the body, feel the entire body as a whole completely relaxed and at ease. Realize that the body is nothing but organized, concentrated energy. Experience its subtle nature as energy. Feel yourself lose all sensation of weight and mass. Experience the body as an electromagnetic force field floating freely in space. Experience yourself floating in a vast, infinite, shoreless sea of scintillating shimmering white light. See this light interpenetrating, pervading and permeating every atom and cell of your being. Now focus all your attention on the third eye center in the region of the pituitary gland and see a star of brilliant white radiance there. Experience a reciprocal flow of light, energy, sound and consciousness between this point in the center of your head and the entire universe including the sun, moon, planets, and stars. Consciousness is floating from the center of your head to them and from them to the center of your head. If you prefer, imagine this center of light in the heart instead of the head and follow the same procedure. Remain in this state for at least 5 minutes. Feel that you are tuned in to an infinite reservoir of love, wisdom and power that will enable you to live joyously, happily and successfully. Experience all the divine virtues present in you already. You have only to let them operate. These qualities exist in omnipresent consciousness. When the mind, emotions and personal ego are quieted and stand aside, the divine attributes will flow through you.

When you wish to end the relaxation, slowly become aware of your body; become aware of the floor under you and the physical surroundings. Stretch and get up slowly. Go forth into your daily activities renewed, refreshed and directed by the God-consciousness within you. This is an excellent procedure to use in bed before you go to sleep at night. It is especially effective for insomniacs and people who have difficulty getting to sleep. Not only will you go to sleep sooner but you will sleep more soundly and efficiently. The constructive suggestions and the relaxed state of your body will continue during sleep.

HOW TO SLEEP

Rest is suspension of the moving activity of the mind in a state of homogeneous balanced vibration. While resting one should reside in the belief that no new disturbing forces are coming into the subtle bodies. If rest is done with self-observation on the level of consciousness, or pure awareness, it is meditation. Without self observation, rest becomes deep, dreamless sleep.

For all people, with the exception of high adepts, sleep is a necessary process to regenerate the body and to reestablish equilibrium in the emotional and mental bodies. The principal of consciousness never sleeps, not even in the deepest states of dreamless sleep. By remaining in the state where consciousness is aware of itself, you can remain in full conscious awareness even while the body rests and all emotional and mental activity is at a standstill. This kind of sleep becomes a meditation.

The point in time just before falling asleep at night and just before waking up in the morning are especially valuable and significant. At these times you are still consciously self-aware, but the activities of the mind and emotions are in abeyance. Because you are conscious, but the attention is unoccupied with any particular thought or perception, you are able to receive intuitive impressions coming from the higher levels of spiritual consciousness. This state is very much akin to the states achieved in meditation. You should try to make the period between waking and sleeping longer and longer until it includes the entire time during which you sleep.

Always be careful to make the last thought in your mind before you go to sleep a positive and spiritually uplifting one. Since this is the last thought to go into the unconscious mind before sleep, it acts as a very powerful suggestion which will continue all night in the deeper levels of mind while you sleep. Likewise, when you awake in the morning, start your day off with a brief period of meditation and then proceed into your day's activities, operating from the higher level of consciousness established in your meditation upon awakening. To facilitate this process, it is often good to read a few pages out of some sacred book or to go through a few mantras either mentally or out loud.

RAJA YOGA

"He who is not happy with nothing, will not be happy with everything; he who does not cherish the little things, will not be thoughtful of the great things; he with whom sufficient is not enough, is without virtue, for the physical body of man lives only from day to day; if you supply it with what it actually needs, you will still have time to meditate, while if you seek to supply it with what it wants, the task is without end."   LAW OF BUDDHA

Raja Yoga is the yoga of meditation. There is a difference between prayer and meditation. In prayer we say, in effect, "God, listen while I talk." In meditation, we say, in effect, "God, speak while I listen." We must ask ourselves who has the most valuable things to say. Once we have, so to speak, focused our attention or tuned ourselves in through prayer, we should quietly await the answer from our inner consciousness by means of meditation.

Meditation is the process by which we experience pure consciousness. By means of meditation higher octaves of spiritual energy are made to flow through the subtle bodies and the mind; emotions and body are harmoniously attuned to the vibratory rates of higher consciousness. Mental and emotional activity are brought to a standstill so that the astral and mental bodies are capable of reflecting, without distortion, the love, wisdom and power which come from the plane of pure consciousness. Thus the subtle bodies are able to receive the vibratory imprint of spiritual energy and act as transmitters and receivers of the energy of consciousness. Only through meditation can higher states of consciousness be directly experienced.

Meditation is a universal process that goes on in all of life's activities; it is the simple focusing of attention to accomplish any particular act. In Spiritual Meditation this natural process of the mind is directed toward the discovery and experience of mind and consciousness or the Ultimate Energy of the Universe in which everything is manifested. It is directing the attention back to the level of causality rather than to the level of effect.

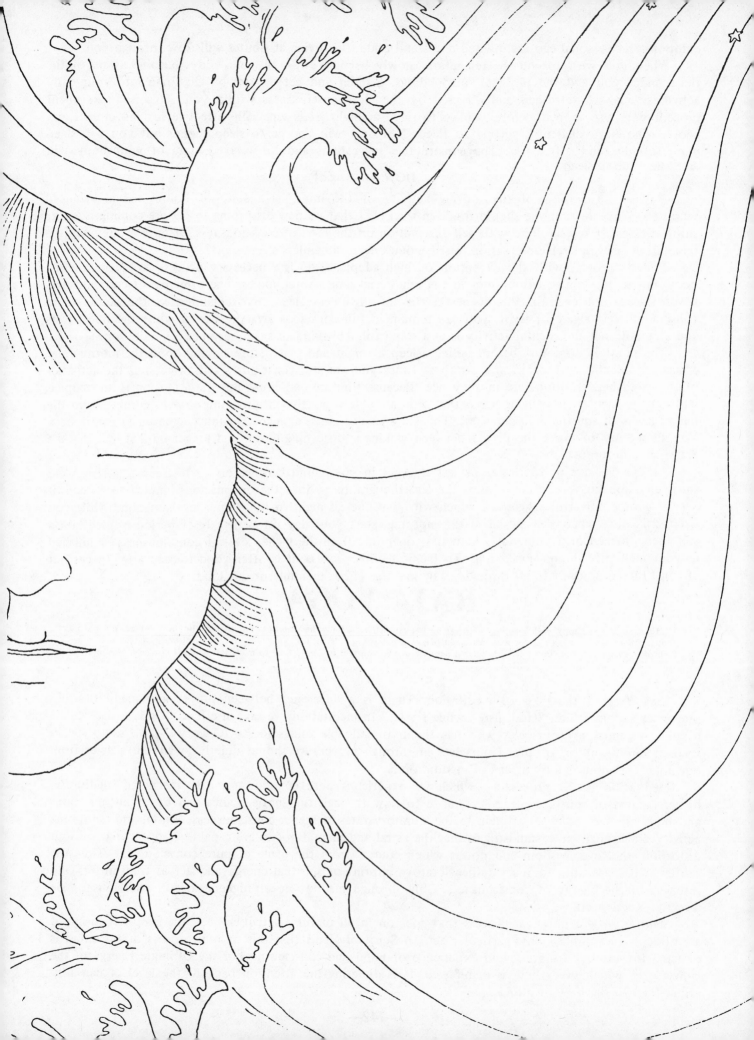

It is good to have a quiet place in your home for meditation where you can build up the right atmosphere in the room and charge it with spiritual vibrations. This is the real meaning of home. Home is where you can relax and be your real self! It is where you can always return for peace and inner contemplation. Eventually you will reach a stage in development where you consider the whole universe your home.

There are certain physiological conditions which are also conducive to meditation. Anything which increases the subtle activity of the cells will make it possible for the body to harmoniously attune itself to higher rates of vibration on the subtle planes of spiritual energy. Heat, produced by meditating in front of a fire, will increase cellular activity, as will hatha yoga, breathing exercises, and strenuous work. The natural stresses induced in the body by being outdoors in extremely cold or extremely hot weather, will also increase cellular activity. It is always good to meditate during or just after exposure to any of these conditions.

By the practice of the meditation techniques described in this chapter, the subtle bodies are interpenetrated by the vibrations of higher levels of spiritual energy. This spiritual light contains tremendous energy which dissolves and shatters any inharmonious tendencies existing within the mental and emotional bodies.

Any thought forms or energy patterns existing within the etheric, astral and mental bodies which are out of harmony with God's evolutionary plan are broken up by the strong spiritual vibrations induced by meditation. The energy contained in these inharmonious patterns is released to be repatterned for a constructive purpose. Through the process of meditation the personality nature is perfected as an instrument through which spiritual consciousness can work in a clear, effective, and undisturbed manner.

All beginners and even most experienced meditators, to a greater or lesser degree, experience difficulties in meditation caused by various thoughts, emotions and sensory perceptions which distract the attention and interrupt the continuous flow of concentration. It sometimes seems that the more we fight these distractions and try to overcome them, the more they bother us, the more the process of fighting them itself becomes a distraction. It becomes obvious that a wrong approach in dealing with distractions is in use. To say that I must not think of something is to think of it even more with a negative qualification added.

To overcome distractions we must stop thinking about them and also stop thinking about not thinking about them. This can be accomplished only by bringing the attention back to the original process of meditation. If the attention wanders again, bring it back to the thing being meditated upon whether that is a sound current, watching the breath, the light in the head, or any of the other meditation techniques described in this chapter. Keep bringing the attention back as many times as necessary to make it stay on the topic of meditation.

Another method is to place the attention on that consciousness in you which is experiencing the distracting thoughts, emotions and perceptions.

A third method is to observe the breath. The rhythm of the breathing is the regulator of the flow of vital forces within one's being. This technique simply consists in observing the process of your breathing without trying to change it or interfere with it in any way. This practice eliminates distractions of the mind and the emotions. The quiet state which it induces makes it possible for intuitive knowledge and impressions from deeper levels of consciousness to present themselves to conscious awareness. It is a good technique to practice at the beginning of a meditation session before engaging in one of the other meditation techniques.

As you intently observe the rhythm of the breathing process without trying to change it in any way, you will notice that the breathing naturally tends to become more slow and rhythmic until it seems to stop in a steady state of complete relaxation where you neither inhale nor exhale. You will feel that you are breathing light and energy through every pore of your body. All restless activity of the emotions and mind will come to a standstill and you will feel yourself resting or suspended in the presence of pure light and consciousness. Do not be afraid of this state as it will regenerate the entire body, vitality, emotions and mind. Your whole personality nature will be purified and flooded by the light of the Supreme. The body will automatically breathe again when the cells demand more oxygen. This period of rest and quietude is the suspension in the ocean of prana.

SOUND CURRENT MEDITATION

Go to a quiet place where you will not be disturbed and sit in a comfortable meditation posture with spine erect. Close your eyes and listen in the center of your head with full attention for whatever sounds present themselves. Gradually, with practice and concentration, you will begin to hear a steady sound within the head. It may sound like the roaring of a river, like a low hum, like the roll to thunder or like a high sustained note of an organ. Keep your attention steadily on the highest pitch that you can hear. In the beginning the sound may seem to be in the right or the left ear. It should not be listened to in the left ear, since this can lead to sensual attachments and distract you from the spiritual disciplines. With practice the sound should be centralized in the center of the brain and expanded until it successively includes the whole head, the whole body, the surrounding space and ultimately the whole universe. This sound is perceived directly by the brain and the subtle bodies and does not come through the physical sense organ of the ears.

This sound is the sacred word, the AUM vibration. It is the vibration of spiritual energy as it flows through the physical and subtle bodies of the meditator. Its source is omnipresent cosmic consciousness. By meditation on it, one is lifted up into higher states of consciousness and united with the supreme spiritual reality.

By placing your concentration on the sound current, you will direct your individual consciousness back to its source in omnipresent cosmic consciousness, creating a complete circuit from cosmic, supreme existence through your personal instrumentality of the subtle bodies back to God or cosmic consciousness. The flow of the consciousness through the meditator floods the subtle bodies with light and brings about an automatic burning or transmutation of destructive tendencies within the subtle bodies. Any patterning of energy within the subtle bodies which is out of phase with the rhythm of the universe is consumed in the light manifested in meditation and the energy contained in them is released back to the unqualified spiritual energy substance of the plane from which it was originally organized into the destructive pattern.

In listening to the sound current you may hear several different pitches or tones. These are the various harmonic overtones of the vibration of pure consciousness which correspond to the various subtle bodies. By listening to the note of the highest pitch, you will attune yourself to the higher octaves of spiritual energy which will then automatically harmonize the lower octaves.

Meditation on the sound current is considered one of the highest forms of meditation and it should be practiced by every serious student of Yoga. This form of meditation is directly related to the highest chakra, the sahasraram or thousand-petalled lotus at the top of the head.

The sound current is the language of consciousness. The more you practice meditation on the sound current, the more your mind will be filled with direct intuitive knowledge of truth. This knowledge will manifest as an instantaneous pure concept or knowledge which can later be enclosed into language for the sake of communicating it to other people.

MEDITATION ON THE LIGHT IN THE HEAD

The Third Eye Center, which is also called the agna chakra, is located on the forehead, rooted in the pituitary gland which is in back of the root of the nose, or in back of the joint just above the bridge of the nose in the center of the forehead.

To practice this form of meditation, close your eyes and concentrate on the point in back of the bridge of the nose while observing your inner field of vision. The light will begin as a point of illumination which will expand until it includes the entire visual field. With ever-increasing absorption in concentration, you should observe this field of light with your attention brought to a single point within the center of the visual field. A more intense light on a higher plane of vibration will then burst out from this point and fill the entire visual field again. By repeating this process over and over you will go through veil after veil and experience higher and higher planes of vibration until your being is flooded with the light of God consciousness. By this practice, the capacity for spiritual vision is developed.

In the course of this practice, you may begin to see the workings of various chakras of the body; you may see geometrical patterns, thought forms, scenery, visual memories and other visual phenomenon. This is the content of the subtle bodies revealing itself to your awakened spiritual vision. When this faculty of internal vision is highly developed, you will be able to move this visual point of observation to any place within the body or outside the body to which you direct your attention and see exactly what is happening there on whatever rate of vibration you are perceiving. By adjusting the rate of vibration and the point to which the attention is directed, ultimately anything in the universe on whatever plane of manifestation it exists, can be seen.

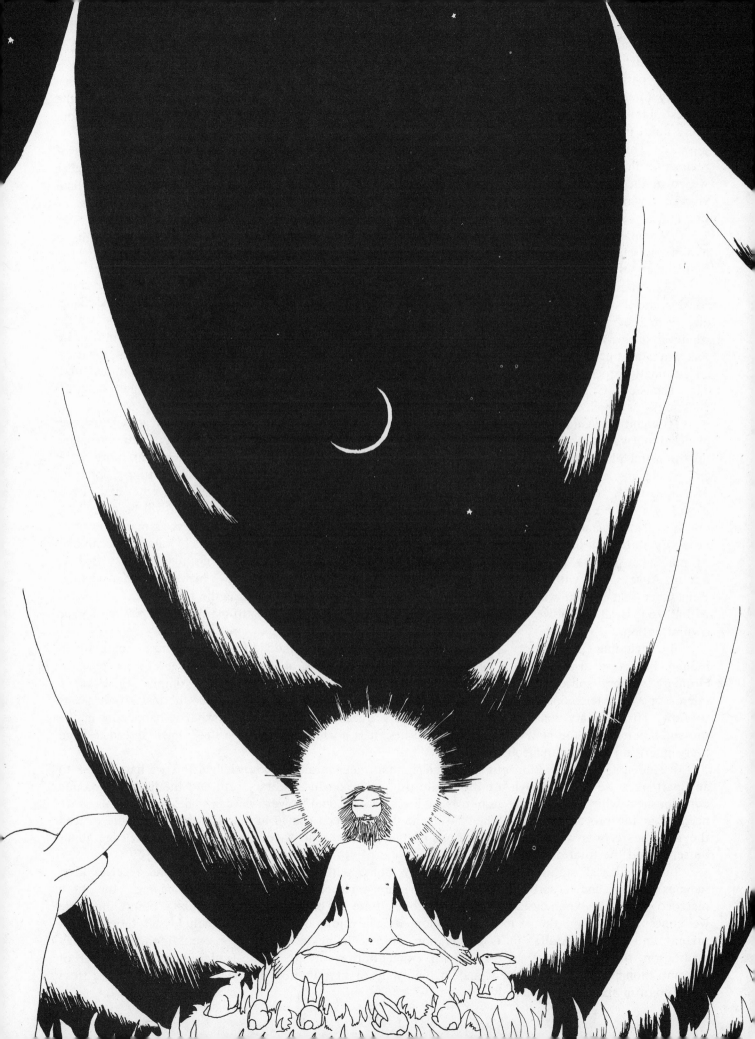

As this ability is developed, omnipresent consciousness will use you as a spiritual lighthouse to shed healing spiritual illumination on all who come within your sphere of influence. As this practice is gradually perfected, time, space and direction will become less and less a barrier until you are able to see in every direction simultaneously from any point in space you will to direct your attention to. In the highest state of God consciousness you will, as the soul of the universe, radiate and receive light from every point in space simultaneously.

The Third Eye Center is the easiest place to begin to see this light, but in the higher stages of realization the capacity for vision is not restricted to any special   location within the body. The higher we go in the experience of faster rates of vibration, the more all the senses are merged into one sublime vibration which is perfect seeing, hearing, and feeling all rolled into one. This is the awareness of omnipresent consciousness acting on itself.

With practice of this form of meditation, you may in your normal state with eyes open begin to experience clairvoyant phenomena such as seeing auras and thought forms. These are merely the by-products of meditation and should not be sought as an end in themselves.

There are certain subsidiary techniques to meditation on the third eye center which deserve some consideration. One of these is the technique called Spontaneous Energy, which is a technique investigated by Dr. William J. Pinard. His method is simply to observe the field of vision and watch whatever images present themselves there in the same manner as one would passively watch a movie. In this way, the unconscious mind presents its own visual symbols before the conscious awareness, creating an automatic process of catharsis by which repressed psychological problems are recognized, understood and dismissed. Gradually this brings about an inner purification and produces a higher state of consciousness which Dr. Pinard calls Superconscious Mind.

It would be valuable to describe in more detail a technique by which a meditator goes from one plane or octave of vibration to a higher one. Let us use a specific example. Suppose you are perceiving on the astral plane and you wish to perceive on the mental plane. In order to perceive the more rapid and subtle mental plane rates of vibration, pick any point as small as you can visualize within your field of vision. While on the astral plane concentrate all of your attention within that small point and pierce it with your concentration. When the point expands out again in a burst of light you will be perceiving on the mental plane or a higher subplane of the astral plane. Continue this process as many times as necessary until you have reached the level of vibration you wish. This is an especially valuable technique to remember if you find yourself trapped in the perception of thought forms ugly or distorted in nature. Always deal with such seemingly evil forces by transmuting them to a higher octave of energy. Remember that hidden within your own concentration or attention, which is the force of consciousness within you, is all the power in the universe. You have only to learn how to manifest the power of your own attention.

By including all vibratory phenomena in meditation, the individual consciousness operating in human beings is also expanded and made to experience its oneness with supreme consciousness. Ordinary sensory space perception is merely a limitation of attention; even a simple device like a microscope or a telescope can distort it. The more consciousness is reflected in us the faster time seems to flow. The ordinary sense of boredom is merely a lack of observation of what is happening in the present moment. In the state of pure consciousness it is possible to hear, see, feel, smell and taste from every point in space simultaneously.

We do not contain within our individual human mechanisms all knowledge. But we have access to any part of it we need through intuition. Intuition is like having a library card and the library is cosmic consciousness which has infinite resources of love, wisdom and power; we can make withdrawals as we need to in the process of living. When sufficient skill has been gained in meditation, we are able to read the Akashic records which are the memory of the universe and to discover timeless knowledge about ourselves and the total of creation.

In the highest states of meditation, every point within the meditator gives and receives love, radiates energy and absorbs radiations. The more microcosmic our attention becomes, the more macrocosmic is its experience. The more we concentrate all of our attention within a point, the more we concentrate within the exact present moment; the more our awareness includes all time -- past, present and future. Meditation is observation of and living in the exact present moment. Through meditation the will, which is one-pointed concentration of attention, is developed. The point of concentration becomes omnipresent and in that state of illumination one sees the entire universe from every point in space simultaneously.

Without attention it is impossible to sit in a Guru's presence. It is possible to attain enlightenment by paying close attention to what a great Guru says. The dedicated student who does not have a Guru will soon find one. As the old saying goes, "When the student is ready the teacher will appear." This is true also for the Guru within the student. When the mind is purified and held steady in concentration, higher consciousness will automatically manifest itself. We must learn to extract wisdom from everything by realizing that the whole universe and every experience of life is God in manifestation teaching us. We merely need to be fully awake to experience and participate in the school of life.

As you improve in meditation you will not only develop vision and hearing on the subtle planes, but you'll develop the higher aspects of the other senses as well. The sense of touch will not be limited to just the physical body. You will feel the presence of energy and of material objects as densifications of energy everywhere in space.

The circulation of mental energy within the body and outside it will create feeling sensation anywhere in space where your consciousness is present to observe it. This faculty of clairsentience will begin as a feeling of soothing electricity or tingling sensations in various parts of the body; you may feel waves of heat and cold; a rhythmic pulsation may appear that will make you want to rock your head in rhythm with it. Feelings of weightlessness and flying in space or feelings that the body is rotating, when in fact it is still, may also present themselves. Just remain steady and observe the manifestation of these forces. At certain times you may perceive perfumes or scents to which you can ascribe no physical cause. These also indicate the awakening of higher faculties. They are merely the byproducts of the flow of consciousness within the meditator.

Once you have established new constructive habit patterns by purifying and reorganizing the subtle bodies, meditation will become your natural state twenty-four hours a day. In meditation there is a natural tendency to want to talk or think about the inner experiences that come in meditation. This tendency should be restrained, until after you finish your meditation because if allowed to operate it will interfere.

Only after you have finished your meditation should you think, write and talk about what you experienced. It is a good idea to keep a diary of your spiritual experiences in order to trace your own progress and to remember your higher realizations.

LAYA YOGA

Laya Yoga is the science of using the chakras to bring about higher states of spiritual realization. Laya Yoga links and harmoniously attunes the physical, etheric, astral and mental bodies to each other and to consciousness by developing the chakras.

The word chakra means wheel. The chakras are revolving vortices of spiritual energy existing in the subtle bodies. They relate to major nerve plexuses and glands in the physical body. The agna chakra or the brow chakra, for instance, is related to the pituitary gland and to the subcortical area of the brain.

The chakras are the interchange points of energy between the physical and the superphysical aspects of human nature. They link the subtle bodies and project energy into and receive energy from the outside environment. They act on the astral and mental planes as sort of whirlpools or revolving funnels of energy. By focusing the attention of any one of the seven chakras within the human body, the flow of energy in that chakra is increased and the psychic and physical functions associated with that chakra are intensified in their activity. This is the inevitable working of the law: wherever attention or consciousness is focused, energy is generated and manifested at that same location.

In laya yoga each chakra harmonically resonates to and is vibrated by the appropriate frequencies of sound and light. In this connection, colored light and music are often used for purposes of healing, meditation, or inducing certain states of emotion, mind and consciousness. The power of art, music and drama over people's minds and emotions is based largely on the above laws.

The planets, astrologically considered, are the chakras of the solar system; and the chakras in people are harmonically attuned to them, "as above so below." The zodiac is a vast twelve-petalled chakra with its center in the sun. There is an interlocking harmonious unity pervading all levels of the universe.

Music can play a tremendous role in humankind's evolution. The harmonies and rhythms present in music heal and stimulate the subtle bodies of people. Music has a direct effect on the chakras. Music is truly medicine for the soul. Music induces emotional states by creating certain vibrational activities within astral and mental bodies. Emotional recollection is examination of an emotional vibration pattern in the desire body by conscious energy. The great musicians of the past have tuned in to the music of the spheres and have recorded what they heard so that people could reproduce it and be uplifted by it.

There are seven major chakras in the human body to correspond to the seven subplanes of each plane, and the seven major notes in the musical scale. The locations and functions of these chakras are as follows:

The sahasrara chakra or thousand-petalled lotus, is located on the top of the head and is related to the pineal gland and the cerebral cortex. It is the doorway to cosmic consciousness and relates to the highest experience of cosmic consciousness. The sahasrara has twelve inner petals and 932 outer petals.

Meditation on the sahasrara chakra stimulates those brain activities which the cerebral cortex controls, namely those of higher intuition. The activity of will and sense of pure existence are increased. This chakra is particularly associated with the sound current; therefore, the faculty of clairaudience will be stimulated by meditation on it. The activities of the pineal gland will also be increased which will make the body more sensitive and receptive to spiritual forces. The individual self is united with the cosmic self through the activity of this highest chakra which is our ambassador to the infinity of God consciousness.

The agna chakra is located on the brow slightly above and between the eyebrows. It has two inner petals and ninety-six outer petals. It is the center of the third eye or clairvoyance. It is also the center of willing. By meditation on the agna chakra which is related to the pituitary gland and the subcortical areas of the brain; the personality structure is integrated and brought under the control of the will. The activity of the pituitary gland is stimulated. The hormones which the pituitary gland secrete regulate the other glands in the body, including the thyroid, adrenal glands, gonads, as well as other glandular functions. When the pituitary gland functions fully, the entire glandular system of the body, which has so much effect on our physical health and emotional states, is brought into harmonious balance. When the activity of the third eye center is awakened, the entire body is flooded with light and sight is developed.

The visauda or throat chakra has sixteen petals and is located in the area of the thyroid gland. It has to do with speech and the power of the spoken word.

Meditation on the throat chakra stimulates the thyroid gland and increases the spiritual creative vibratory power of the spoken word. The faculty of speech is made more powerful, clear, precise and meaningful. The artistic and creative faculties of the individual are also stimulated. The throat chakra is intimately related to the practice of mantra yoga.

The anahata or heart chakra is located in the heart and has twelve petals. It is the seat of the divine spark, or soul nature. It is related to the higher spiritual emotions of love, bliss joy, compassion and sympathy.

Meditation on the heart chakra stimulates the higher emotions and develops the faculty of clairsentience, or divine sense of touch, whereby you can feel the presence of any object or energy force anywhere in space within the body or outside of it. Meditation on the heart center floods the subtle bodies with divine love and makes one aware of the flow of vital energy within the body.

The manipura chakra is located in the solar plexus. It has ten petals and is related to the emotional desires, the functioning of the digestive center and vital energy. Meditation on the solar plexus chakra increases the metabolic or digestive process. This chakra is related to the astral and emotional levels of vibration. Improper meditation on it can stimulate lower psychic and emotional tendencies.

The muladara chakra has four petals and is located at the base of the spine. It is related to the principle of the will to live and is the seat of the kundalini power. Meditation on this chakra arouses the kundalini force which can then be raised through the spinal cord or central nervous system called shushumna to the sahasraram. This process vivifies and stimulates all the chakras and greatly intensifies the regenerative and spiritual power of the yogi. This is an advanced technique which should not concern the beginner.

The Swadhisthana chakra or sacral center is located about three or four inches above the muladara chakra. It has six petals and is related to the sexual functioning of the body and to the adrenal glands. Meditation on this chakra by a properly prepared and instructed yogi can give control over the sexual forces in the body and increase the physical vitality.

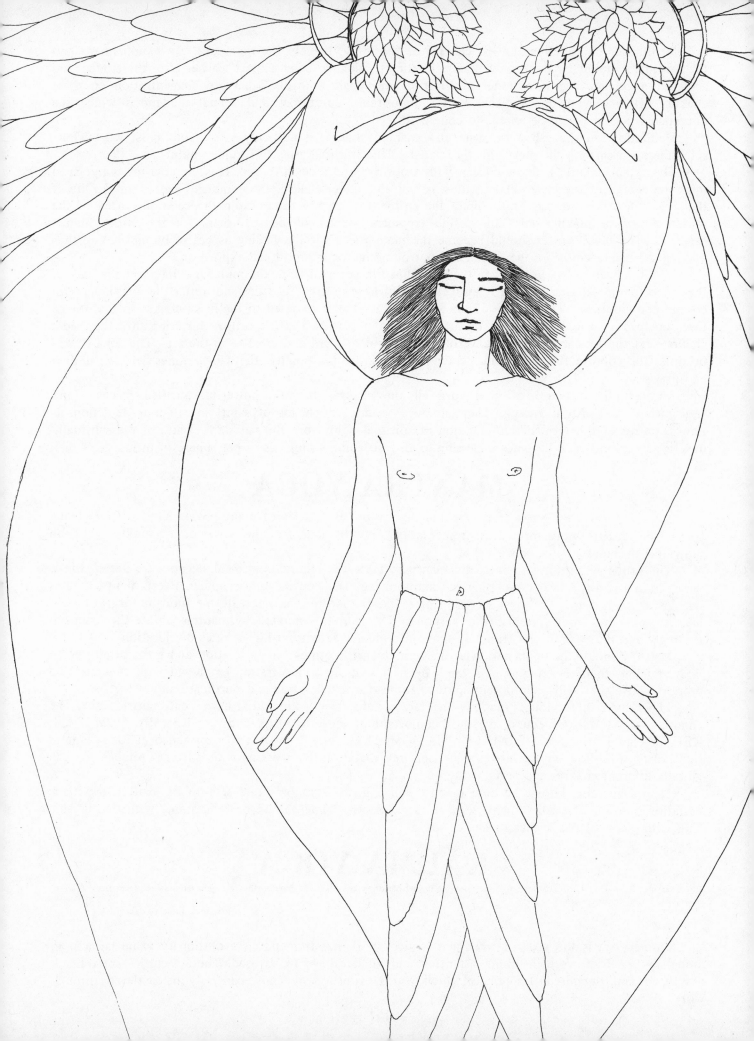

Meditation on the three lowest chakras of the body, namely the manipura, the swadhisthana and the muladara should be done only under the direct guidance of an expert teacher after the student has achieved a certain degree of inner purification and yogic control. Otherwise concentration on these chakras below the diaphragm can arouse undesirable emotional and sexual tendencies which the unprepared person would be unable to cope with.

Meditation on the sahasrara, agna and anahata chakras is not only safe, but most worthwhile, since these chakras are the most directly related to the spiritual aspect of human nature.

The spinal column is like a magnet with a positive and a negative end. It is the goal in laya yoga to raise the energy of the lower chakras thus making the higher chakras the command center for the life of the yogi. The ultimate aim is to direct the entire flow of life forces from the cerebral cortex or the sahasrara chakra making this chakra the command center of consciousness for the entire human organism. The heart center should become the main focus for the feeling aspect of human nature thus making the higher emotions the dominant controlling factor in emotional expression.

In the advanced stages of Yoga the kundalini fire is raised from the muladara chakra at the base of the spine to the sahasrara where it awakens the highest spiritual faculties and unites the individual with cosmic consciousness. The energy of the solar plexus chakra is raised to the heart chakra so that divine love supercedes desire. The energy of the sacral center is roused into creative expression thru the throat chakra, and the human becomes powerful in the spoken word and creative in the arts. The agna chakra becomes the coordinating command center for the entire personality; the will becomes decisive, unified and powerful.

Through the practice of laya yoga all the chakras become powerful, purified receivers and transmitters of spiritual energy. The halo seen around the heads of saints in religious depictions is representative of the tremendous radiation of spiritual light from the sahasrara chakra of the spiritually developed person which becomes a blessing to all who come within his or her sphere of influence.

MANTRA YOGA

Mantra yoga is the yoga of prayer and invocation. By means of mantra yoga, God or pure being speaks the creative word through instrumentality. Thus by means of the power of the spoken word the individual becomes co-creator with God.

The sound vibrations generated by mantras vibrate the etheric ocean and set up wave patterns in it which have a constructive, stimulating and harmonizing effect on the subtle bodies. Every mantra creates its own thought form. The most sacred mantras like the giotre mantra create the thought forms of great beauty, symmetry, and universality of response. The sounds generated by mantras vibrate the tissues in the body and the chakras and stimulate them into greater activity at higher rates of vibration.

Mantras should be spoken slowly, deliberately, with utmost concentration and great attention on understanding their meaning as they are spoken. The more concentration employed with their use the more effective they will be in potent spiritual forces for regeneration and purification.

In addition to the longer mantras there are certain vowel sounds that have great mantric value. The chanting of AUM is of course the most important of these. Other sounds are RA, MA, OOM, RAM, KEE, or combinations such as AUM-RA-MA-OOM. These should be chanted over and over for as long as one breath will allow with great resonance and reverberation. By working with different pitches you can vibrate different chakras and parts of the body.

Names are also known to have mantric value. Each word or sound sets up its own characteristic vibration pattern. The vibration pattern of each person's name should be in harmony with that person. This is the basis of the science of numerology.

KARMA YOGA

"Look at me, Arjuna! If I stop working for one moment the whole universe will die. I have nothing to gain from work; I am the sole Lord. But why do I work?"

KRISHNA, BHAGAVAD — GITA

Karma yoga is the yoga of work and service. Work has tremendous evolutionary value because in doing any kind of work the mind, attention and vitality have to be used. These faculties are trained, developed and organised. Experience, upon which evolution depends, can only be achieved through work.

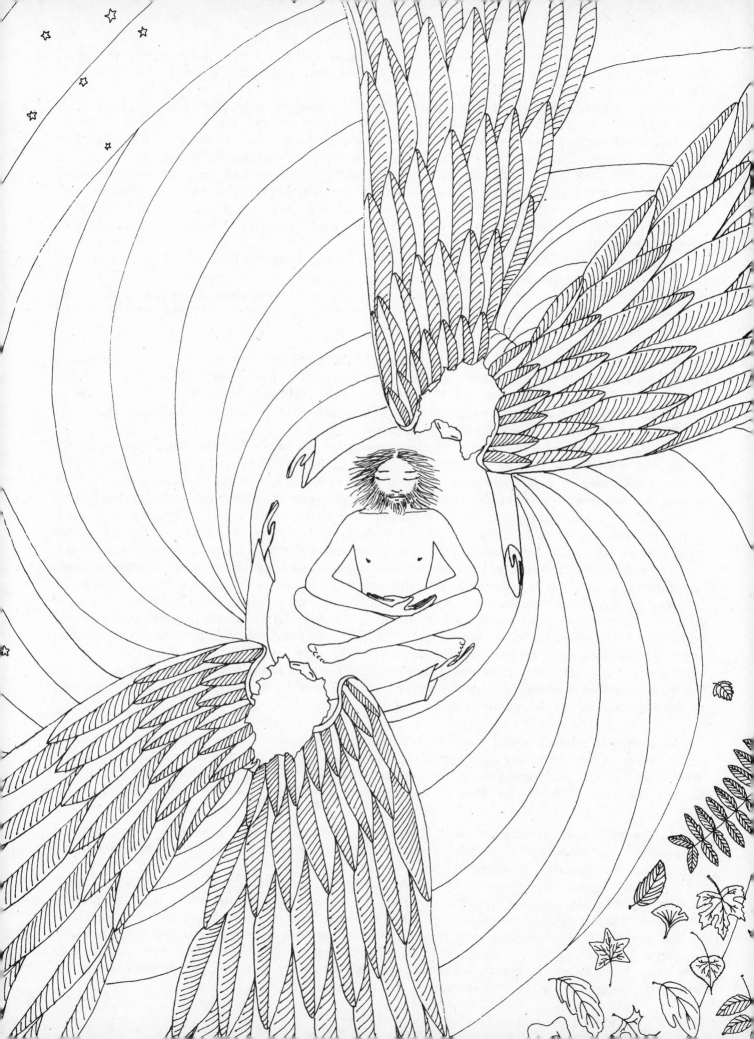

Work is the very nature of existence. All existence is in motion and work is the activity of motion. Work is the inevitable activity or harmonic flow of God or pure existence on all levels of manifestation. It is the power of life in expression.

Stress is conducive to work and evolution because the organism under stress seeks to protect itself and maintain its equilibrium. To do this it must do work to overcome the stress.

True work never makes us tired. It is only worry, anxiety, negative emotions or any disharmony that makes us tired. When we learn to work with love, in harmony with the rhythm of the universe, we will never feel tired. We will be able to work indefinitely with complete ease, joy and relaxation. Relaxation is not lack of activity; it is a state of balanced activity brought about through concentration.

When we see everyone as a manifestation of our own self, then we will work to protect and serve all. When enough people reach this level of awareness, civilization becomes a self-protective, self-sustaining entity and world peace will be established.

Love is work and work is love. To begrudge work is to begrudge love. By means of work and discipline, we express our love of God and our love for our fellow humans who are also God in manifestation. Happiness is work with awareness. Unwillingness to work comes from lack of awareness. A person is unhappy only if he or she refuses to work for what he or she wants. Creativity is work, and creation is the result of work.

Love is the perfection of work. Work creates well organized vibration patterns which manifest as beauty. Because all life works, all life ultimately manifests beauty. Work is the music of the spheres. It is the cosmic flow of life rhythms. To love someone is the willingness to work with that person, to contribute to his or her awareness and to share awareness through work. Our best friends are the people we work and create with. Work is beauty, love and joy.

We should work for the joy of work. In karma yoga the means and the end are the same. We should find our fulfillment in the process rather than in its fruits. When we take this detached attitude, the fruits will come of their own accord; we need not seek them. Karmic law always sees to it that we receive that which we have rightfully earned. From the viewpoint of enlightened consciousness, there is no such thing as individual possession or ownership. Everything in the universe including one's mind, body, and senses, is a manifestation of God and is therefore owned by the totality of God. When the realization of the unity of the individual self with the universal self is achieved, the yogi understands that he or she owns the entire universe, and as relative body, mind, and senses, owns nothing, not even his or her self. Once this is understood, all selfish cravings and desires for relative things comes to an end. The enlightened person according to the path of karma yoga, performs his or her practical material duties in the world with an attitude of detachment, realizing that he or she is participating in and performing functions in the cyclic flow of universal harmony. They become instruments in the hand of Supreme Consciousness, performing the intent of the supreme. This kind of action leads to enlightenment and liberation. They realize that in all their actions in the relative universe it is really the Supreme Being that is acting. Through the proper performance of karma yoga, civilization progresses and all the physical needs of the human being are met.

Meditation is the highest and most difficult form of work because it requires the most one-pointed concentration. In this sense, all yoga is karma yoga. Raja yoga is merely a more advanced form of karma yoga. Work is yoga and yoga is work. Work is the process of evolution. The higher the rate of any vibration the greater is the work it does. To really work is to really meditate and to really meditate is to really work.

The perfection and salvation of every human being is inevitable, because nothing in existence can escape work. Pure consciousness has infinite capacity for work, which expresses through the vastness and eternity of our evolutionary unfoldment.

Once an organism is created on the lower octaves of manifestation, it becomes like a storage battery for attracting, containing, and transmitting the higher vibratory rates which it is harmonically attuned to. When such an organism is evolved to the human level by its work and the work done on it by the processes of nature, awareness or consciousness arises in it to a greater and greater degree. Awareness arises in perfected instrumentalities or manifestations which have been perfected through their work. Work creates awareness. We should not wait for energy with which to do work. We should employ the energy we have to work in order to generate more energy.

If everyone were busy doing his or her own work there would be no war and no fighting but, rather, peace and harmony. Peace comes from the willingness to work, to create harmony. War arises out of a lack of awareness, a lack of appreciation for the work of others through neglect of one's own work. To work is to participate in and to partake of life.

We are of no use to God or to ourselves until we have learned the lesson of honest hard work. Even God cannot help the person who is not willing to work. God says, in effect: "I exist in you. Ask me for anything, and I will give it to you in the form of your own strength and discipline." It is through our work that we become a divine instrument in the hands of God. We must always realize that it is God who is the real worker in us, who in the form of our own consciousness is the creator and sustainer of all our activities.

BHAKTI YOGA

"Stand ready and watch the heart... It is not easy to love, as do the great ones, with a pure love which requires nothing back; with an impersonal love that rejoices where there is a response, but looks not for it, and loves steadily, quietly, and deeply through all apparent divergences, knowing that when each has found the way home, the home will be found to be at-one-ment."

INITIATION, HUMAN AND SOLAR, ALICE BAILEY

Bhakti Yoga is the yoga of love sometimes called the Path of Devotion. Bhakti yoga is worship of God in all of God's creations. It is seeing everything as divine in its innermost essence. In its most highly developed form, bhakti yoga is that perfect love which can give everything and ask for nothing because it is everything and it gives only to itself. In so giving it perfects all manifestations created out of itself. The individual is perfected as one of these creations, until the realization of oneness with Pure Existence comes and then he or she becomes a perfect instrument through which God's love expresses itself.

To the bhakti yogi the happiness of all beings is his or her happiness. Their joy is his or her joy, their fulfillment is his or her fulfillment because the bhakti yogi sees his or her self as being the self in all. The bhakti yogi has perfect patience. He or she recognizes love as a process of helping other people and beings to manifest their evolutionary expressions. The bhakti yogi's identification and happiness goes beyond his or her own personality to include all life. In dealing with fellow humans, the bhakti yogi recognizes love as a process of experiencing together. The experience is the one consciousness working through both people or human instrumentalities. Love is recognizing yourself in another person or being. The bhakti yogi recognizes love as being and acting in harmony with another person. The bhakti yogi understands that as soon as we are ready to give in love; God, as our own self, supplies us with infinite love, wisdom and power and all resources to express love.

We have not to receive love but to become love. Love is the creative power of our own immutable existence. It is the practical expression of our oneness with God and the whole creation. Love should not drive us in the form of desire, it should emanate from us as the expression of God's eternal presence in us and in all life. Love is a state of experiencing your consciousness inside other people and beings, helping them to grow and express outward, to present their gift to the world.

Love is also the state of total joy and happiness. Even the sense of being unhappy implies a concept of what happiness should be which shows us that we already contain happiness and happiness is our real nature. As a manifestation of pure being, we must create happiness rather than try to seek it outside ourselves. It is work to be unhappy. All work has evolutionary value. Therefore all unhappiness must eventually lead to happiness. Evolution starts with existence and is consummated in love. Love is the highest product of the evolutionary process.

Love is experiencing the beauty and goodness in every detail of life. Love is a universal force that expresses itself on every plane of manifestation. On the highest level it is the complete harmony and intercommunication between all the points in the universe. Without this detailed appreciation there is no enrichment or experience. Even wisdom, great as it is, is only the skeleton of life, the evolutionary blueprint. Love is the accomplished fact of the cosmic harmony, the flesh on the skeleton of cosmic law, the life of the universe. In the presence of love, all beings give up their enmity and live in peace and harmony. Love is God's highest gift to humankind, the force which gives meaning and purpose to existence.

The practice of bhakti yoga is the best means of organizing and perfecting the desire or astral body. But it is a universal power that will transfigure every aspect of the human being. When the highest love incarnates in the human being, obedience to God is inevitable. In that state human will and God's will become identical.

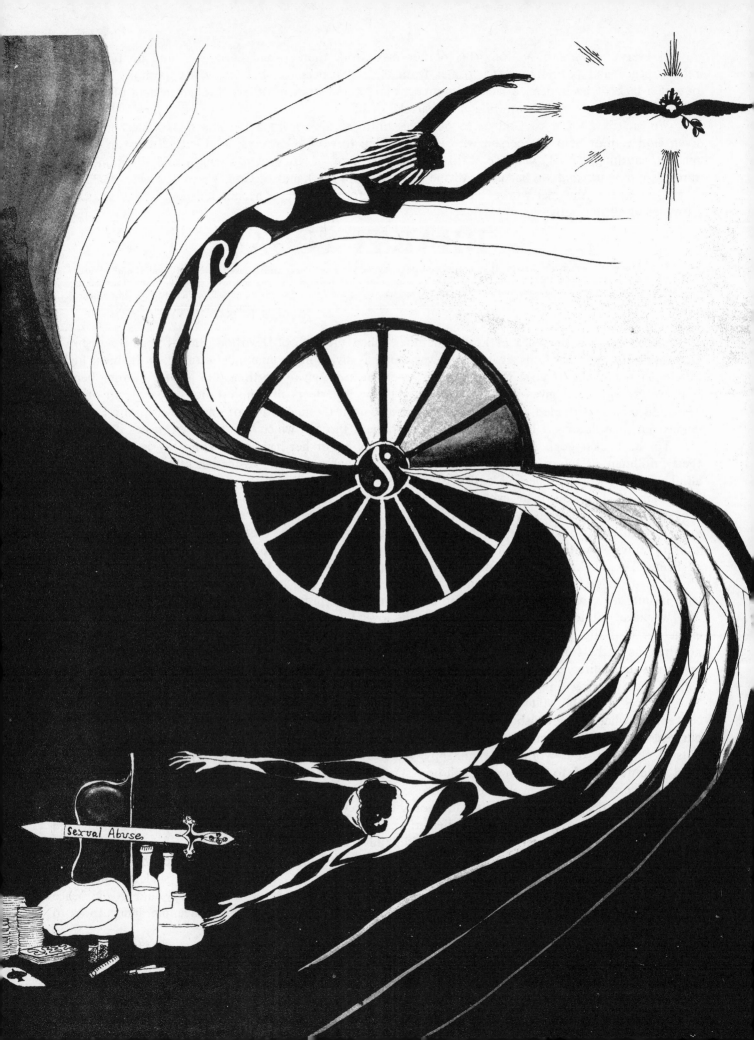

TANTRA YOGA

The union of man and woman is like the mating of Heaven and Earth. It is because of their correct mating that Heaven and Earth last forever. Humans have lost this secret and have therefore become mortal. By knowing it the Path to Immortality is opened.

SHANG-KU-SAN-TAI

Here in this body are the sacred river; here are the sun and moon, as well as all the pilgrimage places. I have not encountered another temple as blissful as my own body.

SARAHA DOHA

If a man makes love without ejaculating, his vital essence is strengthened, his body becomes harmonized and his subtle hearing and vision will become acute. Although such a man has repressed his passion, his love for the woman will increase; it is as if he cannot get enough of her.

YU-FANG-PI-CHUCH

The Knower of Yoga should always worship the female power, according to the revelation of the Tantras. One should worship mother, sister, daughter, wife and all women. During this kind of worship there should be contemplation of the essential unity of Wisdom and Means, the female and male principles.

ADVAYASIDDHI

The Goddess resides in all women and the Lord abides in all men.

JVALAVALI VAJRAMALA

Tantra is probably the most misunderstood of all the yogas. It is the Yoga of Total Experience of Every Aspect of Life. The main premise is that every basic or natural activity of life is fundamentally divine and will lead to self-realization if engaged in with detachment, devotion and awareness.

It is the primary philosophy of tantra yoga that matter can ascend to spirit as well as spirit ascend to matter. The interaction of energy upon itself on lower planes of manifestation can create higher harmonic overtones as well as lower ones. Tantra deals with the process of transforming sensory energy into spiritual energy and sensory experience into spiritual experience by sufficient concentration of attention on the functioning processes of our lower sensory energy patterns. These patterns become so charged with energy that they begin to manifest higher octave pattern imprints of themselves, thus reproducing sensory patterns on the higher octaves of spiritual energy. By this process the senses are spiritualized through fulfillment and brought under the control of spiritual consciousness. At the same time a means of manifesting spiritual values and forces on the material level is developed. It is the contention of tantra yoga that we must take the body with us in meditation and transform its energy into spiritual energy. The body thus becomes a means of expression for the spirit rather than an obstacle to the experience of spiritual states of consciousness. Tantra yoga teaches how to evolve. It is the method of the will within people which bends matter to its purpose, rather than discarding it, and thus conquers all obstacles to spiritual unfoldment. It is a combination of love and power. It overcomes matter by fulfilling it and molding it instead of trying to deny it. In tantra yoga the body is used as a road map for evolutionary development. Tantra yoga brings every aspect of life into mutual harmony and leaves nothing out.

Lower levels of experience can only be transcended by fulfilling them. It is impossible to renounce something you have not had.

Tantra yoga is usually associated with sex, but sex is only one aspect of the total practice of tantra yoga albeit a very important one. The philosophy and methods of tantra yoga can be applied to any sensory experience or practical activity of life. In tantra every note in the harmony of life must be sounded including sex. It is recognized that the body is an instrument of experience and that love through the body is a process of self love. Sex should lead to a lack of tension through union.

Because the total amount of energy in the universe remains constant and energy can neither be created nor destroyed, in sex no energy is wasted; it is merely transformed. By means of proper attention to the process of sexual union, sexual energy can be transformed into spiritual energy of expanded awareness. In tantra yoga it is necessary to register the vibration patterns of the sexual partner in order to properly match and polarize them. This is a good exercise in attunement to another person.

In sexual embrace no one should move for half an hour; just feel the exchange of energies. Then take your time and go about sex slowly, being aware of everything. Maintain sensation at a very high level for a long period and then bring the level of sensation down slowly while remaining in a high state of love and conscious awareness. After sexual union one should not indulge in sleep but should go into a state of meditation. He or she should find out who the experiencer of sexual pleasure is. This leads to expanded consciousness.

Tantra yoga is a great destroyer of hypocrisy. Sex is very important to develop the feeling aspect of our being. If we have not experienced and do not understand human love, how can we hope to understand divine love.

REINCARNATION

In the process of human development, there comes a time when the physical body is worn out like an old suit of clothes and can no longer serve as a useful tool for gaining evolutionary experience on the physical plane. At this time the soul and the subtle bodies must withdraw from the physical body in the process called death. When this happens, there is no energy or guiding principle to sustain the physical body and it disintegrates back into the chemical elements from which it was organized. The soul takes with it in the form of a small compact vibrational energy pattern the complete record of all the experiences of the physical body. This is called the permanent seed atom of the physical body.

One by one the subtle bodies disintegrate, keeping a complete record of their experiences in the permanent atoms. In this way the soul retains all the experiences of each of the incarnations just past as part of its evolutionary development. In the process of dropping each of the subtle bodies, all the experiences which have transpired in those bodies during the lifetime that has ended are reviewed and passed before the person's vision so that the soul may garner the full karmic lessons of those experiences.

For instance, in the astral body the person must live through direct contact with all the astral forces and emotional vibration patterns which he or she has created during the physical embodiment which has just ended. He or she must experience in the astral body the consequences of these forces. Thus the human being records in the memory of his or her soul, the discrimination between harmony and inharmony, good and evil. The human being is thus taught by karmic law to create harmony and happiness and to work in co-operation with the cosmic laws.

Death is not an instantaneous process; it happens by stages. As each of the subtle bodies is discarded the energy of the plane to which it belongs receives its substance. The etheric body is the first to disintegrate, next comes the astral body, and finally the mental body. These subtle bodies are temporary bodies, just as is the physical body. Finally the soul stands naked on its own plane but retains all the experiences of the incarnation just past. The soul remains in this condition for some time until the experiences of the previous incarnation have been fully assimilated and it is ready for a new incarnation. The length of time required to discard each of the subtle bodies will depend on the point in spiritual evolution of the individual involved. If the soul is highly evolved, they will be discarded quickly.

When a time and place providing suitable astrological conditions is found, and the social, family, national, physical and other conditions are in place, the process of incarnation begins again. The soul chooses a time and place suitable for fulfilling the karma incurred in past incarnations and for its further evolution. The process is planned in such a way that any qualities in which the soul is underdeveloped with be strengthened, while mistakes made in previous incarnations can be corrected.

As the process of incarnation begins, the seed atom of the mental body gathers about itself matter of the mental plane which is on the same vibratory rate as the karmic patterns recorded in the seed atom; when this process is complete, the newly formed mental body and the seed atom of the astral body gathers astral substance from the astral plane and molds it according to the karmic patterns recorded in the seed atom of the astral body. By a similar process, an etheric body is organized around the seed atom of the etheric body. The soul and its subtle bodies then await the opportunity to take command of a fertilized ovum in the womb of a prospective mother. The soul having entered the mother's auric field and having taken charge of the fertilized ovum, proceeds to supervise the building of a physical body by making use of the hereditary factors received from the parents and by arranging these to create a body from its archetypal pattern.

There is no final resting place in evolutionary development. In the process of evolutionary change and the cycle of reincarnation, every birth is a death and every death is a birth. All is the process of life in evolution. There is no death because existence is eternal and immutable. Life is always present to experience death. How can there be death when there is life present to observe it? There is only the constant repatterning of life.

Consciousness doesn't need language. Every language and the entire evolutionary process is the language of consciousness. When consciousness communicates to people, it is always in a language they can understand.

"Death is essentially a matter of consciousness. We are conscious one moment on the physical plane and a moment later we have withdrawn on another plane and are actively conscious there. Just as long as death is identified with form aspects it will hold for us its ancient terror. Just as soon as we know ourselves to be souls and find we are capable of following our consciousness or sense of awareness in any form or any plane at will, or any direction in the form of God, we shall no longer know death."
ALICE A. BAILEY, TREATISE ON WHITE MAGIC

The question always arises that if there is such a thing as reincarnation, why is it that we do not remember our past incarnations? This is not universally the case. Many people under hypnosis have been able to recall in detail their previous incarnations and have been able to speak in ancient foreign tongues which they had never studied and had no knowledge of in their present lifetime. Some of the information gained in this way has been checked and verified by historical records.

There are recorded cases of children in many parts of the world who have been able to remember their previous incarnation and give accurate facts concerning it. This often happens when a child dies young due to illness or accident and is immediately reincarnated, sometimes into the same family, and retains the same mental body from the previous incarnation.

The reason that most of us do not remember our past incarnations is because, for the most part, the mental body is the primary seat of memory. As explained above, after each incarnation, the mental body is dissolved and the record of it is maintained in the permanent seed atom of the mental body. This seed atom exists on a higher octave of energy than does the mental plane since the permanent seed atoms are part of the soul. Most people are not in sufficiently good attunement with the soul on its own level to be able to read the permanent records of the previous incarnations which exist on that high level of vibration.

When human beings have fully developed a body of intuition on the Buddhic plane, they will be able to remember all their past incarnations because this body of intuition will remain intact from incarnation to incarnation.

At our present stage in evolution, we would not be able to withstand the emotional pressure and all the mental confusion that total memory of all our previous incarnations would cause. It is a divine mercy that we don't remember them. Such memory at our present stage of development would interfere with the performance of the present evolutionary job at hand. We do not even remember most of the details of our present incarnation. How many of us can remember what we did on May 5th when we were eleven years old? Rest assured that nothing is lost in the evolutionary process. The soul on its own level remembers everything. When we reach a stage in evolution where it is useful for us to remember all of these things, we will remember them.

The psychic, Arthur Ford describes his eyewitness account of the hereafter: "Each person is a continuing entity through eternity. No beginning and no ending... There has never been a time when we were not, and we always will be, even though in constant changing forms and stages, for we are as much God as God is part of us... For if each of us is God, then taken together we are God; we know that another person is necessary to us as our own arms and legs. Each of us is incomplete without the totality of humanity, both living and dead." ("A World Beyond" by Ruth Montgomery, Fawcett Pub Inc, Greenwich, Conn.)

In time, a soul learns the laws of each confining form, assumes control and uses the form for soul perfection. Once he or she has outgrown the form, he or she discards it for higher forms. One progresses always by means of detachment from the form. We have repeated death and birth so many times that we should feel familiar with them. We have died many times and shall die again and again. Even sleep is a form of death, although we return each time into the same body.

Death is a joyous occasion. The soul is released from the bondage of the physical form and is given access to the more powerful faculties of the new form.

When death is unavoidable, a person should be allowed to prepare for it. He or she may wish to invite friends and relatives for a reverent, joyous celebration. Alice A. Bailey suggests the following program for an easier exit into the next world: Let there be a period of silence in the chamber to allow the soul to prepare for departure; when recovery is impossible, orange light focused on the head makes exit easier for the soul; certain notes from the organ, and mantric phrases create peaceful vibrations; the head should point to the east.

GOD IN EVOLUTION

By means of the evolutionary process, God organizes the essence of pure existence from a state of simple homogeneous vibrations into an infinity of organized patterns of energy which exist on all lower planes of manifestations. Eventually, self-conscious intelligent beings are developed through which consciousness can function and directly manifest its will on any plane of creation. The human is one variety of such beings.

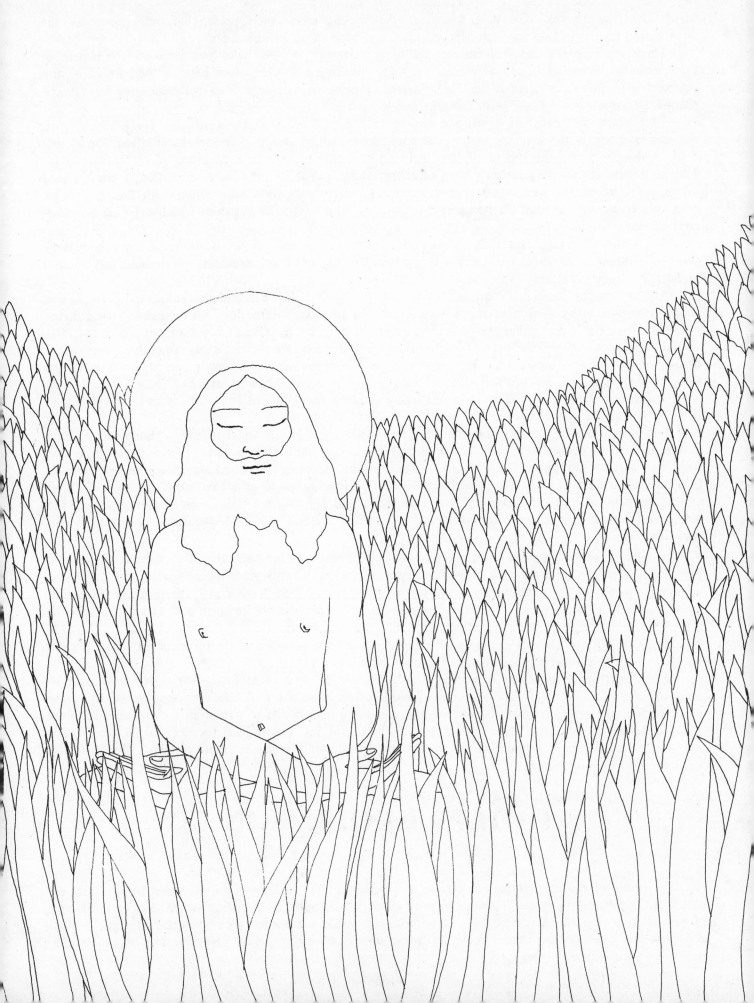

In human evolution, INDIVIDUALISM, must precede UNIVERSALISM. People have to go through the stage of ego identification in order to become organized, independent, self-sustaining entities which can later realize their oneness with cosmic consciousness and be used as divine instruments by that pure consciousness. It is each person's evolutionary individuality of difference which, in the form of the organized subtle bodies, ultimately unites him or her with all existence. Oneness with God is not a state of blank conformity; it is experiencing oneself as the one in all and the all in one. Enlightenment is experiencing oneself as pure existence or consciousness. Nothing is ever lost to pure being or pure consciousness because it can, in the course of evolution, dissolve and remanifest anything at will. We must learn to include everything in our awareness. As pure consciousness, all exists within us. Dualism is transcended by including it in oneness, not by denying it.

Descent of spirit into matter is one phase of evolution. Ascent of organized matter back into spirit is another phase of evolution. FREE WILL of evolving organisms develops as matter returns to spirit, as does the Karmic responsibility of the evolving organism which accompanies the use of free will. As mind is developed in the human stages of evolution, there is the possibility of directing the flow of attention and becoming an independent co-creator with God. An individual's free will operates within certain limits. An individual has free will only when he or she unites his or her individual will with God's will, which alone can know all the infinite indirect causal factors entering into any given situation and all possible future consequences of any action. As long as people are limited in making choices by the finite memory of their own personalities, their decisions are predetermined by the contents of their personal memories and limited knowledge. Only by uniting with omniscient pure consciousness, can all contingencies be accounted for and the best possible choice be made.

There are no mistakes. All seeming mistakes are only relative. They become our teachers and thus lead us to perfection. Thus, in the long range, all-inclusive view of God; no action is evil action; all is part of God's evolutionary process. Evil actions serve the useful purpose of teaching via the law of karma. Evil actions are only evil in the sense that they lead to perfection more slowly than virtuous actions. By virtuous self-discipline or good action, a person's evolution can be speeded up. From the point of view of an evolving organism, good actions are preferable because only through perfecting oneself in harmony with all can oneness with God or pure consciousness be experienced.

There is no choice for us whether to learn or not to learn. We have only a choice of what means to learn by. We can learn by our mistakes through the process of karmic retribution, or we can learn by obeying the command of our own inner consciousness which is the presence of God within us. We cannot avoid participation in the process of the universe which is an educational and perfecting process. Through consciousness, all mistakes become our teachers, and are transmuted into wisdom.

Education is largely a process of developing the human instrumentality by perfecting the subtle bodies. A person is not capable of receiving any more truth than his or her subtle bodies are able to tune in on. Evolution is a process of perfecting organisms or instrumentalities for consciousness to function through.

By meditation on the process of evolution, we learn how to act in total harmony with the rhythm of the universe and all the forces in our circumstances. Only then does suffering cease. Suffering is the safety check system by which evolution warns any evolving organism that it is stepping out of line with God's evolutionary purpose. Thus the evolutionary process is kept in order.

In a state of harmony everything relates constructively in a manner conducive to the evolution of everything else. At the highest level this becomes the state of the one in all and the all in one. The motto "one for all and all for one" is the best guide for spiritual living if it is applied universally so that no one and no thing is left out. The will of the illumined person is identical with God's will and the person simply acts as a vehicle of expression of that cosmic will.

It is possible to change future events by erecting a new image on the level of pure consciousness and letting it precipitate into manifestation. It is possible for a person who is not fully illumined but who has developed some occult powers to condition future events on the physical level by operating from the faster time scale of intermediate planes of spiritual energy such as from the astral or mental planes. Such powers will be limited, however, and will lead to swift karmic retribution if they are used for selfish purposes because the person using them wrongly will have to cope with his or her own miscreations.

The progress of evolution is not a straight-line progression. Evolution accelerates as it progresses. The more we grow the more we have to grow with. Evolution proceeds in an exponential spiral, higher forms of energy evolving faster because their rate of vibration is more rapid. Salvation, or perfection in harmony, is inevitable for all beings. God gives us everything we need so that we can become one with the divine. Giving and receiving are the same thing, because the giver and receiver are both creations of God and manifestations of the same essence.

Enlightenment for any individual is a process of organizing a vehicle of experience and expression on the superconscious plane. This body must be organized out of the energy substance of the plane that comes above the mental plane in vibratory rate. Enlightenment or living in the eternal now is a state of perfect timeless patience. In that state the person experiences his or her self as all existence. He or she who fully experiences God becomes God.

If, at present, the human is an imperfect being, he or she is also an unfinished being. People will be perfected in the fullness of the evolutionary process. This knowledge should not lead to laziness however. At the human state in evolution, we are responsible for deliberately and consciously taking a hand in accelerating our own evolutionary progress. We must participate in evolution in a practical way on every plane of manifestation including the physical plane.

Indian culture, while it has made the greatest contributions in understanding the nature of pure being and the higher spiritual forces, is behind in technological development because in the past it has ignored evolution on the practical, physical level. Indian culture has concentrated too much on being and not enough on becoming. Western civilization has made the reverse mistake and has concentrated too much on practical becoming and not enough on spiritual being. The principles of both being and becoming need to be understood and incorporated into our daily life. Eastern and Western civilizations have much to teach each other. When this cultural cross-fertilization has completely taken place, a more noble world civilization will emerge which will incorporate the best qualities of all the world cultures. At the present time no one nation or culture is capable of adequately leading the world. The various nationalities, races and cultures must all learn from each other. Each has its own specialized contribution to make. Need is evolutionary process yet to be accomplished. Our needs show that evolutionary experience is yet to be fulfilled. There is much need in the world and much work to be done. The greatest need is also the greatest promise.

ETHICS OF YOGA

In the course of studying yoga, we hear a lot about the problem of overcoming the personal ego. The purpose in yoga is not to destroy the ego but to transcend it by including it in a larger synthesis. The part of ego which we must overcome is considering oneself a separate entity apart from the rest of life. We must swallow the ego by including it in our consciousness along with the rest of the universe.

Humility which seeks to become nothing and less than a worm is false humility. In it a tremendous egotism is hidden. Such pretenses at saintliness usually reveal a tremendous pride in one's supposed meekness and humility. True humility does not seek to make a person less than the marvelous being that he or she is, but rather recognizes the infinity of God and God's creation and is ever mindful of the tremendous amount of evolutionary unfoldment that still has to take place before the human is a perfected being. The person of real humility recognizes his or her shortcomings, is honest with his or her self and other people and does not pretend to be something which he or she is not.

The humble person recognizes that what he or she has achieved thus far is nothing compared to what is still to be achieved and the work that is still to be done. Humility arises out of honesty and willingness to see things as they are. The humble person is always a practical and realistic person. Hypocrisy is evasion of truth through refusal to honestly recognize what is. The most humble thing is usually the most beautiful.

We should always be frank about our limitations. Honest ignorance is always better than dishonest pretense. One should always admit that he or she doesn't know something if he or she is ignorant of it. This way we do not mislead others and fool ourselves. We can then recognize what knowledge has to be gained and set about acquiring it.

Liberated person is the person who does not get caught up in his or her own self-imposed limitations. Such limitations usually arise out of selfishness in one form or another. Selfishness is a refusal to recognize and endeavor to be in harmony with other people and other forces in life. We must recognize our total environment as another manifestation of our own consciousness and work in harmony with it by following the guidance of our innermost intuition. This is called living according to divine grace. When one functions according to guidance from the soul he or she works in complete harmony with the rhythm of the universe. It is our duty to discover and obey those universal cosmic laws which are made by God. Human-made laws are the sickness of our culture. Living according to divine grace requires discipline in the beginning, until the correct habit patterns become ingrained and automatic. Through discipline we express our love for and oneness with God. The consciousness in us is the creator of discipline. Eventually people will manifest perfect discipline because it arises out of the infinite, pure consciousness which is the innermost essence of our being.

The aim of Yoga is to create happiness for ourselves and others. Each person's happiness is the happiness of all. People cannot be happy in an environment which they have made unhappy. The way to be happy oneself is to make other people happy. This is achieved by means of service performed with an attitude of detachment. Through this kind of service we express love.

The person who helps other people is accepted by other people. As soon as a person works to make other people happy, they will supply him or her with everything he or she needs to carry on that work which is making them happy. We should seek only that happiness which makes all people happy. To make anyone unhappy is against the nature of consciousness. It is also important to accept the gifts of other people graciously because it helps other people in their evolution. Some of the greatest emotional harm is done by the refusal to accept the gifts and services of other people. It is a denial of love which often leaves a deep scar in the psyche of the giver.

At the same time it must be remembered that service must not be used as a way of bargaining with other people. Love can never be bought by service, especially when the service is not asked for. Such hypocritical service is not real service but service with strings attached which is almost always resented. Real service is performed so joyously that it induces no sense of obligation, guilt and debt in its recipients. We must let karmic law decide from what source our payment comes.

Moral precepts can always best be taught by example. The moral laws of God are present in our innate nature because we also are a part of the rhythm of the universe and the economy of nature. When we see good, we will naturally imitate it. Love can be expressed and accepted but it can never be forced. A person is either evolved enough to accept it or he or she is not.

Evil can only exist on the lower octaves of manifestation because on the higher octaves energy patterns interact with each other so fast that any inharmonious vibrations that are out of phase are immediately cancelled. Therefore, by functioning from a higher level of consciousness we can overcome evil and create order in our lives.

Peace is more than just the absence of war; it is constructive activity for good. Peace is a active dynamic quality of harmony or well organized and ordered interrelationship of the parts of any organism or grouping of people. Harmony is a dynamic process with the element of order introduced into it.

Desire for things we don't have keeps us from enjoying what is at hand right now. The richest person is the one who is satisfied with what he or she has and who does something useful with it. Much of suffering comes from the inability to disengage the mind and emotions from inappropriate objects of attention.

In order to have peace, we must have self-confidence. The mere fact that we exist means that we are accepted by the universe. We do not need to strive to be appreciated. As consciousness we already exist as everything that we wish to be loved for. We only need to appreciate ourselves and our self in all manifestations and all people.

War and conflict arises out of discontent which is restlessness of mind and lack of perception of the opportunities which are right at hand. The important spiritual work is to enlighten as many people as possible starting with ourselves. Then peace will manifest automatically. We have no right to ignore anything in our environment. We must learn to live at peace with all beings. We must contribute as much to life as we take out of it. War and conflict can be overcome by doing one's own constructive work to create peace. Trying to stop violence and evil by means of violence only creates more violence and evil. Efficiency in life is not enough. We must ask, efficiency for what purpose? The greatest discoveries of science, if applied with the wrong motive for the wrong purposes, can be the means of our destruction.

When a person has self confidence, he or she does not need to fight to prove his or her self. We must overcome all fear because it is the root of all hatred and conflict. The spiritual person fears nothing because he or she does not fear his or her self. By identifiying with the pure consciousness in us, we become invulnerable to death and all forms of fear and danger. It should be remembered that those who fear death never really live.

A person's evolutionary development may be measured by what a person is afraid of since one cannot be afraid of anything that can be encompassed by one's own consciousness. An enlightened person has become one with all-inclusive consciousness and thus the entire universe is that person's self in manifestation. Such a person sustains his or her fellow beings by awakening awareness or consciousness in them which creates the energy necessary to cope with the problems of life. As consciousness, he or she is the self of all. Only at the level of consciousness can we feel exactly as another person feels. It cannot be experienced through physical, etheric, emotional and mental activity alone.

A teacher will sometimes enlighten and purify the subtle bodies of his or her students by interpenetrating them with his or her own consciousness and then radiating out from inside the student. A Guru is a teacher who teaches for the sake of teaching. He or she is interested in truth; he or she does not look for rewards.

Because all praise and blame must be filtered through one's own mind, one's opinion of one's self is what matters for happiness. Our own inner consciousness must be the final judge of our lives and guide for our actions. If one is overly concerned about other peoples' it shows that one is not relying on one's self for happiness.

Contentment comes from a willingness to receive the evolutionary value of whatever experiences life presents. In the state of dispassion or spiritual detachment we neither feel compelled to possess anything or to get rid of it. Much of suffering comes from wanting something before it's time or holding on to something after it's time. In the state of Oneness, there is no attachment because one cannot be attached to one's self. Existence simply is.

We should not desire anything more than we desire experience of consciousness. This is detachment. There is no need to pursue anything because consciousness as the creative principle is omnipresent in us. We must create what we need out of ourselves.

We must learn to enjoy our evolution so that we will be motivated to participate in it more intensely. This is the value of the development of love, or bliss, aspect of our nature. Impatience is a lack of awareness of what is going on right now.

We must love and respect all people. From foolish actions we can learn what not to do. Respect is gratitude to other people. It is appreciation of other people and the work they do. To feel this we must observe the activity going on around us. To observe people's activity leads to constructive participations in it.

We must be willing to work hard for what we get. Karmic law demands of us, as human instrumentalities, that we contribute as much to evolution as we receive from it. Our destiny is up to our use of our own free will. We are constantly creating ourselves in the image of what we say, think, and do.

We should be satisfied with what we get in life because that is what we have given. We have no right to demand anything which we are not already. It must be earned by hard work. Strength is peace; it is resting in one's own being. From that inner center or power we can create what we need.

We should never seek to impose our preconceived notions and dogmas on other people. The blind missionary spirit is a very dangerous thing. The missionary is so irreligious that he or she does not realize that everyone is God.

It is possible to do violence to the psyche by offering a person truth which he or she is not capable of understanding. This is so because the emotional thought forms and repressions which the person has in his or her subtle bodies will react violently and throw the subtle bodies out of harmony. This is especially true when such subjects as psychedelic drugs, sex, religion, and politics are involved in the discussion.

Pain is stress greater than an organism can bear easily. Pain serves to intensify experience but it can also be destructive if too intense. We should avoid undue pain to ourselves and others. Sometimes we must wait for the development of harmony with other people so that we can fully share our experiences with them and give and receive love in the fullest sense. This is especially true in regard to personal love relationships.

Above all, it must be remembered that love is the most important thing in life. We should seek only that happiness which is the happiness of all. As soon as we are ready to give in love, then God as our own innermost self manifested as a karmic law supplies us with unlimited power and resources.

To aid us in realizing "God is within," we may seek the help of a living teacher (God personified to teach the science of the Spirit), interpretations of esoteric scripture, texts of ancient teachers above all needed is discipline, discrimination, silence, study and meditation. The books will aid, the teacher will aid, the environment will aid but in the end we are alone. We will be treading a path, if we are sincere and humble, which love of God has prepared for us uniquely. The crown of glory will come when we have mastered self, and have transformed the ego into a flame of love to warm the hearts of others.

As our meditation advances, we will know that we are on the path. For more and more joy will come in the hours that we spend listening to the divine symphonies, the sounds of cosmic creation. We will discover that there is no death, our body will become just one of the places where we spend our time in order to prepare the spirit for advancing. It will become easier and easier to leave the body, at will, to communicate by E.S.P. and to read the Akashic Records. As time passes more and more of the perfection of the divine self will become integral to our being.

Suggested Reading

1. Course in Miracles (Coleman Graphics, 1 Huntington Quadrad, Huntington Station, NY
2. Stalking the Wild Pendulum, Bentov, Bantom Books, N.Y.C.
3. Death of Ignorance, Dr. Fred Bell, New Age Holistic Awareness Publ, Laguna Beach, CA

available through OMangoD Press.

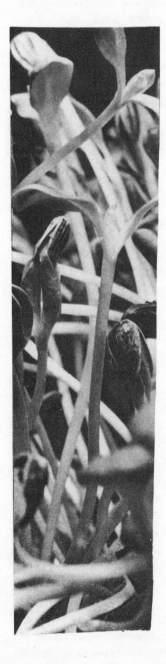
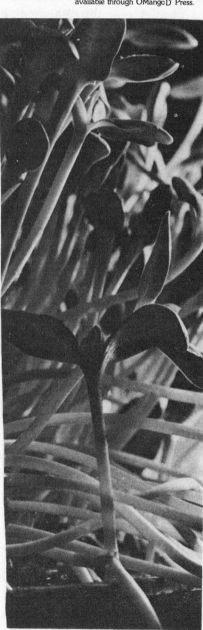
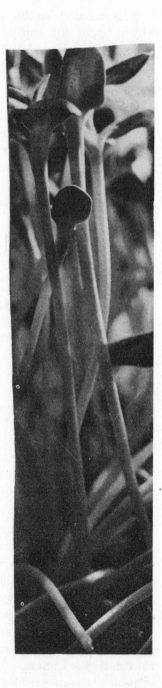

MOTHER, FATHER AND CHILD
THE RIVER OF LIFE

If a man engages in the sex act just once without emitting semen, then his vital essence will become strong. If he does so twice, his hearing and vision will become very clear. If three times, all bodily diseases will disappear. If four times, an inner peace will become attached to his spirit. If five times, then his blood circulation will be greatly improved. If six times, his loins will become very strong. If seven times, his thighs and buttocks will increase their power. If eight times, his whole body will become shining and radiant. If nine times, his life expectancy will increase.

YI-FANG-PI-CHUCH

"And the Lord God commanded the man saying, of every tree of the Garden, thou mayest freely eat; but of the tree of knowledge of good and evil thou shalt not eat of it, for in the day that thou eat thereof thou shalt surely die."

GENESIS 2:15-17

"He that believeth on me, out of his belly shall flow rivers of the living water."

JOHN 7:38

Conservation of the sexual fluid is requisite to abundant health, vitality, maintenance of youth. It is indispensable for the highest spiritual development. Sexual energy may be transmuted to vital energy which opens the spiritual centres and enables one through meditation to commune with the Cosmic forces.

Dr. Bernard shows aging, which starts at puberty, is the direct result of diet:

"In Smith's opinion, the gonads produce their physiological effects by withdrawing certain substances from the circulation, thereby stimulating the production of these substances in excess, with the result that they must be withdrawn from the blood by the sex glands in greater amount; and this withdrawal produces the symptoms of puberty and other affects attributed to a positive action of the gonads in supplying internal secretions to the organs.

"Changes that occur in the male at puberty, such as the sudden growth of the bones, the appearance of hair on the face and the change of voice, can be explained on the basis of the theory of chemical withdrawal through seminal emission which produces a deficiency of certain minerals as calcium and phosphorus in the blood and leads to compensatory super-excitation of certain endocrine glands, as the adrenal, thyroid and pituitary, as well as to the degeneration of other glands, as the pineal and thymus." (242)

"The pubertal crisis, rather than being natural and necessary, really constitutes a pluriglandular disturbance and mineral deficiency produced by chemical withdrawal from the blood of certain substances by the gonads, which they elaborate into secretions that are given off from the body at this time. Without such genital excretions (nocturnal and other seminal emissions in the male and menstruation in the female), there can be no puberty. Instead, the gonads will continue their function of glands of internal secretion, which they performed since the time of birth and during the prenatal state, in a manner similar to that of the thyroid and other endocrine glands. It is an error to believe that the gonads commence to produce sex hormones at the time of puberty and that previous to this time they did not. If they produce more hormones at puberty it is not due to any awakening to a higher development but to the super-excitation produced by the hormone deficiency caused by loss of vital substances through seminal emissions in the male and menstruation in the female, the end of the pluriglandular upheaval that then results being a loss rather than a gain.

"In the male, many of the symptoms resemble those of castration, as do the sudden elongation of the bones, which is not a natural condition; and in the female, the sudden fattening of the body resembles the obesity that follows ovarian degeneration or the ovarian overactivity that occurs in women after marriage, when they tend to become fat. Since it is the function of the ovarian hormones to oxidize fat, as is that of the thyroid hormone thyroxin, the accumulation of fat on the body after puberty, like the elongation of the bones of the male, must be viewed as a castration symptom of gonadal weakness as a result of overactivity and temporary deficiency."

A classic experiment (243) of Dr. Francis Benedict of the Carnegie Institute on the influence of low protein diet in controlling sexual tendencies and eliminating nocturnal emissions from the evidence he supplied leads one (242) to conclude "sex in its ordinary manifestations among civilized human beings is not the product of natural instinct that it is generally supposed to be but is a chemotropism evoked or conditioned reflex (in Pavlov's sense) evoked in response to aphrodisiacal stimulation by foods and beverages, especially animal proteins, alcohol, coffee and also tobacco. This tropistic reaction, in both its physical and psychological aspects, is subject to voluntary control through diet, an alkaline-forming, low protein vegetable diet reducing it, while an acid-forming high protein diet increases it."

"Professor Sajaus, the greatest endocrinologist since Professor Brown — Sequard, like the latter, defends the doctrine of continence on physiological grounds, claiming that the semen contains hormones or internal secretions of the sex glands of nutritional value (such as lecithin, phosphorus, calcium, iron and vitamin E, as well as human cholesterol) to the physiological economy and is not a worthless excretion that can be lost with impurity . . . chemistry of the semen proves it to be very similar to that of nerve and brain tissue." (242)

Sexual fluid loss is a contributing factor in every form of disease. Its composition is similar to that of nerve and brain tissue. These organs are the first ones to be affected. Since the body is totally dependent on nerve energy levels, the loss has an effect on the whole body. Indigestion, emaciation, shortness of breath, nervous debility, constipation, premature old age, epilepsy, paralysis, senility, may be caused by this daily drainage. When seminal loss was corrected in the experiments of Drs. Steinach and Vornoff, all symptoms of many diseases disappeared; the body regained its former vigor and rejuvenation took place.

Dr. Bernard discusses the tremendous mineral loss which takes place in the sexual act:

"Ross and Scholz found that when the thyroid gland is overactive, much phosphorus is eliminated. On the other hand, underactivity of the thyroid causes such elimination to be lessened. In order that phosphorus be properly assimilated it is important that the thyroid be neither over nor underactive. Lorand points out that overactivity of the sex glands is associated with abundant elimination of phosphorus and calcium. While both puberty and castration produce similar deficiency of calcium and phosphorus in the blood, resulting in elongation of the bones, in the former case they are both suddenly withdrawn through seminal emission, while in the latter case the influence of the sex glands in facilitating their utilization is removed.

"According to Marshall, the retardation of the process of ossification by the loss of calcium and phosphorus which then occurs produces the elongation of the bones at puberty, a true castration symptom, due to chemical withdrawal through the semen and not to hormone action. Havelock Ellis notes that persons given to lascivious behavior tend to be short rather than tall. The failure of the young organism to attain full development when castrated or as a result of masturbation is likewise due to a disturbance of calcium and phosphorus metabolism thus produced.

"MacCallum and Voegtlin found that withdrawal of calcium from the nerve cells leaves them in a state of hyperexcitability, which can only be made to disappear by supplying the body with calcium. TETANY, they state, may be regarded as an expression of such hyperexcitability of nerve cells, due to calcium deficiency, and may be overcome by administration of calcium. Since seminal emissions involve an abundant loss of calcium, we can thus account for the nervous symptoms that follow them: the tetany-like symptoms of the sexual ORGASM, followed by extreme fatigue. The nervous symptoms of puberty and the "awkward age" have a similar origin. The same is true of the loss of phosphorus through seminal emissions, which is essential for the nutrition of nervous and brain tissue and whose deficiency produces nervous and mental symptoms which, when pronounced, can manifest as actual neuroses and psychoses." (242)

Beside the wasting away of precious seminal fluids through voluntary sexual intercourse, there are other involuntary, semi-conscious and unconscious acts during which the seminal fluids escape from the body.

Nocturnal emissions take place at night during amorous dreams. Spermatorrhea is the flowing out of seminal fluids without voluntary effort.

Spermatorrhea originated at the time when the human being ignorantly changed from natural food to a diet of nuts, cereals, animal flesh, dairy products, fish, tea, coffee, salt, alcoholic beverages and tobacco.

The first effect of these irritating substances is to overstimulate the sexual function by causing localized invigoration and potency. This may lead to excessive intercourse or masturbation and sooner or later ends in the weakening of the organs. At first, the involuntary night emissions are attended by erection and pleasurable dream sensations; but, as the sexual organs become weaker and lose their tone, the emissions also take place in the day when urine is passed and when the bowels are moved. In extreme cases, the precious seminal fluid is running away without intermission.

The seminal vesicles are sandwiched between the urinary bladder and the rectum. When the bladder is filled with urine and the rectum (lower colon) with fecal matter, these organs become distended and press upon the seminal vesicles. This forces the seminal fluids into the urethra, to be evacuated via the urine. In a state of health, the ejaculatory ducts open into the urethra only during the sexual act. Because of an unnatural, irritative diet and pressure from a filled bladder and rectum, the ducts are kept in a continuous state of tension until they become relaxed to let seminal fluid pass while urinating or defecating or, in more serious cases, during the slightest exertion.

When semen escapes with the urine there will be a sensation in the urethra as if something heavier than usual is passing, giving a slight prickling, tingling sensation. The urine will look cloudy, with floating globules resembling dissolved gum arabic. During defecation, the penis will be covered with glutinous, sticky fluid. Occasionally, mucus from prostate or bladder will be discharged, consisting of only a few drops of transparent fluid which thread when touched. Such losses are especially apparent during detoxification. Semen is much thicker in quality and more opaque than mucus. Sometimes the semen is so diluted in the urine that its loss escapes detection, outside of causing a slight pleasurable sensation and a few spasmodic jerks of the bladder as the last drops of urine are passed.

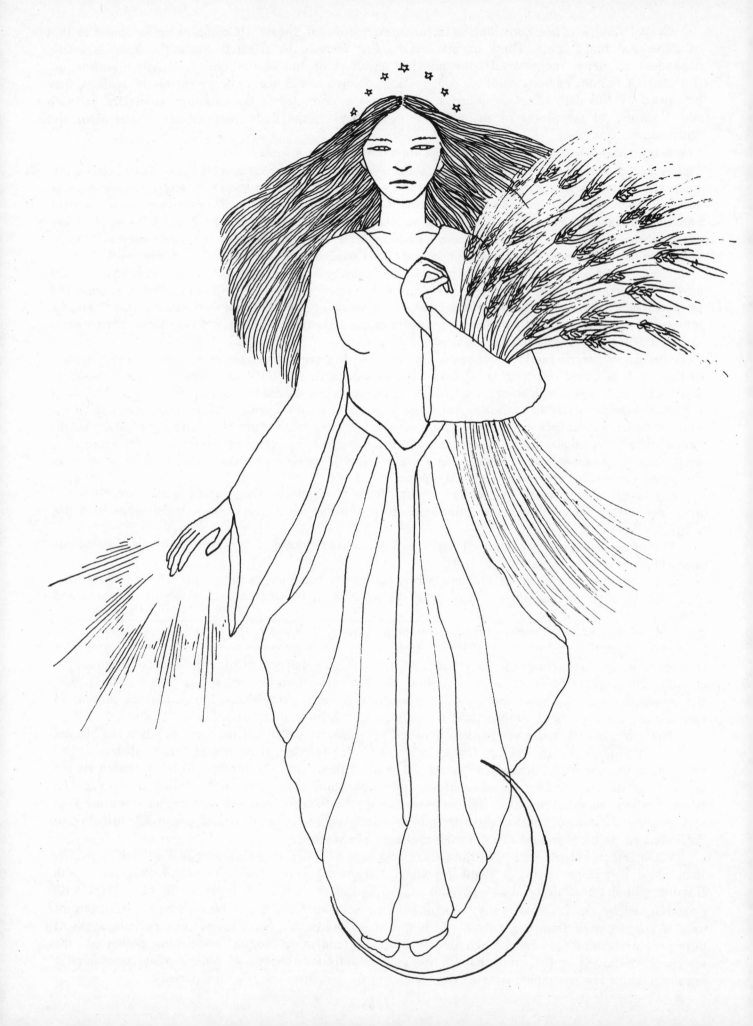

HOW TO REJUVENATE THE FOUNTAIN OF YOUTH

1. Abstain from high protein foods — all animal products, seed, nuts, grains, legumes. Avoid spices and processed foods.
2. Reduce, then gradually eliminate, losses due to intercourse.
3. Reduce pressure on seminal ducts from the eliminative organs:
a) At bedtime, autosuggest that the subconscious wake you whenever baldder or colon needs evacuation.
b) Eat no later than 6 p.m.; reduce food and fluid intake in the afternoon.
c) If constipated, take nightly enemas.
d) At night, sleep on the side instead of the back.
e) Under supervision, take a three to four day liquid diet.
4. Exercise. In morning and afternoon; nude sunbathe; expose abdomen and sex organs to the sun's rays.

BIOLOGICAL SUPERIORITY OF WOMAN

"For freedom Christ has set us free stand fast therefore and do not submit agin to a yoke of slavery." Galatians 5:1

"It seems strange that the Mother of the race should be made the Slave of the Fruits of her Womb. It appears peculiar that she should have no privileges except those received through her son. It seems illogical that the God Principle of the Universe, in its infinite wisdom, should endanger the existence of the Race by making the Mother of it the weak, cringing underling of her husband." HILTON HOTEMA

"There is a parallel resemblance in the sexes that proves and shows their conformity in essential parts to some remote ancestor or progenitor, which preceded them before division of the sexes." CHARLES DARWIN Origin of the Species

"Mellaart's report, written in 1966 before the completion of the excavations, shows that Catal Huyuk, whatever its name may nave been ten thousand years ago, was not only a matriarchal but a utopian society. There had been no wars for a thousand years. There was an ordered pattern of society. There were no human or animal sacrifices: pets were kept and cherished. Vegetarianism prevailed . . . the supreme deity in all the temples was a goddess." ELIZABETH GOULD DAVIS THE FIRST SEX

"All female animals yield their regular ovulation, but it is not accompanied by waste or loss [of vital fluid]. Woman only is cursed this way. But let the female brute lose the control of her procreative function as woman has been deprived of hers [under male rule], and let her be subjected to the unbridled passion of the male, as woman is [Gen. 3:16], and she will soon begin to feel the curse. It is through woman's freedom only, and her resumption of her natural queenship in the domain of sex that she and man can be redeemed. Where is the female animal that wastes her life away at every changing moon? There are none such, save perhaps among the monkey tribes, and the fact exists there for the same reason that it does in woman. No animal that has intercourse for reproduction only, is cursed as woman is." VICTORIA WOODHALL

EFFECT OF DIET AND LIFE STYLE ON MENSES

Throughout nature, the biological superiority of the female is evident. Only the civilized female "seems" to be inferior physically to the male. This condition is brought about largely by the debilitating effect of the menstrual hemorrhage.

The increased consumption of animal protein (doubled in the last 25 years) and of processed foods by civilized humans is causing the menses to appear earlyer each generation and to last longer. According to Dr. E. L. Wynder, president Am. Health Foundation, "diet is related to the increasingly early age of menarche, the start of menstruation - six months earlyer among girls every decade since 1850." (Boston Globe, Dec. 5, 74, p. 50). In my practice I have met girls who started menses at ten and the flow lasted for as many as 15 days.

Because of more natural living, low protein diet and seasonal sexual practices, menses is less of a problem to the uncivilized woman.

Among many of the primitive races and in technologically undeveloped countries, females work side by side with males; many employers have shown preference for female laborers because of their superior endurance and strength.

In the United States, in spite of the menstrual and social handicap, female longevity exceeds that of the male; a larger proportion of females reach the century mark. Hardening of blood vessels and high blood pressure are more common among men than women. There are fewer miscarriages and stillbirths of females than males; the female brain has a finer texture and more complex organization, and, relative to body weight, is 25% heavier than that of the male; her thyroid gland, which has three lobes, is larger than the two-lobed one of the male.

During childhood, female physical size and performance in school exceeds that of the male. This phenomenon is well known to school teachers. With the onset of menstruation and the great loss of essential body fluids, the rapid development of the female is brought to a premature slowdown.

Loss of calcium, which is so essential to develop bone and muscle and to stabilize the nervous system, result in slowdown in skeletal growth. Loss of iodine, lecithin and vitamin E has a detrimental effect on brain development. Loss of hormones, which are more concentrated in menstrual discharge than in the bloodstream, speeds the aging process. Many females are anemic because the monthly hemorrhage causes a reduction of hemoglobin, the oxygen carrier. This has a significant effect on further brain development and nerve activity. Were it not for menstrual losses, the initial superiority of the female would persist in all later stages of physical development.

Historically, menstruation appeared in females after the family unit had migrated to a cooler climate and/or adopted an unnatural diet and increased sexual activity. The development of the family in an unnatural environment involved many hardships. Males very readily used the services of females to do the most unpleasant, monotonous, physically strenuous tasks, while they engaged in the arts of hunting, philosophy, war and religion. The female was the first slave of the male. Often a man kept a large flock of slave wives to perform all necessary chores.

Organized religion, with its male-dominated priesthood, has successfully convinced woman that she must have committed some "basic sin" (Gen. 3:6) for which she must enslave herself to the male: "Thy desire shall be to thy husband, and he shall rule over Thee"(Gen. 3:16). Centuries of inculcation of this dogma have helped to make the female subservient to the dictates of the male.

Through false medical and religious teachings on menstruation, the male-dominated society has managed to keep woman in a slave-like position by insuring her persistent weakness through biological ignorance. Men have claimed mental superiority because of a seeming deficiency in production of great works in philosophy, art or science by the female.

There were times in history when women were not suppressed, and had equal cultural, educational and economic opportunity to achieve their potential. There are instances recorded where pagan women achieved high excellence and superiority over males.

The Pythagorean school produced at least fifteen historically outstanding women. The last was Hypatia of Alexandria, who was murdered by a band of fanatic monks led by the jealous Cyrus, archbishop of Alexandria. The great Greek philosopher, Socrates, had studied under Aspasia, the young female Delphic Oracle. Ammian and Diodorus comment that the women of ancient Gaul were stronger than the males and fought the Romans. Strobo mentions that Gallic women were taller than men. Skeletal remains proved them to be seven feet tall.

Havelock Ellis remarks that all outstanding women in history were relatively free from menstruation. They either menstruated slightly or not at all as was the case with Joan of Arc, proven by medical records during her trial for witchcraft. The well-known ninety-year-old Frenchwoman, Ninon de L'Enclos, who continued to look like a young woman to the end freed herself from menstruation through a special diet. Wallace states: "Some females of robust constitution and right fiber are called viragoes. These, from constitution, menstruate sparingly or not at all."

It has been proven by Bernard, Ehret, Haig and other experimenters that a low protein vegetarian diet leads to a progressive diminution of the menstrual flow until it is replaced by a bloodless discharge as occurs in female animals. Through dietary control and avoidance of erotic excitation of the ovaries, this mucous discharge can also be made to disappear, leading to regeneration of blood, producing new body and brain cells. (242)

In our culture many pathological states are considered natural just because they are normal and prevalent. For example, it is "natural" to die from heart attack; doctors predict that by the year 2000 one of the most "natural" causes of death will be cancer. Actuarian reports state that to be at least 20% underweight increases health and longevity, however doctors and friends consider slim vegetarians sickly because they are not "normal" in weight.

During menses it is considered "natural" to bleed, to have headaches, cramps and back pain; however, these problems seem to exist only in sickly females and domesticated or civilized animals and are non-existent in healthy primitives or wild animals.

LETTERS FROM GIRLS WHO STOPPED THE .

I have known many instances in which menstruation ceased in three to eight months after an improvement in diet. The following letters are representative of some new experiences for females on raw food diet.

MENSTRUAL PERIOD IT IS NEVER PAINFUL, BUT OFTENTIMES I SIMPLY DON'T HAVE THEM. So I'm wondering whether it is normal for women to have menstrual periods? And what has been the experience of other women on raw food diets? (I'm 27 years old.) I remember Ehret talked of women ceasing to have periods. And another woman who lived for years on a raw fruit diet said she only menstruated once every 6 months.   Donna W., Berkley, Feb. 72.

Dear Viktoras: I wrote to you some time ago; at that time I was alarmed because I had missed three months' menstrual and had only been eating basically raw foods for exactly that period of time. I have still not menstruated once since commencing this regime, I feel no monthly discomfort, physical or mental, to speak of and in general I can attest to the fact that MISSING PERIODS IS NO LESS THAN A JOY. However, I still wonder how easily I should accept this phenomenon, whether or not I SHOULD WORRY ABOUT EVER HAVING CHILDREN, whether I am going to experience some unforseeable malady in the long run. These are all things which my friends when hearing about my condition become alarmed over. I myself generally have belief that my body is doing better than ever but occasionally the words of these friends make me question again this peculiar diet.

After so much anxiety and urging, I finally went to a doctor of obstetrics and gynecology at the Stanford Medical Center in Palo Alto. There I had a kind of review with a Dr. L. to whom I mentioned the Hippocrates Health Institute and Professor Ehret. Having seen several other women with cases much like mine, and as he was in the process of writing a paper on the phenomenon, he was reasonably interested in my case. He either has written or will write to your Institute in Boston for further information. Of course in diagnosing me, he felt my diet was lopsided; but he also seemed to believe that I was in fine shape and there at least has been no damage incurred in the short run. Well, I could have told him that. He urged me to begin eating high protein foods and that if I did so I would most likely begin menstruating again, although spottedly at first. It was a harmless visit but I didn't really learn too much. What I think I want to hear more than ever is that other women perform (or react) as I am and that I may still be able to reproduce. I have heard you say that you know women whose flow ceased and that is mostly the reason why I am not very worried about all this. I'll be interested to hear from you when your time permits.

Sincerely,
Mary R., Aromas, Calif., Dec. 1971

Dear Viktoras: Finally received a copy of Love Your Body. The book inspired me to get back to raw foods. Every day I freak out with one of your delicious recipes. It makes it so easy to stay on this "strange" diet. I have moved again and have new friends. They're into yoga and meditation. I join them several times a week. They have seen your book (L.Y.B.) and were so delighted that someone can make the subject of nutrition so simple. I have been preparing some of your sauces with sprouts at the ashram. Now everyone wants your book. So cash enclosed, rush me two dozen copies.

Life is one of change. WHILE WORKING AT THE INSTITUTE, I had withdrawn from dexamil and other stimulants after 8 years of being hooked. I found that the raw food and juices provided me with more energy without the 5 p.m. letdown. Also, MY MENSES REDUCED TO A CLEAR, SCANTY FLOW, LASTING ONLY FEW HOURS WITH HARDLY ANY BLOOD LOSS. Those five months with you at Hippocrates were some of my most memorable moments into body and spirit awareness.

After returning to secretarial work, I SLIPPED BACK TO EATING WHATEVER WAS AVAILABLE — generally one meal a day, using dairy products, fruit and vegetables and occasionally meat, plus lots of coffee and cigarettes. The loss of energy brought me back to the occasional use of dexamil. MY MENSTRUAL PERIOD BECAME DIFFICULT, LASTING 4 TO 7 DAYS.

Five months ago, I took your advice and replaced dexamil and coffee with several cups of Ginseng tea. The results were marevlous — feeling high without letdown. Now I have even given up the use of the tea, except for special occasions.

Since I returned to the raw life, I feel the new me. Presently, I'm preparing a photo portfolio — I think I'm ready for the fashion world. Summer is here and the raw food is easy. My period has practically disappeared. I hope I will be able to handle the diet in winter. Thank you for your kindness.

Love,
A.K.

Results from considerable research do answer the questions these young women have asked: Is monthly bleeding natural? Can non-menstruating women become pregnant? Is cessation of menses due to good health or extreme poor health? How may menses be eliminated?

WHAT IS MENSTRUATION?

The beginning of the menstrual flow occurs actually at the end of the menstrual cycle. It represents the climax of twenty-eight days, plus or minus, of preparation of the body for conception.

The menstrual cycle is governed by hormones produced by the pituitary glands and the ovaries. Estrogen and progesterone are the substances that the ovaries naturally manufacture under the direction of the master gland, the pituitary. With ordinary amounts of these hormones in the bloodstream, the pituitary gland signals the ovaries to release an ovum every month at the midpoint between the menstrual periods. When hormone levels are a little higher, as in pregnancy, the pituitary does not direct ovulation.

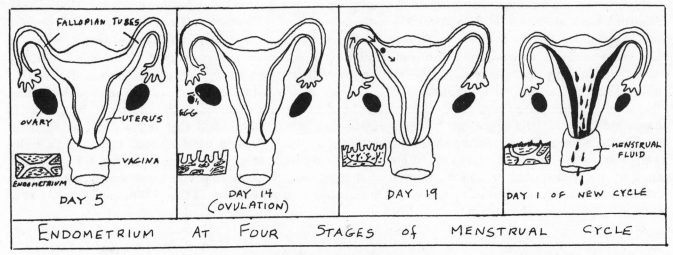

ENDOMETRIUM AT FOUR STAGES OF MENSTRUAL CYCLE

DO ANIMALS MENSTRUATE?

Undomesticated animals do not menstruate, but they have periodic mating seasons known as heat, rut or estrus which usually occurs several times a year, generally in spring and autumn. In the normal state, during ovulation, the genital organs of females of lower animals are slightly congested and are moistened with mucus.

However, after the non-menstruating animal is captured, the estrus becomes transformed into a bloody flow, manifesting as the menstrual hemorrhage. This results from an unnatural diet and artificial living conditions. This occurs with the cow, donkey, mare, bear, pig, cat, rabbit, dog and monkey. Monkeys menstruate five times a year. This has very little to do with fertility, since they rut only twice. The cow has a discharge, sometimes quite bloody, every three weeks; yet it ruts only once a year.

MONKEY MENSES

Dr. Rhodes, professor of obstetrics at the University of London, discusses the difference between menstruation and estrus.

"The lining of the uterus is the endometrium, which is under the control of the hormones of the ovary. Since these are produced in waxing and waning cycles the endometrium waxes and wanes in time with the hormone secretions from the ovary. THIS IS TRUE FOR ALL MAMMALS, BUT ONLY IN THE PRIMATES IS THE PHENOMENON OF MENSTRUATION SEEN. This is the periodic shedding of the endometrium from the uterus which is seen as a bloody discharge from the vaginal orifice . . . the physiological significance of menstruation is not known . . .

"In the lower animals estrus occurs in regular cycles depending on the species and its environment. The vaginal bleeding which is seen in the animals at estrus is not comparable to menstruation as bleeding is associated with ovulation in the estrus cycle, but the vaginal bleeding of menstruation occurs only after the death of the corpus luteum approximately fourteen days after ovulation. EVEN AMONG THE PRIMATES MENSTRUATION IS NOT UNIVERSAL AND IN THE NEW WORLD MONKEYS OCCURS ONLY SPORADICALLY, BUT IN THE OLD WORLD MONKEYS AND THE ANTHROPOIDEA MENSTRUATION IS THE RULE."

A probable explanation for the difference in menstrual pattern of the Old and New World monkeys is that the monkey of the Old World (Europe, Asia and Africa) has been contaminated with processed food through many years contact with these civilized countries. The New World monkeys have had very little contact with factory-made food. Even now, the New World is far more uncivilized and primitive than the Old World.

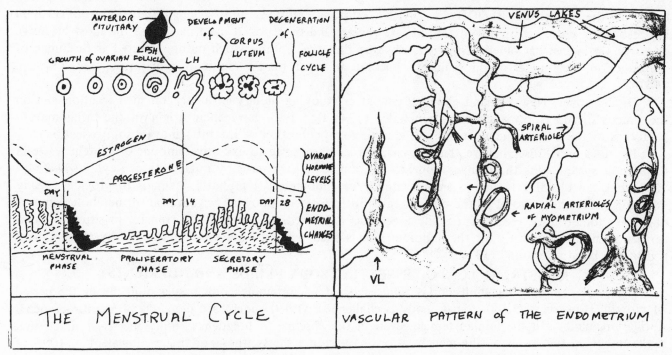

THE MENSTRUAL CYCLE

VASCULAR PATTERN OF THE ENDOMETRIUM

Menstrual bleeding in Old World monkeys is associated with congestion in the arterioles located in the uterus lining. New World monkeys (Cebus, Ateles, etc.) have periodic cycle of bleeding, microscopic in nature and associated with minimal tissue loss. Goodman, Wislocki and Kaiser have pointed out that THERE ARE NO COILED ARTERIOLES IN THESE FORMS. Dr. Rhodes writes: "The spiral arterioles are the key to the phenomenon of menstruation for they have been observed to contract and relax in the few days before the menstrual flow. During contraction the endometrium blanches and during relaxation becomes congested. This observation was made by Markee . . . constriction of the arterioles is intense and so probably leads to anoxia . . . the vessels break too and this is responsible for the bleeding." (126). The spiral arterioles are equivalent to varicosities in veins, which result from ingesting mucus-forming processed foods. The Old World monkeys have ready access to this diet from their civilized cousins whereas the New World monkeys have to be satisfied with bananas. Gilman and Gilbert (202) showed that menstruation is not natural for the Old World monkey. They observed that when female baboons were fed on a vegetables only diet, menstruation cycles ceased.

MENSES AS A TOXIC REACTION

Dr. Bieler, in the informative bood, "Natural Way To Sexual Health" (125), discusses menstruation: "The female suffering from a state of toxemia, with her liver failing to filter as it should, places a burden on the natural menstrual functions . . . this function is turned into a sort of garbage filter, resulting in chronic inflammation of the womb.

"When toxic blood seeks an outlet through the womb via the menstrual function, the resulting inflammation and irritation to the delicate mucous membrane throws the organ into spasms which are registered as pain or cramps. If the toxin is milder or more dilute, the patient simply feels heavy or congested in her pelvis. Once the flow has started, nature pours out as much toxic material from the blood as possible. This inflames the deeper layers of the womb. What should be a normal flow develops into a hemorrhage, sometimes lasting for days and reducing the patient to a state of anemia. The womb weakened after such chemical poisoning is easy prey to harmful bacteria (125, p. 174).

"Toxins that have been temporarily sidetracked into the body tissues and into such organs as the lymph glands, spleen, liver, subcutaneous tissues, skin, muscles, and bones are mustered and thrown into the bloodstream. They seek vicarious elimination through the menstrual flow. The patient feels heavy and congested in the pelvic area. There is a slight rise in temperature, which means that the adrenal glands have increased oxidation in an effort to burn some of the toxic material. The pulse becomes rapid; the palms sweat; nervousness and insomnia follow (125, p. 175).

"The QUALITY OF THE MENSTRUAL BLOOD varies according to the chemistry of the toxic material. BRIGHT RED, profuse, odorless blood accompanied by severe uterine cramps comes from improper digestion of starch and sugar. The offending toxins are acids such as lactic, acetic, pyruvic, oxalic and formic which have not been completely oxidized to carbon dioxide and water. On the other hand, if the menstrual BLOOD IS DARK, odorous, clotted, and stringy, the toxins of protein indigestion or putrefaction are present. Eggs, cheese, and overcooked meat can cause the most offensive odors in the menstrual blood. Thus it is obvious that the womb, which nature selected as the organ of reproduction, can, under chemical duress, become an organ for the elimination of putrid waste (125, p. 176)."

Dr. Schroyer, New England gynecologist, after studying dietary influence on menstruation and on the mucus discharge of leucorrhea, concludes (134) that both have their origin in the inflammatory condition of the uterine mucus membrane due to toxic condition of the intestines (autointoxication).

Reynold and Kaiser believe that menstrual bleeding is due to excessive amount of protein waste in the lymph system plus the damage done to the lining of the uterus by putrefaction. Reynold suggests: ". . . that the bleeding is due to an inadequacy of endometrial lymphatic channels to provide a ready mechanism for the removal of the protein catabolites formed following withdrawal of metabolic support of the endometrium" (135). These substances, as expressed by Kaiser, ". . . remain in situ and cause further tissue destruction until the endometrium is shed down to the area maintained by the capillary bed of the basal arterioles" (131).

MENSTRUAL LOSS OF ESSENTIAL BODY FLUIDS AND NUTRIENTS

The male on attaining adulthood is concerned with maintaining body tissues built during the period of growth. However the adult female body is challenged with the increased demands of nutritional needs during pregnancy. In the human female, even in the absence of pregnancy, it has been estimated that replacement of the losses during menstruation may require the synthesis of tissue equivalent to 100% of her body weight (122).

Among the nutrients lost are lecithin, calcium phosphate, sodium chloride, alkaline lactates, sodium bicarbonate, potassium chloride, cholesterol, albumin, mucin, vitamins A and E, amino acids.

Dr. Frank, New York gynecologist, says that menstruation involves a very high loss of female sex hormones. In the menstrual blood there is six times the number of sex hormones concentrated than in blood in general circulation. This periodic loss of sex hormones in a period of thirty to forty years of menstruation brings on the menopause, effecting loss of youth (137).

CESSATION OF MENSTRUATION DUE TO POOR HEALTH

There are many cases where menstrual flow has stopped due to a highly toxic diet. The body is weakened to a point where it loses its ability to carry out the monthly cleansing process. As toxins continue to build up, unless there is a change in life-style, the female will develop some chronic disorders.

With cessation of menstruation during pregnancy, a toxic woman experiences many new discomforts when she is forced to hold onto her poisons. Morning sickness, edema, vomiting, dizziness and rapid breathing are some of the visible symptons. Toxins are excreted via channels other than the uterus, but pain and illness result when these organs are already overtaxed.

When a woman never menstruates, it may be due to some malformation, such as an imperfectly formed hymen, atresia of the vagina or imperfect development of the vagina, uterus or ovaries. It may be due to a general disturbance in the quality and quantity of nutrients as well as to disorders of the endocrine system, including ovarian tumors.

Temporary cessation of the menstrual cycle may occur with a change in routine or in climate, a long journey (especially to ocean or mountains), change of residence from country to city or vice versa, extraordinary joy, grief, anxiety or exciting work, exams and study, entering a new occupation, financial troubles, a love affair, difficulty in home life, obesity (138).

When the female starts to improve in health due to improved nutrition, if the disorder is not a structural one, she will start to menstruate, quite often profusely. As the months progress, menses will become painless. If the female is healthy enough, menses will cease. This time it will be to her benefit.

CESSATION OF MENSTRUATION DUE TO SUPERIOR HEALTH

Professor Evans, in experiments with animals, showed that by reducing the protein intake one can delay the appearance of the first estrus and lengthen the resting period between successive periods. Reduction of caloric intake leads to similar, but less marked results (123).

Comparing the modern woman to the less sophisticated one, we note that menstruation is less a problem among primitive peoples (124): "One is astounded at the apparent cleanliness of the vagina in Navaho women who know nothing of douches and personal hygiene. Few Navaho women wear undergarments and the great majority apparently do not use perineal pads during menstruation."

In a detoxified woman, the bloodstream has all the material needed to build healthy tissue; as a result her uterus is made of strong tissue, and, with the monthly increase in blood pressure, blood will not be forced through the uterine tissue.

The toxicity of menstrual blood has been well substantiated. Mach and Lubin (136) showed that the blood plasma, milk, sweat and saliva of menstruating women contains a substance that is highly toxic to protoplasm of living plants. This toxic substance is not present during the intermenstrual periods.

The presence of toxic matter becomes obvious when one discovers that "during the first three days of menstruation the leukocyte counts in the discharge were generally higher . . . on the first days it was three times higher than normal values for venous blood." Leukocyte count goes up only when there is poisoning of the body.

Dr. Bieler, M.D., in his excellent book, Natural Way To Sexual Health, 1972, observes that: "Among one primitive people in the Australian bush country, WHO LIVE ENTIRELY ON FRUIT, THE MENSTRUAL PERIOD LASTS ABOUT TWENTY MINUTES; approximately a tablespoon of blood is expelled . . . The women of the American Indian of the Great Plains who lived on a simple diet and were exceedingly active, had a short uncomplicated menstrual period, scarcely noticeable" (125).

If menstruation were a natural function, it would be present in all healthy women. However, investigations show that unhealthy women experience the longest menstrual period, and, as health improves, menstrual discomfort diminishes. If a woman has not degenerated too far, chooses her diet wisely, abstains from sexual activity, follows an exercise program in fresh air, menstrual losses will continue to diminish and, in some cases, disappear altogether.

Dr. George Starr, M.D., claims menstruation is unnatural and pathological. He has cured thousands of women of this discomfort so that their periods were no longer bloody. He writes: "Nothing influences a woman's monthly flow more than diet. Sometimes a woman who flows profusely can be cured entirely by cutting down the diet and living on raw food. Often persons will skip one or two months when changing from heavy cooked food to raw food but they need not worry about it" (139).

Havelock Ellis writes about a woman who suffered painful and profuse menstruation on a meat diet and found menstruation and pain almost completely vanished when she changed to vegetarian foods. Ellis quotes her: "Food too makes a difference. I find that if I take two meat meals each day during the previous twenty-four to twenty-eight days, the next menstrual shows more blood. On two occasions I have lived on a vegetarian diet for three weeks and the flow has decreased — almost ceased in fact."

Dr. Schroyer feels that to reduce and end these discharges (menstrual and leucorrheal) it is necessary to detoxify the blood and the intestinal tract, which is best accomplished on a low protein, strictly vegetarian diet. This leads to re-establishing the intestinal flora. Dr. Schroyer believes that menstruation is a product of pathological inflammation of the endometrium (mucous lining of the uterus) (134).

Arnold Ehret claims that menstruation is due to a toxic condition of the blood. He found that a low protein diet, mainly raw vegetables and fruit, caused menstruation to take place at progressively longer intervals until it finally disappeared. Ehret writes: "If the female body is made perfectly clean through this diet, menstruation ceases . . . every one of my female patients reported their menses as becoming less and less — then two, three, four month intermission, and finally disappeared."

This method of reducing menstruation works best in a female who lives in chastity, free from uterine hyperemia caused by sexual activity which can induce menstruation, regardless of diet. However, as she rebuilds herself nutritionally through the mucusless diet, and limits intercourse to a minimum, bleeding completely ceases.

DIET, MENSTRUATION AND FERTILITY

There are quite a few studies of recovery of the potential for reproduction after a period of inadequate nutrition. In protein-deprived adult male rats, the seminal vesicles soon returned to normal after the rats were fed a diet containing casein (127). Ovarian maturation and function inhibited by underfeeding was renewed by increased feeding, with a resultant return of reproducing capacity (128, 129).

Dr. Alexis Haig writes on his experience with humans: "Excessive loss at the period has been greatly influenced by the patient going on a uric acid free diet. A remarkable and very interesting point with regard to one or two of the cases was the tendency for the flow at a period to be missed out all together. These last cases have since married and had children without any trouble. Can it be that by living on a more natural diet woman would have her periods correspond then with those of other mammals (which are bloodless)" (130).

Dr. Israel, M.D. writes that in his practice he has run into some cases where the females do not menstruate but do conceive. He writes: "It is absent in the few WOMEN WHO NEVER MENSTRUATE BUT NEVERTHELESS BEAR CHILDREN and show on repeated biopsies, cyclic endometrial changes identical with those of menstruating women" (131).

The following are studies of larger scope. "Severe general under-nutrition may produce amenorrhea (cessation of menstruation) and infertility. In Rotterdam during the period of gross malnutrition from Dec. 1944 to May 1945, fifty percent of the women had amenorrhea and the weekly conception rate fell from a prewar figure of 206 to 93" (132). However, the difference in fertility could have been due to war and the absence of men. Millis, in another study, found no evidence of reduced fertility in Singapore during a period of general under-nutrition in 1947 (133).

The conclusions one can draw from these two studies is that general undernutrition does not necessarily lead to infertility. As a matter of fact, a diet adequate in vitamins, minerals and sunshine, though low in protein, fat and carbohydrates, can provide all nutrients needed for the birth of healthy children. The Hunzas, Georgians and Equadorians who eat a diet low in protein, but otherwise adequate, have been around for thousands of years and show no loss in fertility.

MENSTRUATION, FERTILITY AND WAR

Whitacre and Barrera state: "During war and in other situations where starvation conditions existed, amenorrhea is common" (138).

Hommberg found that before the war, out of 1356 patients observed, only 9 percent of the cases were amenorrhea. In 1917 there was a rise to five percent and in 1918 to nine percent. German physicians attributed this to "defective nutrition, underfeeding, physical starvation, exposure to cold and wet, enforced celibacy."

Rubner, in his report on under-nutrition in Germany during the World War blockade stated that on reduced rations, (31 gm. protein), a cessation of menstruation occurred with many women. Strickel found that, during 1917, cases of amenorrhea were seven times more frequent at Charite Frauenklinic, Berlin than before the war.

MENOPOUSE

If a woman has taken steps to stop the monthly loss of body fluids at an early enough age, the ovaries will continue to function throughout life with reproductive capacity persistent into centuries. In a healthy woman, menopause occurs, if at all, quite late in life.

Dr. Bieler writes: "The normal menopause in the healthy woman is almost symptomless. But the toxic female who has had relief from the burden of her poisons through menstrual channels truly suffers as a whole series of new ailments arise: menopausal hot flashes, extreme nervousness, headache, arthritis, neuritis, gastric and intestinal indigestion, weakness and prostration, irritating vaginal discharge, palpitation of the heart, shortness of breath" (NATURAL WAY TO SEXUAL HEALTH, p. 176).

"For the patient suffering from milder disturbances of menstruation and menopause, much relief can be offered . . . by limiting the diet for one or two days just before the period begins. Urine tests will indicate whether the toxins are protein or starch and sugar related. If the latter, then the appropriate antidote is an acidic cleanser consisting of diluted fruit juices taken every hour. If protein acids are the offenders, an alkaline base such as diluted raw vegetable juice or vegetable soup (without meat) is prescribed" (p. 180).

TO BECOME A MOTHER

"Teach us to create in sacredness
Noble thoughts of children
Wrought in Thy Image."

SWAMI YOGANANDA

"You are the bows from which your children, as living arrows, are sent forth."

KAHIL GIBRAN

Nature is orderly; there are fundamental universal principles governing all aspects of reality. Individuals with outstanding physical, mental and spiritual qualities have been produced because certain requirements have been met either due to chance or conscious effort. When a man and a woman are joined in spiritual union, they have taken on a mutual responsibility for their own growth. When you include a child in this union, you are expanding the partnership.

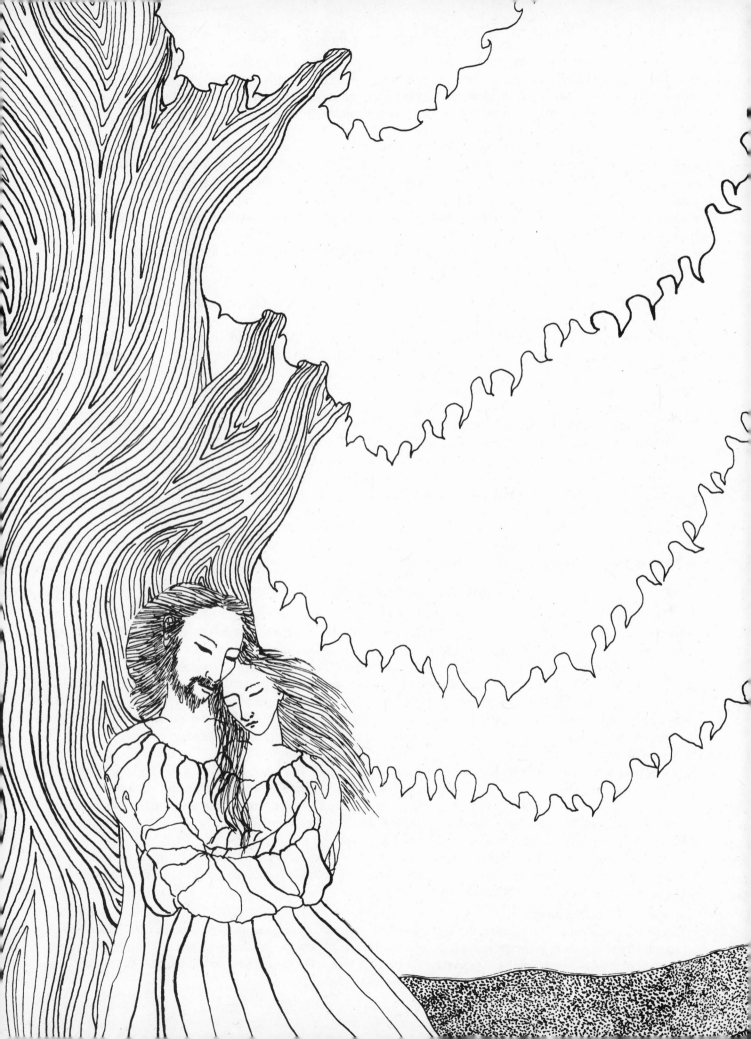

PREPARATION FOR PREGNANCY

To create a superior child, you need an environment filled with love, consideration, harmony and spirituality. Education and wealth are no guarantee of health and happiness. Parents are the soil from which a child blossoms. Quality of genes, personal cleanliness, continence, positive emotional attitudes, a spiritual life-style, astrological and karmic influence as well as physical environment, play a role in determining what soul will enter the impregnated female.

Prepare your consciousness for birth. Have the greatest desire for a child. Have visions of what it is going to be like. Let the baby be as real as if he or she were already with you. Study scriptures, the works of the ancient wise ones and inspirational writers and poets of all ages. Study the lives of great people. Spend time in nature. Find joy in the little things of life. If you become satisfied with less material goods, then you will become more imaginative and will discover how much you really have and how few your true needs really are.

It is best to improve the nutritional pattern at least six months prior to conception. However, at any time during pregnancy you may begin to improve the spectrum of nutrients in the diet by adding sprouts, indoor greens and juices.

Do not make any radical change in diet after conception. Do not try a detoxification regime or a fast of more than twenty-four hours. Any pronounced variation in the level of body toxicity could trigger cleansing reactions harmful to the fetus. For example, do not switch from a cooked food to a fruitarian diet or vice versa. A change from a concentrated diet to the lighter, juicier raw fruits permits the body to eliminate toxins stored in the tissues. On the other hand, if you have thoroughly detoxified your body, the bloodstream would be flooded by the toxins produced from the body's efforts to metabolize cooked foods.

To minimize the damaging effects of such poisons during pregnancy, you may switch gradually to an organic vegetarian diet and avoid a rapid weight loss. This will prevent a quick release into the bloodstream of DDT and other chemicals stored in body fat.

Above all avoid drugs, including cigarettes, alcohol, spices, strong soaps and smog. Since the placenta does not filter out these substances, they can damage the fetus.

Nor should your mind be poisoned by stress from competition in the business world, tension from driving in heavy traffic, violence on television or movie screen, arguments, excessive noise.

If you take wheatgrass juice, sprouts, seed, nuts and cooked vegetables, live naturally and are happy during pregnancy, you will give birth to a healthy child.

COMPLICATIONS OF PREGNANCY

Dr. Dieckman, in the American Journal of Obstetrics and Gynecology, observes that eclampsia and toxemia, which account for twenty to forty percent of maternal deaths in the United States, are practically absent in the underdeveloped countries. He notes that the incidence of eclampsia is 450% higher among Mohammedans than among the Hindu. "The most likely explanation of the greater incidence is that the diet of the Mohammedan contains meat in contrast to that of the Hindu who eats no meat." Additional statistics show that the incidence of eclampsia in Charlotte, N.C. was 2000% higher than in Bombay (Journal of Reproductive Medicine, Aug., '69). Considering that Americans are the leading consumers of animal and adulterated foods, the results are not surprising.

Hauch and Lehmann in a study of eclampsia in Denmark observed, ". . . The decreased occurrence of eclampsia during the war in Germany and also in Denmark has been attributed to the lack of protein and fat in the diet and the increased work of the women, resulting in better oxidation of food."

"Various authors in discussing the etiology of eclampsia have stated that the disease is uncommon or low in the tropics. The majority have ascribed the low incidence to the low protein diet which they assumed to be mainly carbohydrate," states Dr. Dieckman.

Fields and Davis, obstetricians, demonstrated from the records of 1503 multiparas, that: ". . . excessive weight before pregnancy . . . is associated with greater incidence of prolonged labor, cesarean section, maternal complications, prematurity and toxemia."

Another doctor, Dr. Cowan says:

"A too early consolidation of the bones of the fetus is one of the reasons for dangerous and painful childbirth . . . if the woman . . . abstains from . . . graham and white flour, beans, peas, barley and all farinaceous substances, and milk, butter and cheese; in the place of these using only fruits and vegetables . . . the child born under these conditions will be softer and smaller than usual, but soon will grow in strength and beauty." (The Science of a New Life)

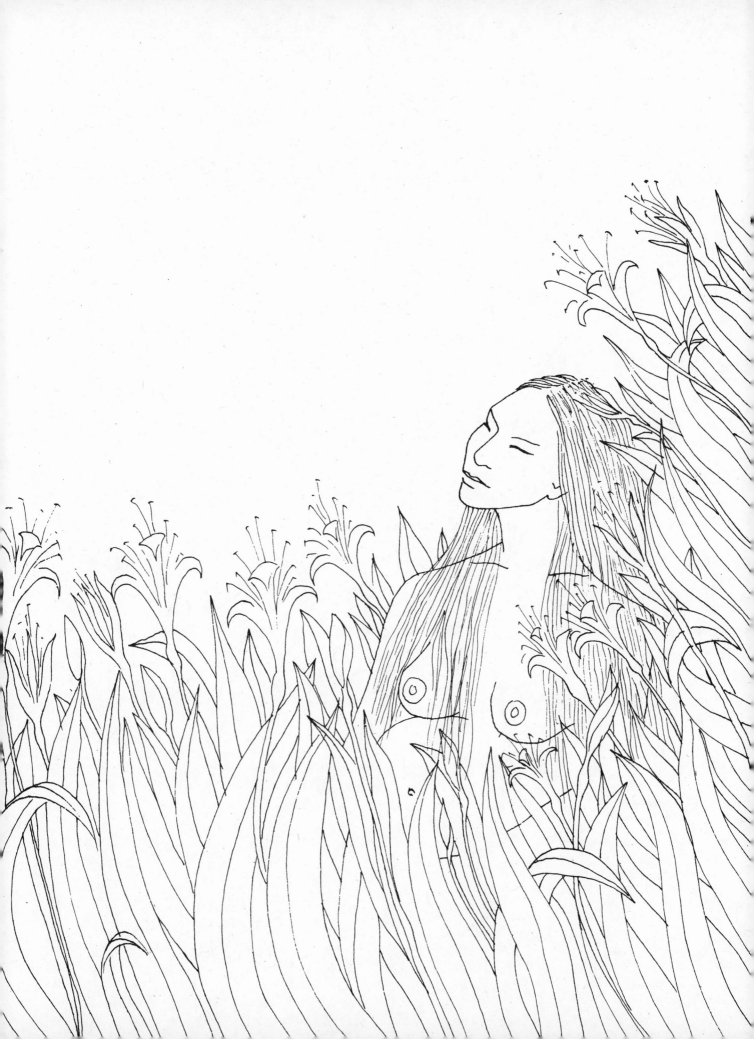

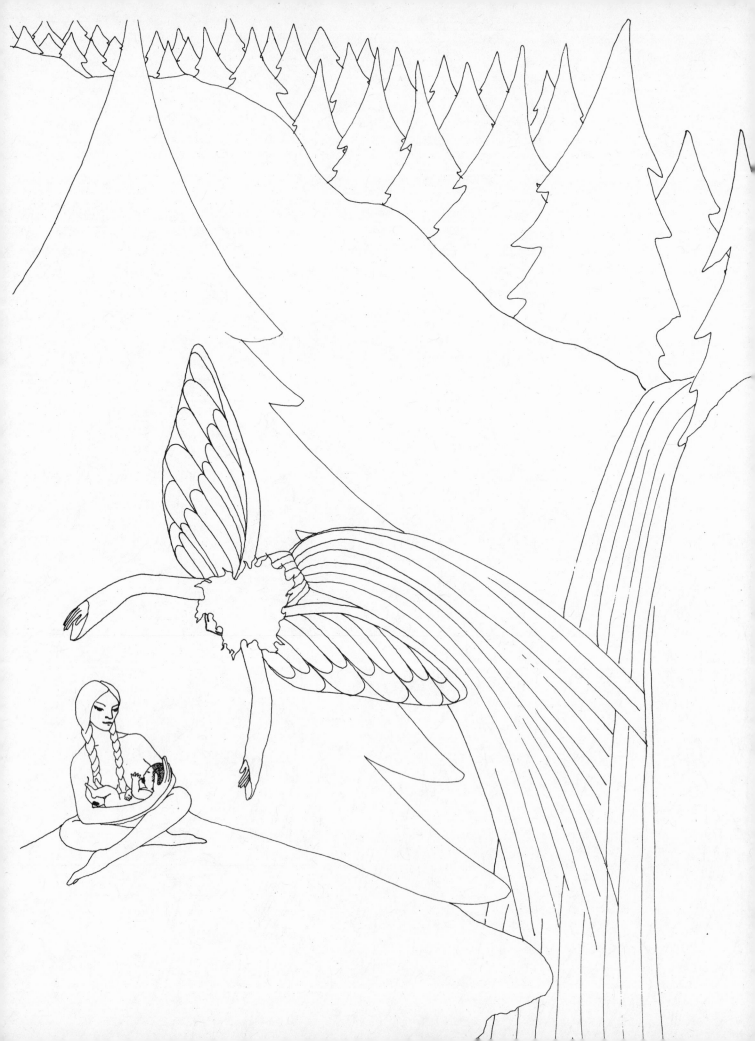

A pregnant woman in a perfect state of health does not need extra food. Overeating leads to a large, fat baby and a painful childbirth. The birth is also painful for the baby. It is its first introduction to pain and a response of fear is registered in its subconscious. Some brain damage is done because the skull bone is still relatively soft and exerts pressure on the delicate brain cells, as the baby exits from the mother.

Adopting a more natural life-style, once the transition is past, will effect a complete absence of fatigue, clear-headedness, and improvement in appearance and unsurpassable health. Because you will become much slimmer, birth will be painless.

NATURAL CHILDBIRTH

If properly prepared for, natural childbirth will be a beautiful experience. You may benefit from specialized exercises to prepare your body for easy delivery. There are classes in such exercises which may be attended by both parents. Or they are described in books on natural childbirth (see Appendix).

During the first delivery, it is wise to engage the services of a physician, midwife or nurse. Wherever it takes place, for the best health of the baby and yourself, refuse all drugs and anesthetics. Too, you will be awake to help the baby come into the world and to experience the joy of his or her arrival.

SUPERBABY

BREAST MILK FIRST FOOD

Give baby nature's perfect food — breast milk. Most nursing mothers have not had the benefit of an organic raw food diet; as a result their milk contains a large amount of DDT and other chemicals. However, this should not discourage them from breastfeeding. The composition of mother's milk is complex and precise, varying in nutrients and concentration in each species of mammal. Noone can create an equivalent substitute.

Dr. Goran Lofroth (Department of Radiobiology, Royal University of Stockholm) states: "I personally believe that human milk, when available, is superior to formula milk — and consequently the solution of the problem is not to abandon breastfeeding and human milk but, instead, to decrease and eventually stop the use of DDT and similar persistent chemicals."

If mother's milk is inadequate in quality of amount, there is no need to look for a substitute. Increasing the consumption of sesame seed, sprouts and juices will correct the condition.

According to La Leche League (an organization for the encouragement of breast feeding of the newborn), there is really no woman who cannot breast feed. The following story reported by the La Leche League testifies to the truth of the matter: "Lorraine B. tried unsuccessfully to nurse her first two babies. Her next two babies were not nursed at all nor was her fifth baby, David. Shortly after birth, however he developed a severe diarrhea and an eczema condition, and by the age of eleven weeks he could not tolerate any kind of formula or solid food. As a last resort, the doctor prescribed breast-milk. Jean P. a nursing mother who lived in the vicinity, offered to nurse David and he responded immediately.

"After the first breastfeeding, the baby slept all night for the first time in his life and thereafter his difficulties quickly cleared up. At this point the mother telephoned La Leche League for help. They suggested that she start nursing David for two minutes on each side about eight times a day, increasing the sucking as the nipples became less tender. From time to time while he was at her breast, she gave him, with an eyedropper, a little breast milk donated by nursing mothers to encourage his effort. After eight days, Lorraine's milk began to come, slowly at first; but, by the end of a month of concentrated effort, she alone nursed the baby."

FOOL PROOF MILK FORMULA

The makers of baby formulas cannot duplicate the changes in composition or volume that takes place weekly in mother's milk as the human body makes adjustments to adapt to the hormonal and nutritional needs of the growing baby.

Dr. Pamela Davies at the Institute of Child Health at Hammersmith, London says that babies bottle fed with cows' milk may suffer from hardening of the arteries and high blood pressure in later life, leading to coronary heart disease.

The Jelliffes discuss some of the problems arising from cow's milk formulas: low blood calcium in the newborn, overload on the infant's kidney from having to expel waste products of excess protein, diarrhea, respiratory infections. They state: "In the early weeks of life the intestinal wall of the infant allows 'foreign protein' to pass through. This increases the possibility of long-lasting allergies, including milk-induced colitis and possibly sudden 'cot death' from an allergic reaction to cows' milk." They furthermore recommend fruit as the ideal weaning diet: avocado, papaya, mango, banana, pears and apples (World Health Organization Chronicle, 25(12):537,1971).

CHILDREN SICKEST IN USa

In the United States, a deformed child is born every five minutes — one in every ten families. In this country alone, we are producing yearly 250,000 deformed infants (equivalent to a city the size of Dayton, Ohio). Many babies are born diseased. Even most of the apparently healthy are so toxic at birth that their opportunity to develop health is severely limited. In the United States, according to the World Health Organization:

"Nearly half a million children are affected by rheumatic fever.
Ten million boys and girls under 21 have defective vision.
A half million have orthopedic or spastic conditions.
Two million have impaired hearing.
Seventeen thousand are deaf.
Four hundred thousand have tuberculosis.

Seventy-five percent have dental defects.
Three out of every 100 draft registrants have heart trouble.
Three out of every hundred have a mental disease.
Two out of every 100 have a neurological difficulty.
Ten out of every 100 have defective vision.
One out of every 40 have defective hearing."

These statistics indicate only the observed and reported conditions.

TOXIC BABY REBORN

Dr. Bieler states that unless the mother is detoxified "the baby comes into the world . . . full of toxins from the mother's blood and an intestine full of meconium (black bile). The baby is, in fact, so toxic that even with the best care it usually takes three years to eliminate his or her inherited birth poisons" (Food Is Your Best Medicine).

Chronic and acute diseases of childhood result from toxicity of the mother's body and the diet of the child. Dr. Bieler states from personal experience that excess protein intake during infancy and childhood, depending upon concentration, can result in leukemia, cancer, rheumatism, polio, skin disease or tonsillitis. Heavy starch and mucus-inducing foods (all dairy products, grains, sugar, breads) bring on serious respiratory disorders (asthma, pneumonia, measles, chronic runny nose). Toxemia, stemming from an excess of fatty foods, expresses itself as acne, boils or styes. A child born of properly prepared parents will not develop these or other serious disorders.

Uninformed mothers, with the best of intentions, often feed infants "baby food." This is a misnomer. Highly overcooked food with additives, seasoned to suit the adult taste with salt and/or monosodium glutamate, is sold in glass or tin cans at a very high price. Such concoctions have little nutritional value. They overtax the child's digestive organs with the toxic products of indigestion in addition to the poisons contained in the food.

No cooked food may be considered baby food. A baby is sometimes fed cooked starches (pablum, cream of wheat, cookies) as early as three weeks of age. And yet, the baby's digestive organs are not developed to handle starches until the teeth are fully developed.

Nor are synthetic vitamins fit substance for a baby. They are not a food; they are simply no substitute for vitamins from mother's milk, live foods and sunshine. In addition, they may be toxic to the child.

For example: Dr. Isobel Jennings of the University of Cambridge, England, (VITAMINS IN ENDOCRINE METABOLISM, Charles C. Thomas), writes: "In many cases synthetic vitamins are now available which may be identical with the naturally occurring substance or only closely related. The close relations, although useful in many ways, pose some problems in that they may have only a fraction, whether large or small, of the biological activity of the natural product. They may substitute for several, but not all, of the functions of their natural counterparts so that it is essential to use extreme care in their use."

"D2 is structurally different from D3 in having an unsaturated side-chain. It is prepared by irradiation of ergosterol, a vegetable sterol present in ergot and in yeasts. D2 varies in its antirachitic (anti-rickets) potency in various animal species and is rather more toxic that the naturally occurring animal vitamin."

Vitamin D2 is alien to our bodies. Commercial milk is fortified with synthetic vitamin D. Natural vitamin D3 is produced by the body under the action of sunlight. It is necessary for absorption of calcium into the bloodstream through the intestinal wall, for the release of bone calcium when the blood serum calcium is low, and for building of bones and teeth. Synthetic vitamin D fails to regulate this delicate calcium balance, and when taken in large doses can be a factor in kidney failure, mental retardation, dental abnormality and heart murmur.

After weaning, even a toxic child will gain natural purity on an organic live food diet. During the periodic cleansing reactions (fever, diarrhea, boils, colds, vomiting), give the child dilute vegetable and fruit juices (see Appendix: Shelton, Wigmore, Bieler).

If, occasionally, the detoxified child develops skin rash, fever, diarrhea, cold or flu, it is the result of some error in the current diet. Quite often it is caused by a diet high in starch, protein or fat, or inorganic, processed food. Other causes could be food that is spoiled, under-ripe, over-ripe, cooked, badly combined. Generally place the child on a fluid diet: fresh juices diluted with water, liquid of unseasoned soup or water.

All disease symptoms are corrective mechanisms to eliminate the cause of bodily disorder. Do not try to check them with food or medication. Dr. Bieler says: ". . . a good rule to remember is that the bowel can be cleansed of toxins (by enema or physic) in twenty-four hours; the blood in three days; the liver in five days, providing no food is taken."

The child's bloodstream should under no circumstances be filled with poisons from vaccination or inoculations. The medication, if it does not kill one or maim one for life, can shorten the life. If illness is due to inadequate diet and sanitation, vaccination may produce a 'favorable' short term effect — suppression of a healing acute disease, which, if doctored incorrectly, can cause death — at the expense of permanently weakening the constitution, and permitting a continuing build-up of toxins which eventually manifest as chronic disease.

For those who follow natural health ideals, childhood diseases generally never develop. If symptoms manifest, stopping all food intake and taking only water or alkaline fluids, will cause them to pass quickly, leaving the body stronger.

If vaccination is mandatory, object on religious grounds. Necessary documents are available from Rising Sun Christianity, Christian Science, Unity, the National Health Federation. Insist that the temple of the living God cannot be defiled with filth. If all fails, take the child with you into an area where you will not be persecuted for your belief.

FOR SUPERIOR BIRTH NO SEX DURING GESTATION

The Talmud condemns coitus during pregnancy, and declares copulation in the first three months after conception deleterious both to pregnant mother and the fetus, while intercourse later in pregnancy is characterized as an action which is destructive of human life and equivalent to feticide. The Koran also prohibits sexual intercourse during the whole gestation, as well as during lactation and menstruation. In China, total abstinence during pregnancy is one of the first medical laws.

The findings of Masters and Johnson (Human Sexual Response, Little, Brown, 1966) showed that orgasm is associated with rapid heart rate and oxygen deprivation. Dr. L. Strean (The Birth Of Normal Babies) warns of the danger of anesthetizing women during childbirth because "lack of oxygen even for a short period could produce damage to the fetus."

Another Masters and Johnsons finding was the physiological tracing of the source of uterine orgasmic contraction. Limmer says orgasm "resembles the patterns of first stage of labor contractions." He cites Dr. Javert's (Columbia physician) study of 213 pregnancies of women who habitually miscarried. Dr. Javert found 90% were able to bear children when they abstained from intercourse after conception. Thus it is quite certain that in some women, coitus during pregnancy causes premature birth; sometimes labor pains begin a few minutes after the act.

Dr. Shirley Driscoll, M.D., Harvard Medical School, says infection, for example congenital syphilis and toxoplasmosis, rank among the most common cause of prenatal death. Infection may also cause mental retardation or neurological defects among survivors. Dr. Driscoll hypothesizes that infection may be transmitted to the fetus via the mother's blood, the amniotic fluid or from the father during intercourse.

Dr. Tilden, M.D. in his "Diseases of Women" says: "The stockman, as well as the humane society, would prosecute anyone ignorant and stupid enough to allow the males of any breed of animals to tease and sexually excite the pregnant females, but this health-destroying practice is permitted without protest among human animals."

Mother's resentment, anger and frustration of being forced into intercourse produces toxic blood from the hormones secreted by emergency oriented ductless glands.

Mother has great responsibility toward the future generations by controlling the events of her body. The perfect child will be the result of pure diet, continence and happy thoughts.

The fetus is the result of an egg, which is many hundred times larger than the impregnating sperm. The fetus develops for nine months under the constant environment of mental stimulation and nutritional fluids of the female. The mother's hormone balance, intelligence and nutrition are of much greater importance than the genetic contributions of the father. The male can make the greatest contribution to the growth of the new being by providing a loving, safe and happy environment for the mother.

CONTINENCE DURING LACTATION

Ideally a mother does not resume menses until the baby stops nursing. Sexual intercourse during lactation quite often induces premature menstruation, vitiates the quality of the milk and induces termination of the nursing period. In continence, the gonad secretions are lymphatically absorbed and carried by the blood to the mammary glands, stimulating secretion of milk.

Gonad secretions are very rich in phosphorus, the element required to build brain tissue. Loss during orgasm reduces the quantity of phosphorus in mother's milk and may well retard brain development in the child (Creation of the Superman, Dr. R. Bernard).

"Continence or non-secretion of the genital glands causes conservation of lecithin, while the activity of these glands, as a result of sexual indulgence, causes loss of lecithin which is the chief constituent of their structure" (Dr. Raymond Bernard, Prenatal Origin of Genius).

Prof. A.B. McCallum of John Hopkins University writes: "The importance of lipoids in mammalian nutrition is illustrated by the fact that the growth of the brain is directly proportional to the lecithin content of the mother's milk."

Dr. Bernard concludes that genius, of superior mental power, originates during gestation and results from superior development of the embryonic brain and endocrine glands. He doesn't believe that a lecithin supplement to the diet is sufficient, because other important substances are lost, especially the hormones from endocrine glands.

After sexual intercourse, putrefying seminal fluids may be absorbed through the vaginal wall into the lymphatic system of the lactating mother. Ensuing protein toxemia makes her milk toxic to the infant. Such milk is especially damaging to the baby if the father smokes, drinks or takes drugs. Often, however, the newborn rejects such breast milk.

To conclude, continence during gestation leads to superior embryonic growth, while continence during lactation produces lecithin-rich milk, necessary to the brain development of the infant.

LITTLE ONE'S DIET

Don't overfeed; let the child dictate to you how much, what food and at what time to serve it. Three or four feedings a day are adequate. Do not feed the child at night. Crying doesn't always indicate hunger. Feed the child enough to insure growth. You are overfeeding a child if superfluous secretions are discharged from his or her eyes, nose, ears. If a child has gas, it is because of the food eaten, air pollution or emotional factors.

Today doctors are beginning to recognize that overfeeding of children predisposes them to ailments. Dr. Roy Walford, UCLA Medical School, raised his rats and mice on a diet which contained only one third the calories of a normal diet, but all the vitamins, minerals and essential nutrients. The test animals lived 50 to 100 percent longer than animals fed on a full diet, and developed 10 to 60 percent fewer cancers. He believes humans would live much longer if caloric intake were decreased in the very young, "the effect is less pronounced when you start in maturity" (Sunday Boston Globe, Nov. 7, 1971).

Dr. Paul Dudley White, former physician to the late President Eisenhower, told members of the Oregon Heart Association that children as young as two and three years old are showing signs of atherosclerosis (fatty deposits in arteries) "The main reason . . . is that Americans are overfeeding their children with wrong foods and not encouraging them to get enough exercise."

Dr. White says that offending foods are large amounts of eggs, whole milk, cream, cheese, butter and meat. "Aside from containing too much fat, some of these foods also contain large amounts of cholesterol, which is very bad for the circulation . . ."

Dr. Jack Soltanoff strongly objects to the feeding of starches and pasteurized milk to baby, instead he advocates fruit (227):

"... solids given to baby should be dates, figs, raisins, persimmons, well-ripened bananas, etc. rather than starches or cereals. Fresh fruit in summer and dry fruits in the winter are best. Many of the troubles that children suffer from are in large part due to the practice of feeding them starches, cereals, sugars and pasteurized milk. This is a serious error as up until the end of the second year these foods are swallowed without being chewed or salivated sufficiently, and are eaten by an infant or child whose digestive juices have not yet developed enough to digest and assimilate starchy foods."

For the first year, milk from a healthy mother is usually sufficient food for a child. At the age of a year, the child may start taking fresh fruit and the juice of vegetables, greens and sprouts. The child knows its body's needs better than the parent knows them and should be given the natural food he or she likes best. If the food is rejected or the child shows signs of fever, diarrhea, nausea, skin eruption, especially soon after a meal, you can be sure that the food caused it. Discover which of the foods eaten within the last twenty-four hours was the causative factor and eliminate it from the diet.

While traveling, it is very important that no sudden change in diet takes place. It can result in severe diarrhea. If diarrhea occurs, stop intake of all food. Dilute citrus juice and soup broth may be fed until the child's condition improves. It is very important to give the child only fruit which is fully ripened and organic. If such fruit is unavailable, substitute indoor greens, weeds, sprouts and grass juice. Eat local organic seasonal fruits and vegetables.

Don't give baby any nuts or seed. A baby born from detoxified parents has a highly permeable digestive tract (almost like a sieve). Undigested protein can enter the system, causing allergic reactions. Avoid all starches and fats. Protein should be taken in the form of amino acids from fruit, grass juice and delicate sprouts (mung, alfalfa, buckwheat, sunflower). When your child is old enough to chew food thoroughly, he or she will thrive on the same live food diet which you eat and will be spared "childhood diseases", "colds", and trips to the dentist.

Give the child plenty of sunlight (midday sun rays are too strong except in winter), fresh air, zone therapy on the feet, massage of body, especially the abdomen and plenty of love. Exposing the child to the light from a 40 watt red bulb for thirty minutes, will help him or her to pass gas.

I cannot over-emphasize that for her milk to provide a complete food for the baby, the nursing mother must be in excellent health. During lactation she must follow a very careful, nourishing diet and refrain from ingesting any contaminants. This is not a time to institute a strenuous cleansing diet or fast. The following letter attests to this fact:

Dear Viktor,

Back in December, my wife, Pam, and I did something very foolish. We both started a fast, but the only problem was that Pam was nursing our baby girl, Nirvana, (at that time she was nine months old). Well, it caused Pam's milk to become deficient as a food for Nirvana. To aggravate things, our lives were so uprooted that we failed to notice any change in her until her weight loss had become quite severe (to the point that the doctor we brought her to said that she was starving to death). God, what a shocker! Of course, the doctor recommended giving her cow's milk and eggs, but did "let" us try to wean her according to our diet under the "threat" of taking her away from us if she did not show marked improvement. Well, we first started giving her sprouted wheat milk and sunflower-sesame milk but then leaned heavily on cooked grains (cereals and stews) under the pressure of putting weight on her quickly. And she did gain weight and was more lively. So we continued a heavy grain diet for her.

But she started developing a heavy mucus condition which would not go away. At this point I decided to put some faith in the raw foods diet that was working so well for me, as a good diet for Nirvana. We started and are now feeding her fruit and fruit juices, vegetables and vegetable juices, seed milks and nut cheeses. She is thriving and the mucus is virtually gone. And she is gaining real weight not just a bunch of shit in her colon.

Love,
Rich, Jersey City, N.J.

During the first few months, the baby may sleep most of time — follow the lead of the child. Do not disturb the sleep with schedules or with unexpected visitors. The child will cry only when hungry or when sleep is disturbed. As the child grows, he or she will discover the exciting things missed because of sleep and will want to stay up later, but parents should initiate an hour for sleep which will make enough rest possible. It is a good practice to put the child to bed after meals, just as all animals do.

Have a definite time for bed in evening; enjoy a chat and read stories that will leave the child in a serene state. Better to read to a child stories of adventure, biographies, nature and travel stories than tales of Santa Claus or Snow White. Let the child tell you goodnight stories which he or she recalls from past incarnations or has created from the day's adventures. Give a child intellectual material for ethical and mental growth. Read favorite stories many times. Act out some of them. Let the whole family share in this evening "read-in" as the last meeting for the day.

From the period of conception onward, the child is storing in the brain information from the environment and trying as much as possible to relate this information and make sense out of it. Do not fill the brain with silly baby talk, as many parents have a tendency to do. There is no need to invent new words for sexual organs or to imitate the child's manner of speaking. Remember, the child is trying to imitate the language patterns of the adult. As the child develops, he or she will drop the baby talk.

The brain of a baby, at birth, is already half as large as it will ever be, whereas the body has a lot of growing to do, so that from birth onward the intellect is much easier to work with. In conversation, answer questions thoughtfully and seriously. If you don't know the answer, look it up as soon as you can. Keep the child's quest for information satisfied. The Chinese prepare the child early for the adult world. They talk to the child from birth onward as if he or she were already an adult; as a result the child's brain develops much earlier than it otherwise would.

During the early years, provide a safe, protected environment, minimizing danger. Hazardous objects should be out of reach of the child. In nature, there are fewer dangers, but still a child needs guidance in the art of survival.

Encourage creativity. Avoid factory-made toys, unless they are designed to develop imagination and skills to help the child to understand the natural world. Nature has much more to teach and recreate than most toys.

Of all synthetic pacifiers, television is probably the most pernicious, instrumental in spiritual, mental and physical deterioration of the growing child. Materialistic commercials equate love with food, possessions and sensuality. Children are bombarded with details of violence, drugs, drunkenness and war. All too often this view becomes the children's real world, distorting, even forming, their values and separating them from emotional involvement with people, creating a perverted view of God and nature.

When excess television viewing replaces outdoor life and creative activity, it can weaken the body and dull the mind. Watching the flickering screen can damage the eyes. It has even induced convulsions in some individuals. Red has proven the color most potent in inducing convulsions; it is ten times as effective as green or blue. It seems quite probable that color television has played a part in the recent increase of epilepsy in America. (149)

Potentially, radiation can affect even future generations by altering the chromosomes of the growing child. I repeat, television can be dangerous.

Do not indulge the child. Independence of character and imagination and the capacity for love are built in a positive environment in which natural food is eaten and living is frugal. Hardship, participation in home chores, imaginative play and devotion to spiritual exercise will temper the spirit for heightened aspirations.

Let your family life reflect a morel principle. It is best held together by love for the sake of love. The good life can be best developed in the company of those who love and let you be yourself. Practice more and teach less. Allow no violence in your hearts or your homes. Violence and cruelty are not part of love. Instruct with love and reason, never by punishment. Train your children in the beautiful laws of God so that they may grow up emotionally secure with the wisdom to face all ordeals. Free your homes from all crossness, all harshness, all sarcasm. If you see a fault or weakness in anyone, do your best not to judge, or mention it to others. For by talking about it, we give it power. Rather, discuss the problem with the person concerned when the time is right. Maintain a sense of loyalty to the family or group.

A poet has stated:

A child who lives with criticism learns to condemn.
A child who lives with hostility learns to fight.
A child who lives with fear learns to be apprehensive.
A child who lives with pity learns self pity.
A child who lives with encouragement learns confidence.
A child who lives with praise learns to be appreciative.
A child who lives with acceptance learns to love.
A child who lives with recognition learns to have a goal.
A child who lives with fairness learns justice.
A child who lives with honesty learns what truth is.
A child who lives with friendliness learns that the world is a nice place in which to live.

Let your child spend the growing years in nature not in a polluted city. The youth of today cannot afford to repeat the patterns of their parents. We are starting a new age.

Let us advance the concept of a tribe, learn to extend our boundaries beyond the possession of two individuals entangled in the chains of matrimony. The future lies in group marriage — people joined to express common values, love and respect for one another.

The joy of having many brothers and sisters is already being practiced in many of the city and wilderness communes. Children are not anyone's property. A poet has expressed that the parent might house the body of the child but not the child's spirit. Give your love freely but not your thoughts, for the child lives in the world of tomorrow, which may not prove accessible to you, unless you can become as the child — pure and open. Be willing to learn from a child; the child is your teacher as much as you are the child's and maybe more.

Let children grow within the framework of the tribe, with the rights and responsibilities of the adults. Let them be free of control by two parents. It is their right to develop within their own subsociety of peers. All the men will be their fathers and all the women their mothers. This way a child can grow, unhampered by possessive parents and may love and be loved freely. The child will be able to identify with several others instead of just physical daddy or mommy and will learn independence and self-reliance very early in life. There will be no childless couples or individuals. There will be no urgent need to reproduce in order to have a child with whom to share your life.

It seems to me most important to carry on the most intimate growth in the garden of two lovers in a natural environment within the framework of a larger society where the communal struggle will evolve into a ritual of meaning. A life-style similar to that of the Essenes might be a good model.

Whether in context of tribe or other family setting, you will continue to act as guardian angels of the child. Yours will be the subtle responsibility to see that the child will have the environment to grow through the karmic longings in the vehicle it has chosen within your protecting guiding atmosphere.

When man and woman are joined in a spiritual union, they have taken on a responsibility for their own growth. When you include others — children — into this union, you are expanding the partnership. You will be the guru of the child and the child will be your Master. There is a good reason for every relationship formed and for every individual that you will encounter in your life. God has entrusted you with a particular child, not just any child. Just as much as he needs your guidance, so also you need the guidance from the child. You are special. Your child is special. You are all together for a special reason. God has plans for every family.

Make the family an experience of inner unfolding. Do not set up any emotional traps. Be an open channel for perfection. Family is a very important vehicle for greater self mastery and discovery. Do not forget that you are not alone when you live in a family, share the joys as well as the frustrations, fill the home with laughter and adventure.

Let us in the future build our roofs under trees, permeable to the light of God, and in the shadow of the family, each member unfold daily another petal of the perfect lotus so that we would give beauty and fragrance to the lives that surround us, and at the same time dwell in the mirth of our brothers and sisters. Our mission within the next few generations to bring heaven back into the temples of our bodies, so that we would not know death, only planar transition, in the continuous evolving plan in the good universe where we can partake in the divine music.

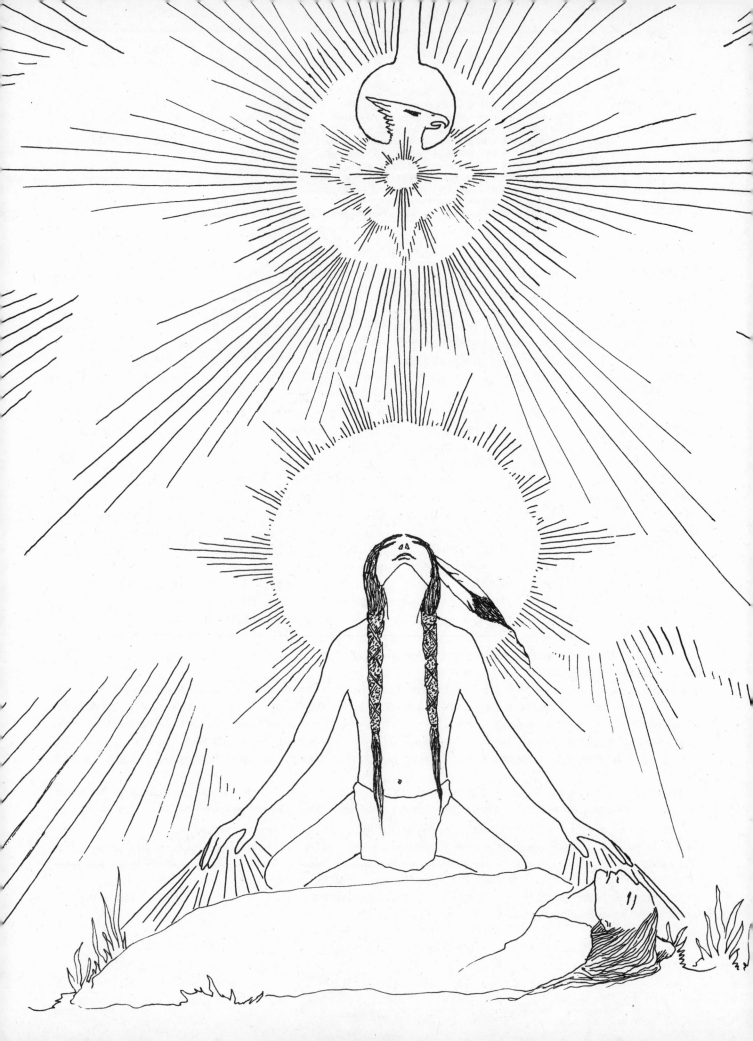

HEAL AND BE HEALED

"Your first duty is to make the body healthy. Without health, nothing can be achieved. Not only higher goals, but even worldly success is based on your health, your condition. Whatever you want to do, spiritual, social, national, you have to do it with your body. Your thoughts are manifested only through your body. You can fulfill desires only through your body."

SWAMI SATCHIDANANDA

TO BECOME A HEALER

Those of you who are drawn to helping sick humanity will be confronted with many legal problems. Currently, not all healing systems have equal opportunity under the law. In most countries outside the USA, all doctors who are licensed to practice have equal privileges before any court with the same responsibilities and the same limitations. In the USA, the court system looks for AMA approval.

Initially, drugs were defined as poisons, and their use was under the control of a medical monoply. Doctors knew how to use these poisons to "combat" sickness. However, in framing the 1938 Federal Food and Drug Law, the word "drug" became anything used to treat, prevent, diagnose, mitigate or cure a disease as well as "articles other than food intended to affect the structure or function of human or animal." With this law, the AMA was able to wipe out competition from osteopathy, chiropractic, naturopathy, homeopathy, acupuncture and color and nutrient supplement therapy. It took years of legal struggle before some of these professions were given legal status. Today the AMA union is still the richest and most powerful in the country; however, the new breed of doctors are not holding it sacred. This year (1973) was the first time that less than half the graduating interns joined it.

In many states a person may be charged with practicing medicine without a license if anything he says or does can be construed or interpreted as diagnosis or prescribing.

Many who are knowledgeable in the healing arts, for self-protection, when asked for specific instructions, will answer with qualifications as "I heard J.Q. used this method...", "Someone sent in this testimonial, and here is what he did...", "If it were me, I would do...", "There is no disease, only a polluted temple; if it is cleaned out and given proper nourishment your body can heal itself; follow the laws of Nature. Sin no more."

There are at least three paths to choose to pursue the healing arts as a profession.

One can study for an M.D. degree and experiment with natural methods on the side. This can be very hard on the mentality and conscience. A person would have to waste thousands of hours in the study of drugs and surgery and never use such tools except in an emergency. The financial investment can run as high as 50,000 dollars.

A far better approach is to pursue osteopathy, chiropractic, homeopathy or acupuncture. They will give you professional training and quite often legal protection. You will then be in a position to guide people on the path to health. Europe and Asia are far more advanced in these fields; hence, study outside the USA may be preferable.

The third path is that of the self-taught "healer." Such a person has studied widely and self experimented with juices, dietary supplements, herbs, fasting, diet, healing crises, zone therapy, iridology, physiognomy, color healing, tchiatsu, massage, acupuncture, meditation, yoga, and psychological and spiritual disciplines. Generally, such a person has studied in many centers, traveled extensively and has helped many people, however, this person is without recognized status.

I have met many in the second and third groups, few in the first, who were in trouble with the law for helping the sick to become healthy. Some have been jailed. Quite often they have made claims of cures; some have been framed; others broke the legal terms of the word "drug." A chiropractor, who used zone therapy, was arrested for malpractice. However, many of the states are becoming quite lenient—especially those on the coast—as the demand for natural methods becomes more prevalent.

The following guidelines should be helpful:

a) Never make any claims of cures. The body heals itself; it is never cured.
b) Never threaten or try to scare anyone into becoming healthy.
c) If you are a professional be active in your professional organizations.
d) Influential people when healed can act as your protectors.
e) Become ordained in some church. You will be awarded a Doctor of Divinity degree. It can be obtained with only several months of training at cost of under $100. You might want to start your own church. You will help to build temples of God. Have each patient join your church. Incorporate the healing practices as part of the religious services. The law will not dare to interfere with religious practices.

Don't go into healing with great financial expectations. Healing is a sacred profession. Work as God's helper. God will determine the reward. You might ask for donations from the well-to-do as required to take care of your needs; from the less fortunate, give your service as an offering to God.

Do not waste time with people who are not willing to cooperate with Nature's Law. Be loving. Offer suggestions that they would be willing to practice. Don't make life too difficult for anyone, unless absolutely necessary, and then only for a short period of time. Always offer hope for a better future. Inform the person that with Nature's methods the healing process may bring on acute symptoms; and complete recuperation may take a long time.

Experiment on yourself. Observe others. Study the books of many practitioners. Be very cautious when giving advice on hearsay or regarding phenomena which you have not experienced or observed.

Psychology plays a very important role in healing. Love God. Love self. Serve others with love. People are sick because of the filthy state of the digestive tract, especially the colon. They are also constipated mentally; love energy does not flow freely. Love them, show them how to clean up. Increase their energy through live juices, massage, zone therapy, exercise, yoga, rest. Increase their nerve energy through positive attitudes, silence, prayer, song, unlimited amount of rest, loving service, devotional duty, fun and joy.

When dealing with the sick, you will have to inspire confidence to obtain the quickest results. Ability to foresee an ailment, before it ever develops force, will help many people to bypass severe pain if they institute a self-healing regime. Avoid naming diseases; for some patients the label will be just another worry. Such labels only name symptoms anyway.

Diagnosis is a complex art. In the West, it is practiced generally through pulse-pressure examination, blood, urine, tissue analysis and many painful techniques which require the use of surgery.

Jesus, Teresa Newman (Catholic Saint, breatharian), Edgar Cayce and many other healers could read a person's past, present and future, just from his or her auric vibrations. They healed the sick by recharging them with the missing body-spirit vibrations or else instructed them how to heal themselves.

The East has developed many techniques of diagnosis that are being spread throughout the West by the Macrobiotic Community. Some of the techniques are found in acupuncture, Do-in, tchiatsu, physiognomy and the twelve pulse test.

Fasting a person for three days will give you a great deal of information on the state of that person's health. The more toxic a person is, the more discomfort he or she will feel. It will take longer for hunger to disappear, the urine will be dark and much mucus will collect on the tongue. There may be headache and nausea. General health may be estimated by pulling a hair from a person's head. If the hair comes out easily and painlessly, it indicates malnutrition with an overacid condition. Split ends indicate protein deficiency and poor food combining.

Palmistry, graphology and astrology can give a great deal of data about past lives, current status and future ailments. Today, palmistry is becoming the "helping hand" in some doctors' offices. When properly interpreted, certain lines and changes in lines, may be warning signals that can alert a doctor to the oncoming of a severe disease. Dermatologlyphics, or palmistry, is presently being taught at the University of Minnesota. Likewise, iridology can tell the whole history of your body and can be used in the same way as palmistry.

The pulse-dietary technique, as developed by Dr. Coca, allows you to determine which foods you are allergic to. These foods can be responsible for asthma, hay fever, diabetes, high blood pressure, migraine and tired feeling. Basically the test consists of observing the pulse count after ingestion of commonly eaten foods. If there is a dramatic increase after eating a certain food, it generally indicates your body has difficulty metabolizing it. (The Pulse Test, Coca, University Press, 1956).

When determining the state of the person's health, observe the ear lobes, hair line, skin tone, body structure, and weight, facial lines, posture, and appearance of the eye. Topics that should be explored are the following: complete diet, past ailments, current complaints, bowel movement, sexual habits, occupation, emotional status, food combination, quality of teeth, exercise and social forces. The determination should be a silent one. It is illegal to diagnose. If you suspect, from observing facial lines, congestion of the liver, you can ask questions to verify this: "Have you had liver problems in the past? How is your protein digestion? Do you have gas?"

Every practicioner should consider at least the following causes in the history of disease:

1. Work — Things one comes in contact with; check out: chemicals, ventilation, tobacco smoke, noise, physical activity and social setting.

2. Bath — Does the patient use too hot baths, how frequently? Steam? Salt?

3. Exercise — How often? Strenuous infrequent exercise can be dangerous. Yoga, gardening, swimming and walks are best for health. What sort of posture?

4. Diet — What is the main food the patient lives on? Is it properly prepared, combined and balanced for physical needs? Is there time for mastication and mental rest after the meal? What are the cooking utensils made from (best is porcelain or glass)? How much seasoning or salt? What kind of water is used? Is the food organic? Is there at least one bowel movement daily?

5. Sleep — Is the room dust free, well ventilated, warm, silent? Electric blanket, detergents and strong chemicals in blankets can be harmful. Direction of patient's lying in bed can make a difference; for example, lying with one's head north is considered ideal. Does one meditate, and/or rest during the day? Does one relax before going to sleep? What sort of activity is pursued for relaxation?

6. Clothing — Does coloring run on skin? Is the clothing too warm or cold; does it produce skin irritation or restrict circulation? Is it of the right color for healing and personality?

7. Light — Is kerosene or gas light used (can be very harmful)? Does the patient get adequate sunshine and fresh air every day?

8. Mental — Find out what factors influence happiness and anxiety, produce worries, bad temper. Does one relate well in family, friend or social setting?

9. Environment — How bad is air pollution in the area? Is there a nuclear power plant in the vicinity? Is the home located in the vicinity of a commercial farm, airport or heavily traveled road? Is the house heated by gas? Is it being filled with fumes from a pilot light? Is the ventilation adequate? How many hours daily exposure to t.v. radiations? Is it a color set?

10. Excesses — They can be very destructive. Does the individual excess in alcohol, sex, eating and/or work?

With a good picture of the sick person's background and habits, you are now in a position to be helpmate and friend, as the two of you work out a program which will effect healing for a happier life.

The treatment will be a long term program individually worked out for the person. A diet consisting of two to six meals a day, should be written up, guided by the person's digestive ability. The simplest meals are best. A cooked vegetable diet program might be used. A juice regime and bed rest might be required by those of low energy. Daily evacuation must be ensured, even if it means the use of enemas. Control of "crises" must be delicately observed, to ensure that no mistakes are made. When needed, other healing professions should be consulted. In time the person will understand the meaning of "Be Your Own Doctor."

For best results, the person should be advised:

1) Not to discuss his or her new diet or therapy with friends and relatives until positive results have been obtained. They might be discouraging.

2) To take a reasonable length of time to experiment with the diet before deciding whether it works. An average of four months (three weeks at the absolute minimum) is necessary to show conclusive results. It may have taken twenty to thirty years of sloppy eating and unnatural living to produce the symptoms of disease. The healing process usually takes less time.

3) That the new living habits will be difficult at first, but, with perseverance, they will be easier to maintain because life will become more enjoyable as the person becomes healthier.

4) Healing takes place most rapidly when one is happy and not worrying over symptoms. The mind should be kept busy with reading, meditation, a hobby or gardening.

5) Rest is central in healing. When tired, the person should not be pushed — it is time for bed rest. At least once a week, the person should take time out for uninterrupted rest—to sleep and rest for ten to twenty-four hours.

TEMPLE OF GOD

"Know ye not that ye are the temple of God, and that the Spirit of God dwelleth in you? If any... defile the Temple of God, (that person) shall God destroy; for the temple of God is holy, which temple ye are?"   I COR 3:16

"I tell you truly, should you fail to keep but one only of all these laws, should you harm but one only of all your body's members, you shall be utterly lost in your grievous sickness, and there shall be weeping and gnashing of teeth. I tell you, unless you follow the laws of your Mother, you can in no wise escape death... She shall heal all... plagues, and you shall never become sick. She gives ... long life, and protects you from all afflictions; from fire, from water, and from the bite of the venomous serpent."   ESSENE GOSPEL OF PEACE

The human body is constructed of a hundred trillion cells. The vitality of the body is the total energy of individual cells. The function of organs and tubings is to insure the integrity of the fluids in cells, with no single constituent varying more than few percent. As long as the nutrients (solar energy particles) are internalized in the right quantity and proportion and waste is eliminated, the life of cells is insured. Overnutrition leads to toxemia from putrefaction or overstorage of nutrients; undernutrition leads to energy loss, starvation of cells, causing cell functioning to fail.

The body maintains the constancy of the internal environment through the activity of organs and ductless glands. They have the capacity for processing fuel of different densities: solid, liquid, gas, and radiation.

The digestive system is well adapted for processing solid and liquid fuel. Teeth grind food into fine particles and mix it with saliva. The combined activity of mouth, stomach and small intestine break food into micronutrients which can be absorbed into the blood and lymph systems for transporting the fuel to the cells. The liver and endocrine glands, and some other organs, act collectively in intermediate metabolism which further break down nutrients into forms directly utilizable by cells. The ductless gland system supervises the body's functions for survival emergencies, dictates growth, reproduction and many phases of metabolism. When the body is perfectly balanced these glands act as coordinators of soul and energy forces. The kidney maintains the delicate balance of fluid electrolytes, excretes over 90% of the waste products of protein metabolism, as well as the ingested non-nutrients.

The internal tides are centralized within the circulatory system of heart, blood and lymph vessels. The circulatory system keeps the fluids surrounding the cells continuously mixed. Every part of the body is bathed by fluids from every other part of the body within any 10 to 30 minutes of time.

The blood vessels (of which there are about 30,000 miles in body) carry on rapid transport of oxygen, nutrients, waste and red blood cells.

The lymph system consists of lymph fluid, vessels and nodes. It acts as the major food transporter and is the home of the white blood cells. Lymph fluid, is similar in composition to sea water. This body of water is continuously, but slowly (relative to blood), on the move.

Lymphatic vessels or capillaries lie beside blood capillaries. They are extremely porous so that they can collect large particles — such as old debris of dead tissues, undigested protein and dead bacteria — from tissue space fluid. Small filters, lymph nodes, digest protein particles (quite often they leak out from capillaries) and return them to the lymph stream in the form of amino acids.

The main lymph trunkline proceeds upward in each leg, each arm and from the digestive system, all finally coverging in a single tube— the thoracic duct— emptying into the large vein near the heart.

The two large lymph nodes located at the start of the digestive tract (tonsils) and at the end (appendix) act as filters and warning devices. The condition of the tonsils indicate the amount of mucus in the body whereas the appendix warns of protein putrefaction. When inflamed —enlarged due to overwork — tonsils make it unpleasant to eat, a fast is indicated. Appendicitis and tonsillitis have been treated perfectly successfully through fasting, cold compresses and enemas, as well as with acupuncture. If toxemia is allowed to progress to an extreme level, leukocytes will increase to protect the body; their great number can create symptoms of acute disease. If no change is made, eventually leukemia may be diagnosed.

The respiratory system deals with the gases in the body. It receives oxygen from the air and, via the blood, transports it to tissue space surrounding cells and picks up carbon dioxide, plus many other gases, to be expelled through lungs. Many ionized elements are absorbed through the lungs; these energy-charged particles can act as a basis for the creation of nutrients.

The energy system is centralized in the skin and chakras. The sensitivity of the skin to solar energy and the penetrating quality of solar rays in a completely detoxified individual enable the internal organs to act as assimilators of the breatharian diet. The hemoglobin carries on the same functions as chlorophyll.

The skin, exposed to consistent solar activity, becomes pigmented insuring that the correct amount and right quality of electromagnectic waves are absorbed to give optimum energy to the body.

The skeletal and muscular systems provides movement toward sources of food and pleasure and avoidance of danger. This skeletal movement can be controlled in many directions. Because of bad diet, unbalanced occupational posture, accident or emotional tension; the spine, muscles and joints become distorted, damaged or misaligned. Yoga postures, exercise, chiropractic,   osteopathy, rolf massage and/or zone therapy may help to correct these conditions.

The adjustments will have a functional effect on the nervous system (brain, spine, and peripheral nerves), which controls bodily activity. This system has two separate divisions: the sensory: which reports and analyzes the immediate environment; the motor, which controls the muscles and some of the glandular secretions via the autonomic nervous system. If the skeletal system is unbalanced by poor posture, impingement of a nerve can interfere with the flow of its impulses to associated organs, thus impairing their function. Furthermore, a distorted skeleton and weak muscle tone result in crowding and displacement of internal organs. Poor dietary habits can produce enlargement of organs which then press on the spine, causing backache.

From abnormalties of the vertebrae may be diagnosed diseased conditions of the body which can be checked by further examination. The following is a list of the vertebrae with parts of the body affected by them:

Organs and Parts	Spinal Nerve Centres
Head	1st to 6th cervical
Heart	3rd cervical to 5th dorsal
Intestines	9th dorsal to 5th lumbar
Kidneys	11th dorsal to 5th lumbar
Legs	12th dorsal to 5th sacral
Liver	6th to 12th dorsal
Lungs	1st to 9th dorsal
Larynx	1st and 2nd cervical
Pancreas	9th and 10th dorsal
Phrenic Nerve	2nd to 5th cervical
Peritoneum	1st and 2nd lumbar
Prostate Gland in males	10th dorsal to 5th lumbar
Spleen	9th and 10th dorsal
Trachea	5th and 6th dorsal

(Central diagram of the spine with handwritten labels: HEAD, HEART, INTESTINES, KIDNEYS, LEGS, LIVER, LUNGS, LARYNX, PANCREAS, PROSTATE, SPLEEN, TRACHEA. Handwritten captions: "CHIROPRACTIC RELEASES THE POWER" and "THE SPINE IS THE HUMAN BIO-COMPUTER SWITCHBOARD CONTROLLING ENERGY FLOW AND VIGOR")

For best posture and elimination of backaches, sleep on the hard floor, earth or on a ¾ inch plywood board on the bed. Add a few layers of blanket to simulate sleeping on the soft earth.

HAIR CUTS CAN BE DANGEROUS TO YOUR HEALTH

Hair, too, is an important organ. On a natural diet, hair grows to a certain length and stops. No animal need cut its hair. There is a fixed length of hair for armpits, skin, genitals, face and head.

Shaving and haircutting is health-destroying. Frequent male haircuts may speed balding(females rarely go bald). A child resists with fear the acts of barbers. After a haircut, one may feel the drain on the mental faculty, quite similar to the feeling after loss of sexual fluid. Not only is the hair lost, but also the hair shaft bleeds repair fluids at the cut ends. Nutritional loss due to haircutting affects the brain. In school, other factors considered, long-haired girls are the best students. Hair is the receiver and transmitter of divine emanations--it makes you receptive to spiritual forces. Saints and sages instinctively let their hair grow.

Hair is like a plant which grows out of rich soil. The scalp is your garden. If it is robbed of nutrients through frequent harvest; if the entrance of nutrients into the scalp is prevented by the clogging effect of mucus foods; if the diet is so overacid it causes scaling of the scalp with dandruff and destruction of hair roots--then you can anticipate loss of hair.

At age 27, I was losing as many as 400 hairs a day. My scalp was covered with dandruff and itched constantly. I had many gray hairs. For several weeks after I improved my diet, hair loss and dandruff increased. This was part of cleansing. In time, hair loss stopped and gray hair disappeared. Eventually, after several years, most of the hair grew back.

A low protein diet will keep the hair healthy, if other health rules are observed. Balding and receding hairline need not be a cause for concern. A healthful diet and hygienic living can promote renewed growth of hair at any age.

PHYSIOGNAMY

"The shew of their countenance doth witness against them; and they declare their sin as Sodom, they hide it not. Woe onto their soul! For they have rewarded evil onto themselves."

ISA. 3:9

"For we are made a spectacle unto the world, and to angels."

1 COR. 4:9

"Everything in our appearance, from our posture to the structure of our navel, speaks of our health, past and character. The person who understands this language penetrates the deepest human mysteries at will. This is the key to self-knowledge, to social judgement, and to true health. Without it we are doomed to analytical techniques which must end in failure; people being whole, must be judged as such and cured as such."

"Before we learn to judge, however, we should realize that no one is without sickness. If such people existed, they would not be worth having for friends. They would know nothing about life, for without sickness there is no health, without lower judgement, there is no way to become higher . . . Those without sickness will never understand the meaning of freedom, for our sickness comes directly from our own abuse of our free will. The true meaning of freedom can only be learned through failure . . . To see others we must begin by seeing their dreams, their idea; we must try to acquire a total view of them . . .Next, we should see a person's vibrations, which are manifested in their words, expressions - all their actions."

THE TEACHINGS OF MICHIO KUSHI, Vol. 1, P. 36-54

PHYSIOGNOMY is the art of analyzing facial features to determine the state of health and character of an individaul. The sins committed on the body manifest in the face as lines and sagging tissues. With ill health or emotional problems, wrinkles begin to appear. As the internal quality of the body improves, so does the beauty of the face. The only way to remove wrinkles, is to remove the cause of wrinkles, which has very little to do with age. Being happy, eating right, rest, clean environment and service are the true beauticians.

(follow chart on following page):

1) Congestion of the liver.

2) Degeneration of the liver and gall bladder from too many acid-forming, processed foods.

3) Chronic indigestion from excessive eating, badly combined foods resulting in degeneration of the intestine.

4) Nervous system is breaking down from acid, spicy foods and drugs.

5) Circulation is poor from muscus-inducing foods.

6) Expansion or advanced degeneration of the liver.

7) (a) Advanced degeneration of the duodenum.

(b) Widespread degeneration involving duodenum, liver kidney. Reflects a life-style filled with excesses. Quite often there is retention of water in the tissues.

8) Loss of sexual drive.

9) Pouchiness, purplish dark color and/or illness. Kidney dgeneration from over-acid condition. Forerunner to sexual drive extinction. Kidney may be enlarged; pressure may be causing lower backache. Prostate malfunction. Intestine is clogged due to food excess. Insufficient rest.

10) Lung degeneration. May appear as hills, valleys or ravines. Rosy cheeks indicate expanded capillaries in the lungs; extreme pallor indicates extreme degeneration – lung cancer or emphysema – or severe indigestion.

11) There is a strong link between kidneys and ears. Kidneys control the electrolyte balance which determines energy of cells as well as vitality of the total being. Dr. Paul Peters (Univ. Texas, Austin) explained that important stages of development of both ears and kidney take place in the embryo at the same time. If one organ is abnormal, the other may also be defective. Large ears with long lobes, close to the head, are signs of birth from a healthy mother. Such a child has greater potential for health, happiness and long life. No lobes (the majority of today's children) indicates birth from an unhealthy mother. Unless they observe hygienic laws, they will have much sickness, and die at an early age. I have acted as nutritional consultant to Mr. New England, 1970. He has hardly any earlobes, was born sickly; but because of a strict regime of physical culture and diet, he has developed into a physically healthy giant. Similarly, seemingly healthy individuals of advanced age, though drinking, smoking and eating all the junk of our civilization; almost always have very long earlobes, which indicates a very strong inherent constitution and a body that can withstand a great deal of misuse. Their children have shorter earlobes; their grandchildren no earlobes; in another generation sterility occurs. Sometimes, at an advanced age, once-long earlobes shrink and develop lines (may be as many as 4). This change in earlobes indicates an extreme misuse of the body, often the result of coffee, stress, alcohol and sex.

In Dallas at a 1974 Am. Heart Assn. annual convention, Dr. Jack Sternlieb of the Mayo Clinic reported:

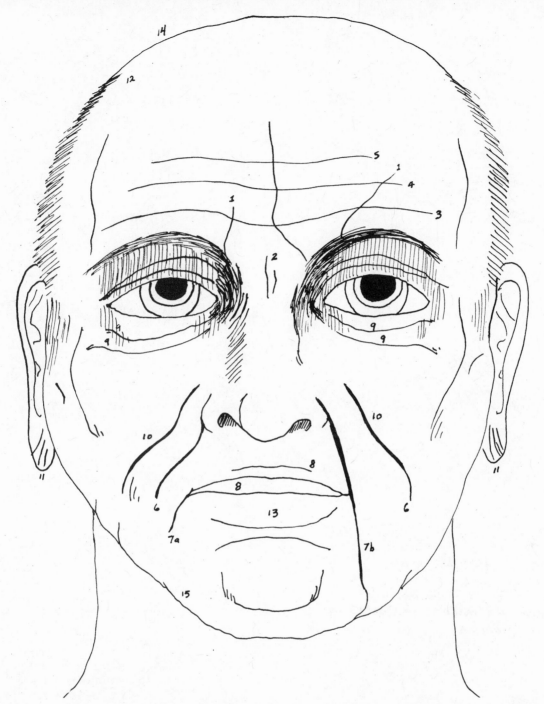

12) Baldness or dandruff. Over-acid condition from too much protein, fat, coffee, salt, sugar or dairy products. Too many haircuts.

13) Swollen lower lip indicates weak muscle tone of the colon or chronic mild indigestion from bad food combinations. Some authorities claim such persons to be passionate; instead they are suffering from an unclear head, indigestion or constipation. Such a condition, if not corrected, will lead to an expanded large intestine. The upper lip indicates condition of the stomach: if swollen, bad indigestion. If allowed to persist, it can be the cause of heart attack. If lips are bluish, circulation is very bad.

14) Upswept eyebrows indicate an aggressive, highly active person whose mother ate a predominantly animal food diet. Down-slanting eyebrows indicate a gentle, philosophical being whose mother's diet was mainly vegetables during pregnancy. Furthermore, the mental attitude of the child could have been created by the life style of the mother, her thoughts, ambitions, desires, which could have transcended dietary limitations.

BAD FOOD DEGENERATION

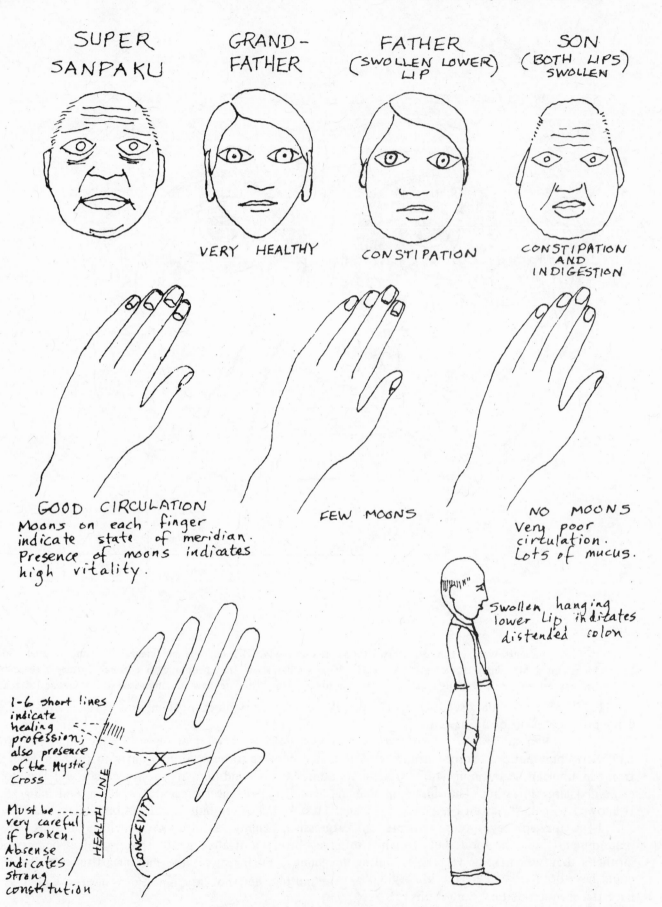

SUPER SANPAKU

GRAND-FATHER

FATHER (SWOLLEN LOWER LIP)

SON (BOTH LIPS) SWOLLEN

VERY HEALTHY

CONSTIPATION

CONSTIPATION AND INDIGESTION

GOOD CIRCULATION
Moons on each finger indicate state of meridian. Presence of moons indicates high vitality.

FEW MOONS

NO MOONS
Very poor circulation. Lots of mucus.

Swollen hanging lower lip indicates distended colon

1-6 short lines indicate healing profession; also presence of the Mystic Cross

Must be very careful if broken. Absense indicates strong constitution

HEALTH LINE

LONGEVITY

15)Head Shape: Carrot shaped (top wide, narrow chin): thinker, critical, negative; Fig shaped (top narrow, chin wide): activist, optimistic, aggressive; Mango shaped (top wide, chin medium curve): balanced, understanding, peaceful.

Other characteristics (not shown on chart) to look for are:

1. Gray hair from too much salt, over-acidity, hot cooked foods, coffee, sexual excess, enzyme deficiency, anxiety. To correct condition, change your habits — use sprouts and grass juice.

2. Bulginess, sagginess or looseness of chin and cheek area indicate too much protein, fat and beverages.

3. Moons on fingernails indicate good circulation. The presence of a moon indicates the vitality of the organs in the corresponding meridian. Pink fingernails indicate good quality blood. Horizontal white lines indicate a period of halt in nail growth due to menstrual drain on the thyroid (calcium loss). Vertical ridges, a long period of anxiety.

4. A red, veined, bulbous nose indicates high blood pressure; purplish color: low blood pressure.

5. Flaring, wide nostrils indicate good lung capacity.

6. Color of face: extreme pallor indicates bad lungs or severe indigestion; yellowish color (with or without dark brown spots on body or face, especially if yellow color appears suddenly) indicates a bad spleen; greenish tint indicates cancer; red indicates high blood pressure and overworked heart; purple indicates very sick, near death.

7. The skin is the largest eliminative organ. Generally its activity does not leave tell-tale traces. When the body is very toxic, one needs soap and deodorants; also, blemishes appear. These symptoms warn of disorders of internal organs. Some observations about the skin: (a) offensive orders: bad food combinations, processed foods, excess animal products; (b) dry scaly skin: too much mucus, body is starving; (c) broken capillaries and varicosities: too much animal protein, excess food; (d) moles: fried food, excess protein. (Note: moles start as little pools of red toxic blood in the skin surface, then become isloated from the life stream, eventually coagulating into black spots); (e) blackheads: too much processed oil, starches, fried food or animal protein; (f) pimples: persistent indigestion, leading to toxic blood, caused by diet rich in processed starches which are quite often combined with sweets or fruit; or unwise food combining, fried foods and dairy products; (g) birthmarks and beauty marks are signs of the mother's ill health and emotional problems, plus astrological influences. They can be used to interpret the character and fortune of an individual. Quite often, they indicate the presence of overtaxed eliminative organs in mother or offspring. (h) measles: indicates body vitality is quite high; organism makes a dramatic attempt to expel a large amount of toxic matter, using the skin of the entire body; (i) tumors: too much protein; (j) leprosy: breakdown in digestion, especially in weak individuals, who are eating putrefactive animal protein in a very   warm climate.

8. Lacklustre eyes indicate many long-standing ailments, often the result of much seasoning, coffee and meat. White, cloudy irises indicate a large dairy product consumption. Clear, sparkling eyes are a sign of good health and circulation.

Dr. Maria Papazacharieu, at a recent international medical congress on sterility, reported that a woman can determine pregnancy by looking in a mirror while holding a magnifying glass in front of her eye. If there are three small red dots on the pupil she can be sure she is expecting a child. Furthermore, if in the iris (the colored circle of the eye) small crystal -shaped dots form near the pupil, it will be a boy. If the dots are nearer to the white of the eye, it will be a girl.

Sanpaku is a condition in which the white of the eye can be seen between the pupil and lower lid — an indication of a grave state of physical and spiritual illness and high susceptibility to disease, accidents, and tragic death.

Recommended reading:

1) Oriental Diagnosis, What Your Face Reveals by Michio Kushi, $4.95 ppd., East West Journal, 233 Harvard St., Brookline, MA. 02146.

2) A Doctor's Guide to Better Health Through Palmistry, E. Schermann, M.D., $6.95, Parker Pub. Co. Inc., West Nyack, N.Y., 1969.

IRIDOLOGY

Iridology is defined as follows by Dr. J. Haskell Kritzer, M.D.: "Iridology is a science revealing pathological and functional disturbances in the human body by means of abnormal spots, lines and discolorations of the eye."

This definition is amplified by Dr. Bernard Jensen:

"The eyes reveal structural defects, latent toxic settlements and inherent weaknesses in organs of the body including the presence and the source of acids, catarrh, prolapsus, anemia, nerve tensions and other troubles. Toxemias and where located, activity of each organ, glandular conditions and drug poisonings are accurately identified. Chemical balance, miasma, congestion, constitution and the power of get well all show in the eyes. Iridology does not name diseases. The purpose of Iridology is to determine the location of inflammation, the stage of inflammation, how it was caused and the steps necessary to overcome it." (182).

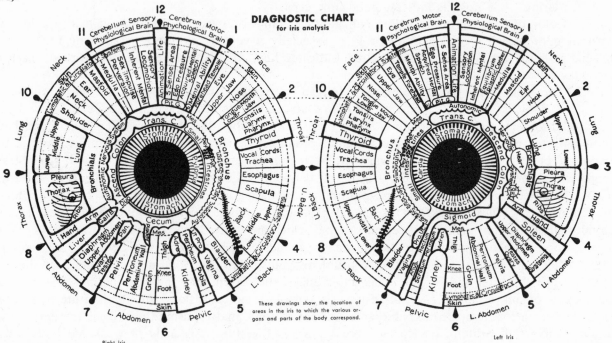

DIAGNOSTIC CHART for iris analysis

These drawings show the location of areas in the iris to which the various organs and parts of the body correspond.

Right Iris   Left Iris

Eyes mirror the condition of the body. The iris is a center for countless tiny blood vessels, muscle fibers and nerves (imbedded in the four pigmented layers of the iris), which are linked with every part of the organism via the autonomic nervous system. In an unhealthy body, toxins are deposited in the iris, irritating the nerve endings and leaving a record in the iris of the condition of overworked organs: Signs of ill health are visible as cloudy patches, dark spots and lines.

An explanation for changes in the iris is as follows: Each organ acts as a transmitter. The iris is like a TV receiver tuned into signals from each organ, which are mapped onto the iris screen. The vibrations from a continuously overworked organ lead to changes in the four-layer structure of the iris.

The power of iridology as a diagnostic tool is illustrated by Dr. Jensen's photographs, chart and analyses (182):

SECTION 1 – Left iris, brown with some blue showing through.
Density 3. Colitis. Boils. Gas. Mental retardation.

A.–Psoric itch spots.   B.–Scurf rim.

C.–Heavy Catarrh.   D.–Gaseous bowl pockets.

SECTION 2 – Left iris; blue. Density 2. Lymphosarcoma of bronchial tubes.

A.–Murky blue

B.–Drug spot (sulphur and iron), bronchial tube.

C.–Drug settlement, gastro-intenstinal tract.

D.–Heavy congestion, intestinal tract.

E.–Black scurf rim. F.–Good texture.

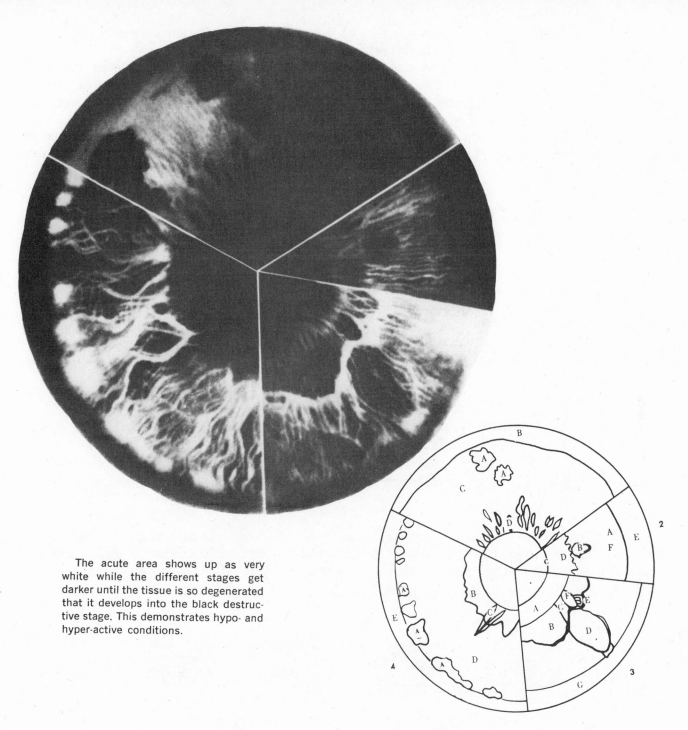

The acute area shows up as very white while the different stages get darker until the tissue is so degenerated that it develops into the black destructive stage. This demonstrates hypo- and hyper-active conditions.

SECTION 3 — Left iris; blue. Density 3. Extreme gas pains half-way down descending colon. Heart flutter and arythmia.

A.—Chronic acid stomach.

B.—Very toxic bowel. C.—Bowel adhesion.

D.—Closed tension, lower lung.

E.—Heart lesion.

F.—Bowel pockets, causing heart pressure.

G.—Scurf rim.

SECTION 4 — Left iris; blue. Density 4. Vaginal and sinus discharges. Glandular enlargements in groin.

A.—Lymphatic congestion throughout (zone 6).

B.—Inherently weak bowel structure.

C.—Settlement of sulphur and iron in bowel.

D.—Heavy Acidity. E.—Scurf rim.

In Section 1 of Color Plate the white part of the brownish discoloration shows extreme acidity. This is the acute sign of acidity and catarrhal settlement.

In Section 3, discoloration of inner ring shows that acid condition of stomach has been there many years, aggravated by taking certain drugs. Autonomic nerve wreath shows up extremely well; you can differentiate the gastro-intestinal tract area from the organ areas. There is a direct relation between the large closed lesion and that portion of the intestinal tract area opposite the lesion.

Section 4 shows clearly the 6th zone, containing the lymphatic rosary and the 7th zone on the periphery, which is the area of skin and circulation. Note that that lymphatic rosary goes through the circulation area."

THE RETRACING PROCESS...the right way to get well

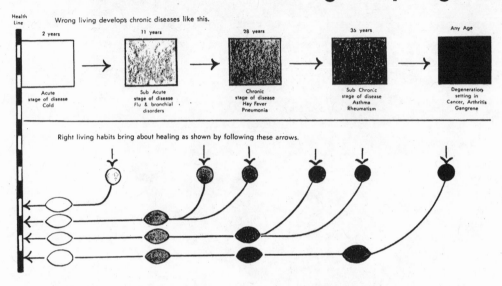

The different stages of disease of any organ can be determined by the color value in a specific area of the iris. In acute disease, the area is white; in sub-acute, light gray; in chronic disease (asthma, diabetes, heart disorders), dark grey; eventually, in sub-chronic disease, the area becomes black.

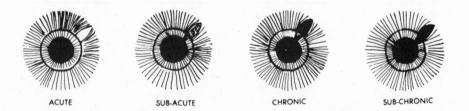

The iris mirrors the progress of internal healing and effectiveness of therapy.

As the body regenerates, the iris changes in color value. Abnormal spots gradually change from dark or black to a progressively lighter color. With this change in color, you may anticipate healing crises which can manifest as symptoms of acute disease. With healing, the natural color will return. The whole iris may become lighter in color.

It takes years of study to achieve mastery in diagnosis. The novice should first become familiar with the following areas: autonomic nerve wreath, lymphatic rosary, digestive tract, kidney, liver, lungs and thyroid. Those who plan to reach any level of expertise should consult Dr. B. Jensen's book, "The Science and Practice of Iridology" (182).

One of the greatest joys which a practitioner may anticipate is to help someone to regain the perfect iris. The perfect iris is flawless — no distortion of fibers, no spots, no cloudiness. Its natural color is blue, green or brown.

ZONE THERAPY AND ACUPRESSURE

"Take good care of your feet
Better watch out what you eat

Better take care of your life
Cause noone else can."
THE BEACH BOYS

Healing with the hands is as old as aches and pains. It was known to the Ancient Egyptians, Chinese and Grecians, and probably to the inhabitants of the continents of Atlantis and Mu.

They recognized that the human body is a symphony of vibrations. The internal organs orchestrate energy from sun, earth and planets to give our body the life force. Lymph, blood and nerve impluses can flow freely only through unobstructed channels. If they are blocked we become sick. We are not in harmony with the laws of Mother Nature and Father Sun.

Zone therapy, foot massage, spot therapy, acupuncture, reflexology and contact healing have a common feature — through manipulation and/or applied pressure, pain can be relieved and health restored to any part of the body. The most attractive element of such therapy is that you can heal yourself and others through the use of your hands. The results are often visible after a single 20 minute application.

Touching healthy tissue produces no unusual feeling. However, we instinctively rub or press a sore spot; often the pain disappears after this applied pressure or massage. A severe headache may have no relation to the head; instead the source of trouble may be the stomach or the colon.

One wise doctor reasoned: "If pains or other pathology are referred to distant sections, could we not influence the diseased area by treating some of the referred areas?" He proved correct. In 1913, William H. Fitzgerald, M.D. discovered that "there are ten invisible currents through the body." He described ten longitudinal zones, five on each side of the body, extending from the head, through the

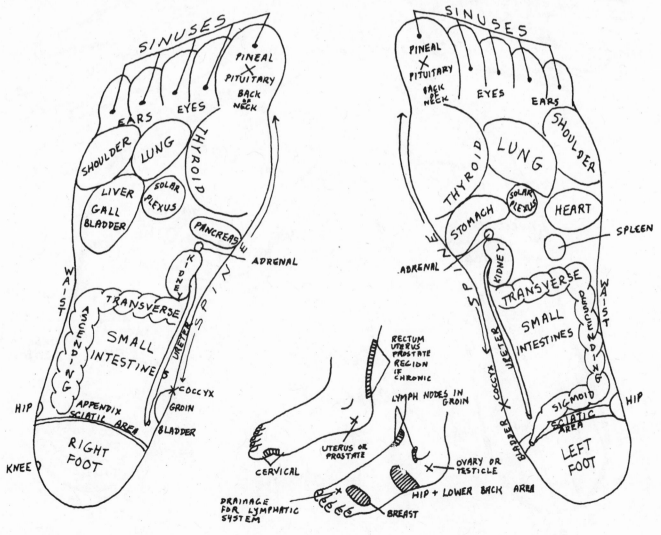

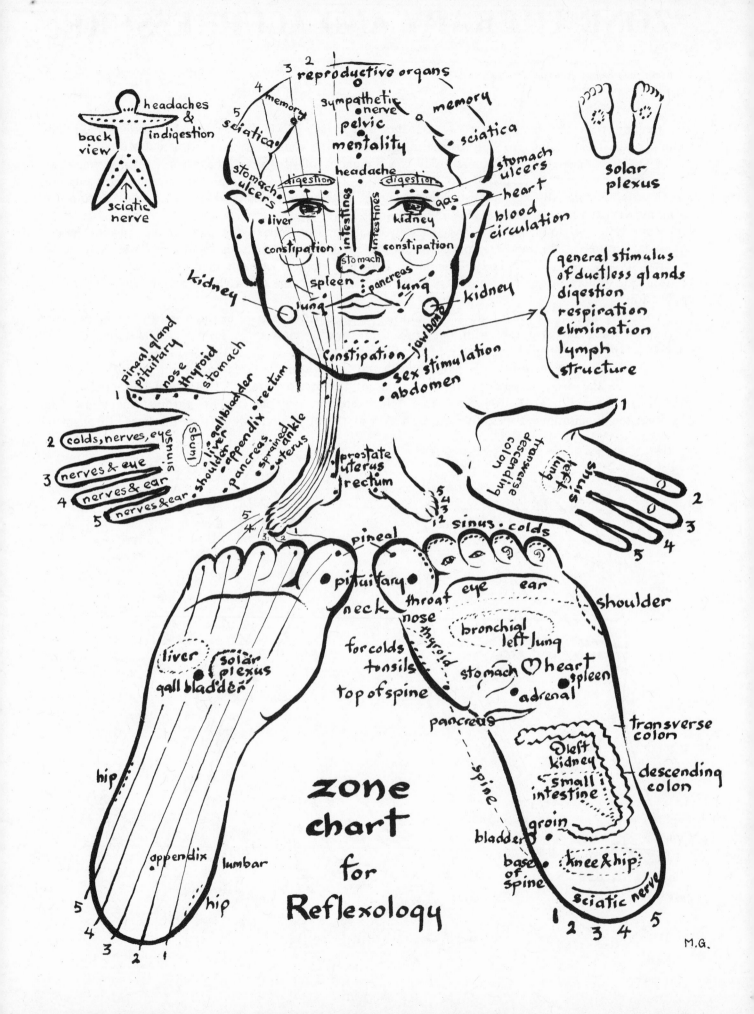

zone
chart
for
Reflexology

trunk, to the toes and fingers (see chart). He found pin-point areas on the surface of the body tender or painful to touch. Pressure on these areas can break up crystalline waste deposits, increasing nerve and blood supply to relieve congestion in corresponding areas in the same zone. However distant the affliction from the area where pressure is applied, it can speed the detoxification process and strengthen internal organs.

Stimulation of a reflex point will normalize function in the associated organ, i.e. digestive juices will pour more profusely or stop; peristaltic action will become more or less vigorous; hormone secretions will be more or less active.

Dr. Fitzgerald, discusses the theory behind zone therapy. "It is certain that control centers in the medulla are stimulated . . . their functions may be carried out by the pituitary body through the multiple nerve paths from it. We know that when inhibition or irritation is continuous, many pathological processes disappear. We are certain that lymphatic relaxation follows pressure. People are admittedly of chemical formation controlled by electrical energy or electric vibrations" (Zone Therapy).

Drs. J.S. Riley, E.F. Bowers, and G.S. White were among the untiring pioneers and practitioners in zone therapy.

Later, Eunice Ingham Stopfel perfected compression massage of the feet. She feels that since there are reflex points in the feet corresponding to every part of the body, it is sufficient to work on the feet alone. She says, "You are increasing the circulation and raising the body vitality, and as the vitality increases, Nature has the strength to overcome and throw off the poisons of the system" (Stories The Feet Can Tell).

A detoxified individual, after eating badly, will notice in zones related to the stomach, digestive tract, and pituitary areas, a ticklish-itching sensation, followed eventually by pain, then cessation of sensitivity, unless finger pressure is applied to these zones. By discovering which zones are sore, you can follow the effect of your lifestyle on your organs. For example, when I returned to polluted city air after several weeks in the mountains, zones to the liver and kidney were very painful for more than an hour. Eventually, the nerve endings become so filled with toxins that they became desensitized. Furthermore, at a distance of about 30 miles from the city, reflex points related to the lungs started itching, then became painful. Eventually the sensation stopped and hurt only on application of pressure. Living constantly in polluted air, we become unaware of the damage it does to our bodies.

During the detoxification regime, you can anticipate many reflex points, related to eliminative organs, to become sensitive or sore to touch. These organs are laboring very hard to eliminate toxins released from tissues. Zone therapy, by increasing circulation, will give them additional energy.

At the start, in some cases, only temporary relief can be anticipated. Pain will persist until its cause — congestion — has been eliminated. Some conditions will require many months of work before one can obtain the desired results (defects in the eye or ear, or body paralysis). Seldom is only one organ ailing: generally it is a total response of the body where one organ is affected more than others. When doing zone therapy, always treat reflexes for the whole body, with special emphasis on the very sore spots.

As your hands develop sensitivity, you will be able to feel small granulations (generally crystals of uric, lactic, purine or carbonic acid).

In my work, I have found reflexology extremely helpful in relieving backache and shoulder pain, constipation, headache, toothache, tension, over-worked kidneys, and gall bladder problems due to overeating. I work on related reflex areas on the feet; sometimes also on the hands, face, and back or press directly on the area over the affected organ.

Many points on the back and neck are apt to be sore; the application of a tolerable amount of pressure for five to twenty minutes can result in a tremendous increase in strength of the internal organs. Tchiatsu techniques, or those found in Zone Therapy (Dr. Fitzgerald) are highly recommended.

COMPRESSION MASSAGE OF THE FEET

While giving zone therapy, insist upon silence. Concentrate your attention on your work. It is good for the recipient to abstain from food for at least two hours prior to treatment.

You may, if you wish, first soak the feet for five to ten minutes in hot water. Scrub the soles gently with a stiff brush.

When working on your own feet, a comfortable position is semi-reclining with the foot to be worked on resting on the opposite bent knee. When working on another's feet, you may be seated directly in front as he or she lies on a bed or in a semi-reclining chair. If the person's legs are slightly elevated on a pillow, the feet are easier to grasp. With one hand, hold the foot in a comfortable position.

Using the other hand, apply steady pinpoint pressure to the reflex spots with a rotating motion of the inner corner or tip of the thumb, ring, middle and index fingers together; individual knuckles or heel of the hand. You may also use pinching and squeezing. Rotating the toes and fingers is very effective. If you have weak hands, the smooth end of a ballpoint pen or toothbrush can be used as a tool to exert the desired pressure.

Start the treatment with the big toe, applying pressure to the top, sides, front, and bottom. Work down all of zone one to the heel (see chart). Then give a general quick massage, noting crystallizations and sore areas. Return to the toes and work down the rest of the foot to the heel. On the digestive tract start with the stomach area. Follow with the small intestine area, then the colon. Next work on the back of the heel and the sides of the ankle, followed by the top of the foot. Don't limit yourself to specific mapped-out spots. Explore the whole foot. If any area is sore, it should be treated. Special attention should be given the ductless glands (pituitary, thyroid); this will aid rejuvenation of the body.

If a person feels pain in any zone, you know that the corresponding area of that person's body is sick. Repeated application of pressure will, in time, relieve local tenderness and heal illness.

Let your instinct guide you as to how long you should apply pressure. Generally five to twenty seconds is long enough for a single application of pressure. Release the pressure and re-apply. Intermittent pressure is especially good for very painful spots.

Watch the person's face for signs of extreme pain. Reduce the pressure if it causes too much pain. Return repeatedly to the sore spots, intermixing pressure with a general foot massage. If a spot is unbearably painful, work on the surrounding area, the other foot, or on corresponding hand areas.

If the feet are very sore, be gentle; limit your first few sessions to a half hour foot massage, pressing each sore spot for only ten to thirty seconds. Zone therapy can release a large amount of toxic material. When it enters the circulation, it can tax the eliminative system, causing a great deal of discomfort. So initially, with very sick people, do not overwork the sore areas. You might even have to skip a day to allow the body to catch up with detoxification.

A rule of the thumb for the length of a zone therapy session: if person is chronically ill, with eliminative organs and detoxifying organs affected, it is a good practice during the first 3 sessions not to work on feet for more than ten minutes; in all other cases one can work 20 to 30 minutes without overtiring the feet. Initially light to medium amount of pressure. If trying to relieve or assist an acute condition, or headache, indigestion, pain, then apply as much pressure as will be tolerated for up to 30 minutes. The problem generally disappears in 5 to 30 minutes. If condition should reappear at a latter time , repeat the process. If zone therapy is overdone, the person receiving the treatment will experience great deal of tiredness for next two days. Rest and enemas should be used.

Before breakfast, one should do a self diagnosis. Press on eyeballs with moderate amount of pressure. If sore it is best to skip breakfast (and stop having late suppers) until hungry or else have something salty, cellery juice beet, carrot, cellery and green juice. Check also "hoku" point on hands, as well as on the feet areas for liver, kidney, digestive tract and pituitary. If any of them are sore, skip brabreakfast (this does not necessarily apply to hypoglycemia),or else have rejuvilac, or same as for eyeball test. In every case, one should do at least 15 minutes zone therapy plus deep breathing before drinking the liquid. If digestive tract not empty, especially the stomach, having a breakfast will increase toxemia and produce a tired feeling for the rest of the day.

After the first two weeks of treatment, everyone — healthy or sick — should have zone therapy for at least five to ten minutes daily.

After doing zone therapy say "I release you" shake your hands vigorously and wash them. Let the recipient rest or sleep after a session of zone therapy.

PEBBLES AND BALLS Place large marbles, golf balls, or pebbles one or more inches in diameter in a pan of warm to hot water. Sitting or standing, immerse your feet in the water, pressing them firmly against the pebbles for fifteen to twenty minutes. For a milder treatment, cover the balls with a towel, with or without the basin of water. Spend as much time as possible walking barefoot in sand, ocean water or grass. Never wear rubber soled shoes. Because rubber does not breathe, it insulates you from earth vibrations and it interferes with the elimination of waste through the soles of the feet.

Add chick peas or small pebbles into shoes for continuous zone stimulation. Use avocado pit to step on to stimulate the intestinal tract and colon for constipation.

FINGERS AND HANDS

COMB CRUSH Press a dull-toothed metal comb firmly into the palm of the hand and the soft tissues of the fingers. Maintain the pressure until you feel relief from the condition you are treating for.

Pressure applied in the webbing between the first finger and thumb can end headaches, insomnia, constipation, as well as diarrhea and induce a feeling of well being that lasts for days. This point is one of the most vital centers and is called Ho-Ku. It has a direct effect on the intestine and nerves. Because of the conjested condition of civilized digestive tract, Ho-Ku is very painful when pressed. One finds this point mentioned in karate for disarming an opponent through application of hard pressure. In therapy, apply as much pressure as you can tolerate.

BRISK BRUSH: to tranquilize   Clip spring clothes pins to all the finger tips or in between the fingers. To tranquilize or achieve blissful relaxation, using a natural or steel bristle hair brush, starting with the finger tips, stroke the top of the hand and arm to the shoulder for two to fifteen minutes; stop before it becomes painful. Or brush gently over the whole body for at least ten minutes; it will give you restful sleep. Don't use enough pressure to bruise. Avoid if you have poor skin tone.

To anesthetize   either the left or right side of the mouth for dental work, clip clothes pins on the finger tips of the corresponding hand. In fifteen minutes the nerves to the teeth should be numbed. Acupressure for control of pain can be learned by dentists in a few hours (Zone Therapy, Dr. Fitzgerald).

Dr. George Weaver and Dr. Edmund Casey (President of National Medical Association), both of Cincinnati, Ohio; also, Dr. Howard Hall of Covington, Ohio use acupressure — applying finger and thumb pressure to block pain in dental work. Dr. Weaver states: "I can teach any dentist to use acupuncture pressure in less time than it takes to play nine holes of golf." He has taught the method to 26 dentists and he asks them to pass the knowledge on to their colleagues.

To revitalize :   For relief of motor or sensory paralysis, stroke the affected area as well as the feet, hands, face and vertebrae with a steel or natural bristle brush. A diet of sprouts and grass juice is revitalizing. It may take two to six months to get results.

SPINE AND BACK

The spine is made of twenty-four vertebrae, cushioned by discs, held in place by a muscular structure. Through it flows the major nerve supply. Rigidity or curvation of the spine can interfere with the flow of electric impulses and blood supply to every part of the body.

The following are methods to increase the flexibility of the spine.

BALL BED : A metal bar installed in a doorway is best. Otherwise grasp the upper edge of the door frame and hang loosely for at least thirty second. Stretch out the tense muscles. Do not tense the body by lifting the feet if they touch the ground. Swing the body to the left and to the right. Twist the shoulders to the left and right. Keep the back erect afterward.

ROCK AND ROLL   (If you have osteoporosis or severe back problems, do not practice this exercise without consulting a physician. Instead, do zone therapy).

Obtain a 20 by 30 inch rug. Roll it very tightly. Fasten it with string or strong rubber bands. Cover it with sponge carpet padding 20 by 15 inches. Fasten it. Place it on the floor. Lie on the back with the roll under the shoulders. Movement one: Interlock the fingers behind the neck and let the arms touch the floor. Twist the portion of the back (above the roll) to the left and right. Do the adjustment a few times only, without strain. Movement two: With the hands interlocked behind the neck bring the elbows as nearly as possible together. Rock up and down across the roll. Be gentle so as not to arouse any severe pain. Move the roll down the spine about 1½ inches and repeat both movements. Repeat this pattern the full length of the spine.

HANGING : Lie on the floor on a rug or blanket. Place a ball under any painful area (not spine) and lie on it to relieve backache. Large balls (softball, tennis ball or baseball) may effect temporary relief of sciatica or muscular rheumatism (be sure you are on a low protein, vegetarian diet) and aching in the lower back or buttocks. Many have obtained relief from sciatic nerve pain within five to fifteen minutes. (Sciatica is often the result of an acid condition from many years of chronic indigestion or spinal impingement). If you cannot bear pressure at the site of pain, move the ball to the surrounding tissues. Small balls may be used to relieve pain in the upper back. You may combine several balls during the treatment.

MIGRAINE HEADACHE ususally originates in the colon or stomach. It is a sign of indigestion due to excessive eating, allergic reactions, fermentation of starch and/or putrefaction of protein, producing in the stomach a wide range of toxins. The resulting detoxification activities overwork the liver and kidneys; the endocrine glands attempt to direct the toxins to other eliminative organs. This hyperfunction can cause them to swell. As the pituitary gland enlarges, it presses against its bony enclosure, sometimes causing the severe pain of migraine headache (Food Is Your Best Medicine, Bieler).

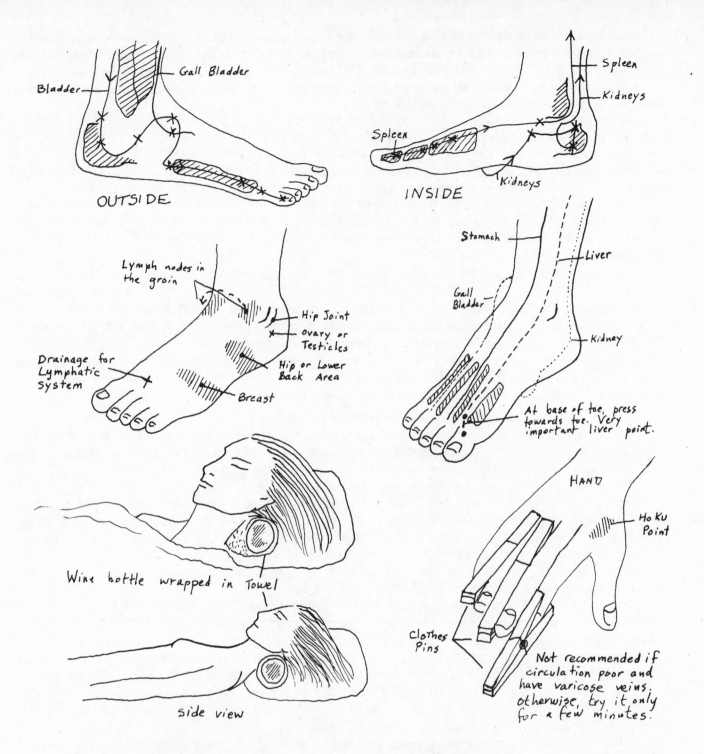

OUTSIDE

Bladder
Gall Bladder

INSIDE

Spleen
Kidneys
Spleen
Kidneys

Lymph nodes in the groin
Hip Joint
Ovary or Testicles
Hip or Lower Back Area
Drainage for Lymphatic System
Breast

Stomach
Liver
Gall Bladder
Kidney
At base of toe, press towards toe. Very important liver point.

Wine bottle wrapped in Towel

side view

HAND
Ho Ku Point
Clothes Pins
Not recommended if circulation poor and have varicose veins. Otherwise, try it only for a few minutes.

To prevent headache, start zone therapy at the earliest sign of indigestion: anger, tightness in the neck, pain in the eyeballs, especially when pressed, soreness (or ticklishness) in the reflex areas related to the digestive organs. If the condition is caught early enough, two to fifteen minutes of zone therapy will prevent development of headache. Apply as much pressure as you can tolerate to reflex areas on the face and feet.

Clip clothespins to the fingertips, leaving them on as long as you can bear it. Starting with the thumbs, move one or more pins from one finger to the next, on both hands simultaneously. Clip pins between fingers as well.

For the quickest results (two to five minutes), obtain 12 ounce soda bottles which may be filled with hot water, or hard balls or stones 2/3 to 3/4 inches in diameter. Stand on them barefoot, rolling them under the arch on the reflex areas related to the digestive tract and the spine. Apply as much pressure as you can bear. You might have to repeat the process several times during the day before congestion is totally relieved.

If the headache is the result of protein indulgence, sometimes the juice of 1/4 lemon in 1/4 glass of water, fresh pineapple juice, dilute apple cider vinegar, or hot miso soup broth with cayenne pepper can aid in flushing toxins from the stomach.

Most severe migraine headaches I have observed may be relieved in one to three hours by applying one or more of the following techniques.

1. If you feel nauseated, regurgitate. If you have weak lungs, be careful; violent vomiting may tear the surface of the lung. It will heal in a day, but can be very painful. Try to induce vomiting. Drink two to four glasses of warm water. Add enough sea salt to give it salty taste. But not more than 1 teaspoon altogether.
Breathe deeply. Expand and contract the stomach at least 10 times. Tickle the back of the throat with the fingers. Regurgitate. If the content of the stomach is bitter and yellowish, it is excessive spilled-over bile. Take several enemas. Rest or take a warm salt bath.

2. Roll your feet hard across a coke bottle to stimulate the digestive tract. This is very effective for relieving dizziness. Press and massage all zone areas on the chin, eyebrows, eyeballs, back of the neck and feet. Use clothespins on the fingers.

3. Place on your pillow a carpet roll or wine bottle rolled in a large towel. Lie on your back so that it is under your neck. If you have poor circulation do not use this technique for more than a half-hour — the neck might become numb. Go to sleep with the light on (the red end of the color spectrum radiated from any incandescent lamp is a strong energy source for the nerves and the digestive tract). If you wake with a headache, do zone therapy again.

4. Don't eat or drink until really hungry. Start with a very small amount of dilute grapefruit or celery juice or rejuvelac. In severe cases, drink only juice or broth for a period of 24 hours.

5. Sickness is never fun. Follow the health rules (Appendix). Then heads will be for brains, not for aches.

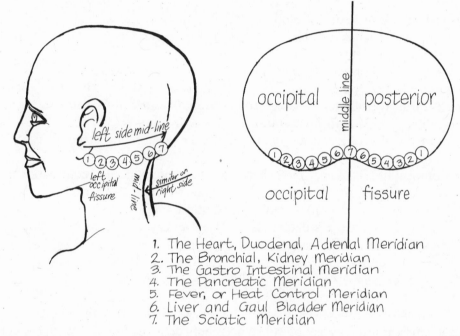

1. The Heart, Duodenal, Adrenal Meridian
2. The Bronchial, Kidney Meridian
3. The Gastro Intestinal Meridian
4. The Pancreatic Meridian
5. Fever, or Heat Control Meridian
6. Liver and Gaul Bladder Meridian
7. The Sciatic Meridian

CONSTIPATION: Work on all reflex points on the face and feet, spending 90% of the time on points corresponding to the ascending transverse and descending colon, the small intestine, the stomach.

In addition to finger pressure, stand on a 12 ounce bottle, rolling it under the arches. After a twenty minute application, there generally will be a bowel movement within the hour. Severe cases are apt to be temporary unless one is eating live food.

SLEEPLESSNESS AND TENSION : This is a sign of indigestion, constipation, severe cleansing reactions or emotional stress. Work on reflex points as for headaches and constipation. Apply pressure and firm massage to the forehead, eyebrows, eyes, back of the neck and shoulders. After five minutes of intensive work, you will probably fall asleep. Otherwise follow with a body massage of brushing the skin with a natural or steel bristle hair brush.

MASSAGE

"Work with your hand, as we commanded you."   I THES. 4:11

Massage is a loving thing to do. A loving massage is always therapeutic, especially if you ask for the highest energy flow through your hands and the recipient's body. Above all, it should make the recipient, and you, feel good. If you don't love to do massage, don't do it.

If you wish to obtain a license, you can go to a massage school. Or you can learn from someone who gives a good massage.

To learn to give a good massage, you must practice. Your hands will become sensitive to the needs of the recipient, especially if you completely give yourself over to what you are doing. You can invent your own strokes, or you can read George Downing's marvellous MASSAGE BOOK for an exact description of each stroke, accompanied by an accurate drawing. He even gives you the rudiments of anatomy.

Do massage only when your vitality is high, when you are rested and happy. Then good vibrations will flow and you won't pick up any sick or tired vibrations. It is natural to feel exhilarated, never tired, after giving a massage.

You can give a good message on the floor — just remember to keep your back straight, and work from your hips. whenever possible. Ideally you can work at a massage table. Then you can use your whole body, leaning into the strokes — it's like dancing.

If you need an incentive, there are now available many massage workshops, inexpensive, but intensive enough to get you started.

THE BENEFICIAL EFFECT OF MASSAGE

*Massage dilates the blood vessels, improving the circulation and relieving congestion throughout the body.

*Massage increases the number of red blood cells especially in cases of anemia.

*Massage acts as a "mechanical cleanser," stimulating lymph circulation and hastening the elimination of wastes and toxic debris.

*Massage relaxes muscle spasm and relieves tension.

*Massage increases blood supply and nutrition to muscles without adding to their load of toxic lactic acid, produced through voluntary muscle contraction. Massage thus helps to prevent buildup of harmful "fatigue" products resulting from strenuous exercise or injury.

*Massage improves muscle tone and helps prevent or delay muscular atrophy resulting from forced inactivity.

*Massage can compensate, in part, for lack of exercise and muscular contraction in persons who because of injury, illness or age are forced to remain inactive. In these cases, massage helps return venous blood to the heart and so eases the strain on this vital organ.

*Massage may have a sedative, stimulating or even exhausting effect on the nervous system depending on the type and length of massage treatment given.

*According to some authorities, massage may burst the fat capsule in subcutaneous tissue so that the fat exudes and becomes absorbed. In this way massage, combined with a nutritious but calorie-deficient diet, can be an aid to reducing.

*Massage by improving the general circulation, increases nutrition of the tissues. It is accompanied or followed by an increased interchange of substances between the blood and tissue cells heightening tissue metabolism.

*Massage increases the excretion (via the kidneys) of fluids and waste products of protein metabolism, inorganic phosphorus and salt in normal individuals.

*Massage encourages the retention of nitrogen, phosphorus and sulphur necessary for tissue repair in persons convalescing from bone fractures.

*Massage stretches connective tissue, improves its circulation and nutrition and so breaks down or prevents the formation of adhesions and reduces the danger of fibrosis.

*Massage improves the circulation and nutrition of joints and hastens the elimination of harmful deposits. It helps lessen inflammation and swelling in joints and so alleviates pain.

*Massage helps to reduce edema (or dropsy) of the extremities.

*Massage disperses the edema following injury to ligaments and tendons, lessens pain and facilitates movement.

Massage makes you feel good.

ELLEMENTS OF MASSAGE

1) Harmonious environment (personal cleanliness, quiet, freedom from interruption.)

2) Energize and center yourself (concentration).

3) Assist the recipient to a comfortable position. Ask whether he or she has any physical ailments. It may be necessary to avoid certain areas. For example, avoid pressure on badly varicosed veins, brusies or new scar tissue.

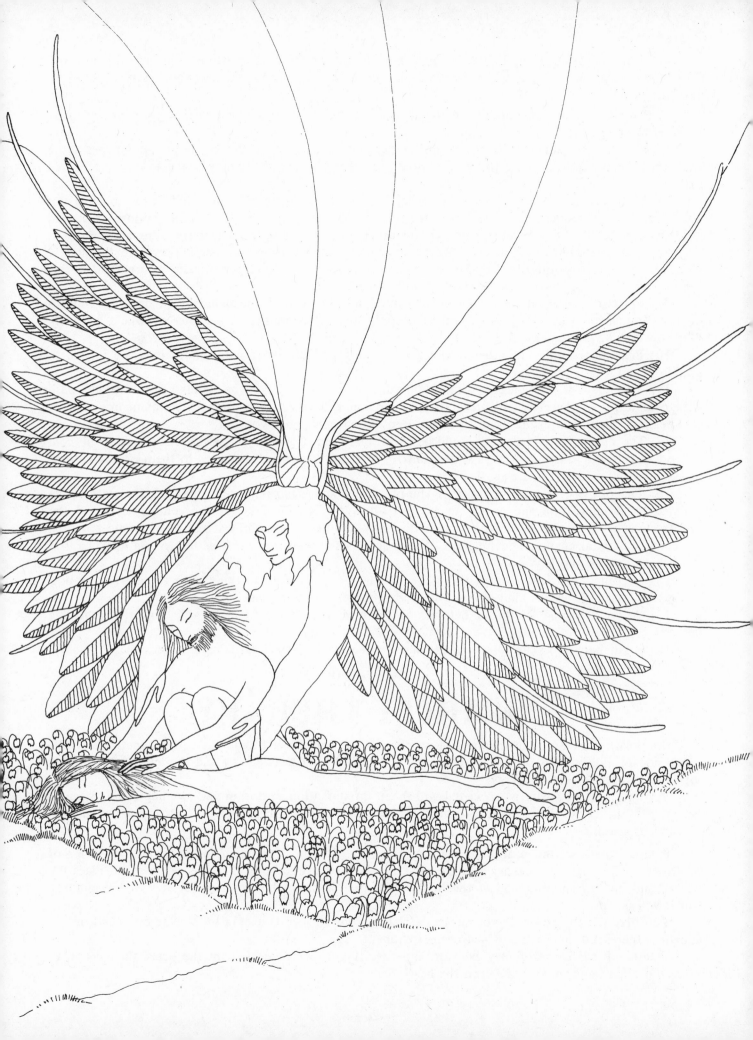

4) Visualize the recipient in a state of well-being and yourself as a channel through which energy flows. Remember, the recipient may be tired, asking for help. You are the recipient's servant. Do well unto the person.

5) Place the hand momentarily on the recipient (usually the shoulders) so that your presence may be accepted before you begin.

6) Work on the aura. Palms downward, stroke the hands through the air about three inches above the recipient's body from head to foot   slowly, so that you feel the energy transfer. It may feel cold or hot.

7) Resiliency is a potential quality of every part of the body. Work slowly and firmly to bring this about. Jerky or sudden movements by the operator might cause the recipient to lose trust and consequently the freedom to relax. Upon completion of an area, smooth its corresponding aura.

8) Tense areas are often tender. Work very slowly; concentrate on energy flow into the area visualize blue-green soothing-healing for the area. Let the area rest and periodically return to it during the massage. Often more than one treatment will be necessary.

9) Injury or inflamed areas in general should not be worked mechanically   or only under a doctor's guidance. Auric work is helpful as is application of vitamin E, grass juice or wheat germ oil. Work on the corresponding reflex area.

10) Beginners should not attempt work on persons who are ill or with whom they are unable to establish rapport.

11) Terminate the massage by smoothing the entire aura. Shake you hands vigorously and wash with cold water to the elbow to break the psychic connection. Again picture the recipient in a state of well-being or silently offer prayer or blessings. Center and re-energize yourself.

12) The duration of a massage should be about one hour. Coconut oil, safflower or sesame oil, cold pressed and organic, may be used as a lubricant for massage. You may add herbs to them or a few drops of essential oil.

13) The purpose of massage is to psycho-physically and electro-magnetically alter the state of the body so that circulation and energy exchange pathways are opened up at the cellular level and the proper state of ionization is created so that the body will have continuous access to its innate potential for control of vital energy. The function of massage is essentially the same as that of Hatha Yoga, but through an external agency.

14) Become proficient from working on healthy people before working with those who are not. Always be loving, generous, kind channel of energy. Surrender to the task.

15) A juice regime 24 hours before and after massage helps to make it a powerful purifying process.

16) A salt bath and sleep following the massage make it a perfect revitalizing experience.

POLARITY THERAPY

In polarity therapy, the therapist views the human body as a balanced electromagnetic field. The right side of the body is considered charged with positive sun heat energy and the left side, the carrier of cooling moon receptive energy.

An excess of positivity is associated with heat, inflammation, irritation and swelling of an organ or an area of the body. Excess of receptive energy is associated with the cooling effect of poor circulation, tension or spasm.

Polarity therapy can return the body to a balanced state. For example, to reduce an excess of positivity, place the left, negative-charged hand on the area of the body that needs treatment. Place the other hand on the opposite side of the body. Hold the hands in this position for at least ten minutes. Relief will come.

You may tap the power of your heart (probably your strongest) chakra by placing one hand over it and the other hand on the area which needs treatment.

Treatment of the torso may be more effective if you place one fist on the back, then lie on it. Place the other hand opposite it or on the heart chakra.

COLOR HEALING

Just as the root or plant that cannot catch the sunlight becomes a stunted, faded, undeveloped organism; so the individual who is cut off from the White Light of the Spirit becomes ill. The flow is stopped usually through wrong thinking or wrong action, with the result that a blank area, so to speak, is formed which swiftly becomes the breeding ground of negative or undivine thoughts and elements which work themselves out as disease conditions of all kinds.

Color treatment is based on the principle that all healing is a change of mental attitude or belief. Color in itself does not do the healing; it merely gives the body the spark of power to perform its own healing processes. Application of color increases the vibratory rate of the physical and etheric cells. In a higher vibratory state, the physical body becomes more sensitive and receptive to the healing force which flows. Each person benefits from the use of color, or any type of healing, according to the measure of his or her own ability to respond to and use the power which is received.

RED RAY: The red ray is a heating, vitalizing and stimulating vibration with direct effect on the etheric center governing the physical vitality. It is excellent in all blood-deficiency diseases, but should be used with care. Red stimulates the liver and builds the red principle of the blood. In the form of food, it is best represented by red or cayenne pepper. Red increases the circulation and warms the entire body and helps to clean out mucus and waste from the body. Vitamin B-12 is red and Vitamin E is scarlet.

ORANGE RAY: The orange ray stimulates and builds the lungs. It relieves gas, convulsions, and cramps — including menstrual cramps — throughout the digestive system. Orange relieves spastic and sluggish colon and small intestine and helps to cause vomiting when food is not being digested. Most all spices come under the orange color. Vitamin B-complex is orange.

YELLOW RAY: Yellow cleanses and purifies the whole system, assisting in loosening calcium and lime deposits. It stimulates the liver and activates all organs except the spleen, increases the appetite and aids in assimilation of food. Yellow has a tonic effect on nerves and builds nerves and muscles and activates them where other systems fail. Yellow influences the higher mind and soul.

In the **LEMON COLOR** are found more elements than any other color and many of these elements are solvents, thus making lemon most effective in all chronic conditions. Lemon loosens and eliminates mucus throughout the entire body and stimulates and builds the brain for clearer and more positive thinking. Vitamin C is Lemon.

GREEN is a vibration of harmony and balance, hence it is of fundamental importance to the nervous system. Soothing and sympathetic, it does not excite, inflame or irritate. Restorer of tired nerves and giver of new energy, it is nature's master tonic. Green stimulates the master (pituitary) gland for better control of other glands and organs throughout the body, dissolves blood clots, and builds muscles. Green represents the chlorophyll or cleansing principle. Start all schedules of color healing with one or more green exposures.

BLUE RAY is an "electric ray" with a calm, peaceful, cooling vibration. It is useful to induce sleep and relaxation and to relieve the effects of stress. An astringent, it may be applied to relieve inflammation, inward bleeding and nervousness. The oxygen of blue increases perspiration to relieve fever.

INDIGO RAY Influences the central part of the head in the region of the pineal gland. This ray exercises dominion over eye and nose and is of great value in the treatment of certain forms of nervous and mental disorders. It is secondarily of use in lung diseases. Vitamin K is Indigo.

VIOLET RAY'S main province is the brain and the mental and spiritual nature. Much harm can be done by improper and indiscriminate use of the violet ray. Because of its very high vibrational rate, it is not suited to the undeveloped or retarded mind, and thus should be used with discrimination. It is the stimulator of the crown chakram and controls the pituitary gland. Violet is best suited to the artistic temperament and to those with a great desire to express themselves on the creative plane of mind. Vitamin D is Violet.

The healer should bear in mind that the two basic colors used in color healing are red and blue — the thermal and the cooling. These two colors form the basic vibrations in every human being. The main physical signs of a lack of Red Ray are seen when the person is deficient in energy, rich blood, appetite, or suffers from constipation. Secondary indications are sleepiness and generally inactive disposition. When the Blue Ray is lacking there are signs of overactivity, fussiness, irritability, feverishness.

To obtain health, vitality and pure blood, use the rose-red and the orange ray; for rebuilding health after illness, tune in to the green, blue and violet rays. For depression, loneliness, frustration, we let the mind vibrate to all Seven Rays. The more we think of the inexhaustible Color Forces surrounding us, the less lonely and despondent we will be. Clear Golden Yellow is one of the most powerful forces against depression and limitations of every kind. For prosperity, success and progress, the Cosmic remedy is the Green Ray. For mental development and mind power, harmonize with the Golden Ray of Mind. The yellow ray has a healing effect on digestive troubles, stomach disorders, and complaints of the circulatory system.

To do color healing, the ray is directed to the chosen area of the body. The rays may be: 1) radiated from a lamp or reflector (many hardware stores carry color floodlights) or from a large flat bottle of water stained with the appropriate color from water paints, juice, flowers or herbs. Permit a floodlight or sunlight to shine through the bottle, projecting the color onto the etheric body; (2) projected thought images into the mental body; (3) inhaled as air exposed to colored light; (4) absorbed into the body from the elements contained in certain foods and light-charged liquids.

A further aid to healing is color massage. The healer having first washed his or her hands in tepid water, bathes them from three to five minutes in the full rays of the color lamp, them rubs them briskly together and gives massage for ten to fifteen minutes.

For further information on methods of color healing, read S.G.J. Ouseley's Color Meditation, and The Power of The Rays.

One of the best papers published on the response of humans to color stimulation is the work by Robert Gerard, a psychologist. He reported that "red", "blue", and "white" light stimuli, equated for brightness, produced consistent bodily and emotional responses in 24 normal adult males. The following variables were observed: (1) brain wave patterns, (2) respiratory movements, (3) electrical acitivity of the heart, (4) frequency of eyeblinks, (5) blood pressure, (6) palmar skin conductance (a measure of autonomic arousal based on reaction of the sweat glands in the palms of the hands). In all physiological measures except heart rate, here was significantly more arousal with "red" than with "blue". Intermediate levels were obtained with "white" light. Brain waves tracings showed least arousal with "blue" The subjective responses paralleled the physiological data. The subjects reported a feeling of greater over-all well being, greater relaxation and calm, and less hostility and anxiety during "blue" than during the other stimuli. Under "red" illumination there was more tension and anxiety, excitement and sexual arousal (Gerard: "Differential Effects of Color Lights on Psychological Functions Ph.D. Thesis U.C.L.A. Ap. 1958).

Ott has reported on the effect of pink fluorescent lamps in human behavior. The staff of a St. Petersburg, Florida, radio station replaced the white fluoescent lamps in the control rooms with F-40PK pink tubes in an effort to brighten the surroundings. Within 2 months, personal relations had deteriorated to a noticeable degree: poor performance on the air, widespread irritability and disputes between employees and managers. Two employees abruptly submitted their resignations with the reason of dissatisfaction with themselves and their co-workers. One of the staff said that if the pink tubes were not removed he would "go out of his mind". They were quickly replaced with the original white tubes. Within a week a noticable change occurred: tempers ceased to flare, congeniality and cooperativeness began to reappear, the resignations were withdrawn, and performance on the air improved noticeably, with mistakes at a minimum (Ott, Optometric Weekly, Sept. 5, 1968).

MEDICINAL HERBS

Chairman Mao's latest brilliant thought is that doctors should not prescribe new drugs until they have exhaustively tested them on themselves. Thousands of Chinese women doctors are now testing a new contraceptive injection, taken quarterly, to see how it works. Chairman Mao thinks doctors are best qualified to detect and describe side effects experienced first hand, to be more responsible for drugs given, and to encourage revolutionary medical gains.

[THE DAILY NEWS, 2/12/73]

"The Superior doctor prevents illness; the mediocre doctor cures imminent illness; the inferior doctor treats illness."   CHINESE PROVERB

Herbs (including roots, seeds, tree leaves, barks, etc.) can be prepared in different ways. They can be dried, converted into powders or the fresh juice can be pressed and taken in its natural state. The oils and essences can be obtained thru maceration in wine. The best way to extract the mineral salts, vitamins and other soluble substances such as gums, sugar, extract and portions of the essential oils and resinous matter is by the process known as infusion. Infusion is the process of steeping (without boiling) certain substances in water for the purpose of extracting their soluble elements.

To extract all the valuable elements from herbs, roots, barks, leaves, etc. without destroying their vitamins and disorganizing their mineral salts do as follows: (1). Grind or cut in small pieces the herb, root, etc. and put in cold distilled water and let steep for several hours. It is important to use distilled water because it contains practically no mineral matter or other substances. It has a powerful affinity for the salts and other elements of the herbs and extracts these elements from them. Let the herbs steep in the water for three to twelve hours. Then strain and keep this precious solution and, instead of throwing away the herbs, add a little more water to them, set on the fire and let come to the boiling point. Allow them to stand for 30 minutes and strain again. Finally, add this boiled decoction to the unboiled portion and it is ready to take. It is very important to do this because if you boil the herbs before separating the soluble salts and vitamins thru infusion, you will destroy the life element of the herb, kill the vitamins, disorganize the mineral salts. On the other hand if you infuse only the herbs, then those elements which can be dissolved only at high temperatures will remain in the herb. (2). These infusions or teas should be taken hot, at about 115 to 120 degrees F. However, if the weather is warm and the patient feels a desire for something cooling, these teas can be taken cold. Teas can be sweetened with honey, but never with refined sugar. (3). Usually, the best time to take the tea is 30 to 60 minutes before meals. When taken at this time, the tea will not interfere with the process of digestion. In about 15 to 20 minutes it shall have either been absorbed from the stomach or passed into the duodenum. It will have cleansed the stomach and prepared it for the reception and digestion of the next meal. It will also supply the blood with the precious mineral salts so valuable for the secretion of digestive juices and neutralization of acids. (4). However, in the case of the carminatives (those herbs which have the property of expelling gas from the stomach and bowels) they should be taken hot when troubled with gas and heartburn. DOSE: The average dose should be from one fourth to one half teaspoonful of the herb, root, bark, etc. for each cup of water. Buy a grinder and grind the dried herbs as fine as possible so that the distilled water may penetrate and dissolve the nutritive elements.

ALTERATIVES

Under this heading are those herbal medicines which effect a gradual correction of a general diseased condition without producing visible effects such as purging, vomiting or sweating. The tea from these herbs may be taken when there is chronic disease accompanied by lack of appetite. These teas can be taken hot or cold not less than 20 to 30 minutes before meals, twice a day. Take them 20 minutes before meals if hot or 30 minutes before meals if cold. You should not sweeten the teas under this heading. The following herbs belong to this group:

Papaya-Mint, Golden Seal root, Yarrow herb, Bittersweet herb, Sarsaparrilla root, Barberry root, Sassafrass bark, Buckbean leaves, Black Alder bark. DOSE: One half to one teaspoon of the ground herbs, roots, leaves, etc. for each cup of water, twice a day before meals as explained above. In making these or any one of the following teas, you may use just one or a combination of two or more herbs. Never use more than one teaspoonful of herbs to one cup of water unless specified.

ANTHELMINTICS OR VERMIFUGES

These are herb medicines which cause the expulsion of parasite worms from the small and large intestine such as the tape worm and ascarid. The following are the best known remedies for the expulsion of these intestinal parisites:

Pumpkin seeds. These common seeds are a very effective remedy for the expulsion of the tapeworm and other intestinal parasites. Proceed as follows:

Fast for from one to two days. Cleanse the colon with two or three enemas. The day you break the short fast, get three or four oz. of pumpkin seeds and grind them or crush them thoroughly. After the seeds are thoroughly ground dissolve them in a cup of water, drink it very slowly. Two hours after, take one and one half oz. of castor oil. Within two to four hours, and almost without any pain, the parasite is almost invariably expelled. There are other plants which also have the property of expelling the tapeworm, ascarids and other parasites. The herbs most used for this purpose are wormwood, tansy and malefern. They should be taken as follows: DOSE: mix one half to one oz. of the ground herb with honey and take in the morning the day you break the one or two day's fast. Children should be given proportionately smaller doses.

Many years ago I read in the Essene Gospel of Peace about a way of getting rid of the tape worm. This consists in having the patient fast for two or three days. After the bowels have been emptied by means of enemas and there is no food for the tapeworm to eat, it naturally feels hungry and goes up and down the intestines in search for food. At this time, the victim of the tapeworm sits in a vessel of warm milk at a temperature of about 102 degrees. The tapeworm seems to smell the milk and comes out via the mouth to appease it's hunger with milk. When it's head is out of the body it is seized with the hand and the whole body of the tapeworm is extracted. I have never had occasion to trick the tapeworm out of the body in this way but I have been told that it works. So you might try this method first.

ANTILITHICS

To this group belongs the herbal remedies which have the property of preventing, dissolving and eliminating urinary calculi or bladder and kidney stones and other calcareous deposits of the body, such as those which cause arthritis and gout. The following herbs belong to this group:

Wild carrot, wild radish, plums and prunes, onions, parsley, gravel plant herb, golden rod herb, wild violet leaves and buchu leaves.

DOSE: one fourth to one half teaspoonful of the ground herb to each cup of water. Take it hot or cold three times a day, no less than one hour before nor less than three hours after meals. These teas may be sweetened with honey.

ANTI-RHEUMATICS

These are those fruits, vegetables and herbs which have the property of preventing and correcting rheumatism. To this group belong all citrus fruits such as lemons, grapefruit, oranges and pineapple. Also the following herbs:

Sassafras root, licorice root, horseradish, dandelion root, yarrow, bittersweet twigs, black alder bark, and black willow bark. DOSE: Of the citrus fruits you can take from one to two pints of orange or grapefruit juice daily for a week. After this preliminary treatment, you may take one cup of tea of the above herb at 11 a.m., one glass of citrus fruit juices at 4 p.m. and another cup of herb juice at 8 p.m.

DOSE: One half teaspoon of ground herbs in 10 oz. of distilled water. Drink it hot one hour before meals.

Abstain from those foods which produce much uric acid such as eggs, legumes, nuts and seeds.

ASTRINGENTS

To this group belong those herbal medicines which have the property to tone up the relaxed tissues and make them firmer and solid. Their effect is to contract the tissues and prevent excessive discharges such as excessive menstrual flow, bleeding from the nose etc.

The following herbs are indicated to relieve and correct these disorders:

Sage, willow, shepherds purse, wintergreen, blood staunch herb, pilewort leaves, oak bark, and blackberry root. DOSE: As before, grind and infuse one half to one teaspoonful of one of these herbs in 10 oz. of water and take two cups of the tea one hour before meals.

CARMINATIVES

These are those substances which allay pain and dispel wind or gas from the stomach and bowels. The principal carminatives are the following:

Aniseed, caraway seed, cardamon seeds, cloves, sweet fennel, ginger, peppermint, thyme and parsley. DOSE: One half teaspoonful of the ground herb in one cup of distilled water. Drink it very hot whenever you are distressed with gas in the stomach or intestines.

If suffering with colic pains due to distension of the intestinal walls, caused by gas, you may do as follows: DOSE: Mix one half teaspoonful of ground aniseed, one half teaspoonful of ground peppermint and one half teaspoonful of ground fennel seed. Now put in one pint of water and let it boil for five minutes. Take one cup of this decoction very hot. If the pain does not disappear within half an hour drink another cup of tea. Unless the pain is due to a very serious obstruction, it will be relieved within ten to thirty minutes. It very seldom fails.

DEMULENTS

These are very important substances which have the property of soothing and relieving an inflamed mucus membrane; also for protecting it against irritation. These herbs are very useful in cases of irritation of the mucus membrane lining, the respiratory, digestive and genitourinary tracts. The following herbs are the best:

Licorice root, slippery elm bark, fenugreek, mellow leaves, coltsfoot leaves, flaxseed, marshmallow root and comfrey plant. DOSE: One teaspoonful to every cup of water, sweetened with honey and taken hot. Abstain from food for one or two days, cleanse the bowels and drink one cup of tea every two hours. The irritation will disappear very soon if these rules are followed.

DEPURATIVES

These are substances that dissolve and eliminate toxic matter from the blood.

Some of the very valuable herbs of this group are the following:

Sarsaparilla root, buckthorn bark, linden flowers, marsh rosemary root, dandelion root, figworth herb and burdock root. DOSE: One half teaspoonful of ground herbs in one cup of distilled water. Take it hot or cold one hour before meals, three times a day.

DIURETICS

These are substances which, when taken internally, increase the flow of urine. They are indicated in cases of dropsy and in disorders of the kidneys due to excessive irritation. The following herbs are the principal ones of this group:

Shave grass, juniper berries, dandelion, parsley, strawberry, sarsaparilla, horsetail, broom herb, golden rod herb, whortleberry leaves, borage, asparagus, parsley, horsetail and honeysuckle, watermelon juice. DOSE: One half teaspoonful of the ground herb to each cup of water, sweeten with honey and drink hot twice or three times daily, thirty minutes before meals.

EMETICS

These are substances that cause vomiting. It goes without saying that these medicines which cause vomiting should be used only on very rare occasions after having eaten some poisoned food or after having eaten beyond the power of digestion in order to prevent serious indigestion and distress, also when there is obstruction in the intestinal canal and defecation cannot take place.

Under these conditions it is necessary to resort to the lesser of two evils, that is to force vomiting of the fermenting and putrefying mass of food, or the poison taken, thus producing quick relief and perhaps save the life of that person. The best known emetics are the following:

LOBELIA. This is one of the best emetics. In small doses it acts as an expectorant. In doses of six to eight grains it acts as a vomitive.

DOSE: Take 8 to 20 grains of the powdered leaves dissolved in one cup of warm water.

MUSTARD. The black seed is the one that should be used and not the yellow seed mustard.

DOSE: Take from 50 to 100 grains of the ground seed dissolved in one cup of warm water.

In case you do not have these emetics on hand you can use common salt to produce vomiting. Dissolve half a teaspoonful of salt in a pint of warm water and drink it, not hot, but just warm.

EMMENAGOGUES

These substances promote and stimulate menstruation. They are indicated when the menstrual flow is very deficient. However, provided that the state of health is good, there is no reason to worry about scanty menstrual flow or even about no flow at all, because healthy women who live a natural life and eat natural food do not menstruate, or if they do, it is very little. However, if the menstrual flow is scanty and accompanied by pains it is advisable to take a tea of the following herbs:

Misletoe herb, pennyroyal, bloodroot, and rue.

DOSE: From 30 to 50 grains (one half teaspoonful) of the ground herbs in one cup of hot water. Abstain from meat, fish, eggs and denatured cereal products, and let your diet consist of fruits, nuts and vegetables.

EMOLIENTS

This name is given to those substances which have the property to soothe irritation and soften the tissues. These should be taken in the form of teas to allay internal irritation and in the form of poultices applied to sores, boils, suppurating wounds, and to promote healing. Use the following herbs in the form of teas when there is irritation and catarrh of the mucus membrane lining of the air passages, the intestinal tract and the genitourinary organs:

Mallow, marshmallow, flaxseed, prickly thistle, onions, borage, comfrey, licorice and fig juice, raisin juice and prune juice, (meaning the juice of these sweet fruits which have been soaking for ten or twelve hours).

If affected with boils, sores or other external growths, apply to the affected part a poultice made of ground flaxseed, fenugreek or a finely grated raw potato. Any of the above mentioned herbs is very beneficial to soften growths or to allay irritation when applied as a poultice.

EXPECTORANTS

These are herbs which cause the expulsion or expectoration of mucus and phlegm from the mucus membrane lining of the throat, bronchial tubes and lungs. They should be taken when there is acute or chronic catarrh of the mucus membrane of these organs. The following are some of the herbs which produce this effect:

Coltsfoot herb, liverwort, horehound, marshmallow leaves, fenugreek seed, asthma weed, flaxseed, aniseed, older roots, elecampane root and wild sage leaves.

DOSE: One teaspoonful of the ground herbs (or whole seed) in one cup of hot water. Take one hour before meals or three hours after meals, three times a day. Fast one day and then go on an eliminating diet.

HEPATICS

These are those remedies that promote the action of the liver and increase the flow of bile. The following herbs belong to this group:

Rhubarb root, dandelion root, liverwort and barberry bark.

DOSE: One half teaspoonful of the ground herbs in one cup of distilled water three times a day, one hour before or three hours after meals.

These herbs are useful in cases of jaundice and other liver disorders.

NERVINES

These medicines allay, soothe and calm irritated nerves. The following herbs belong to this group.

Nerve root, crampbark, rosemary leaves, rueherb, and valerian root.

DOSE: One half teaspoon of the ground herbs, root or bark in one cup of hot water. Take when irritated or nervous.

NEPHRITICS

These are remedies which are useful in affections of the kidneys. The following herbs belong to this group:

Whortleberry leaves, uva ursi leaves, juniper berries, buchu leaves, and gravel plant leaves. (Juice: watermelon, wheatgrass.)

DOSE: One teaspoonful of the ground herb in one cup of hot water. Take it two times a day one hour before meals. Abstain from uric acid foods as listed above.

STIMULANTS

The following herbs produce a natural stimulation due to the fact that their valuable salts and vitamins are quickly and easily absorbed into the blood stream thus giving strength and vigor to all the vital functions of the organism:

Dong quai, gotu-kola, Fo-ti-tieng, ginseng, sarsaparilla root, strawberry leaves, linden flowers, rosemary leaves, wild cherry bark, yellow dock root, pepermint and spearmint. Dose: one teaspoonful of the ground herb to one cup of water. Drink three or four times a day.

SUDORIFICS AND DIAPHORETICS

These are substances that produce perspiration. The only difference between these two is that diaphoretics produce a slight perspiration, while sudorifics produce a more powerful perspiration, laying drops on the surface of the skin.

This class of herbs is very useful in promoting elimination through the pores of the skin and in relieving internal congestion. Teas from these herbs should be taken often, especially preceding, during and after the hot sweat baths..

LAXATIVES

The following laxatives are non-irritating substances which produce a natural bowel movement.

Figs, raisins, prunes, flaxseed (ground), psyllium seed (ground), juice: 6 oz. carrot, 1 oz. beet, 6 oz. spinach, or wheatgrass, lactobacillus culture, cherry. A few herbs can produce a mild evacuation of the contents of the intestines. These are:

Chinese rhubarb root (5 to 10 grains), cascara bark, 10 to 20 grains.

It is always better to depend upon the enema, in cases of constipation, than to depend upon laxatives, purgatives and cathartics, even if the cathartics come from the vegetable kingdom.

In conclusion, I want you to remember the following facts: (1). Do not expect that herbs, however beneficial they be, are going to cure you of a chronic diseased condition. Their virtue consists in conveying to the body in a more concentrated form, those elements which are deficient or absent in our diet. They also supply the blood with substances which dissolve or neutralize toxic matter and render it easier for elimination. (2). Never depend upon medicinal herbs alone. They can be considered as an addition to and not as a substitute for the other health measures such as diet. They are the compliment of a defective diet, supplying the mineral salts and vitamins which are deficient in our ordinary foods. Hence, herbs should be considered as foods and not as medicines.

(3). Do not commit the mistake of thinking that if a cup of herb tea is good, two or more cups will be better and hasten the process of healing. An overdose will perhaps produce the contrary effect and retard the curative process.

(4) Live herbs are best for healing. The dew of grasses or plants may be used also. Run your palms over the grass; rub the dew on your body and face. Roll in the dew or collect the dew in cotton cloth during the early hours of morning. Squeeze out the essence. Apply it externally. Collect healing herbs, extract the juice and mix it with two parts grass juice. The herb juice will provide the specific stimulating vibrations for healing the chosen area or system of the body; whereas, the grass will supply the complete nutrition to build, rejuvenate new cells and insure the heaing to be long lasting. The grass vibrations seem to tame some of the undesirable side effects of some of the wild plants when taken inappropriately or in too large of a quantity (see p. 57)

CAUSE OF DISEASE

"Today germs are not our principal enemy. Our chief medical adversary is what I consider a disturbance of the inner balance of the constituents of our tissues, which are built from and maintained by necessary chemicals in the air we breath, the water we drink and the food we eat."
DR. TOM D. SPIES, late Professor of University Medical School, J.A.M.A. June 7, 1958

"Every so-called DISEASE is a crisis of Toxemia; which means that toxins have accumulated in the blood above the toleration point, and the crisis — the so-called disease — is a vicarious elimination. A cold is driven into chronic catarrh, flu may be forced to take on an infected state; pneumonia may end fatally if secretions are checked by drugs."
J.H. TILDEN, M.D., Toxemia Explained

Over-eating and anxiety are the most popular forms of suicide. Toxemia and enervation are the underlying causes of all disease whether acute or chronic. Toxins in the body originate from wrong choice of food, worn-out body cells, drugs, unloving thoughts, polluted air and water. Enervation comes from overactivity, noise, radiation, extreme climate, overeating, sexual excesses, vaccination, toxins, stress or rapid detoxification.

In most degenerative disorders, the body is enzyme-exhausted and nutritionally deficient. Lack of enzymes leads to incomplete metabolism. The undigested food must be eliminated as toxins. Waste accumulates from infancy because of toxemia and enervation, eventually, to a level which may interfere with the functioning of the body.

How long it takes to become sick depends upon the constitution inherited from the parents and how much toxemia and enervation one's lifestyle generates. The stronger the inherent constitution and the more one adheres to the health rules, the longer it takes to pollute the body. The weaker the inherent constitution and the more abuse the body receives, the less time will it take to become sick.

To be "healthy, happy and holy" is a total commitment to a natural lifestyle in a natural environment. Unless one obeys all the health rules (See Appendix) one will eventually become sick.

ACUTE ILLNESS,   (colds, mumps, measles, open sores, typhoid, flu . . .) is an attempt of the body to remove accumulated toxins by increased elimination through the skin, lungs, nose, eyes, ears, colon, kidney. If there is sufficient vitality and the eliminative process is not hindered by food or drugs, the body is capable of restoring itself to good health.

Germs do not cause disease. We have at all times in our body germs of typhoid, tuberculosis and diphtheria. The rapid increase of bacteria during illness is the result of excessive mucus-inducing, incompletely metabolized food which provide the germs with a perfect diet. Also, the congested bloodstream inhibits passage of phagocytes; hence, germs multiply. New germs can be formed every 12 minutes. In 24 hours, several trillion can be created from one germ. Germs secrete many toxins.

Pasteur, in the end, conceded: "Bernard was right: the microbe is nothing; the terrain is everything." The terrain is the body. The germs multiply very rapidly when the body is congested and polluted.

CHRONIC AILMENTS   result from repeated suppression of acute cleansing crises. As long as the body is able to eliminate toxins through acute illness, there will be no chronic disease. However, if there is no change in lifestyle, inherent vitality can diminish to the point where an acute, eliminative illness will not occur.

Waste continues to build up in the colon, joints and organs with associated discomfort and offensive odors (see Fasting). A microscopic examination of an unhealthy body reveals uric acid and calcification in many of the cells; accumulation of fatty non-reproductive cells; adherence of excess mucus to the mucous membrane, precipitation of acid crystals into the muscles; degeneration of elastin in connective tissues into collagen which stiffens the body; formation of tumors from cross-linkage of incompletely metabolized protein with free radical molecule (acid salts, insecticides, heavy minerals) and nucleic acids.

When the accumulation becomes extensive enough, an examination will reveal it. The diagnosis will be leukemia, cancer, arthritis, asthma, heart disorder, arteriosclerosis, Bright's disease, rheumatism. The name given to the disease is determined by the quantity and nature of stored toxins, as well as the location of the congestion.

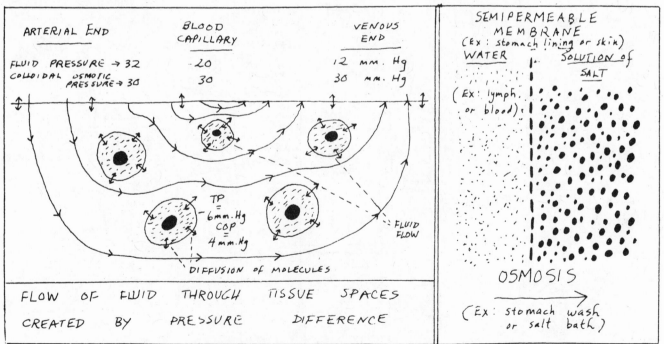

OSMOSIS AND THE ECOLOGY OF DISEASE

Everything in the universe is in a state of dynamic equilibrium which is pulsating with the cosmic rhythm of growth and decay. The same principles operate in astrophysics, microchemistry and cellular biology. The mechanics of cleansing, toxemia and food assimilation are best observed at the cellular level.

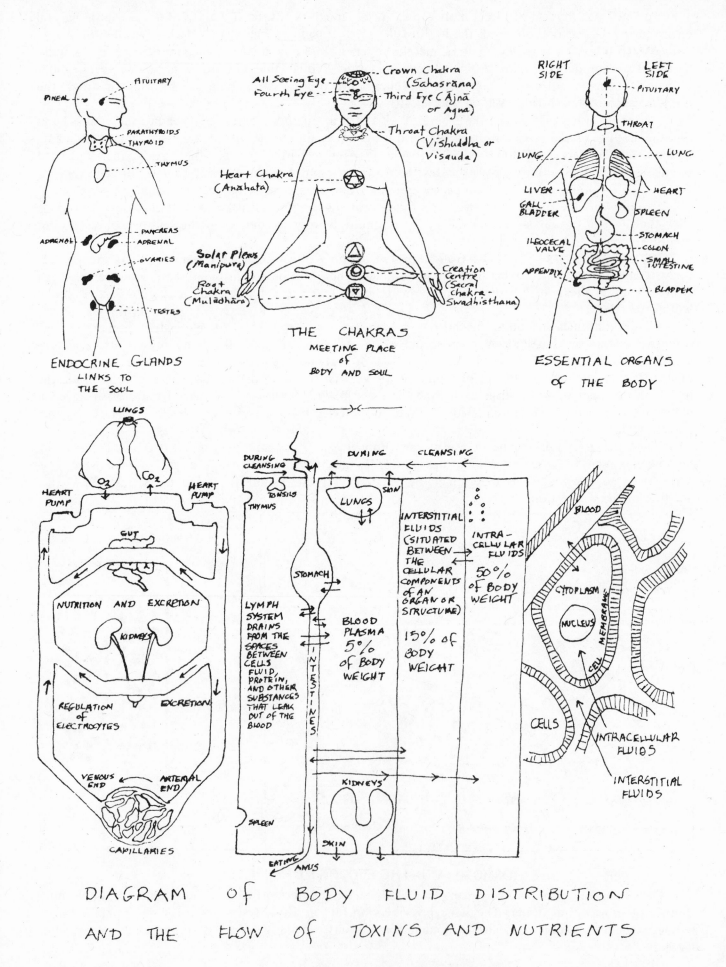

ENDOCRINE GLANDS
LINKS TO
THE SOUL

THE CHAKRAS
MEETING PLACE
of
BODY AND SOUL

ESSENTIAL ORGANS
of THE BODY

DIAGRAM of BODY FLUID DISTRIBUTION
AND THE FLOW of TOXINS AND NUTRIENTS

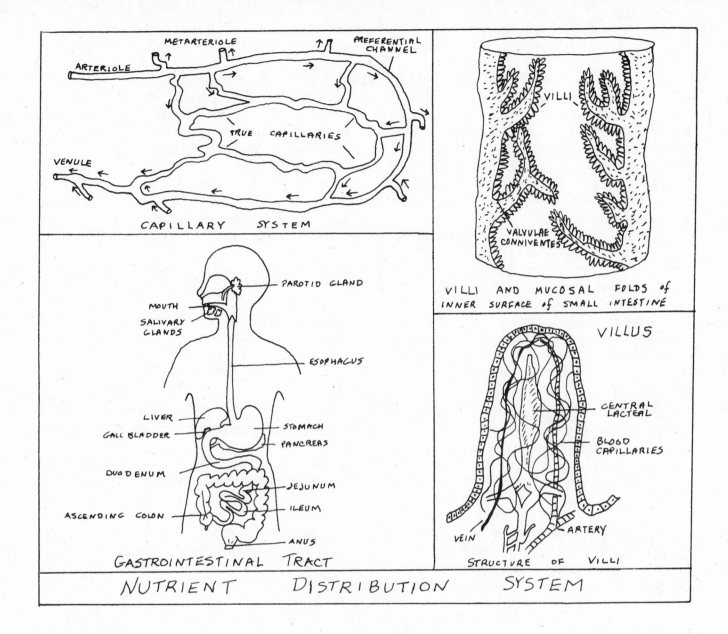

NUTRIENT   DISTRIBUTION   SYSTEM

In any living organism, osmosis, diffusion and filtration are responsible for the transfer of substances in the body to maintain the dynamic equilibrium of life. Factors influencing the movement of substances across the cell membrane are size of molecules, solubility, electrical charge, viscosity of the blood and degree of mucus congestion of the cell wall.

If two solutions (content of digestive tract and blood or lymph system) of different concentrations are separated by a semi-permeable membrane (cell wall) which will pass both water and the dissolved substances, the solute (toxins and nutrients) will pass from the side of higher concentration into the solution of lower concentration, while the solvent (water) will pass in the opposite direction until the solutions have established a dynamic equilibrium.

After a meal, nutrients and toxins flow from the intestinal tract into the blood and lymph system. Through the action of osmotic pressure, the nutrients and toxins next pass into the interior of the cell, the cytoplasm.

All cells have a common feature. The cytoplasm has an alkaline reaction (negative) and the cell nucleus has an acid reaction (positive). This creates an elctro-voltage potential between the cytoplasm and the nucleus. The potential determines the vitality of the cell. If the potential is reduced low enough, death takes place. In the bloodstream most toxins have an acid reaction, which eventually neutralizes the alkalinity of the cytoplasm.

If the concentration of the toxins in the bloodstream is higher than in the cells, toxins will continue to flow into the cytoplasm. Eventually the toxins precipitate as crystals. Periodically, during periods of heightened vitality, the body tries to correct this condition through acute healing crises (disease). After many years, failure to improve one's habits will result in chronic disease (retention of toxins).

During therapy, diet change and fasting the intake of toxins into the digestive tract is reduced to a minimum, hence, also, in the blood and lymph system. In a sick body, the concentration of toxins in the cells is much higher than in the blood or lymph. Because of osmotic pressure, the toxins flow from a concentrated area to one that is less concentrated; that is, they are absorbed into the lymph, bloodstream and digestive tract. Then the toxins are filtered out by kidney, liver, lungs and lymph nodes and are eliminated by way of lungs, skin, kidney and colon (see diagram).

The rate of cleansing will be slowed if the toxins have already crystalized or formed cross-linkages with cell molecules. Enzyme-rich juices from immature greens (such as grasses) and alkaline fluids help to speed the cleansing.

To provide optimum energy for detoxification without additional strain on the eliminative organs, all physical activity should be reduced to a minimum.

The best doctors are those patronized by animals in nature. This team of doctors is available to you: sunshine, pure air, live food, exercise, relaxation, good posture, continence, fasting, God-consciousness, happy heart and loving thoughts.

There are many natural therapies that employ these doctors. They all include some form of dietary restriction. The less food and fluid taken, the more severe the cleansing reactions. Each person, from knowledge of his or her vitality level, should determine the best therapy (see Fasting). Introduce gradual changes. No matter what one's level of vitality, one can always benefit from juice therapy. Any improvement in diet will lead to improvement in health.

Body vitality can be increased through dietary restrictions and natural living. It will give you the strength to follow even more rigorous cleansing programs. Each new stage of purity will increase your strength, youthfulness and joy in living.

Following is a list of diets in ascending order of speed and effectiveness of detoxification and severity of cleansing reactions: diet restriction and nutrient supplements, kosher, macrobiotic, vegetarian, live food, mono diet of raw vegetables, mono diet of fruit, live vegetable juices, wheatgrass juice therapy, fruit juices, water fast and dry fast.

Eventually, whatever diet or therapy you choose, the cells will attain a state of dynamic equilibrium. There will be no more cleansing reactions. If one maintains this equilibrium, the diet is referred to as balanced. It takes some individuals years to reach this stage. In the long run, the juicier the diet, the less food you eat, the cleaner your body will be and the stronger you will feel. You should anticipate periods of weakness until the cleansing is complete. In yoga philosophy, it is said if you become completely pure and strong enough, you can live on fruit, then fluid and finally on solar radiation.

How soon you regenerate your body and regain health and vitality depends on your inherent constitution, karma, nature and quantity of toxins deposited in the cells. Operations, drug therapy and radiation treatments limit your regeneration. The programs suggested will prevent further development of chronic disease and, in most cases, will reverse chronic ailments and improve health.

For a more extensive study of how the human organism uses the eliminative organs, respiratory system, ductless glands, nerve networks, digestion, muscles, liver, blood and lymph to give maximum purity to each cell under toxic conditions due to diet and polluted environment, read books on human anatomy, physiology and metabolism.

Highly recommended: TOXEMIA (Tilden), THE BIBLE, FUNCTION OF THE HUMAN BODY (Guytom), FOOD IS YOUR BEST MEDICINE (Bieler)

CRISIS

"All cures start from within out and from the head down, and in reverse order as the symptoms have appeared."
HERRING'S LAW OF CURE

Crisis is a turning point in a disease. There are two kinds. One is forced upon the apparently healthy body by the accumulation of foreign matter beyond the current toleration point. For example, eating more than usual of mucus-inducing foods will generally result in the cleansing process of a "cold" within three days. Another type of crisis develops when, due to hygienic living, vitality increases sufficiently to discharge, partially or totally, stored toxins which cause chronic disease.

All chronic disorders must be brought to an acute state and eliminated from the body through the mechanics of crisis. Every part of your being participates. It is the cooperative effort of the physical, mental and spiritual faculties.

Every eliminative process (healing crisis) which has been suppressed in the past through the use of food, drugs or overwork will have to be relived. Generally, after adopting a cleansing regime, a child reaches a crisis in three to fourteen days. In adults it can take up to three months. You will know when it is near because you will feel wonderful. When dark or black holes in the iris start becoming very white, the crisis is near (see Iridology). Occasionally, temporary lines or swelling of facial features, especially of the lower lip, may appear (see Physiognamy). Zone therapy meridians become sensitive, especially those related to eliminative organs.

Crisis can take the form of open sores which continuously discharge pus of poisoned blood, boils, excessive menstrual discharge, fever in the form of flu, itching (which may persist for months), diarrhea (a beautiful 85 year old lady had it for 6 weeks), coughing, frequent urination, vomiting, extreme exhaustion and symptoms of past ailments. Elimination through eyes or ears can cause the organs to stop functioning for several days.

Emotional purification is part of the general detoxification. Relived hatred, old stress and anxiety will come to the surface. You will have to confront the psychic reasons for your ill health. You will discover why you are addicted to food and why you desire to be sick. Allow yourself to cry, scream, hit objects (not people) to let off steam. Keep a daily diary of your psychic rebirth. You will see increase of lovingness toward others as you become more forgiving and loving toward yourself. Memory will improve — you will have less to hide and to repress. Daily, increase your consciousness through practice of faith, hope, generosity, charity, love, aspiration, patience, sympathy, non-interference, kindness, courage and duty.

A healing crisis usually lasts 3 days. It will come and go as often as necessary until all poisons are removed from the body, provided there is enough vitality to eliminate these poisons.

During the crisis, it could be reassuring to be under the care of a doctor or a friend who is versed in the laws of nature.

The following suggestions will be helpful:

1. Don't eat until fever, pain or inflammation has subsided. If symptoms last longer than 5 days, grass juice implants may be administered. Use Rejuvilac when available.
2. If thirsty, allow as much cold or warm lemonade as desired. If urine is thick and viscous drink water even when not thirsty.
3. Keep warm. Use more covers. Keep windows open for continuous fresh air. Have a tray of wheatgrass next to the bed.
4. If possible, flood the whole body or area causing discomfort with the appropriate color (see Color Therapy).
5. Keep record of temperature. If it goes over 103, rub down body with cold wet towel only until fever reduces to 101-102; it is undesirable to suppress fever. After the fever abates, a warm bath should be taken to wash away released toxins.
6. Do zone therapy to keep vitality high.
7. When the toxic waste, which has caused this acute disease (crisis), has been eliminated, fever disappears and hunger returns; begin drinking dilute citrus juice for the first two days. If digestion is good,   you may include pulp with the orange juice.
8. Daily enemas during crisis are suggested. If after three to seven days the bowels have not moved, take a small olive oil enema with a hand bulb syringe. It will prevent laceration in the rectal wall when hard fecal matter is expelled.
9. When you have an opportunity, stay in unpolluted air; take short sun baths.
10. Following a crisis, take an eliminative diet consisting of acid fruit; green juicy raw vegetables; indoor greens.
11. Rest will ensure quick recovery with milder symptoms. You may need to stay in bed 12 to 22 hours daily.
12. **If headaches present, do stomach washes first. Do zone therapy on acupressure points related to stomach, liver and kidney.**

WARNING: Use the detoxification regime with caution if you are highly toxic and/or if your nervous system, liver, kidneys, lungs or other organs are in a weakened state.

You can easily give youself a quick examination with the aid of physiognamy and iridology — it will reveal the state of the internal organs. The level of toxicity will be indicated by the markings around the border of the iris (the lymphatic system). The star shaped or circular colored ring around the border of the pupil will reveal the state of the digestive tract and nervous system.

Too rapid detoxification can bring about dramatic loss of calcium from teeth and bones which could take years, if ever, to replace. The eliminative organs can be so overworked that a year of rest may be required to regenerate them.

If you are very toxic and go on a total cleansing regime of juices and/or a low protein diet of fruit, sprouts, and vegetables for longer than three days, you should permit yourself time for unlimited bed rest and several enemas daily.

If you are unable to rest, you should follow a program of slower cleansing. During the day, take about two quarts of fluid (rejuvelac, watermelon and vegetable juices) plus several ounces of juice from indoor greens and sprouts. Daily take one, but no more than one, three ounce portion of seed or seed ferment. Blend all your sprouts and vegetables — Mix no more than three types. Quite often during the day it is good to chew on the indoor greens and spit out the pulp.

The process of recovery can be uncomfortable, but it leads to the health and happiness which come with the joy of well being. You will become more childlike in mind and body, recover a sense of innocence and zest for living. You will know detoxification is complete when you discover that urine and sweat have the fragrance and taste of the fruit just eaten. Your eyes will be clear.

HOW TO KEEP YOUR TEETH PAINLESSLY

Dr. Francis Pottenger, Jr. (73) performed a ten year study involving 900 cats, which demonstrates the effect of cooked food on teeth and bones. A cooked protein diet began to effect an unhealthy condition in the mouth within three to six months. Pregnant cats showed these changes more quickly. "The permanent teeth are, in general, more irregular in size and alignment than the deciduous teeth. Gingivitis persists, gums become spongy, and abscesses gradually develop. It is through this process of secondary infection that most cats on a cooked meat diet lose their teeth."

More than sixty percent of Americans wear dentures, and most children wear braces on their teeth as a consequence of our cooked protein and processed carbohydrate diet.

Tooth decay is the result of overacidity from eating grains, sugar, honey, dried fruit, seed, animal products, cooked and processed food.

When starting on a vegetarian diet, there were many small cavities in my teeth which needed the attention of a dentist. The gums were continuously sore, occasionally bleeding. Some of the teeth were so loose that I could easily move them about. After a year on a vegetarian regime, all these problems vanished. Some of the the exposed nerves were covered with a solid mineral layer, all pain ceased and I could eat acid fruit without discomfort.

A dentist found my teeth to be in excellent shape, in spite of the fact that I brush them only a few times a year, usually when fasting. He said that new cavities were impossible, since my saliva was alkaline.

I resumed eating dried fruit, honey and processed foods; all former problems returned in a few weeks.

Fillings have fallen from two huge cavities. I'm waiting for fillings to drop out of three other teeth. Metals used in fillings are conductors, and can set up a high voltage, through coupling (you can test this with an E-meter or voltage meter). This has been shown to be a factor in mental disorders.

Furthermore, dissolved metal from fillings is circulated in the bloodstream, acting as an irritant, inhibiting the action of vitamins and enzymes. (Read: Super Health From Super Foods, Dr. Bernard).

Fillings can be made from non-toxic porcelain or quartz.

To relieve toothache:

a) Remove food particles with a toothbrush and alkaline paste or sea salt. Use a toothpick daily to clean out the cavities. Never use commercial supermarket toothpaste. It will destroy your gums.

b) For quick relief from toothache: rinse the mouth every ten minutes with sea water or grass juice, apply zone therapy to the knuckles of fingers and toes in the same zone as the aching tooth.

c) Correct the overacid condition of the body: abstain from all food and fluid for one day, especially when toothache is triggered by indigestion. Use several enemas during the day. Follow with a program of alkaline juices, sprouts, sesame seed and sea vegetables. This regime can correct an overacid condition within a few days and in time may reverse decay.

d) I overcame the most extreme pain resulting from overacid body condition and chipped tooth by chewing on grass. The toothache subsided and disappeared in five minutes. Prior to that, I had tried acupuncture, zone therapy, salt mouth wash and enemas without any relief. Over the years I have discovered grass (any kind) is excellent for the relief of all painful problems. Chew the grass, then apply it as poultice on insect bites, lacerations, injuries and blows to the body. The immersion of crushed finger immediately after injury into grass juice for 20 minutes prevented the appearence of pain or black and blue marks. 24 hours later, at the start of pain, I immersed my finger for another 20 minutes into grass juice. Pain was relieved never to return.

Dental decay may be a reversible process in which developing cavities are actually chemically repaired, according to Dr. Stephen Wei of Iowa's College of Dentistry.

He subjected freshly extracted teeth to a weak acid for forty hours to demineralize and soften the outer enamel. He then immersed the teeth in a specially prepared solution for five days.

Cavities in their early stages were almost completely remineralized. Calcium and phosphorus were almost completely recovered in the remineralized enamel, and the end product closely resembled that of normal enamel in chemical composition. The microhardness of the enamel was also partially restored.

It is possible to achieve this result with diet. In my own case, after one year on an alkalinizing diet — indoor greens, sesame seed and vegetable juices — soft enamel was restored to hardness.

Dentists studying the primitive Yanomami Indians in Brazil discovered that they have incredibly healthy gums. Dr. Cleber Pereira, head of the expedition, concludes it is because the Indians don't use toothbrushes, depending instead on the cleansing action of the hard fruits and roots they eat.

Newspapers have reported cases of people who, because of a simple natural diet, have grown several new sets of teeth, after the age of fity, seventy and one hundred: "In Arabia, Dr. Weber noticed an old woman who ate but once a day and then consumed only a few dates. She was a strong woman and Weber thought she was about 40. He was extremely surprised to learn she was 198, despite her miserable diet. She told him that when she was 156 her teeth were renewed for the third time, and all her symptoms of rejuvenation always appeared after a prolonged fast. . . . In 'Believe It or Not' Ripley states that Numas DeCugna of Bengal, India lived to be 370 years old. He grew four new sets of teeth, and his hair turned from black to gray four times. He died in 1566." (Man's Higher Consciousness, Hotema).

REGENERATION OF THE EYES

The eyes are a sensitive barometer of the general health. Indigestion makes the eye painful, especially when slight pressure is applied to the eyeball. Damage done to the internal structure of the body is vividly displayed in the iris. Eyes cannot be healed until the internal organs have been rejuvenated.

The biggest culprit in destruction of the eye is pasteurized dairy products (other mucus-inducing foods also play a role) plus lack of sunshine, smog, salt, and a nutritionally inadequate diet. Encrustation on the eyelashes in the morning is a tell-tale sign of the use of the eyes as an eliminative organ during the night's fast. These excretions can accumulate and eventually harden on the lens to create a cataract. The eyes can be rejuvenated if you make dietary changes, do eye excerises, zone therapy and discontinue the use of eyeglasses. Rejuvenation will take at least four months.

Eye Exercise: To strengthen the eye muscles, do these exercises daily. Follow an imaginary diagonal line without moving your head as far as you can stretch those eye muscles. Do this five times and repeat in the other direction. Do likewise with a horizontal and vertical line. Rotate the eye in a wide circle, clockwise five times, then counterclockwise five times. After each set of five, blink rapidly several times, squeeze the eyes tight shut, then completely relax them. Do not overstrain. Gradually increase each exercise up to fifteen times.

Eyewash: Use wheatgrass juice in the eye cup. Be sure to strain the juice to remove sediments.

Eye Energizer: Apply zone therapy on the feet and hands in areas related to the eyes to break up crystallizations. This will increase nutrient supply to and waste elimination   from the eyes.

Mental Exercise: Close the eyes and send energy to them by imagining a red color bathing them. The best time to practice this is during a headstand or shoulderstand or on a slant board while doing deep breathing exercises.

Morning Greetings: Look at the rising sun, briefly, only when it is just appearing red on the horizon. Ask for good eyesight. Think of good reasons why you need it. Also sun your eyes in the daytime, looking into the sun with closed eyes — you will see a red color.

Sun Bathing: Spend as much time as possible in the sun, sand, water, grass. Walk barefoot, wearing as few clothes as the law requires. Use eye glasses only when absolutely necessary. They filter out some essential rays needed for complete health.

WHEN SOMEBODY FAILS TRY GRASS

People often seek the path of natural healing when all else has failed to heal them of arthritis, diabetes, cancer and other symptoms of degeneration. Though we do not treat or "cure" a "disease" once advanced sysmptoms of toxicity manifest, we may adapt our basic healing techniques to relief of these symptoms.

DAIRY PRODUCTS AND ARTHRITIS

Arthritis is diagnosed at an advanced phase of general deterioration of health. The most visible symptoms are stiffening and/or inflammation of body tissues, especially in joints and tendons.

In 1972, Prof. Nanna Svartz, head of the King Gustav V research Institute in Stockholm, (203) reported that, after thirty years of study, she and her team identified the cause of rheumatoid arthritis as a germ found in milk.

"Tests conducted on people suffering from rheumatoid arthritis have revealed the presence of milk bacteria in eighty percent of cases." She declared the germ was found in pasteurized milk from America, Canada and six European countries.

Though correlation of milk and arthritis is conclusive, the germ is not the causative factor. The germ exists there only because of appropriate mucus from a dead food diet to feed it.

Dr. Francis Pottenger Jr. (73) made a study implicating cooked food and milk in the development of arthritis. "The male cats fed on metabolozied Vitamin D. milk (from cattle fed irradiated yeast) and raw meat showed osseous disturbance very like those on pasteurized milk. Young males did not live beyond the second month and adult males died within ten months. The most noticeable fact was that there is a tendency for the calcium phosphorus ratio to become unbalanced, approaching 2.5 to 1 as compared with normal of 2 to 1 . . . The cats fed pasteurized milk as their principal item of diet, and raw meat as a partial diet, showed lessened reproductive efficiency and some skeletal changes. Cats fed evaporated milk showed even more damage. The most marked deficiency occurred in the cats fed sweetened condensed milk." No such problems occurred with cats on a raw food diet.

The underlying cause of arthritis may be overacidity of the body due to toxemia or to long periods of stress. Overacidity causes dissolution of bone calcium. This calcium plus ingested inorganic minerals are carried by the bloodstream and deposited in areas of poor circulation.

Mucus from processed bakery and pasteurized dairy products (wheat gluten and milk casein are used to manufacture some of the most potent water-resistant glue) deposits in tissues, clogs the blood vessels and deposits on vessel walls, decreasing the velocity of the blood.

Cooking or heating converts organic materials in plants into inorganic minerals. Since inorganic minerals are highly insoluble, they enter the bloodstream in unassimilable form and tend to deposit out in areas of slow blood velocity (highly congested tissues).

Organic sodium has the property of increasing the solubility of inorganic calcuim. Some of the best sources of organic sodium are lemon, grapefruit, spinach, celery and dandelion. Juice from vegetables may be taken with carrot or wheatgrass juice. Daily one should consume at least one quart of juice. The day may start with a pint of grapefruit juice. Wheatgrass juice will produce quick minimization of pain. Extraneous calcium and other minerals will be filtered out by the kidney and excreted in the urine.

To become and remain free from arthritis, processed foods must be eliminated from the diet. At the initial phase of regeneration, there may be periods of increased pain and stiffness and/or its appearance in new areas due to circulation of an increased amount of minerals released by the dietary regime. Many arthritics have reported freedom from pain after following the live food and juice regime for only a few weeks.

THE SWEET LIFE OF A DIABETIC

Diabetes is due to a deficiency of insulin. Inititally, the shortage is nearly always created by excessive demand due to high intake of processed carbohydrates (sugar and starch) and to a mucus-forming diet which clogs the insulin-secreting glands (islets of Langerhans), thus reducing the volume of insulin entering the bloodstream.

Dr. Douglas Coleman, senior staff scientist at Jackson Mammalian Genetics Research Institute, Bar Harbor, Maine, says, " . . . overeating could be the most important factor in individuals with hereditary predisposition to diabetes . . . The second possible cause is high blood sugar causing abnormal insulin secretion that in turn increases appetite."
(Boston Globe, No. 22, 1973)

The secretion of insulin into the bloodstream is an endocrine function of the pancreas. Insulin controls the rate of transfer of glucose through cellular membrane. In the absence of an adequate supply of insulin, the blood glucose is incompletely metabolized, hence unavailable for energy. To supply energy, the body then rapidly metabolizes fats, causing a highly overacid condition leading to coma.

The impossibility of perfect control of insulin through injections brings on excess of cholesterol deposition, this leads to atherosclerosis. This degeneration of capillaries can cause blindness, deafness and hemorrhaging in the extremities. (Clogging of the internal mucous lining and tubings greatly diminishes the entry of all hormone secretions into body fluids. This impairs general health and contributes to all forms of mental disorders.)

If the islets of Langerhans are intact, diabetes can generally be corrected in two to four weeks. Guided by the test for sugar in the urine, the diabetic gradually reduced insulin intake. Generally after the third day of live food diet, there is a sharp reduction in the need for insulin. Every few days thereafter, there is a need to decrease the amount of insulin by about five units. Some individuals who try to detoxify too rapidly, may develop insulin shock. After calling a hospital emergency ward, an attendant should work on the zone in the feet related to the pancreas . Upon recovery from shock, the indiviudal may resume the dietary regime.

THE TIRED HYPOGLYCEMIC

The civilized countries because of stress and increased consumption of processed foods have been producing a weaker species of human each generation. Dr. Warren Guild of the Harvard Medical School states that 97% of all adult Americans fail to pass the minimum physical fitness test.

The "in" diseases have shown deterioration of every organ. Ulcers were "in," heart disease was "in," lower backaches (kidney disorder) was "in;" now, hypoglycemia is the "in" disorder with status. It is a disease of insatiable hunger. One may have a full stomach and not be satisfied. More and more people are afflicted by hypoglycemia because of the continuous use of processed foods.

Hypoglycemia is a disorder of too little blood sugar, which provides the fuel for all the cells. Various authorities have estimated that anywhere from 10 to 100 million persons in America are suffering from this condition. According to Dr. Harry M. Salzer of the University of Cincinnati College of Medicine in Ohio.   The following symptoms exist for hypoglycemia:

(1) Psychiatric symptoms: depression, insomnia, anxiety, irritability, lack of concentration, crying spells, phobias, forgetfulness, confusion, asocial and anti-social behavior and suicide tendencies. Might be diagnosed as schizophrenia or manic depressive.   (2) Neurological symptoms: headaches, dizziness, trembling, numbness, blurred vision, staggering, fainting or blackouts,   muscular twitching.   (3) Somatic symptoms: exhaustion, fatigue, bloating, abdominal spasm, muscle and joint pains, headaches, muscle cramps,   convulsions.

Since hypoglycemia is a malfunction of the fuel supply, it affects every organ. As the sugar level drops the basic metabolism of every organ is decreased. This is why hypoglycemia can mimic any physiological or neuro-psychiatric disorder.

The most pronounced symptoms of hypoglycemia are hunger of the most insatiable kind, chronic fatigue during the day with uncontrollable yawning and restlessness during the night. These symptoms can be due to indigestion, which is quite common among hypoglycemics, due to frequent eating. This problem can prolong indefinitely the healing of hypoglycemia unless an effort is made to eat slow, small meals, stay away from sweets, chew food thoroughly and follow other of the health rules (see appendix).

The brain is nourished exclusively by glucose and oxygen. A drop in blood sugar reduces concentration bringing about depression, anxiety and irritability.

The sugar level in the bloodstream is monitored by the ductless glands, especially the pituitary (which is a master gland that recognizes body emergencies) and adrenal (which commands the blood sugar level to increase).

The liver increases the availability of the sugar from storage. The heart pumps it to all the cells. The kidney eliminates the waste products and the lungs provide the oxygen for the sugar burning. We can see now why the aging process is greatly speeded up in hypoglycemia, since it produces complications in every organ; the eliminative organs especially become backed up with waste, bringing on chronic diseases.

The physiology of hypoglycemia is most thoroughly investigated by E.M. Abrahamson M.D. He explains the carbohydrate metabolism and how it is related to hypoglycemia and diabetes. Under healthy conditions of digestion, all carbohydrates (starch, sugar) are converted into glucose. During a meal, the increased sugar level causes the Islands of Langerhans to produce insulin. The liver, under the stimulation of insulin, stores glucose as glycogen thus keeping blood sugar to a proper level. After the meal, adrenal cortical hormones monitor the liver on how much sugar to release to satisfy the energy requirements of the body.

In diabetes the liver is unable to remove enough glucose, causing it to overpour into the urine. In hypoglycemia, due to overproduction of insulin, we have the liver converting too much sugar into glycogen resulting in an inadequate sugar supply in the bloodstream. The Islands of Langerhans overproduce the insulin because they have been oversensitized due to stimulating foods, sugar and stress.

Stress can be emotional or physical. Examples are poor diet, infection, pain, overexertion, child bearing, lactation, burns, fractures, business or domestic worries and drugs.

The worst villain in this disease is sugar. On the average an American consumes in a single year over 102 pounds of sugar. Processed starches contribute greatly to the increased blood sugar level. One slice of bread equals about five heaping teaspoons of sugar. Sucrose (commercial cane sugar) is a combination of one molecule of glucose and one of fructose. Very little digestion is needed to break sucrose into glucose. Sucrose produces the high energy rush with associated overstimulation and sensitizing of the Islands of Langerhans.

Too much of this effort to keep the blood glucose level proper will in time exhaust the adrenal glands so that they cannot do their part in bringing the sugar concentration back up to the correct amount. The adrenals are called on to act since the pancreas reacts so fast to the extra glucose load that it secretes excess insulin, thus reducing the blood sugar level too far. Now, weakened adrenals cannot get the blood sugar back up readily and hypoglycemia symptoms result.

Recent research indicates that a common cause of hypoglycemia is adrenal insufficiency. Many infants are born with adrenal glands functioning poorly since the mother has an adrenal problem. She may have had this problem for a long time or may have been under considerable stress during pregnancy or may have eaten a typical American diet high in refined carbohydrates.

Caffein (from coffee, tea, or cola drinks) stimulates the adrenal gland whose hormones induce breakdown of liver glycogen, releasing it as blood sugar which gives you the coffee lift. The increased blood sugar level from coffee's effect on the adrenals is mistaken by the Island of Langerhans as sugar from a meal. The pancreas tries to force the blood sugar to its normal level. Because of this confusion, coffee without sugar gives you a much quicker letdown. Through repeated stimulation, the pancreas becomes oversensitive even to normal food stimulation.

The liver is an important part of our system to maintain proper glucose concentration. It can be damaged in many ways: from excess alcohol, tobacco, smog, infections, toxic substances and meat. Fortunately, if these liver damaging factors are overcome, the regenerating capability of the liver should restore it for the carrying out of its numerous body functions.

Meat and high protein foods indirectly contribute to hypoglycemia. One of the waste products of protein metabolism is uric acid. It is a member of the purine family, just like caffein. Both are stimulants. Both produce the same effect on the body.

Self diagnosis can be done by anyone. The more symptoms of hypoglycemia you have, the more likely you are suffering from this disease. Since it is very likely the liver is affected, one can look for signs of its disorder: yellow color of skin and membranes of the body, accumulation of bile in tissues, little red points on skin with attached fine branching lines, fierce itching, excess fluid in abdomen. Keep a record of symptoms, frequency, what foods and quantity relieve the exhaustion quickly. For those who are medicine oriented, there is the glucose tolerance test to demonstrate the body's ability to handle carbohydrate sugar.

If you feel you have hypoglycemia and follow the suggested diet, it has been observed that within a week or two, the major mental and physiological symptoms disappear. Within a period of several months, you will discover that you can eat less frequently and be more relaxed with the diet without the occurrence of hypoglycemia symptoms again.

The program centers on removing all stimulating foods; this reduces the sensitivity level of the Islands of Langerhans. During the period the diet is planned out in such a way as to prevent the drop in sugar level by having frequent small meals which are low in the quickly absorbed carbohydrates. It is extremely important to eat by the clock.

The high protein diets with fruit and vegetables, although effective in short term results, have undesirable long term effects (see: protein). Instead, it is best to eliminate all foods (sugar, processed starches, alcohol, coffee, high protein meals) which were contributing factors and centralize on diet and lifestyle which will assure both quick recovery and no future complications.

Instead of high protein, the emphasis is on predigested high protein foods which come in the form of amino acids and enzymes, thus eliminating the stimulating effect of uric acid. A similar program is advocated by the Hippocrates Health Institute.

When complete bedrest and supervision is available, I have witnessed some cases of hypoglycemia on a regime of wheatgrass juice and watermelon fast make a complete recovery within a period of 3 to 4 weeks.

For food preparation instructions see index and recipe section of book.

On Arising — Juice from medium ripe orange, half grapefruit or 4 ounces of water with ¼ lemon.

Half hour later — (4-6 oz.) Rejuvelac, papaya-mint or comfrey tea.

Breakfast : Melon, subacid or acid fruit — no more than a pound. Or juice: Carrot (5 oz) with apple (5 oz); carrot (10 oz); carrot (8 oz) with beet (2 oz) and optional spinach (2 oz) or dandelion (½ oz).

1 to 2 hours later: 6 oz of green drink — sprouts, indoor greens, indoor greens and leafy vegetables; and/or wheatgrass juice (1-4 oz) — drink it first.

1 to 2 hours later — sesame sunflower milk (4 oz) or amino acid electrolite broth (12 oz) or seed yogurt & Rejuvelac (8 oz).

Lunch: Indoor greens, sprouts, sea and land vegetables with fermented seed dressing (1-3 oz) or green sauce (4 to 6 oz). Or green sauce meal (6 to 10 oz) or yogurt (3tbs) with rejuvilac (6 oz) .

3 hours later — green drink (4 to 6 oz) or 4 oz sesame sunflower milk or amino acid electrolite broth.

1 to 2 hours later — vegetable juice (6-10 oz) and/or wheatgrass; sprout — indoor greens juice (4 to 6 oz); or amino acid electrolite broth (6-10 oz). Juices are to be at least 30 minutes before dinner whereas broth or seed milk at least 60 minutes before dinner.

Dinner : salad with fermented seed sauce or green sauce.

3 hours after — same as just before dinner.

Every 1 to 2 hours — till bedtime: rejuvelac (4 oz), ½ grapefruit, lemon juice with water (6 oz) or juice from celery and carrot (6 oz).

During the night: lemon with water, piece of grapefruit, comfrey tea, rejuvelac or the amino acid electrolite broth. Choose one item for the night. Take something whenever you wake up. Keep it next to the bed.

All juices should be thoroughly strained with a fine stainless steel strainer or bamboo strainer or cheesecloth. Pulp can be irritating. Drink the juice very slowly; masticate it. Don't eat by appetite — it is not reliable during the early management of hypoglycemia. If you get a headache or other symptoms, take some nourishment, especially the broth and take an enema. Then rest. When traveling or going out, take with you: seed milk, broth, grapefruit and/or apple.

No-Forever Foods

Sugar, flour products, ice cream, dairy products, fried foods, animal protein, coffee, stimulating teas, alcohol, drugs, vinegar.

No-Now Foods

Wheat cereal and all grain products, lentil and chick pea sprouts, honey, molasses, maple syrup, sweet dried fruits, sweet fruit (banana, persimmon, grapes), starchy vegetables.

O.K. Foods

All non-starchy vegetables — raw or slightly steamed; mushroom, sprouts, weeds, indoor greens. Fruit: sub-acid or acid fruit, apple, peach, apricots, berries, melons, avocado (1/6 per serving). Seed or nuts (1 to 3 oz per serving): almonds, sesame, pumpkin, sunflower. Teas: fenugreek, alfalfa, comfrey, mint, papaya. For clearer head, or the occasional need for extra strength, a cup of ginsing or gotu-cola may be used. All sea vegetables are to be used in moderation for seasoning. Foods are o.k. only when properly combined, eaten in small quantity and in a relaxed atmosphere.

CANCER COMES FROM BAD EATING MANNERS

"If I came up with a cure for CANCER tomorrow, half the people at the National Cancer Institute would commit suicide, and the other half would be out chasing me with a machine gun. The jealousy is so great." — A cancer research observer.
"King Cancer" by Philip Nobile, Esquire, 6/1973

"It is possible that, once discovered, the mechanism of carcinogenesis will be shown to be absurdly simple and measures of control will readily follow."
GREENSTEIN

"Those who fal to get treatment for cancer outlive those who go the cut, burn and/or chemical route. (This is accordng to Dr. Hardin B. Jones, a cancer researcher). Dr. Jones claims that those who get treatment live hardly three years. Those who refuse it live an average of 12.5 years. Dr. Jones, a physiologist with the University of California Department of Medical Physics, has been studying cancer for more than 23 years. Cancer victims are dying at the rate of 1,000 a day."

Acres USA, Oct. 3, 1976

Nobel Prize winner, Alexis Carrel, devoted an entire chapter to the adaptive functions, stating that the body seems to mold itself on events, and "instead of wearing out, it changes." He continues: "Our organs always improvise means of meeting every new situation and these means are such that they tend to give us a maximum duration. The physiological process always inclines in the direction leading to the longest survival of the individual " (Man The Unknown).

The human bio-computer has been precircuited by a divine programmer for maximum survival under all unnatural circumstances. When the bloodstream pollutants exceed the filtrating capacity of the liver, kidney, lymph nodes and lungs, the bio-computer sends out signals to the different centers of the body to start removing the filth from the bloodstream and to store it in preselected areas. The stored matter is called cyst, mole, tumor, cataract, arteriosclerosis, arthritis, rheumatism or cancer. The disease is named according to where the garbage is stored, the amount of garbage, the type of garbage and how fast it is being stored. If the body did not store some of this debris, it would exceed the filtrative ability of the essential organs, which would be destroyed.

The areas selected by the organism for storing excess nutrients and waste are places which have been weakened in some way in the past through bruising, high radiation and/or some area of the body where the level of toxicity is high. The organism, in storing the toxins, hopes that a time will come when the quality and quantity of poisons entering the bloodstream will be lowered so that the stored matter can be dissolved back into the bloodstream and eliminated in a gradual manner through the filtrative and eliminative organs.

Basic to a breakdown in protein metabolism is failure of the pancreas to perform its digestive functions. Environmental pollutants, emotional stress, excess intake of protein and processed foods clog the pancreas with waste. Deficiency of pancreatic enzymes ensues. Failure of the pancreas overburdens the liver with wastes of incomplete protein metabolism.

Dr. Blond (40), who viewed cancer as a general response of the whole organism, concludes from statistics that 98% of all victims of cancer of the internal organs succumb not to the cancer but to the liver disorder."

Dr. Max Gerson (45) says, "The function of the liver cells is so vitally important to the body that it could be compared with the activity of the chlorophyll of the plants. The liver is regarded as so unique biologically that recently it was called the 'balance wheel of life . But as pollutants persist, and growths increase, the liver eventually gives out.

Cancer is only one of many survival mechanisms present in a live organism. In time the bloodstream of most humans becomes heavily polluted from an unnatural life style, high protein, high starch diet, excessive eating, rancid oils, processed foods, synthetic food additives, long periods of worry, anxiety and emotional stress, radiation, noise, high power transmission towers (TV, radio), pesticides, air pollution, smoking, medication, chemicals and genetic weaknesses.

Unless there is a breakdown in protein metabolism, cancer will not develop; in the absence of this "triggering" mechanism, which would have started the manufacture of cancerous cells, the body develops other disease symptoms.

The studies relating nutrition and cancer split into two directions. At one extreme, we can find that complex nutrients (especially when processed) — protein, starch and sugar, and fats — in excess, encourage the development and growth of cancer. These nutrients were basically absent from the original diet of the tropical human. As a contrast, certain vitamins, enzymes, amino acids, and minerals reduce the likelihood of the development of cancer, and, when induced, these micronutrients can play an important role in the reversal of the condition of cancer. Such micronutrients are found in the natural food of humans — fruits, sprouts, greens and grasses.

Mr. McCoy believes diet can influence cancer: "Since the neoplasm in the body is dependent upon the host for a supply of amino acids, carbohydrates, fats, minerals and a number of co-factors; it is only reasonable that the critical period of tumor development as well as tumor growth can be influenced by the dietary regime and the nutritional status of the host." (53).

Eating a steak may be more dangerous than smoking. One pound of charcoal broiled steak has as much benzopyrene(cancer stimulating agent), as in the smoke of 300 cigaretts (Science 145:53, 1964). Mice when fed benzopyrene developed leukemia and stomach tumors (Texas Reports on Bio. & Med. 25:553, 1967).

Studies of the dietary habits of cancer patients and surveys of life insurance statistics suggest that individuals who overeat and are overweight when past middle age are more likely to die of cancer than are persons of average weight or less (59, 60).

An overweight condition comes from an excess consumption of protein, starch, sugar, or fat, or from water retention due to toxicity (salt, processed foods, chemicals, drugs) in the diet or the breakdown of the hormone system.

A diet adequate in protein, starch and fat, but low in life elements (vitamins, minerals and enzymes) will cause cancer. Dr. Engel and Copeland (55) put test animals on a low mineral, low-vitamin diet of refined foods containing cancer-causing agents. They developed a 90% incidence of cancer within 22 weeks. Control animals put on a diet of natural foodstuffs, unrefined and unprocessed foods, developed no cancer although they received the same amount of cancer causing agents in the same period of time. Mammary tumors occurred in 90% of the animals on refined foods, liver and ear duct tumors in 60% of the animals.

Drs. Engel and Copeland tell you exactly how to induce cancer in animals. Feed them refined foods. They state: "These results emphasize that semi-purified or purified (refined) diets are preferable to diets of natural foodstuffs for the early and consistent production of mammary and other type tumors in young female rats."

The following study (61) shows conclusively the protective virtue of natural diet and sprouts in the history of cancer. The study has its shortcomings, since very powerful drugs were used to induce cancer. Expressed in the words of Hillemann: "Benzperene may be regarded as a massive and unfair insult which, like a lethal dose of snake venom, can cause even the healthiest and best fed animal to succumb." In the experiment three different diets were involved:

"Total of 120 animals were used and divided into 3 equal groups of 40 each. Group C was placed on a deficient diet of celery and enriched white bread. Group B was given a whole diet of 3 whole grains and greens. Group A received a supplemented diet consisting of greens, sprouted grains, whole flours (rye, wheat, oats, buckwheat, yellow corn, soybean), urea, potassium bicarbonate, bone meal, vitamins A, riboflavin, niacin, inositol, betaine, choline, B-12, C and D with naturally occurring associated factors, iron phytate, iron glycerophosphate, colloidal minerals of sea lettuce (dulse) and alfalfa."

Some of the conclusions drawn from the study were:

"(1) Only 37.5% of the animals on the supplement diet developed tumors as against 58.3% and 57.5% in the whole and deficient groups. Thus, group A had a margin of advantage of 20% over group B or C.

(2) The average life span subsequent to neoplasia (from all groups) was 35 days. The tumorous life span was 30 to 122 days, and 1 to 74 days for groups A, B, and C respectively. The average neoplastic life span was 60, 34 and 33 days for Groups A, B and C respectively. Thus a supplement diet appears to have favored Group A in comparison with Groups B and C between which there was no diference. Group A outlived Group B or C by 56%.

(3) At the termination of the experiment, there were only 7.5%, 5% and 1.25% of the animals left as "healthy" survivors in Groups A, B and C respectively.

Thus a diet of natural foods favored greatly the survival period of the animals.

There are many studies which show the relationship between dietary intake of carbohydrates, fats or protein and the development of cancer.

Tannenbaum (74) showed that restriction of caloric intake resulted in a marked decrease in the incidence of every type of tumor studied in mice.

Malignant tumors, in order to grow, need energy. Carbohydrates as well as fats can provide this energy. Dr. Henderson states: "The energy demands of tumors is great, although they do not compare with those of a tissue such as liver, which has a large number of specialized functions " (75).

Sugar can play an essential role in cancer. Cancerous cells (76) have first choice of glucose. When glucose was administered to a tumor bearing mouse, the level of lactic acid (waste product of sugar metabolism) rose in the tumor, but not in normal tissue.

An acid condition of the body reduces vitality and predisposes one to disease. Glucose acidifies your cells, Kahler and Robertson (130) found that the pH of rat hepatoma dropped after the administration of glucose, while the pH of normal liver tissue did not change. Millet (78) found in tumor tissue a much lower pH than in normal tissue.

Fat tissue is a specialized type of connective tissue that has been modified to allow the storage of neutral fat, making up as much as 95% of the fat cell cytoplasm. Cancerous cells seem to have a great affinity for processed unsaturated fats and cholesterol. One might say that cancer cells act as storage units for the excess fats.

Lipide metabolism of tumor bearing animals is greatly disturbed (158, 165). In brief, the lipide content of cancer victims, which is mainly in neutral fat, decreases as the tumor grows, beginning when it reaches about 10% of the total body weight (169, 171). A very high degree of lipemia is present (172, 229). The composition of tumor fatty acids shows a preponderence of highly unsaturated fatty acids (97). Fatty acids are transported in the form of lipoproteins (99).

Haven and Bloor (184) look at the composition of tumor tissue. In general, tumors contain a greater concentration of phospholipide and cholesterol than do the tissue of origin, with a lower neutral fat content. The several kinds of phospholipides found in most tissue — lecithin, cephalin, sphingomyelin, and plasmologen — are also represented in cancer cells. However, unsaturated fatty acids predominate in tumor phospholipides.

Cancer cells retain the unsaturated fats for long periods of time, unlike the normal tissue (197).

Although dietary wrong choice, or an excess of fat and carbohydrates, can play a major role in cancer, the key to cancer study is protein. The fat and starch can cause blood vessel coatings, bringing about cellular asphixiation which can result in cancer, so can protein. The fat and starch can supply the energy for tumor growth, so can protein. However, fat and starch cannot provide the amino acids needed for cancer growth, only protein can.

The high protein requirement for cancer growth comes, as a rule, from the dietary intake of animal carcass.

Dr. Szepsenwol has shown (204) that the incidence of lymphatic cancer and lung adenocarcinoma is as high in the mice receiving egg white as those receiving egg yolk. "In the animals of both groups the lymphoid system of the abdominal cavity is the first to be effected . . . the adenocarcinomas of the lungs whether caused by egg white or by egg yolk, are very extensive, frequently destroying the whole lungs."

Dr. White in an experiment (205) kept mice on a restricted dietary intake of cystine (a non-essential amino acid found in high concentration in animal protein) such that no body growth was apparent. Within a lifetime of 22 months, no mammary tumors developed. However, the controls which had free access to cystine had an incidence of almost 100% of mammary tumors. Furthermore, the mice on the restricted diet in cystine, when they were treated with stilbestrol (common additive to commercial animal feed), had a tumor incidence of 44%.

Dr. Dunning (206) showed that added dietary tryptophane (an essential amino acid which can be as much as 20 times more concentrated in animal meat than in protein from vegetarian sources) increased the incidence of induced mammary gland and liver cancer and appeared to be a decisive factor in the etiology of bladder cancer.

Dr. Babson (207) observed that on a diet high in casein protein (the major source being the dairy products) some forms of cancer grew five times as fast as other forms. Rous and Sweet (208, 209) observed that wheat gluten, which is low in tryptophan, has been found to retard the growth of several transplanted tumors.

It has been observed that the amino acid content of human leukemia patients increases in whole blood (210) and in plasma (211, 212). Furthermore the general pattern of diet affects leukemia incidence.

Dr. Saxton et al (213) showed, in a study, that normal feeding of a leukemia susceptible strain of mice can produce a 6.5 time higher incidence of leukemia than in mice kept on restricted diet. Furthermore, the length of life of these mice was considerably prolonged by underfeeding.

Dr. Midler et al describes tumors as "traps" for excess nitrogen and/or nitrogen from the body metabolic pool without permitting any appreciable return to the pool.

LePage et al (146) confirmed the nitrogen trap hypothesis. They fasted cancerous rats for ten days. During the next five days of the experiment on animals that were fed, tumor protein increased 345%; whereas in animals that continued to fast the increase was only 160%.

The fasted rats lost 31% in body weight. Further experiment showed that protein metabolism in the tumor was essentially a "one way passage and that protein of the tumor was not available to the host for use during starvation."

Drs. Henderson and LePage (145), in a review of studies related to the nutrition of tumors, show that overnutrition has a definite effect on the development of cancer. "Such growths have a priority on the utilization of dietary components, and when their requirements outgrow this supply, they are able to extract these nutrients from the tissue or the other essential nutrients as well — fatty acids, purines and glucose . . . This may proceed until the neoplasm literally eats itself out of its home."

Dr. Frank C. Madden, F.R.C.S., Professor of Surgery, Egyptian Government School of Medicine, Cairo (214) relates cancer to diet: "I believe that I am right that the consensus of opinion among medical men in Egypt is that cancer — more correctly speaking, carcinoma — is never found in either males or females amongst the black races of that country. These include the Berberines and Sudanese, who are all Mussulmans, and live almost entirely on a vegetarian diet. Cancer is fairly common, however, amongst the Arabs and Copts, who form the bulk of the white population of the native Egyptians, and who, strangely enough, live and eat much like the Europeans." Europeans, like Americans, are noted for their high protein, processed food diet.

In a national television program, doctors linked the consumption of beef with the development of cancer. Dr. Marvin Schneiderman (215) a statistician with the National Cancer Institute, gave details about cancer incidence of different people in the world and pointed out that Utah, where there is a large Mormon population eating whole foods and restricting smoking and drinking, has the lowest rate of cancer in the USA (Daily News, May 7, 1973, p. 25).

Wall Street Journal reported that American diet of "meat, etc. is now linked with cancer of the colon and rectum." (Oct. 25, 1973)

Not everybody who eats meat will develop cancer. It depends also on the body's inherent vitality, type of work, state of mind, choice of meat, amount of meat and other poisons in diet and environment.

Dr. Otto Warburg (216) a Nobel Prize Winner, Director of the Max Planck Institute for Cell Physiology in Berlin, gave an address in 1966 titled "Concerning The Ultimate Cause and Contributing Causes of Cancer." He reduced the problem to a single primary cause, i.e. because of some harmful chemical stimulation, or radiation or a weakness or error in metabolism, a particular tissue becomes starved for oxygen. As little as a 35% reduction in the oxygen available to the cells, causes them, in an effort to stay alive, to make a fundamental metabolic switch. A cancerous tumor may result.

Dr. John Gainer (217) showed that "slight protein increases reduce oxygen transport by as much as 60% even though the amount of protein in the fluid would be considered within the normal range for human blood."

Thus a high protein diet can reduce the oxygen-carrying capacity of the blood, which produces oxygen starvation, leading to mutation and cancer.

If one has studied chemistry, one will recall that every chemical reaction is reversible. A sequence of chemical activities creates cancer or other diseases. Another sequence of reactions can be used to make these diseases disappear.

While medical cancer "cure" remains "just around the corner," considerable progress has been made in dietary management of cancer.

Dr. Albert Lorincz (218), professor of obstetrics and gynecology at the University of Chicago, starved cancer cells into submission by withholding protein elements essential to their development. The demand of cancer cells for protein is 1.3 to 11 times the level necessary for normal tissues. Preliminary animal experiments by other researchers had shown that diets deficient in phenylalanine and lysine (both essential amino acids) would inhibit the growth of liver and breast cancer in mice. Further investigation revealed that a low phenylalanine diet permits mice to maintain weight, hemoglobin level and plasma proteins essential to life, while inhibiting tumor growth. Experimental patients were put on a strict diet with limited supplements of certain fruits, vegetables, cereals, fats and carbohydrates. Only these patients beyond help of orthodox medical treatment were placed on this program. Furthermore, some synthetic foods were used. The diet was not optimal. However, after weeks to months, some of the cancer regressed; many patients were relieved of pain; some patients were able to resume normal activities.

A macrobiotic diet in conjunction with acupuncture and other energy-building techniques has claimed partial success. If the vitality of the sick person is high enough, quite often just adopting organic foods of reduced protein value, discontinuing the use of sugar and coffee and embracing a quieting universal philosophy can provide the body with nutrients and energy to heal itself. But, since this diet is mucus-forming, low in enzymes and basically acid-forming; it eventually leads to complications.

Dr. Ernst Krebs has developed the use of laetrile to destroy cancer cells. For enduring success, the substance must be used in conjunction with a low protein diet (Control of Cancer, G. Kittler, Cancer Book House, L.A., Cal.).

Fasting is not the most successful method for healing cancer. Because of existing cell starvation and high toxemia such an approach, especially with weak, elderly people, can be dangerous or deadly. It can be used if the individual prepares for it with a detoxifying organic vegetarian diet and juice fasts. It should be conducted only under experienced supervision.

Dr. Duncan Bulkley, a New York Internist, from 1915 to 1922 published several books which described his forty years at the New York Skin and Cancer Hospital where he used a low protein, low sulphur vegetarian diet in the successful treatment of cancer (On Cancer, Its Cause and Treatment; Cancer, Its Non-Surgical Treatment).

"One Answer to Cancer," (Dr. Kelly) presents a nutritional approach (219) to the management of cancer. A vegetarian diet, dietary supplements, animal organ digestive enzymes and fruit/vegetable juices have produced a high rate of success. However, to sprout all the seed and replace grains with juice from their green shoots would remove the seed and grain mucus forming property, thus increase the efficiency of this regime.

Dr. Max Gerson, M.D. (45) used raw juices almost exclusively in his successful treatment of cancer patients.

J. Brandt's "Grape Cure" has reported many cures. The diet is alkalinizing, low protein, enzyme rich and highly cleansing.

Ann Wigmore uses wheatgrass therapy, sprouts, live food juices and fresh fruit. Her regime is simple, effective and readily available.

A successful program for eliminating cancer must have at least the following tools to work with:
1) Something to destroy malignant cells without damaging normal cells.

2) An intensive nutritional program to provide all the raw materials the body needs. The diet should be alkalinizing with a good supply of enzymes.

3) An intensive detoxification program to eliminate toxins which interfere with body functions.

4) Elimination of potential causes of cancer.

The rejuvenation regime outlined in this book satisfies each one of these requirements. In addition to the daily schedule, one should have, if available, a colonic irrigation once every week for the first two months and wheatgrass juice implants at least twice a day (total of two cups) for four weeks. In addition, take at least four cups of fresh fruit and vegetable juice daily. Reduce the number of implants to two or more per week for at least six months. In extreme cases, an individual might stay on a grass juice regime for at least four months.

Shower at least twice daily. Scrub the skin thoroughly with a loofah sponge or natural bristle brush or use a mild soap of neutral pH. Wash your hair at least three times a week. If you have surface cancer, cover it with a wheatgrass poultice.

Do not eat after enemas, baths, zone therapy or any kind of treatment. Eat only when hungry. The body can assimilate juice much more readily than salads or fruit.

If protein foods should be desirable to slow the cleansing process, then it is best that they be eaten before 1 PM. It is best to eat seed fermented — sesame, sunflower, almond, sprouted soy beans — not more than a few tablespoons per serving. Limit them to one, but no more than two, servings per day.

On a low protein diet, muscle and fatty tissues are consumed. The cleansing process may require a loss of one third of the body's weight (unless one is very thin) before morbidity disappears.

One will be weakened by the cleansing regime; therefore, he or she should be assured of unlimited, uninterrupted bed rest whenever needed. One should under no circumstances go on a binge, eat processed food or break health rules; it can be lethal. After detoxification, the body will increase in weight in spite of the fact that one is on a low protein diet.

If you have any fillings in your teeth, complete recovery might require their removal. Studies have shown them to be toxic; the effects range from psychic disorders to inactivation of many important enzymes.

Once you recover, you cannot go back to old eating habits. Dead food and high protein diet will bring back the disease.

The real "Answer to Cancer" is a low protein diet of sprouts, vegetables, juices and fruit.

For testimonials of those who healed themselves of cancer, leukemia, diabetes, arthritis, rheumatism, multiple sclerosis, read BE YOUR OWN DOCTOR by Dr. Ann Wigmore.

If degeneration has not gone too far, regeneration is possible. Though you may have broken nature's laws for many years, you can start obeying them now and achieve a long, vital life.

For perpetual youth one needs a good genetic structure, a warm climate at high altitude, chastity, spiritual aspiration, a non-polluted environment, a fruit diet, frequent fasting and loving friends.

LETTERS FROM FRIENDS

"Our doubts are traitors and make us lose the good we oft might win by fearing to attempt."   Shakespeare

HISTORY OF SECOND BIRTH

Ms. Amsick is in an advanced state of chronic disease. During her lifetime several disease crises (flu, skin rash, cold, boils, etc.) were suppressed with drugs. Toxic material which was being eliminated was forced back into the organism. Ms. Amsick seems to have been cured but her vitality was lowered. This forced adaptation resulted in degeneration of tissues and certain of her organs became affected with organic lesions. She also noted that her ability to get into deep meditation diminished. It did not worry her for doctors reassured her that all these symptoms were part of the aging process.

Through the years of continued body abuse, Ms. Amsick has tried every kind of medicine to cure herself. In spite of her efforts, she was given up to die within a few months. Not willing to accept this fate, she decided to try nature's way which she heard of through a yogi friend.

The changes that Ms. Amsick has experienced since then are quite similar to the symptoms that are felt by almost everyone who goes on a vegetarian hygienic regime. The symptoms express themselves in varied forms, depending upon the genetic factors and dietary history, plus the overall lifestyle.

Ms. Amsick decided to reform her life entirely. She eliminated one by one all foods, interests and activities which interfered with health and a happy life. She discontinued the use of all processed foods, animal products, smoking, drinking and sexual abuse. She even changed jobs because of the chemicals that were in her place of employment. After a month of improved diet, she started to experiment with juice and water fasts of 3 to 7 days. She eliminated enormous quantities of mucus, hardened fecal matter, bile, acids and toxins through bowels, skin, lungs and kidneys. She never carried the cleansing regime to the end because she was too debilitated and underweight and because business, family and financial conditions did not permit her.

After a water fast, she took several days of acid fruit juices. Occasionally, she did 24 hours of dry fast. When hunger returned, quite often she gained some of her weight, although the weight was composed of healthier tissues. She felt quite well and though she was cured of every disease. To her disappointment, nature wanted her to be completely healed. So more crises.

Usually after a few weeks to several months, additional cleansing crises appear. Ms. Amsick began to lose her appetite, was affected with catarrhal elimination through the mucus membranes lining the respiratory, digestive and genito-urine tract. She broke out with a few skin sores. Her temperature hit 106 degrees F. She became quite sick.

She was losing faith in nature and began to think that her struggle was in vain. This is where contact with a nature cure doctor or other experienced individuals can be invaluable. They can provide reassurance and an explaination of what is taking place during this healing sickness.

The doctor will explain that through natural diet and fasting, her body has increased in "cleansing vitality", stored up an abundant supply of alkaline salts and dissolvers and now has began a serious process of house cleaning. Instead of being sorry, one should rejoice.

Physical energy is low because it is being used for internal purification — one should stop wasting energy; rest and sleep is crucial. Avoid all stimulants in the form of nonherbal teas, coffee or concentrated foods (see: Crisis). After a few days of discomfort the body will get rid of a good amount of pathogenic matter. The skin sores will disappear without a trace. Temperature returns to normal. Now, the energy will flow with less obstruction and one will feel stronger, look younger and be healthier than before the acute reaction appeared.

This explanation inspired Ms. Amsick to perservere. She came to understand that the more toxic matter is removed from body, the higher in vitality and the less abuse the body will tolerate.

After the crisis, hunger returned. Ms. Amsick noticed she could live on less food, digest it better and do work which she had not been able to do for fifteen years. Her meditation improved and she took up yoga again. She felt younger than she did thirty years ago. Her wrinkles have disappeared to a great extent and her steps have the spring of youth.

Ms. Amsick decided to change her name to Ms. Amhealed. She noticed that her body is now more sensitive and intolerant to those foods which were injurious to her organism.

She has become an enthusiastic disciple of Nature Cure. Initially, because of ego oriented motivations, she tried to force her opinion on others, offered advice where it was not asked for, became a "know it all." This made her lose friends and made her feel undesirable anxiety.

She had to learn how to adjust her differences with society. New relationships had to be developed. After all, just because she changed her diet and saw the effect of nature's laws, this was not enough to give up friends and business associates. Instead of evangelizing, she became an example of health. Instead of trying to convince others of the correctness of nature's laws, she offered advice only when asked for or when it could be well received, as in time of sickness or distress.

She approached each person as an individual. Children were offered stories that invoked the laws of nature which kept a person happy and youthful, filled with power for a life of adventure. She told them bible stories from genesis and how animals don't like to be killed, whether they be cows or pet dogs. Wife and husband were shown the economics of food, health insurance, beauty, vitality and complexion.

At business luncheons, instead of making an issue of food; eat salads, fruit or simple preparations. If offered something else just shrug your shoulders and say you're not in the mood for it, you're experimenting with a bunny diet, you're trying to be ecological by eating primary instead of secondary protein foods, your kid is trying to turn you into a raw food freak, "Oh I'm just trying the new vogue Dr. Viktoras diet." Have fun with your answers. Discussion of diet can become quickly very emotional. It is best to switch to a topic that fits the framework of your companions. Arguments never win battles. Slowly you learn that living is much more than food.

Ms. Amhealed joy for life continued to increase. Her sense of humor increased. She took more fasts ranging from 1 to 40 days, ate more and more uncooked vegetables, sprouts and fruit and abstained entirely from animal food. More healing crises appeared in different forms until she welcomed these crises.

Finally at the end of seven years of improved living, Ms. Amhealed felt and looked many years younger than when she began to follow nature's path. Her family doctor found that all signs of degeneration had disappeared in her body, every vital organ was sound. Her nature doctor examined her eyes and saw that all the marks of degeneration and organic lesions which had been in the region of the iris which pertains to the kidneys, lungs, stomach, liver and intestinal tract had been healed. Ms. Amhealed's constitution was now sounder than when she was 25 years old. She has earned her youth and the future long life.

I CHOOSE SURVIVAL

While in college, I pushed myself to experience as much as possible. Born under the Piscean sky, of delicate constitution, this often proved disastrous. My living and eating habits were deadly.

By 1965, I knew all the nurses and doctors at the infirmary. They were very generous with tranquilizers, sleeping pills and pain relievers. These I added to fifteen cups of coffee and two packs of cigarettes per day, plenty of alcohol, chronic over-eating (by age 26 I was a chubby 190 pounds). In spite of many ailments, I always felt that one day I would be healthy.

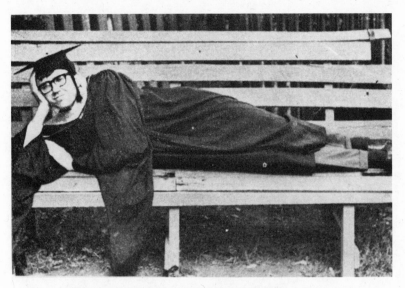

1964 After Masters Degree Weight 195 pounds

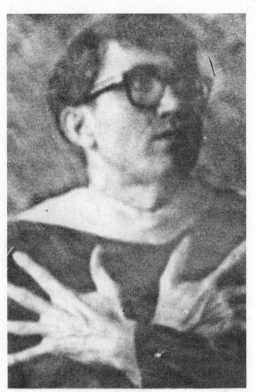

1964 Confussion.

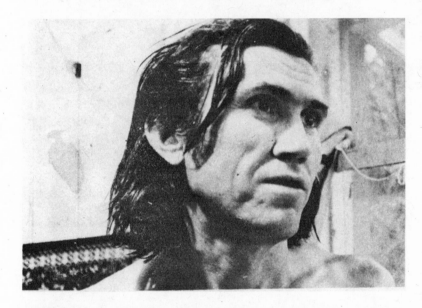

A period of many binges, seasoning and processed foods in 1970. Face lines indicate liver, lung, kidney and circulation problems. Weight 140 pounds.

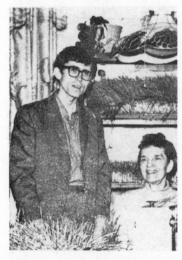

Viktoras and Dr. Ann. V'k is down to 95 pounds in 1969.

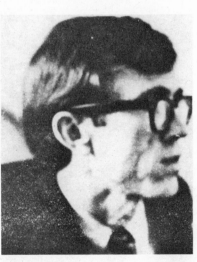

1968 Lots of seasoning, vegetarian Liver and lung marks . 100 pounds

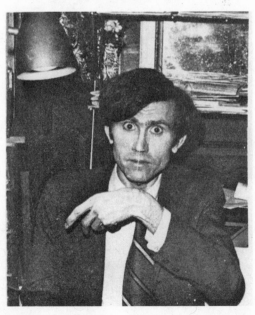

1969 Bad food combinations, lots of bakery products and protein result in tumor on wrist. Very sampaku. Condition disappeared in 1 week of raw food and juices.

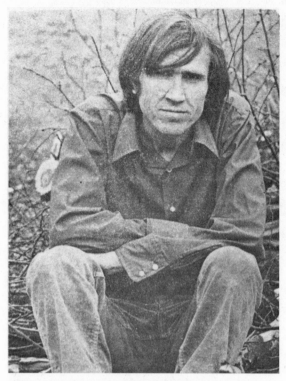

Heavy starch-protein seasoning diet, vegetarian.
Liver backed up. 1971

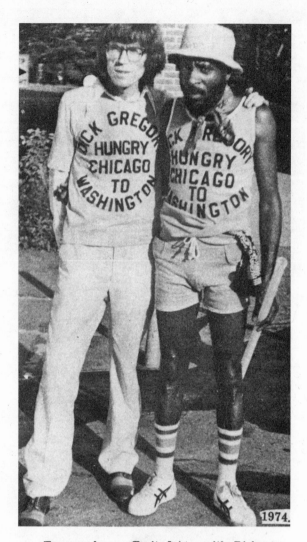

Two weeks on Fruit Juices with Dick
Gregory on 900 mile run to Wash. D.C.

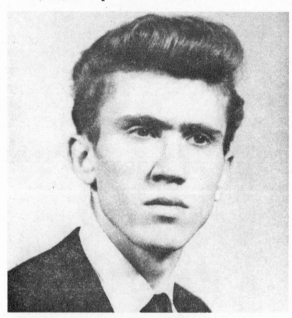

1958 High School

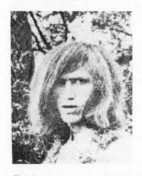

Fruit Diet, Fla. 1972

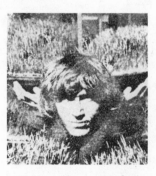

Sproutarian 1973.

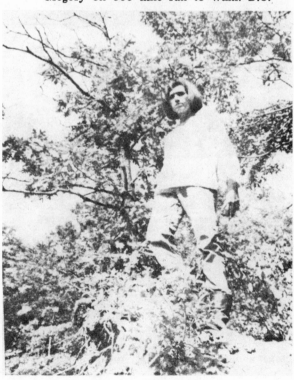

-1973-

A frightening experience shook me from this complacency. I was running up the stairs to a class on the fourth floor. Pain constricted my chest, but I made it to the office, poured a cup of black coffee and started to lecture. My hands were shaking, perspiration poured from my face and armpits. I could not focus my thoughts. The pain in my heart was sharp. I did not think I would leave the room alive. By sheer force of will I managed to finish the lecture.

Suddenly I knew what I must do without delay. I purchased some mild tea, fruits and vegetables. Then I drove to my log cabin, stopping to see my landlord. I told him that I was not well; that if I needed help, he would hear a continuous blast from a car horn which I would rig so it could be triggered from my bed. In that event, he should do whatever he thought necessary for me.

Walking up the two hundred foot incline to my cabin, I had to rest several times because of the sharp pain in my chest. My legs felt like lead. My varicose veins were screaming as if ready to burst.

I went to bed, but could not sleep. Since I was giving up coffee, cigarettes, alcohol, meat, milk and sleeping pills; I vaguely anticipated withdrawal symptoms. I lay clutching the car horn alarm for long distance companionship.

By 3 A.M., my nerves were on edge. I felt paralyzed inside my exhausted body. Headache, cramps and sweat came in waves. The palpitation of my heart increased. It started racing. I clocked it fearfully at 130 at which point I passed out.

I woke at 7 AM, surprised and happy to be alive. I felt well enough to go back to school, but this was illusory; soon I felt exhausted. I went for a five-minute walk. All day, I wondered, what will the night be like? Will I survive it? Outside of knowing that drug withdrawal usually takes about three days, I had no knowledge of fasting, nor had I known anyone who had fasted.

For four days I experienced only minor discomfort, but the nights were sheer torture. However, as the days progressed, I began to feel more certain about my future. I increased the length of my daily walks and by the fifth day fell asleep at 11 PM from tiredness. By the seventh day I was running a few minutes and preparing the soil in the garden. I prayed, thankful to be alive to experience the simple delights of living.

During ensuing experimentation with diet, I discovered that my favorite food, milk (supposedly the perfect food) is a major source of colds and a factor in most respiratory disorders.

Pasteurized milk had been the staple in my diet in early childhood. For the first years of my life, doctors predicted my death as a matter of course. The milk diet (I know now) contributed to disorders of the respiratory and lymph system: tonsillitis, flu, pneumonia, diphtheria, colds, measles, mumps, bronchitis. On several occasions, I developed a high fever accompanied by large, running sores and boils (my body's attempt to cleanse itself). For two months I was semiconscious during a bout of typhoid fever. Family love and strong will to live enabled me to survive.

Doctors continued to predict that I would never be healthy. They said my heart was permanently damaged by a triple dose of diphtheria toxoid given me by mistake. It would have killed a normal child, they said.

The poverty in post-war Germany made it difficult to obtain eggs, milk and meat. I spent much time barefoot in the woods gathering berries, mushrooms, nuts and wild fruit to contribute to our largely vegetarian diet. These simple foods restored my health.

During this detoxification period I had frequent colds and difficulty in eating. Once, within a 24 hour period, I developed a fever of 106 deg. F.; my skin became covered with sores. Because I fasted on liquids and rested, the condition disappeared within 3 days. Much of the past dairy induced mucus was eliminated through the skin in the form of boils which grew into the size of plums taking about 3 to 4 weeks followed by opening up and discharge of pus. Within a period of a year I had 5 such events. This finished my basic body cleansing process.

Arriving in America at the age of ten, I embraced its luxuries: ice cream, milk, soda, white bread, hot dogs, candy, canned foods and processed bakery products. Within a year my skin became pimply, I visited the dentist for the first time and developed severe colds. By the age of sixteen I had varicose veins. At nineteen I had a duodenal ulcer and tumors on my hand. I suffered migraine headache at least once a week. One of the outstanding characteristics of my diet was an excessive use of dairy products in the form of milk (up to three quarts a day), ice cream (on occasion I have eaten half a gallon), condensed milk, swiss cheese. I constantly spit sticky mucus.

Even after the healing crisis in my cabin, I continued this habit. Indigestion was sometimes so bad that I had to substitute lemonade for milk. In a few days my digestion would improve; then the desire to return to milk would become so strong I would repeat the pattern.

In the morning, after a few yoga postures, I would eat a breakfast of milk and cereal. Within minutes the great sense of well-being would vanish, replaced by a fuzzy head, runny nose and lung congestion. Initially I supposed that I had not felt so well as I had thought. However, constant repetition convinced me that the culprit was milk.

I decided to resolve the problem. After three days of lemonade, I tried, on successive days, milk, yogurt, cottage cheese, dried milk, condensed milk. Every one of them induced the same reaction.

Though I was working very hard at this time as a computer programmer, my body was sick. I suffered from insomnia, migraine, stomach ulcer, varicose veins, indigestion.

It seemed time to retire (very appropriately, for at the age of 29 I showed all the signs of old age — my hair was graying and I was losing it quite rapidly).

The books of Ehret and Drs. Walker and Warmbrand gave me hope. I wrote to the authors and met some of them personally. Dr. Warmbrand put me on a vegetarian diet and made chiropractic adjustments. Immediately my digestion improved.

One doctor introduced me to Ann Wigmore. At the Mansion I became acquainted with grass juice and sprouts. The meal, served in famine proportions, looked wriggly; but it satisfied my appetite and agreed with my body. I read 'Why Suffer.' It opened visions of peace in the natural world and the power of the healing strength of grasses. I moved into the Mansion about one month later in May, 1968.

During the early stages of transition into vegetarianism, I had periodic bouts of cleansing reaction. Sweating was so profuse that I had to change my socks four times a day. On two occasions open sores discharged toxins stored for years. At times very irritable, I found the best solution to be silence. Cramps were relieved by massage. Pain and headache responded to zone therapy.

With a cleansing diet my weight dropped, in a period of six months, from 160 to ninety-five pounds. As my body started rebuilding I gained weight and now weigh 135 pounds.

Over the years, I have learned much about health and the needs of the body, but, like many busy people, I have neglected to pay enough attention to my bodily requirements.

One of the most important ingredients of health is adequate rest, which I have never obtained. Under city conditions, sunshine and pure air are not available. There never seems enough time for yoga, fasting, relaxation or meditation. My body has regenerated a good deal on the live food diet, in spite of these handicaps.

Now I have reached a time in life when the longing to be in the countryside is strong. Survival in the city is impossible. Next year, if the country is still intact, I plan to pursue the development of communities away from the city, in the north, the tropics and on islands, for surviving the crisis of this planet. We have little time left to prepare ourselves and our shelters.

However, survival into the 21st century is possible if we center our energies and apply the New Age teachings. This is the only task that has any meaning in our time.

Victor Kulvinskas

Dear Sisters and Brothers,

It has been over a decade since I started experimenting full time with diet, path of simplicity, purification, spiritual search, relationships, and many other aspects of the new age lifestyles.

In the presence of much joy and excitement, I had many setbacks, devastating failures, much pain, binges and suffering, coffee regression and loss of consciousness. I was an addict, full of fear, alone and afraid to reveal and acknowledge my weaknesses. Many have seen me in these struggles, some have judged me and gone back to their old ways. I was not the idol they fantisized, so they rejected the truth in my teachings. One young man, at a meeting ten years later said to me "You know, you were the reason that I did not become a vegetarian." Yet, I persisted on the path. I knew that beyond my addictions, diseased body, sick mind, there was the true me — perfect. And I felt, I would reach that goal in this lifetime.

The "Survival Into the 21st Century" creation was the result of about five years of intense experimentation, endless overwork in research, struggle to become purified and chaste enough to channel a message that I and the whole human race needed to hear. I never doubted the truth that has come through me. I have found no errors during the five years after publishing the book. I feel that the most important message of this book is my earlier preface. Study it and read it often. It will give you comfort. The work has been a struggle, with personal, not theoretical failures.

I came from the Piscean background of a mystic. Childhood was one of sickness, spiritual ecstasy and high energy. Up to age 21, I kept 99% of the time a vigil of silence. I did not know how to communicate. At age 24, in spite of being an honor student, I was classified by my psychiatrist as a catatonic schizophrenic and had a medical record two inches thick at the clinic.

The only thought that kept me going was a feeling from the universe "that there is a better way, there is an answer to my fear, suffering and struggle. The answer will help me to help all others." So, I never gave up hope.

Each year, as I was sliding in desperation and decay, sisters, as well as occassional brothers, have come into my life to pull me out of darkness, and give me the strength to return to the pathways of light. Each time, I made advancements enough so that I never returned to my low levels, instead I took steps in becoming much healthier, stronger, more giving, orderly, cleaner, more loving, open and truthful.

One of the heaviest addictions is coffee. It started in grammer school and in college I was up to fifteen cups a day. My heart began to fail, and so I stopped drinking it for five years. During the three year period where I was into mostly raw food, I drank no coffee. As the detoxification exposed my naked fears, ego, imperfections, programmed self hate and personal doubts, I returned to the coffee for emotional desensitization. It resulted in five years of struggle with coffee, cooked food, binges, vomiting and self doubt — a climax time of shame and self judgement. Those were my darkest years, for I knew the truth and could not practice it.

Only within the last two years, I started seeing the progress that was fantisized in my visions. I stopped hiding and running away. As I started giving of myself more fully, becoming, inch by inch, from moment to moment, more honest with self and others — the universe kept giving me more help.

There have been many events, friends, books and tools that have been important in the overcoming of the causes for the self destructive habits. I would like to share some of the highlights that I recall from my recent past.

First, the acknowledgement of not being well. Eight years ago, a sister secretely volunteered me to be the subject of iris diagnosis in a workshop led by Dr. Bernard Jensen. As a hundred students and friends watched, the kind doctor read all my weaknesses as diagnosed from the iris. My organs and tissues were old and sick. The doctor had not seen such a disaster before. From embarassment, I lost about 10 pounds of sweat during the examination. I was the raw foodist advocate who did not practice what I preached. For some reason they applauded me, I guess for being alive. I felt confused for I thought I was worthy of only censure. A year later, the same sister insisted that I lectured in the nude at the Rainbow Gathering (New Mexico, Truth and Consequences, appropriately named for my task). I, who had barely enough skin and muscle (I was that way before becoming a vegetarian) to cover the mismatched bony structure, was to talk on health, in the nude? No way! I will die in shame. However, I did do it and in the sun, from emotional discomfort, I lost more weight. During the presentation I was not consciously there. As I surrendered to the lesson, I gained spiritual strength and my tongue outpoured a message of love, hope, light and simplicity, of healing. All who were there felt exalted and made one in spirit. These two events led to my gradual acceptance of the condition of my body. With acceptence, I proceeded, in reluctance, to restart the rebuilding of my temple. As I progress, I am still surrounded by the haunting fears of the size of the job and the enticement of old addictions, as well as the threatening, lingering doubts of success.

Second, the recognition that I had no control over my eating and my coffee habit. I was a nibbler, glutton and a vomiter for well over twenty years. My personality and lifestyle was immersed in it. I did not know whether I really wanted to change or was capable of it. I always told myself, ''tomorrow I will get it together,'' instead of facing myself in the now and seeing what I can do now, today, not tomorrow. I did not set out to deal with these issues. It came as a surprise, slowly within the counsels held at All Life Sanctuary, I started to admit publically my hidden, closet junk habits. Within a struggle, I had the information pulled out of me and had no other alternatives but to admit that I was an addict. I shared initially with my companion sister, then with other sympathetic, supportive persons, who likewise were also going through the struggles of overcoming some addictions. Weekly, we used to gather in counsels, or individual partnerships, or emergency calls for support over the phone. As we honestly worked on the issues, the binges dropped in frequency. Likewise, through the study of ''Course in Miracles'', ''Handbook to Higher Consciousness,'' ''Survival Into the 21st Century,'' ''The Thin Book'' (Omangod Press) and the material from local ''Overeaters Anonymus,'' as well as some timely meetings, there evolved some important messages, such as ''confess your sins on to others, or learn from mistakes through evaluation and discussion,'' practice non-judgement and forgiveness for self and others, only truth is real, all else is illusion and will vanish, make all experiences conscious teachers, love self and others as yourself, live in the now — future and past do not exist. Having experienced more than enough suffering, I started to face and deal with the source of anxiety, oversensitivity, impulsiveness, emotional dependence and isolation, irresponsibility, slopyness and so many other non-growth centered traits. In spite of all the advancements, I still experience at times cravings triggered by old desires, but it lacks the intensity of the past or the emotional satisfaction. There are times when my practices are questionable, but I try to acknoledge them with full consciousness, forgiveness and learn to go forward. I lead a less food oriented life than in the past (I try to eat one meal per day, and have a few juice drinks during the day) and make an emphasis on service, teaching, study, yoga, or physical labor, as well as the pursuit of the evasive mental/spiritual/interpersonal frontiers.

I am ending my sixth, seven year cycle, in 1982. This year 1981 has been one of progress and joy, even spontaneous ecstasy at times, as I timidly, with reservations, opened up my heart in trust.

I have the friendship of a beloved sister, who sees through my lies, current and past, who accepts me, shares with me honestly, sees me fail often and yet loves me forever. Its encouraging to be in the presence of such light.

In our All Life Sanctuary community we support each other in our attempt to go through the personal struggles, negative programming and a lack of respect. We opened up gradually in trust and have become closer. Most food indiscretions fell away, size of meals decreased, raw food became our personal choice. In the meeting of hearts in joy, service to one another and the world community, creativity, individuality, respect and love have become the glue of our lives.

I have wished for a long time to share this message, for I felt the readers should know the real story. Brothers and sisters, do not surrender to the ways of the world. Keep up the inner struggle. Persevere in patience and you will find peace. You are being tested and prepared for important work. The struggle falls away as the addictions finish their teaching and lose their pull. Aim for raw foodism and frugal eating, for that is the surest path and tool for spiritual growth, highest mental development, healthiest strength, survival and longevity, with endless love and joy.

I love you and ask forgiveness for delaying so long to say that I am struggling, I am imperfect and I fear in losing your love. I know my spirit is perfect, and in time so will be my ways and my body. Today I see that I am like many others — a student of ''Survival Into the 21st Century.'' The book is also my guide to become Viktorious and to become a servant, lover, and example of truth.

DO IT NOW! (11 Year Old Vegetarian)

Humbly and joyfully,
Love All Ways,

Viktoras
October, 1981

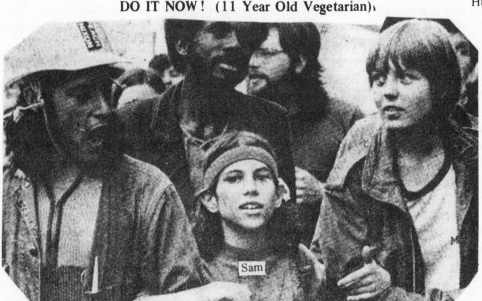

Sam

I was age 11 and I had heard about being a vegetarian because my brother had been a vegetarian for a year or so. So I got to thinking about eating muscles and tissues and stuff like that and I became pretty readily a vegetarian.

My friends said "You need animal protein or you won't grow!" So for the first two years I ate bread and eggs and stuff. Then, at the end of my second year, my brother brought home a book by Arnold Ehret about the mucousless diet. So I started getting into that. "Have to get that mucus out of my body!" Big deposits of mucus started coming out of my nose. It was great!

After reading Love Your Body and getting into raw foods I started drinking a lot of carrot juice and my bad eyes went away. I was wearing glasses. I just chucked them and that was it! One of my favorite drinks is the green juice-carrot-rejuvelac drink you showed me Vik. It's dynamite! I'm heavy on that now.

To continue with my story, I've changed my eating habits entirely. I keep pretty much to a schedule. In the morning, I usually have some kind of fruit. One of my favorites is dried dates or figs with bananas. Or I'll have oranges, organic of course, squeezed and blended with bananas. That really fills me up!

I used to take salads for lunch with me. My Mom would put them in plastic boxes that she used to keep vegetables in the refrigerator; but the salads would get warm and gross and all. So now I take fruit or carrot and celery sticks and sliced cuke with some lemon on them to school about 4 times a week in baggies and a salad once a week. I've made good friends with the school janitor so I can keep my stuff in his refrigerator.

I have to work in this kitchen where the smell of flesh grease is in the air at all times but it's pretty good money at my age: $2.10. I'm going to quit as soon as I can. But, anyway, when I get home from work the first thing I do is take a shower, then I lay around and listen to the radio for a while; then I'll make myself a carrot juice.

My folks like me to eat with them — I don't because they have flesh and everything — but, anyway, I eat with them and I usually have a sprout and green salad with some carrot and beet thrown in. Four months ago, I was having all vegetable salads. I couldn't get the sprouting together. But, before seeing you at the Mansion I was downing tons of greens, so many I couldn't handle them. Then that died off. I couldn't figure out why. Maybe I got lazy. Anyway, I usually have lemon and oil dressing on my salad with spices — dill weed's one of my favorites, so is parsely. I usually have a piece of fruit before going to bed.

One good thing is my father likes watermelon as much as I do, so once a week we'll go and get one. They're pretty expensive now so that's a pretty all right thing for him to do.

About once a month I do a three to four day juice fast. It makes me feel better. If I touch any fermented seeds or even nuts now I feel all clogged up.

That's the food side of it. As far as my social life goes, everything's changed in the way I see things and the way I am from most of the other fifteen year olds. Most of my friends are into dope, nearly 95% of my friends, which is a real drag; but if I want friends, these are the people I will have to put up with.

I'm not trying to be egotistical, but most of the fifteen year olds who I go to school with don't have any direction in life. They don't care about anything. They're so stoned in the morning they can't wake up until 11:00 A.M. When they wake up, they're all disgusting, drink coffee. That's pretty bad for a fifteen year old kid. I can't understand why someone would want to do that.

I go to sleep when I'm tired, usually around 10:30 and get up at 6:45 A.M. It does take a little bit longer for a vegetarian to make lunch. Other people can slap balony in between two pieces of bread and that's their lunch. It's a little more involved.

A couple of years ago I was a girl chaser like most of the other kids. It was the thing — to have a girlfriend. But now I look around me. At least 95% of the girls in school smoke dope, drink. I have no feeling towards them. One of these days I'll find a girl and she'll be beautiful and she'll be a raw food eater and we'll go off to a farm somewhere and you can figure out the rest.

I wish all eleven year olds would switch over to raw foods the way I did. You have more advantage if you start young than anybody. You've got a lot less junk to get out of you when you're young. For any eleven year olds who want my advice out there it's don't worry and don't rush getting into raw foods once you become vegetarian. Becoming vegetarian is good enough for a start. My message is: DO IT. DO IT. JUST DO IT. It's much better for you.

Hey, Vik, I just dug up this picture from when I was a super big peace freak. I though maybe you'd want to use it with this letter. For three years I used to go every weekend down to the Capital and leaflet and help out. There was this group near where I lived called the Washington Area Peace Action Coalition which organized most of the big, huge demonstrations.

Anyway, I was a real super peace freak and I took a training course to be one of the demonstration marshalls.

They were the people who kept order on the lines, directed people, helped people out who were arrested, fainted, got sick. You had to take double training to be a front of the parade marshall. They made sure people didn't break around the front of the line. All the newspaper people were up there in the front of the line taking pictures.

Anyway, on one of these demonstrations in which I was being a marshall on the front of the line this super far out thing happened.

You might recall the newspaper called the Daily World in New York — it might be called the Daily Worker now. Anyway, they got a picture of me in there. They had this whole big article of the peace movement. So enclosed is the magazine picture of me just marching along. I think the objective was "Hey, man, everybody's getting into it." So I hope you'll be able to use it. It's my favorite picture of me.

Well, I got to go now. Got to do my school work. What a drag. School's got me down so bad teaching all those ridiculous, unnecessary things, I'm never going to use ever in my life. So, take it easy.

LOVE YA, Sam

42 DAY FAST; RECOVERY FROM ARTHRITIS, AGE 68, ATTORNEY

"My name is Martin V. Lesser, age sixty-eight, residing at 305 E. 86th. St., New York City. I am an attorney, licensed to practice in the state of New York but inactive for the past two years.

My inactivity and retirement from my profession resulted from ill health. I was suffering from protein deficiency, arthritis, muscular attrition, liver disturbance and osteoporosis of the cervical spine.

The first physician who treated me was Dr. Benjamin J. Hyman, Professor of Surgery at New York Polyclinic Hospital. Under his auspices I was admitted to New York Polyclinic Hospital on August 27, 1969. I remained there five days and he later treated me privately by prescribing synthetic vitamins and advised me to go on a liberal diet with cooked meats, potatoes, desserts.

I followed this advice but my condition became progressively worse. Dr. Hyman died in May of 1970. I then went to a well-known neurologist, Dr. Lawrence I. Kaplan, residing at 812 Park Avenue, New York City. He advised X-rays of the cervical spine which I had taken at Maimonides Hospital in September, 1970. The X-rays showed osteoporosis of the upper cervical area of the spine. Dr. Kaplan prescribed synthetic vitamins and the relief of pressure in the spine by a weight pulley device. The synthetic vitamins and pulley device did not prove effective and I became progressively worse. I lived on the average American diet: cooked foods, abundances of dairy products such as cheese, cottage cheese, ice cream, sweets, whole wheat bread, cooked vegetables, pasteurized fruit juices.

I began to suffer with restricted and painful movements of my shoulders, neck, upper arms and hands; also, I was experiencing post-nasal drip and throat mucus. I went to another physician, Dr. J. Reuben Budd of Passaic, New Jersey. He gave me a thorough physical examination and then gave me NO ADVICE, JUST THAT I WOULD HAVE TO ACCEPT MY CONDITION AS PART OF THE AGING PROCESS. My condition deteriorated further. I then went to see a nutritionist, Dr. Stanley Bass, of Coney Island Avenue, Brooklyn, New York, a licensed chiropractor, in October of 1970. He prescribed a diet of sprouted mung beans and raw vegetable salads and recommended that I also try to obtain some Wheat Grass. Living in New York City, I found it difficult to grow the Wheat Grass and was not able to obtain organic greens for salads. Dr. Bass gave me a book entitled, BE YOUR OWN DOCTOR by Ann Wigmore. I read it and decided to visit Ann Wigmore's establishment, HIPPOCRATES HEALTH INSTITUTE in Boston. It took me over a year to finally leave New York City and go to Boston. I thought I might stay a week in Boston to see at first hand Ann Wigmore's therapy and way of growing Wheat Grass, Buckwheat Lettuce and Sunflower Lettuce, all indoors according to her book. I took a small valise with enough clothing for a week's stay in Boston on November 8, 1971. It being a mild day, I took a light top-coat. After I arrived at the Hippocrates Health Institute and was there a few hours I knew I had been led to the right place for therapy. Despite my lack of sufficient warm clothing I have remained at the Institute for six weeks and followed the therapy advocated.

The following program was suggested: rectal implants of about 8 ozs. of fresh Wheat Grass juice thrice daily every three hours. I adhered to this for 42 days. Occasionally, I chewed some mung sprouts or alfalfa sprouts together with sunflower lettuce or buckwheat lettuce just swallowing the juice and discarding the pulp. This was to appease psychological hunger since I experienced no real hunger while on the fast.

Having been on this Wheat Grass juice fast for 42 days, I am now ready, on December 21, 1971, to return to New York City. I have lost 25 pounds, weighing 135 and I am 5'11" and broad-boned. I am thin but I feel vital. The skin feels firm despite the large weight loss. My pains have disappeared; arthritic signs are almost non-existent. My spine is flexible — without pain. I feel at least fifteen years younger. I intend to get a new series of X-rays to see if the X-rays show any changes in the area previously showing osteoporosis.

I expect to adhere to a diet of sprouted living foods such as: mung beans, alfalfa sprouts, lentil sprouts, and partially sprouted whole wheat berries, together with sunflower and unhulled sesame seeds; also, greens grown indoors plus avocado.

The diet suggested by Ann Wigmore eliminates all cooked foods and all refined, canned, processed foods, together with avoidance of all milk products and meat, fish and eggs. No grains except sprouted grains are used. The diet has shown Ann Wigmore and Victor Kulvinskas to be in superb health and I know it will keep me in good health and correct any other latent conditions of ill-health still remaining.

The atmosphere at the Hippocrates Institute evokes blessings and thanks for all those who have been guests and visited and observed what occurs."

MINISTER, DIRECTOR HEALS PROSTATIC BLOCKAGE

I am a Minister of Universal Unity. Before becoming a Minister or a Brother in the work, I was a Motion Picture Director, Actor, Writer, and finally a Production Supervisor of Instructional Aids at one of the foremost publishers in the United States.

The hustle and constant pushing in the business world makes one become quite unaware of many wonderful things that are available. Thus, my "modus operandi" in the business world was like most people that are out there, trying to make an indentation in life.

This kind of nervous living made me completely disorganized in my food habits, intake of much meats, starches, plus the wrong combination of food. A constant tiredness was prevalent during this time, and when I became a Minister, together with my wife, Roberta, we decided to observe better rules of eating and living. We tryed very hard to understand by purchasing many books on better living, foods and vitamins. Still, this did not give us the complete knowledge of the whole truthful spectrum that is needed to know and further revise the body's function by eliminating all toxins.

In 1971 Roberta and I had the good fortune to meet Victor Kulvinskas, who was in N.Y.C. for certain lectures and stopped at our little chapel in the Hotel Ansonia. From him we did learn of a new health program. This program was the program that is being conducted at Ann Wigmore's establishment, the Hippocrates Health Institute in Boston, Mass.

We observed the small literature that Victor left us and discussed it, but like all things we set it aside for a later time.

During this time I had been suffering with a prostate condition and from the many doctor's visits and prescriptions, I was full of pills and antibiotics. This made me more tired and, having to do a duplex job of conducting a temple, writing a magazine and literature and further sitting for enlightenment classes each evening, with groups of people for Spiritual Science and Music Vibrations, plus the day job at the publishers, it became impossible to continue. I was taken sick with unimaginable pains last year. The doctors prescribed more pills, and nothing was ever said about the cause of my illness, nor the way to conduct my life. More pills, more temporary relief and more weakness . . .and more toxins in my body. In the latter part of June, I was stricken with a complete prostatic blockage, which necessitated having a catheter inserted in my bladder. The doctor said . . "this is it . . . I will send you to a specialist that will observe the whole matter." — This specialist, after putting me through all kinds of agonizing pains . . . finally came to his lucid decision . . ."Operation necessary." This rang a rather sad note. Both Roberta and myself knew than that this was out of the question. Our spiritual sense, plus our Spiritual Science studies . . . and our contact with our Master Teachers, immediately placed a large sign in front of us. Dr. Ann Wigmore . . . and the wheat grass therapy was the solution . . . In a few hours we made all arrangements by phone with the Hippocrates Institute and a dear friend drove us into Boston.

I arrived in Boston at the Institute on Tuesday, with the catheter still in me . . . and discussed the whole matter with Ann Wigmore. I was placed on a program of intense therapy, which consisted of NO FOOD! Each morning, a glass of Rejuvelac (the water that the wheat seed had been soaked in). Then, oral intake of 2 ounces of wheat grass juice . . . two or three times daily - plus 8 ounces of rectal implants of grass juice, twice daily. I continued this therapy for 6 days, then I removed the catheter of my free will . . . And the water from the bladder started to pass. And, slowly within two more days, the pain and the discomfort had passed. During this time I lost 30 lbs. I had arrived at the Institute weighing 190 lbs. — and after 12 days my weight was 160 lbs. I was completely cured. I then started to eat some sprouts and continued the wheat grass therapy. Each evening I would sit comfortably at the dinner table at the Institute and eat moderately of the living food of sprouts. Each morning I would drink watermelon rind juice, which in a short time did remove the cloudy quality of my urine. Within a short span of two weeks, I was better . . no operation was necessary nor will it be necessary, for both Roberta and I have now understood the benefit of the suggested diet of Ann Wigmore which eliminates all cooked foods, all refined, canned and processed foods, together with the avoiding of milk products and meat, fish, eggs, no grains, except sprouted.

We will keep this new regimen — which was given us at the Institute . . . and we will . . . in our walk of life and in our work, suggest this to all.

Our love is perhaps the smallest thing we can give to the people at the Institute . . . who are all working so hard to really bring LIGHT, LOVE and UNDERSTANDING to all humanity, plus saving lives. They did so with mine, with God's help and faith.

For study in color, live food, music and community living please write to me: Charles V. Martignoni, Brothers of Francis of Assisi,
19 Central Ave., Ravena, N.Y.

THE SEARCH FOR HEALTH BY HYPOGLYCEMIC

Dear Victor,

I will begin by saying that I had hepatitis and Anne as a child had many illnesses, appendicitis, chronic infected tonsils, pneumonia, etc., all caused by a combination of drinking contaminated water and eating devitalized foods. Breathing impure air was another factor.

In 1965 I suffered a severe heart attack. At this time Anne started to work in a textile factory; she became very ill and the doctor diagnosed it as hepatitis. The chemicals and fumes had been disastrous for her and she worked until she collapsed. After her recovery (which proved to be partial) she went to work in an office. Some of her co-workers smoked and because there weren't any windows for ventilation there wasn't any fresh air and the effect was very harmful.

Because neither one of us had the good feeling of having healthy bodies we had started to seek ways to help ourselves. We read numerous books written by nutritionists who advocated the natural diet. We purchased whole food, organically grown when possible, and traveled many miles to a Health Food Store. We were faithful to this program. We have believed for many years that people should be healthy in spirit, mind and body. God does not want us to be sick. No matter how diligent we were we couldn't attain the exuberant feeling that comes with good health.

While following the advice of one of the leading nutritionists in the country the results were not as we believed they would be so after reading an article in "Let's Live" magazine about drinking raw carrot juice we decided to purchase a juicer and try it. We felt better and proceeded to follow a raw vegetable and raw food diet as advocated by Dr. Norman Walker.

As it was impossible to have all of our food chemical and pesticide free, we ate oranges that had been sprayed. This was a big factor in our breakdowns. We do not have any professional proof of this but we know it happened. We ate oranges when our energy became low, never suspecting that we were actually taking poison into our systems. I was in a state of collapse and Anne worked under extreme physical stress until she was finally forced to quit.

Before we collapsed we had been seeing a medical doctor regularly and even with repeated tests he would not say it was low-blood sugar or hypoglycemia. I had been in the hospital and had extensive blood tests, gall bladder series, chest X-rays etc. I was released and although I did not have any reserve energy he seemed to ignore this fact. I did not seek another doctor because I vowed I would never go through this testing again. It was horrible!

We were desperate so we inquired to see if there was any place we could go that used the raw juice and raw food therapy. We were given the name of Hidden Valley Health Ranch, Escondido, California.

Dr. Spector who was our doctor at Hidden Valley has degrees in medicine, chiropractic and naturopathic. He was recovering from hypoglycemia and because of his own personal experience recognized what our trouble was very quickly. He questioned me concerning our diet and when I told him about drinking carrot and spinach; carrot, beet and cucumber juice combinations plus raw food he said that we never should have been sick. He believed me without any doubt when I explained about the sprayed oranges. He is the best doctor I have ever consulted.

The important thing was that the doctor (a Naturopath) diagnosed us as having hypoglycemia. He told us to eat bananas because this fruit would bring the blood sugar up slowly, whereas too sweet fruit forces it out. He also advised taking protein before we ate the banana. Yogurt was the choice because we did not eat meat. We could not tolerate cows milk in any form but ate it because he said it was important. We finally told him of the intolerance and were allowed to substitute goat milk instead. He was wonderful to us and helped us to the point that following a stay of one month we returned home. Since we were unable to care for ourselves we went to live with my mother. She lives in the city which was a drawback because we were following this doctor's instructions which included walking and deep breathing. Again the carbon monoxide from automobile exhaust kept us from gaining like we should.

At this time Anne read a leaflet explaining about wheatgrass.

Although weak we started to raise wheatgrass and sprout seeds. About 6 months later we were strong enough to return to our own home . . . we live in the country!

We followed the wheatgrass therapy faithfully for over one year. It was used for implants as well as drinking. We drank rejuvelac, sprouted different seeds, raised buckwheat lettuce, sunflower greens and drank sesame and sunflower seed milk in addition to our other foods. We were gaining but because of going to the city to keep doctor appointments, shopping, etc., the unhealthy fumes were again taking their toll.

Victor, we don't know why we kept subjecting ourselves to carbon monoxide fumes, cigarette smoke etc., except that it meant staying at home, therefore   being with family or friends and we didn't make that decision until forced too. It was difficult to give in and admit that our livers were being continuously weakened and could not function. Finally, the only trips we did make were to the Doctor of Chiropractic.

The first part of April of 1972 after such a trip we were caught in intensive carbon monoxide fumes. From then on was a nightmare. We made reservations to go to the Institute for the 25th of April. We were able to take care of ourselves but the ride to the Airport — the wait in the terminal — confinement on the plane — the ride through Boston (all polluted environments) served to be all that our livers could take. It wasn't long while at the Institute until we could not eat any foods except the greens and sprouts. We drank rejuvelac, and wheatgrass juice but these foods were not enough to sustain us, and we became weaker and weaker.

Upon arrival at the Homestead you served us a glass of raw beet and carrot juice . . . organic! This act proved to be our salvation. I said to Anne — "Organic carrot juice — remember Dr. Walker!" And from then on we drank carrot juice; how well you know this, dear friend.

We were so weak that we could not take care of ourselves. I had been caring for Anne at the Mansion but only because I prayed every step of the way. The 25th of May when we knew you would take us to the Homestead came not one moment too soon. I knew I couldn't make those stairs again.

The carrot juice and the green sauces started the cleansing of the body as well as providing the nourishment we needed and we started to improve. Also, cleansing the colon with enemas were helping to rid the body of so many toxins. You know the benefits of zone therapy and deep breathing and Victor do you realize the value of those beautiful green plants and trees around the Homestead? We cannot find words to express our gratitude for the care you, Renee, Ray and others gave us — only God Bless You.

So to the   present: what we are doing now is essentially the same as in Stoughton. Our diet is raw, of course; however, if the body craves a cooked food we usually bake some onions which takes care of the craving. This doesn't happen too often. We have 1 pint a day of carrot juice. During the summer months we shall have other vegetable juices. Our blended sauces consist of greens and "weeds" and all other vegetables in season. We use olive oil (1 teaspoon each per vegetable sauce), kelp (¼ teaspoon each per day), dulse (washed well, no salt at all) and pure apple cider vinegar (2 to 3 teaspoons with the meal if desired). Also we drink distilled water. The fresh fruits are banana, avocado and Delicious apple, the dried fruits (soaked) are fig, peaches, and apricot which we blend either together or with banana. Remember the banana is the sustainer. We tried to eat fermented sesame and sunflower seeds but cannot tolerate it. We also made sauerkraut (without salt) and find it agrees with us.

About two months ago I read in the "Provoker" a recipe for a whole grain, dried fruit cereal; it is mixed in proportion and allowed to soak 24 to 48 hours. It can be eaten as is but we still must blend.

We take 2 high enemas each day and soak our feet at least once. We walk and do a lot of deep breathing. Besides using the slant board we do stretching exercises and some modified yoga postures as our strength allows. We brush our bodies daily with a natural bristle scrub brush and bathe every day. We get at least 8 hours sleep with fresh air circulating in our rooms and also rest when the body requires it throughout the day. We go outdoors as much as possible.

We have made such good progress but are far from being healed. It will require prayer, time and effort. This experience has been very hard and I cannot explain the bodily discomforts, the complete weakness as well as the emotional feelings that have been part of it. Spiritually we have both gained more than words can express. I understand my fellow man as I never dreamed I could.

We are going to garden! My son wants to raise a lot of food this year — all organically of course. Our land has not had a chemical or pesticide put on it for 25 years — only the organic fertilizers that build the soil plus hay, straw, leaves and sawdust for mulch and the trimmings from our fruits and vegetables.

Anne and I work a little while, rest and do some more followed by more rest. The benefits from the air, sun and working in that soil are going to speed our healing.

One last thing Victor, I am sorry we became so bad after we reached the Mansion. We wouldn't have gone there if we had known that we would not have been able to take care of ourselves, but regardless of rules there is always the chance that someone might need the care that Anne and I received. After all — God works in mysterious ways — and everyone who helped us will benefit spiritually.

I have written this the best I know how, but should you have any questions just write or call.

Peace be with you.   Love, Vernie & Anne

Dear Vernie and Ann:

You certainly have gained in wisdom and love through your healing experiences. I learned much from you while caring for you during your two month stay at the farm. I know your struggle has been persistant and honest. It will take many years to bring the liver back to health, but your progress is evident.

Some comments about your diet are in order. Although it is superior in choice, it is not optimal. Vinegar is too acidy and for a person with hypoglycemia and on a low protein diet, it is highly undesirable. It can lower the hemoglobin level and keep one feeling weak. A better choice is lemon or lime. Figs are too concentrated in sugar for individuals who have hypoglycemia. Most authorities forbid the use of bananas during the healing period — besides the high sugar, they reduce the rate of body cleansing. The introduction of grains, especially combined with dried fruit, is sure to bring on some indigestion, plus the high sugar complications.

I believe that besides the environmental factors and inorganic foods which further impaired your health some of these dietary misconceptions, inspite of an almost optimal program for healing, is extending the duration of your recovery.

Love, Viktoras

HYPOGLYCEMIA HEALED

My Dear Viktoras,   April 20, 1974

I'm sorry I didn't get a chance to answer your last communication — been real busy. Didn't know where I was going to get the time to write you all that you want to know. So car broke down and I'm grounded for 2 days so that's that. Okay. Here goes.

Hypoglycemia, also referred to as low blood sugar, was triggered off in 1966 by 2 major shocks: one mental, the other physical. The first one, my father died unexpectedly; the other, which took place shortly after, was being hit by a N.Y. cab while riding a scooter.

My symptoms were lightheadness, dizziness, headaches, fatigue, depression and inability to remember instructions on the job, which led to my dismissal.

It was while I was on unemployment I got into yoga practice with Swami Satchidananda at the Integral Yoga Institute in N.Y. It was also at the same time that I began medical therapy supervised by Dr. Sacharan of West 58th St. My therapy consisted of a high protein diet, meat 3 times daily, taking salt to bring the sugar up, large massive doses of vitamins and adrenal cortex shots to restore the functions of the adrenal glands, shots to restore memory & to kill unfriendly bacteria in the blood. I also underwent hypnotherapy, actually self hypnotherapy as instructed by Dr. Geandry to get me out of the depression & the suicidal frame of mind I was in — as can be expected under the circumstances.

All was going well till Swamiji lowered the boom by giving a talk at the Institute on the dangers of drug taking and how it can impair not only your physical body but your spiritual body as well.

After the lecture I presented him with my problem. His advice to me was to get off the medical therapy and become a vegetarian, first by eating fish excluding meat, then exclude fish and just eat vegetables and fruit, nuts, etc. I followed this advice with no ill effects.

Then a man by the name of Sri Ravan came to talk at the Institute as a guest of Swamiji's. He had read Dr. Ann's literature while in England and decided to come here and investigate for himself. Consequently he turned me on to her book WHY SUFFER and together we went off to Prospect Park in Brooklyn to gather some soil for our wheatgrass boxes. Using the old meat grinder as she suggested in her book was o.k. for a start, but my system was just lapping this stuff up and I couldn't get enough so I invested in a long distance call to Boston to ask her if I might not come there and work for my therapy. She agreed that I could as she was terribly short of help. Well I dropped everything, packed my bags and off I went.

Well the first 5 days were really rough. I had never fasted before and here I was fasting on fresh extracted chlorophyll from wheatgrass, which has the highest potency of chlorophyll of any living plant. I stayed on this for 5 days; then for 6 weeks I continued drinking 4 oz. at a time, 4 times a day and eating 2 or 3 meals of grapes in between — and not many at that.

Well! Fantastic things started to happen. After about 6 weeks I became the original 100 pound powerhouse. Prior to that I was not much help to Dr. Ann as I was mostly found in a horizontal position, resembling a yoga posture which I believe is called the Dead Man Pose.

However, after 6 weeks, one day I awoke and I felt I had the strength of 10 lions or I should say elephants; lions don't eat grass. I took over the planting of the wheatgrass which was backbreaking work, especially when it got up to 9 or 12 trays (15 to 30 pounds per tray), carrying them down a block long hallway in the basement of the Mansion getting them into a little narrow elevator and to the 2nd and 3rd floor to put on racks in front of windows to let the little white shoots get the light that was to turn them bright green. I took over the post completely to give Dr. Ann an opportunity to spend more time writing and corresponding with people all over the world.

Then glorious spring came and with the instructions of a 60 yr. old lady, a guest from Wisconsin, I broke the soil and planted a ¼ acre garden out at our summer farm in Stoughton. I opened the farm up and made it liveable for guests after it had not been used for 3 years. I rented a machine and cut down all the hay around the property by hand. Took me from sun up to sun down with just one break for a glass of chlorophyll, nature's green magic.

I planted 13 fruit trees and flower bed, cleaned the house from bow to stern, 2 floors, picked up the guests at the Mansion and supervised them to keep them on the program. When the wheat truck came in I was at the Mansion to put away the 100 pound sacks which meant I would be dragging them through that block long hallway to a storage room on the other end next to the planting room, into the room one by one. Then I'd pick them up to stack them on top of each other — 10 to 15 sacks high. After finishing that, I would sweep & mop down the entire basement, go up and start preparation for dinner which consisted of delicious raw food preparations, or I would get out to the farm to do whatever was needed out there. I did all these things with such joy in my heart. Never did I feel the strain of too much work. I had unlimited strength. Gone were the symptoms of low blood sugar.

After not seeing me for about 2 months my Guru's words to me were, "But my child you are so light." He was of course seeing the inner light that comes from a peaceful body free of disease. That's about it Vik. Hope you can use this.

Take care and God bless you. Bhavani.

I met Bhavani about 1 year after her recovery. She had just returned from Mexico. Over 6 months time was spent on a fruit diet, weeks of fasting, yoga, meditation and clean air. She looked 16 years old, although she was well past the age of 30. As I worked with her, I found her to be a dynamo of power, love, charm and beauty. Wherever she lectured, she had followers. Her clearheadedness was shown in her well organized business activities, travels and social life. Six years after her rejuvenation, she is younger and healthier. Her diet is mostly raw food. At the Mansion, the jobs that she used to do alone, have since that time been taken over by 4 boys.

HYPOGLYCEMIA AND SCHIZOPHRENIA

Dear Victor: The lecture you gave in New Haven was a revelation on diet. The stay at Hippocrates Health Institute has changed my life.

Today, I adhere to a diet of greens, sprouts and plenty of spring water. I cannot eat much protein since this seems to disturb me. I have found it best not to consume sugar in any form, including fruit. If I break this rule, I cannot stop eating.

I have found that air pollution has a very disorganizing effect on hypoglycemia. My liver and lungs don't function well in the city and I become very disorganized.

It's been 2 years and 8 months since I've stopped taking tranquilizers after having taken them for 13-1/2 years. I have had approximately 8 electric shock treatments and every tranquilizer available in the market and none really helped me. As a matter of fact because I am hypoglycemic they had the opposite effect on me.

Today I use Alcoholics Anonymous and Schizophrenics Anonymous plus good diet to stay off tranquilizers and all medication, including aspirin. I have taken no pills for two years.

I am in the process of forming a Hypoglycemic group based on natural therapies to help others. Interested parties please write to me. Your friend, Lynette J. Johnson, Apt. 26, 39 Spring St., Htfd, Conn. 06105 (4/7/74)

HYPOGLYCEMIA AND WHAT IS NORMAL

Dear Friends,   1/4/74

Today there is so much confusion about mental illness, its cause, symptoms and cures, I feel it worthwhile to share my experiences with others.

I suffered through schizophrenia intensely over a two-year period. I became a patient at five different mental institutes, all to no avail. I was administered somewhere in the neighborhood of 1500 mg. of Thorizine daily during my stays. All of the various drugs, tranquilizers and psychotherapy made the going rougher.

After experiencing extreme nausea, muscle spasms, frightening states of paranoia and suicide, something had to give. Through a loving friend, I was introduced to megavitamin therapy. Alas, I was returned to "normal" functioning within six months. It was very reassuring, though I missed a true feeling of well-being. I dug deeper, and discovered through various tests that I was anemic, had poor digestion, bromide poisoning, weak kidney and pancreas. Good grief! How do I cope with all this? I'd heard of your wheatgrass therapy and sprout diet. It made sense so I gave it a try. After just a few weeks on this cleansing program and implanting the wheatgrass juice, I woke up with a new look at life. It just hit me one day that I was feeling healthier, like what I used to daydream was impossible.

I tried in vain to share this health discovery with my "normal" associates. BAM! It hit me that what is considered "normal" health is actually sickness. Most all were nursing a chronic disease. Analyzing their diets uncovered a heavy intake of sugar and dead foods. What a set-up for conditions of hypoglycemia!

I went into deep reflection of my past diet and realized I'd been on a collision course since birth.

With every new day now, there is an upliftment in my spirit and well-being. I feel regeneration taking place throughout the body. I have alertness and control over emotions and situations that present themselves. What a blessing your work has brought me. Let's tell the world that "good" health is the normal state. One should strive to reach it.

Thank you and God bless you.

                                                                                    GEORGE SCHMALL

CANCER, ENZYMES AND RAW FOODS

Dear Dr. Wigmore,

Thank you for your letter and pamphlets which I find rather educational and interesting.

The article: "Raw Vegetables Seen As Cancer Curbs" by Mr. Snider is not complete because it is known that there are proteolytic enzymes in raw vegetables which are mainly responsible for the reduction of incidents of cancer with people who eat mainly raw vegetables. It is possible to eat or administer the same enzymes in concentrated form and with this even inhibit cancer genesis more than by eating raw vegetables only. Also the formation of metastases can be inhibited to a great extent which was proven here in Europe in a number of clinical study programs. You may read a book: "Enzyme Therapy" by Dr. Max Wolf and myself (Vantage Press Inc., 516 West 34 Street, New York, N.Y., phone 212/736-1767) in which you will find most of the experimental and clinical data of the value of special proteolytic enzymes in inhibition of carcino-genesis and arteriosclerosis. My research-workers and I have published a number of papers further documenting the value of proteolytic enzymes or uncooked food which contains a lot of proteolytic enzymes, whereas in cooked food most of the proteolytic enzymes are destroyed. I think it would pay if you would incorporate some of these findings in your prints.

I shall be in the United States during most of October and lecture in several cancer research institutes and universities. Maybe there is a chance to meet with you.

                                                                                    Dr. Karl Ransberger

MENSTRUATION

Dear Viktoras: What a wonderful gift I received on my 35th birthday, August 7th--a copy of "Survival Into the 21st Century." I spent my birthday on the beach pouring over the contents in a great frenzy to take in as much of it as possible! I was a patient of Dr. Bieler's until his death almost a year ago, so you can imagine my joy in findng you speaking of toxemia, the detoxification regimens and all the principles I either learned from Dr. Bieler or have come to find out about by myself. Your book has answered so may questions I have had about my remaining health and detox problems--problems I had come to believe were just never going to be solved. Anyway, your book has given me a new jolt of confidence to continue with my own purification process and a renewal of enthusiasm over the directions I am following.

The greatest value of your book for me personally was its lifting of my concern and worry about the cessation of my menstrual periods after a year on my Bieler diet. After a few months on the initial detox diet Dr. Bieler set down for me, all usual symptoms accompanying menstruation (tender breasts, fatigue, nervousness, abdominal discomfort and heavy bleeding) stopped. Then my periods came every other month, every 56 days exactly. This happened for six months. Then my last period--January 1975. I haven't menstruated since. Nothing I read, norr anyone I spoke to, had any answer. Dr. Bieler said simply that my body not "had more important things to do" and seemed to indicate that the menstrual function would return when my glands rebalanced themselves. My good friend, Rob, a young doctor just beginning to practice nutritional medicine here in California (I'll tell you more about him later) was convinced the amenorrhea was nutritionally based and gave me supplements guaranteed to work within four months. Nothing happened. That's where I stood when I got your book--and what a relief. I've thrown out those awful supplements and now know I will never menstruate again and that there's nothing wrong with me. My husband is quite intrigued, and even amused, over this whole turn of events...Optimal Health and Peace, Connie (Calif   1976)

SOUL-STIRRING STORIES
of
Spiritual, Mental and Physical Health Betterment
made possible by the
One Hundred Fifty Year Longevity Society
of the
SEICHO-NO-IE
[Home of Infinite Life, Wisdom and Plenty]
78 Onden 3, Shibuya-Ku, Tokyo, Japan

A few months ago, the details of wheatgrass therapy came into my hands. The simplicity of the whole idea appealed to my commonsense and what its use had demonstrated so conclusively with "incurables" in the United States, agreed fundamentally with what my nutritional investigations had brought to light through the years. Grass is generally considered food for farm animals but I firmly believe that wheatgrass holds within itself a mysterious healing power for suffering human beings that is not found in any other vegetation and which defies analysis to single out. Its superiority cannot be ignored and I am vastly pleased that under the competent guidance of Mr. Hikokichi Sugimura, of "One Hundred Fifty Years Longevity Society" of SEICHO-NO-IE, in the City of Toyonaka, Japan, wheatgrass therapy has been brought to suffering humanity on a scale that has enabled an average of thirty persons a day, for many months, to test its effectiveness on their own bodies. So grateful were the participants of this humanitarian enterprise that they voluntarily forwarded to me their individual testimonials set forth herein and which I am sure will be of tremendous benefit to unfortunates throughout the world.

May the blessings of the Almighty be showered upon you and your activities.

Masaharu Taniguchi, Founder
Seicho-No-Ie

CANCER BREAST. STOMACH TROUBLES.

MRS. CHIYOKO NAKATA. Age 47. Nishinomiya, Japan — For the purpose of receiving medical treatment, she was hospitalized and underwent two operations for breast cancer. After leaving the hospital she was not in good health so she returned there regularly to receive further medications. Meanwhile she was taking a glass of wheatgrass manna each day. In a month, her complexion had cleared up, the signs of the cancer had entirely disappeared and she seemed in normal health.

PLEURISY — ACUTE

MR. INOSUKA NAKATA. Age 62. Nishinomiya, Japan — His condition changed rapidly for the worse soon after he was taken ill in the middle of June and he was bedridden for a month suffering from a high fever. He underwent medical treatment to lessen the water in his body and his doctor advised immediate hospitalization to avoid a worsening of his condition. He rejected the idea because he was convinced that the WHEATGRASS JUICE MIGHT HAVE A REJUVENATING EFFECT and took the mannas regularly twice a day. Although the doctor regarded his condition to be serious the sufferer gradually swung around to bettered health. Finally the danger was over and his chest felt normal. He has returned to work but still takes a wheatgrass manna each day he makes from grass grown in his own garden.

PROLPASE OF ANUS. PILES

MRS. YOSHIKO KUMATANI. Age 50. Amagaski, Japan — For several years she had suffered intolerable pains when she answered the call of nature. Her doctor, after due consideration, told her that her pains would never cease unless she underwent an operation. Although it was not a question of live or die, he advised strongly that an operation be undertaken. During the weeks she was considering his counsel, she had been dipping a piece of gauze into the pure WHEATGRASS JUICE and had applied it to the affected part, leaving it there as a POULTICE DURING SLEEP. At the end of about three weeks, the evidence of piles entirely vanished. No operation was deemed necessary.

ECZEMA — WATERY . . . HIGH BLOOD PRESSURE

MR. HACHIRO KUMATANI. Age not given. Nichinomiya, Japan — Although he had suffered every year for a long period with a watery eczema, the wheatgrass pulp which he applied to the upset condition of his skin was very effective. This was done in addition to his taking his regular drinks of the wheatgrass juice.

His high blood pressure was of long standing. He had taken many types of medication for it through the years but it kept coming back. He found that after he had ACQUIRED THE HABIT FOR WHEATGRASS MANNAS, THE BLOOD PRESSURE WAS BACK TO NORMAL. He discontinued it some little time ago, but the blood pressure remains down.

CARBUNCLE

MR. CHITOSE HARADA. Age 45. Osaka, Japan — During the first part of May, a carbuncle, which appeared on the sufferer's right thigh, put him in a high fever and caused acute pains. Although a medical doctor advised an operation, to let out the pus, the PATIENT STAYED AT HOME AND TOOK SEVERAL DRINKS OF WHEATGRASS MANNA EACH DAY. In six days, a large amount of the pus was discharged as the carbuncle opened of itself. In a week's time thereafter he was back at work.

TUBERCULOSIS

MR. ICHIRO NAKAGAMI. Age 45 Hachoji, Japan — Mr. Nakagami has had direct contact with the activities of the Seicho-No-Ie for approximately ten years as his sister works at the Seicho-No-Ie headquarters. He had enjoyed good health and was in high spirits until sometime during the past spring when he became tremendously fatigued, lost seven pounds in weight for no apparent reason and suddenly developed fits of coughing which brought blood to the surface. A reputable doctor declared him to be a victim of tuberculosis. He had assumed a most important post with a company the preceding October and hard work plus deep responsibility had undoubtedly affected his nerves. Being a pious individual, he did much self-analysis and realized his unfortunate physical condition was the direct result of this new employment. He realized that the tuberculosis had been brought on by his constant worry as much as by some deficiency in his nutrition. He felt that a healing could come through faith so when his doctor suggested hospitalization, he flatly rejected the idea. He remained in his home, devoting his time to spiritual enlightenment feeling that a closer association with the Almighty would rectify matters both mentally and physically. But the coughing up of blood did not cease and early this year, his elder sister, Mrs. Ishii, brought him some wheatgrass manna to try. Following her advice, Mr. Nakagami continued to take the WHEATGRASS MANNA FOR A FULL WEEK EVERY MORNING AND EVENING AND, MUCH TO HIS SURPRISE, THE COUGHING UP OF BLOOD CEASED ABRUPTLY. And, as he continued the drinks, his weight began to increase and three months later an X-RAY EXAMINATION COULD DISCLOSE NO SIGN OF THE TUBERCULOSIS. The doctor was much mystified by THE QUICK RECOVERY WHICH HE SAID WAS UNPRECEDENTED IN THE ANNALS OF MEDICINE.

CANCER OF THE LARYNX

NAME — WITHELD — For reasons that will be explained — The man in question holds a high position in a prominent company in Japan and his wife learned secretly, through his doctor, that he was a victim of cancer of the larynx. The mental attitude of the unfortunate at that time prevented the physician from disclosing the truth to the sufferer. The wife had the doctor use all manner of treatments, including cobalt rays, as the "Time Limit" on the life of this victim was somewhere between a "possible three and six months" unless a miracle happened. The wife came to the Seicho-No-Ie to pray and to obtain cooperative prayers. There she was introduced to the wheatgrass mannas. She induced her husband to use the drink regularly merely as a possible "health measure" while she continued her prayers for his quick recovery. In short weeks she greeted us with the words "a miraculus healing!" Still she kept her secret and it later developed that the cobalt rays had caused ulcers to appear on the throat. She applied the pulp of the wheatgrass to these and continued giving her husband the manna drinks. Recovery — complete recovery - seems assured. But his name cannot be divulged because of the very nature of his work.

HIGH BLOOD PRESSURE GRAY HAIR

MR. HISAKI YAMAGATA. Age 77. Tokyo, Japan — While drinking the wheatgrass mannas, which he extracted from grass he grew in his garden, his GRAY HAIR BEGAN TO TURN TO BLACK — ITS ORIGINAL COLOR. He also discovered, to his great satisfaction, that his high blood pressure had gone down materially. Now that he had regained his health he wanted to share his knowledge with sufferers around him. He came upon the case of CANCER OF THE STOMACH in a man who held a responsible position in his community. This man was taking medical treatment but was dissatisfied with the slow results. Also he disliked the idea of taking drugs so he consented to try the wheatgrass mannas without telling his physician. The results were really miraculous. IN A VERY SHORT TIME, HIS SYMPTOMS DISAPPEARED, THE X-RAY PHOTOGRAPHS SEEMED TO INDICATE A COMPLETE RECOVERY and his physician could not understand the rapid change for the better but gave the credit to his medication which, he admitted, had never before shown such results. We have not as yet the permission of this man to give his name so will include this report in that of his friend.

OLD AGE

MR. ICHIGORO BAN. Age 83. Tokoyo, Japan — At the morning services at the Seicho-No-Ie headquarters, generally gather 13 devout human beings who partake the wheatgrass mannas as a sort of daily ritual. Among them, the eldest of the group, is Mr. Ban who laughingly proclaims himself in this manner: "See, I am quite young." And he certainly looks the part. HIS HAIR USED TO BE GRAY BUT RECENTLY IT BEGAN TO CHANGE BACK AGAIN INTO ITS ORIGINAL COLOR, BLACK. So far, fully one-third of his hair has lost the ashen hue entirely. This transformation has done much to popularize the wheatgrass mannas as the other members of the group have now visual evidences of what it can do physically as well as feel the revitalizing effects in their own bodies.

The other day, a reporter speaking to this little group of 13 gathered together for the morning service made inquiry how the wheatgrass mannas seemed to be benefiting the spirituality, the mentality and physical being of each. "OH, FATIGUE WITH ME USED TO BE A TREMENDOUS PROBLEM," said one. "But that is a thing of the past". Another remarked: "MY SKIN HAS RECOVERED THE SMOOTHNESS I THOUGHT WAS LOST FOREVER." And then the reporter noticed that while the group of 13 would have averaged rather high in ages, THEY ALL LOOKED YOUNG, ALERT, HAPPY AND THEIR SPEECH WAS cheery and hopeful. Mr. Ban, according to the reports of those who had known him for many years, was now younger in looks and far more youthful than as they remembered him a full decade before.

OFFENSIVE BODY ODORS. NERVOUSNESS

WEAKNESS

MISS UMEKO KATO. Age 28. Tokyo, Japan — According to the diagnoses of doctors, Miss Kato was a victim of low blood pressure. She was so weak physcially that the medical men would not risk giving her a "shot" of drugs. She devoted much attention to the teachings of the Seicho-No-Ie and looked forward for divine healing. This gave her mentality a much needed lift. Her spiritual devotion seemed to have overcome much of her nervousness and she considered herself healed in that particular but the weakness of her muscles remained. Last spring, she began using the wheatgrass therapy BY TAKING ONE DRINK OF THE MANNA EACH DAY AND THE RESULTS WERE MOST SURPRISING AND PLEASING. "The weakness seemed to melt away and the 'cobwebs' in my brain vanished as a new alertness made itself felt. The odor of my body, which had been so embarrassing for many years, disappeared and did not return. I found that dipping a piece of cotton in the pure wheatgrass juice and dabbing in under my arms made every bit of perspiration odor vanish. And now let me add something that should interest all women — the wheatgrass drink is easy to take, I like the flavor and it has made my skin soft and velvety."

WOMB CANCER

MRS. KIMIE ITAKURA. Age 49. Izumo, Japan — It was shortly after her 60 days hospitalization for womb cancer, and following the 30-day treatment of the ailment by cobalt rays, when she began to suffer acutely from pains in her womb. This was augmented by a bleeding which made urination every hour essential. The doctor suggested that the cobalt rays MIGHT have caused an ulcer to form which probably had spread to her rectum. This made evacuations necessary almost every hour. BY TAKING THE WHEATGRASS DRINK EACH MORNING, Mrs. Itahura found that the bowel movements became normal, the desire to frequently urinate ceased and the pains gradually abated in her womb. The bleeding ended and it has been many weeks since that deliverance was accorded her with no sign of a reappearance of the trouble. It might be added here that a young lad, known to Mrs. Itakrua, underwent an operation for intestinal ulcer and his body thereafter kept weakening until hope for his life was almost despaired of. THE TAKING OF WHEATGRASS MANAS each morning changed the situation entirely, the recovery was rapid and the boy is now out of danger.

SENILITY

MRS. TERU TAKESADA. Age 84. Tokyo, Japan — She is a senior sister of an artist named Seiei Ogawa, who has an international reputation. Early this year she had been kept in bed because of her senility. Living close to her home was a Mr. Kamegoro Ogata, whom the world might well designate as the senior member of our "One Hundred Fifty Years Longevity Society." Learning about her condition, Mr. Ogata took her some of the wheatgrass manna and encouraged her to take it as a "medicine". She tried the flavor, liked it and remarked that IT TASTED LIKE A "GREEN TEA." SHE COOPERATED WITH THE IDEA THAT THIS MIGHT HELP HER AND INSIDE OF 60 DAYS WAS UP AND around walking on a pair of "getas" — Japanese wooden sandals — which she had longed to do.

LITIASIS IN URETHRA

MR. TOSHI YOSHI HASHIMOTO. Age 44. Osaka, Japan — This sufferer had undergone two operations and still was a victim of acute pains every time urination was necessary. He afterwards tried various types of treatment over the course of many months. In the middle of this June, the calcium in the tubing practically prevented him from urinating at all. The medical doctor advised a third operation but he rejected the idea because of the lack of results from the first two. About this time, the wheatgrass mannas were brought to him by a member of the "One Hundred Fifty Years Longevity Society." TWICE A DAY HE TOOK A GLASS OF THIS LIQUID AND WITHIN THIRTY MINUTES AFTER THE SECOND DRINK ON THE FIRST DAY, HE URINATED FOR THE FIRST TIME 24 HOURS. The swelling in his abdomen went down at once. The two drinks a day for a week seems to have put this trouble to flight.

PYORREA

MR. YASUO AOKI, Age 29, Tokyo, Japan — "I have had several back teeth which the dentists had been treating for years and the trouble seemed to be beyond their skill to rectify. Quite recently, however, these bad teeth seemed to have brought on something even worse, pyorrhea in the teeth along the front of my lower jaw. THIS CREATED AN OFFENSIVE BREATH THAT WAS QUITE DISAGREEABLE TO OTHERS, AS IT WAS EMBARRASSING FOR ME. The extraction of these teeth in the lower jaw was advised by the dentist after a futile effort on his part to treat them successfully. As I am young, I was reluctant to have these teeth taken out and false ones put in their places which I knew would be far inferior to the real ones. I utilized prayer each morning in an effort to find healing. Those supplications relieved my tensions, subdued my worries and I felt that I was on the proper road. After one of the morning services at the Seicho-No-Ie, I was provided with a "breakfast" there. Quite accidentally, I was given an opportunity to try the WHEATGRASS MANNA AND THE NEXT MORNING, MUCH TO MY SURPRISE, THE PUS AND BLOOD WHICH GENERALLY WAS IN MY MOUTH WAS ABSENT. This made me consider carefully what had happened so the second morning I again took the manna. Since then, by continuing the wheatgrass mannas each morning, the signs of pyorrhea have disappeared, my front teeth are tight once more and all talk of extraction by the dentist has been abandoned."

TUBERCULOSIS, INFLAMATION OF
THE BACKBONE

MR. NIKUS KANALI. Age 52. Nishinomiya, Japan — After having spent five long years in a tubercular hospital, receiving the usual medical treatments — without making much progress in health — he returned to his home, hoping that "natural methods" might help his serious condition. It was in the middle of May when his family began growing wheatgrass in their garden. HE WAS GIVEN A DRINK OF THE MANNA EACH DAY WITH THE RESULT OF A RAPID IMPROVEMENT IN HIS HEALTH. Following what he had regarded as a complete recovery, he went to the hospital once more for a thorough examination. NO TUBERCULAR BACILLI COULD BE FOUND IN HIS BLOOD. It was the beginning of June, after he had discontinued the wheatgrass, the lower part of his body became afflicted with terrific pains. He lay helpless on his bed for a full half a month as the doctors tried to determine what caused the miseries. Finally it was determined that inflammation around the backbone was the cause. It was at this point, HE MADE THE DECISION TO TRY THE WHEATGRASS MANNAS INSTEAD OF DRUGS. Again he was rewarded with recaptured health. He is continuing the drink regularly now.

FATIGUE . CHRONIC DIARRHEA. FEVER.

MR. TAKUJI SUGIMURA. Age 15. Toyonaka, Japan — In the beginning of April this boy complained of total fatigue. Then cramps and nausea disabled him as his fever rose to a dangerous point. His doctor suggested that he take a chloromycetin tablet every four hours. But the fever continued and the pain in the abdomen was intense. The family nurse, at this point gave the lad a drink of wheatgrass manna which seemed to be just what was needed to still the fever. His temperature quickly returned to normal, the pain left him and during the following week he returned to work. He continues to use the mannas.

WARTS - THREE ON FINGER,
EIGHT ON THIGHTS.

MISS MIDROI FUCHIWAKI. Age 14. Tokyo, Japan — At the time she entered the junior high school, the warts were small but they soon began to enlarge rapidly. It was in August of this year when she came bursting into the assembly room at the Seicho-No-Ie bubbling gayly that the WARTS ON HER HIPS HAD VANISHED. In answer to questions, SHE ADMITTED THAT SHE HAD RUBBED THE PULP OF THE WHEATGRASS AGAINST THOSE WARTS FOR SOMETIME — SINCE EARLY MAY. SHE ALSO HAD USED THE PULP ON HER HANDS AT NIGHT WHEN SHE WENT TO BED AND DRANK THE WHEATGRASS MANNAS REGULARLY. Those warts also were gone. Her mother, delighted with the turn of events for her daughter admitted that she, too, had been taking the wheatgrass mannas and that HER CONSTIPATION, OF NEARLY TWENTY YEARS STANDING, WAS NOW OVER AND HER BOWEL MOVEMENTS WERE NORMAL.

MENSTRUATION

Dear Viktoras: I've just been reading your book, "Survival Into the 21st Century", and I was really interested in the section on menstruation.

I was a complete vegetarian by the time I was 15 (I'm 18 now). My periods began to cme less frequently (about once every 3 months) and then stopped altogether about 2 years ago. My parents were really worried about this, but I felt better than ever so wasn't too concerned. Mom took me to a gynecologist who did blood tests, etc., and said I was "amazingly healthy". He also said he could put me on the pill and get me started again! NO THANKS!

I was getting around to thinking that since I was feeling so great and not menstruating, perhaps menstruation was a sympton of a "disease" rather than the old "normal, natural process".

I got to thinking that on my natura diet, I had "de-domesticated" myself and that my body was behaving accordngly. So I tried an experiment about 9months ago. I ate dairy foods for a few days to see the effect. Sure enough, I got 2 periods after that. Since then I've becme increasngly confident that not menstruating is natural and that diet is the key. I eat fresh fruit, raw vegetables and sprouts, some nuts and seeds and very little cooked food except for some occasional grains in the winter. Anyway, thanks for the book. It's inspiring andreassuring. Love, Tracey (Australia 1977)

THOUGHTS ON HEALING

The reader will find useful with very toxic persons or those suffering from bad digestion to use dilluted, slightly simmered fresh vegetable juices (or if can tolerate - fresh juices) in conjunction with a diet of lightly cooked, non-starchy, mucuslean vegetables, which may be blended with fresh ones. Green juice mixed with tablespoon of seed yogurt will supply a complete meal and slow down cleansing reactions. The cooked foods should be excluded as soon as the person can handle juices, sprouts and vegetables of low roughage.

BOOKS ON HEALING

The many books that are mentioned are for the expansion of knowledge and experience in the field of healing. The author does not necessarily find agreement with all the matterial contained in the books. If any practice, diet or theory is in conflict with the ideas of "Survival", the reader should give careful thought, study and experimentation. The author feels that the content of survival will not be contradicted.

RECIPES

WHY SEASONING? Fresh organically grown foods are high in flavor, a delight to the palate. You can learn to enjoy them without seasoning.

Inorganic salt is not a food; it is not utilized by the body. Some of it is retained, causing stiffening of the joints, arthritis, hardening of the arteries and kidney disease. Eating grains encourages the craving for salt. In a high enough concentration it inhibits cell metabolism, eventually causing death of the cells. To reduce the concentration of salt, your body will retain an excess of water in the tissues.

Sea Salt may be substituted for the supermarket variety. It, too, is a chemical; so you should use it sparingly.

During the transition, the fermented oriental seasonings (miso, tamari) can add delightful flavors. However they contain sea salt and should be excluded from the diet as soon as possible.

Vegetable seasoning (sometimes called broth powder) is a substitute for salt. But be careful in choosing — it sometimes contains salt, artificial coloring and flavoring and a filler of brewer's yeast and soybeans which might combine poorly with other foods. It may not be made from organically grown products.

Seaweed is the best choice for salty taste. Kelp is a good protective food; it contains all the trace minerals from the sea and has been shown to prevent absorption of strontium 90 and other poisons into the body. Dulse leaves are delicious. Dulse should be soaked in water (this is true for all sea vegetables) to soften it and to wash away the sea salt. Kelp, wakame, nori, kombu, hiziki can be found in most macrobiotic stores. Sea vegetables are food and seasoning. They contain organic salts in an easily assimilable form.

Herbs used with discrimination can subtly enhance the flavor of food. Pick them fresh from your garden. In winter, grow them in pots on your window sill.

Garlic, onion, cayenne, chili and ginger root are noted for healing qualities when one is eating a cooked food diet. They provide flavor for the transitional diet; however, once the body is detoxified, they can act as irritants to kidneys, liver and the mucous lining of the digestive tract.

COOKED FOOD

Cooking: Use only glass, porcelain, enamel or stainless steel utensils. Cook at a low temperature, only long enough to break down fibre or starch. Avoid cooking any seed, beans, nuts or oil-very hard to digest. Never cook green vegetables more than five to ten minutes. Cooked greens can be gas-forming. Best to cook are potatoes, root vegetables and squash. Never eat hot food; always let it cool to body temperature.

Add sprouts to cooked food only the last minute before serving.

Always use distilled water. Rain is water distilled by the sun. Today, due to atmospheric pollution, rain water is not fit to drink. Water may be partially distilled by freezing. Let it thaw. Pour off the water into another container having the precipitated sediment. Freeze again. Each time the process is repeated, the water becomes purer.

You can make a simple solar distiller. Fill a dark bowl with water and place it inside a clean large polyethelene plastic bag. Tie the end of the bag. The sun will cause the water to evaporate from the heated bowl. The vapors will condense on the plastic lining and collect in the bag into a pool of water. Cooked foods may be used sparingly during the early stage of transition to a better diet.

DUTCH OWEN

IRON POT MEALS A cast iron Dutch Oven with a heavy, tight-fitting lid may be purchased at department stores, new age health food grocers or at a second hand store in a variety of sizes. It is cheaper to operate than a regular oven and emits practically no odors. It is ideal for preparing warm food for the student away from home, the lone roomer, the business girl or the couple living on a meagre pension in small quarters. It eliminates hour of drudgery as it only needs to be brushed out once a week.

To prepare the iron pot for the evening meal, line the bottom with flat stones or a grating to prevent vegetables from burning. Scrub all the vegetables carefully with a vegetable brush as the skins should be eaten. Place vegetables in the pot, place over high heat for five minutes, then turn heat low. Baking times will vary.

One Hour: Large beets, carrots, sweet potatoes, plaintain, rutabaga (small or halved), turnip, potato.

Half Hour: Yellow squash, parsnips, peas, beans, sweet corn (husk will turn black).

No more than two cooked vegetables at a meal. Live food should always be the main dish, with cooked food used as a dessert.

COOKED COMFREY SOUP

Lots of comfrey leaves, include stems and flowers. Chop up fine. Cover with water. Bring to a boil. Simmer for few mintues. Cool. Blend and serve over baked potato or with wakame or dulce.

CHOW MEIN

1 cup mung bean sprouts
1 cup lentil sprouts
2 cups sliced onion

1 cup mushrooms
1 cup chopped celery
¼ cup olive oil
Tamari Sauce and sea kelp

Simmer mushrooms, onions, celery in a little water until soft.
Add oil, sprouts, seasoning. Heat but do not cook. Serve over millet or brown rice.

MILLET SOUP

1 cup millet ½ cup onion, chopped fine
1 cup okra or half cup Irish Moss (optional)
2 tablespoons oil

1 teaspoon sea kelp
3 cups water

Wash millet. Soak overnight in 4 cups water. To cut cooking time, blend. Add onion. Simmer for 30 minutes or until there is no starchy taste. Cool before serving. Add thinly sliced okra, sea kelp, oil and sprouts if desired.

GREEN LIFE SOUP

2 cups buckwheat greens
5 tender leaves comfrey
1 cup zucchini

several tomatoes, or 1 cup carrot juice
or rejuvelac
dash kelp

Blend all ingredients. Recommended during wheatgrass therapy for ease of digestion. May be served twice a day, using one to two cups per meal.

SOY LOAF

2 cups soy bean sprouts (lentil, mung, chick pea)
4 medium carrots
4 celery stalks

3 medium onions
herbs, kelp, or veg. powder

Grate vegetables or run through a meat grinder or grass jucier. Blend soybean (other sprouts should not be blended) sprouts with water to a creamy consistency. Mix all ingredients. Use as a salad dressing, soup, form into patties and cook slightly on a skillet or bake as a loaf at 350 degrees for at least one hour (until brown). Eat sparingly — it is very filling.

SEA STEW

6 large leaves Wakambe
1 large leaf Dulce
1/4 cup chopped agar-agar (optional)

1 cup water
4 medium chopped onions

Let the sea vegetables soak in one cup water for about one hour. Simmer onion in ½ cup water for 5 minutes. Add sea vegetables. Simmer for 10 minutes or until the wakambe starts to turn jelly. Cool it. Add sprouted mung, lentil, wheat and or chick peas. Season it, if you like, with Brewer's Yeast.

VEGETABLE POT

Avoid seasoning. Cook vegetables that taste good without seasoning. Combine any three in desired proportions: carrot, turnip, sweet potatoes, butternut squash, potato, oinion. To cook: steam in own jucies or bake in oven.

THE THIRD EYE

SALAD — Choose fruits and vegetables locally in season to save money and to get fresh produce. If you have any indigestion or feel tired after a meal it is probably from eating too much or not combining foods correctly. Limit your salad to a few selections. Start learning to think of your salad as a complete meal.

Arrange the salad so it will be tasty and colorful. Vegetable shredding tools introduce variety of texture and reduce the need for lengthy chopping.

A good quality juicer   and blender (a $20 Hoover is one of the best buys) are a must during the dietary transition, especially for those with poor teeth or a weak digestion. A manual juicer for weeds, grass, sprouts and green vegetables can be a tool essential to survival.

A hand-operated grain mill can be used to grind seed (sesame, sunflower) to a relatively fine powder to mix with water for milk, cream, dressing or yogurt. You can make green vegetable puree by adjusting the mill to fine grind. Though not as efficient as a blender, the mill is useful during emergency or non-electricity oriented subsistence living.

Do not use vinegar, lemon or lime in salads. Many authorities claim the acid partially inactivates chlorophyll. It also slows protein digestion by inhibiting the secretion of gastric juice. It interferes with starch digestion by inactivating the secretion of ptyalin in the saliva. (FOOD COMBINING MADE EASY, Shelton)

Delicious flavoring can be created through the use of rejuvelac, sorrel, dandelion, pepper, onion, garlic, parsley. To thicken sauces, you may use avocado, plain or fermented seed, comfrey, agar agar, wakame, okra, purslane, buckwheat greens or oil.

Vegetables such as pepper, onion, cucumber, after removal of the inner portion, may be stuffed with other foods, such as sauces, for variety.

SPROUT SALAD

6 parts mung beans	1 part lentils
1 part alfalfa seed	1 part fenugreek seed

Mix seed in buckets and soak for 16 hours. Transfer to buckets with holes perforated in the bottom. Grow for three days in a warm room, flooding the sprouts with water at least 3 times per day. During rinsing, many of the seed hulls are skimmed off the top of the bucket. This method is for growing a large quantity of seed with minimum labor. Refrigerated, will keep for up to 4 weeks. Serve with Beet Treat or Seed Sauce.

To produce long sweet sprouts from a mixture of mung, it is very important to keep the sprouting seeds in the dark. The seeds should be covered with a wet cloth and a plastic sheet which gives a tight fit (or dish or lid).

BEET TREAT

6 parts sesame or safflower oil	1 part water
2 parts Biotta beet juice (or 1 lemon and 1 beet)	1 part kelp
	1 part Dr. Bronner mineral seasoning

Shake thoroughly and serve over Sprout Salad. At health conventions, this combination has been our favorite for introducing people to sprouts and living foods. Everyone calls our booth delicious. (Maybe too delicious. This dressing should be used only during transition to a more pure diet).

COMPLETE MEAL SPROUT SALAD

6 parts mung	2 parts alfalfa
1 part lentil	1 part fenugreek
½ part aduki (optional)	1 part sunflower greens
1 part buckwheat lettuce	

The seed may be sprouted in a bucket with holes on bottom. The buckwheat on cotton towels, and the sunflower in jars. Chop the greens. Toss the salad, serve with sesame-sunflower yogurt, which you can dilute with rejuvelac. Add a few sprigs of dulse or a dash of kelp. Note, this meal derives from items that can be stored in quantity for a long period of time. It makes excellent survival food.

GRASSHOPPER SOUP

20 leaves sorrel
20 leaves tender comfrey
10 leaves tender lambsquarters
3 tender leaves milkweed
1 medium zucchini, chopped

1 flower cluster milkweed (optional)
1 large tomato (optional)
1 avocado (optional)
1 clove garlic
2 cups rejuvelac (wheat or millet)

Pour rejuvelac into blender. Add gradually all ingredients. Blend in avocado last.

BEET SOUP

1 large beet diced
½ avocado
1 to 3 cloves garlic

1 cup rejuvelac
1 lemon or lime to taste (optional)

Blend garlic and beet with rejuvelac. Reduce to creamy consistency. Add other ingredients. Blend. Before serving (optional) add two tablespoons homemade sauerkraut. Serve over chopped sunflower greens and a few leaves of dulse.

GREEN FLESH SOUP

1 cup chopped buckwheat greens
1 cup chopped spinach
1 medium tomato

½ avocado
1 to 4 cloves garlic
kelp to taste

Blend and serve.

GUACAMALI

1 ripe avocado
2 diced tomatoes
Seasoning is optional

1 lemon
1 diced red pepper
onion or garlic to taste

With a fork, blend avocado to creamy, lumpy consistency. Combine with other ingredients. Sprinkle tomatoes on top. Serve as a raw sandwich on a lettuce leaf or as stuffing for a tomato or pepper. Variations: 1 small diced spanish onion, freshly minced chili pepper, juice of one half clove of garlic. Combine with celery, lettuce, mung bean sprouts for a complete meal. Russian dressing: Add more water and onion, blend.

SEED MILK

½ cup sesame seed (almond)   2 cups water or rejuvelac

Blend for 1 minute at high speed, ½ cup rejuvelac or water with seed. Gradually blend in remainder of rejuvelac. Strain out pulp. Season to taste with kelp or dulse. Some find the sesame taste too strong, and prefer a 50-50 mixture of sesame and sunflower. You may soak the seeds overnight, then blend. Milk from grains is not recommended. Even after sprouting, they are still rich in starch. After making wheat milk, let it set for five minutes. The glass will be one third filled with white starch sediment. Starch cannot be easily digested in the stomach — it must be thoroughly moistened with saliva. Similarly milk made from mature coconuts can cause indigestion due to the residue of fibre and saturated fat.

COMFREY CREAM SOUP

15 comfrey leaves
2 ripe tomatoes
½ cucumber
1 stalk celery
1 green pepper

1 avocado
1 sprig parsley
1 clove garlic
1 cup rejuvelac
1 tsp kelp

Blend at high speed all ingredients except avocado. With rejuvelac, reduce to desired consistency. Add avocado. Blend. A complete meal.

COLD COMFREY

comfrey leaves
avocado

carrot or other juice
garlic if desired

Place juice in blender. At medium speed, blend in enough chopped comfrey to make a thick sauce; serve over indoor greens. Or reduce consistency to soup.

RAW SEED SOUP

½ cup seed (sunflower, almond, sesame, pumpkin or sprouted soybeans)

2 cups warm water or rejuvelac
seasoning

Soak seed overnight (or grind to fine powder). Blend seed with one cup water at high speed for at least one minute. Add more water if needed. Blend in greens (buckwheat, comfrey, zucchini) if desired. For a more spicy tang, add onion, garlic, chili or dry cayenne pepper. By varying consistency, it may be transformed into a sauce or a party dip.

RICH GREEN SOUP

2 cups indoor salad greens
1 cup rejuvelac or water
seasoning to taste

¼ ripe avocado OR
2 tbs. cold pressed olive oil OR
¼ cup ground sesame or sunflower seed
 – fresh or yogurt

Blend greens, fluid and seasoning. For thickening, add seed, oil or avocado. Buckwheat is best choice for indoor greens. Serve over sunflower greens.

WINTER SOUP MEAL

1 cup indoor greens
1 cup green vegetables
½ cup sunflower seed

onion to taste
cayenne (optional)
hot water

Blend ingredients to desired consistency. Very tasty when prepared from buckwheat greens and/or comfrey. Pour over sunflower greens, mung sprouts and dulse. A warm satisfying winter meal.

For sauce blend indoor green with only one cup water. Serve over sunflower greens, mung sprouts, a few dulse leaves.

GREEN QUEEN

1 avocado
1 cup chopped celery
¼ cup radish sprouts

1 tbs. kelp
juice ½ lemon (optional)
½ cup rejuvelac

Blend ingredients to desired consistency. Serve over sprouts.

GAZPACHO

1 red pepper chopped fine
½ cup sliced celery
2 mint leaves or fresh ginger root, chives,
 onion or garlic if desired.

2 large sliced cucumbers
3 large tomatoes, cubed
¼ lemon (optional)
sea kelp

Blend red pepper and celery with small amount water. Season with mint or ginger root (optional). Add lemon juice and follow with cucumbers and tomatoes, blending at slow speed. Do not liquefy— vegetables must be identifiable as cucumber and tomato. Blend in other seasoning if desired.

BORCHT

2 cups chopped beets
½ cup almonds
1 small green onion

2 cups rejuvelac
½ lemon (optional)
seasoning

Liquefy to desired consistency. Serve over sprouts.

HOT RED SAUCE

3 medium tomatoes
1 cucumber
1 onion or garlic
 curry powder and/or cayenne

¼ cup oil
½ cup water
1 lemon

Blend ingredients. Season to taste. Should be used during transition diet only.

SWEET COMFREY SOUP

15 medium leaves comfrey
1 small chopped zucchini

½ avocado
1 cup carrot juice

Blend ingredients and serve.

FREE COMFREY SOUP

1 small chopped zucchini
½ Avocado (or few leaves of soaked wakambe
    or ¼ cup ground sesame)

6 oz Bista beet juice (or fresh carrot juice)
10 leaves of chopped comfrey

Blend to desired consistency. Add Avocado last.

APPLE SAUCE

2 large diced sweet apples
¼ cup raisins

2 teaspoons lemon juice
¼ cup apple juice

Pour juice into the blender. At low speed, work in raisins, followed with apples, and lemon juice. May blend in a little ginger to give it tang. Raisins may be replaced with ½ cup ground sesame seeds, substitute ½ cup water for lemon. A complete meal.

HEAVENLY CITRUS

3 oranges sliced
1 avocado squashed

2 tangerines slivered
1 cup grapefruit juice

Mix and serve

HERMINT

2 super ripe bananas
1 cup rejuvelac

mint leaves

Blend banana and rejuvelac for 15 seconds. Blend in mint to taste.

PARADISE CITRUS

1 cup carrot juice   ½ unripe papaya
Blend. In minutes enzyme reaction produces most delicious golden pudding.

PRUNEDATE

5 pitted dates (or figs)
3 large pitted prunes

½ cup cold water
¼ cup hot water

Blend fruit in cold water to creamy consistency. Blend in hot water and serve over sliced ripe banana.

COMFREY TEA

Grow your own comfrey. Gather several dozen leaves cutting near soil. Chop stems (crush with bottom of a glass to release juice) and leaves fine. Cover with distilled water. Place on slow fire until heated, but do not cook. Allow to stand until liquid is dark brown. A very refreshing drink. If not used soon, refrigerate to prevent fermentation. Use it to prepare sauces and soups.

Fresh comfrey juice may be obtained by blending comfrey with water, then straining out the pulp.

REJUVENATION NECTAR

1 Cup Chopped Sunflower Greens
1 Cup Chopped Buckwheat Greens
1 Cup Alfalfa Sprouts (or complete meal sprout salad)
2 tbs. Fenugreek Sprouts
1 Clove Garlic (optional)

4 tbs. Sauerkraut (optional)
1 Stalk Celery
1 Sprig Parsley
½ Cup Chopped Spinach
1 Cup Chopped Favorite Weeds (optional)

Run the vegetables through a manual grass juicer. To get all the juice out, run it through at least 5 times, it has salty very agreeable taste. You may sweeten the drink by adding an appropriate amount of carrot juice.

AMINO ACID ELECTROLITE BROTH

1 qt water
2 tsp brewer's yeast
1/2 tsp Dr. Bronner's Powdered broth
    seasoning (optional)
1/4 tsp organic mineral salts
1/2 - 1 tsp dark liquid aminos
    (soy sauce, tamari) or
    Dr. Bronner's or Bragg's liquid aminos.

Pinch of dry parsley
Add at will: unsalted onion powder, savory,
thyme, marjoram, sage, garlic
powder etc. Can use as much
as desired to taste. Or other
dried leafy herbs: basil, a little
oregano.

1/4 tsp kelp or dulse powder

Cook at no hotter than 130 degree temperature. Use cooking Thermometer. Strain and sip cool, hot or cold.

Brewers Yeast is a predigested protein, rich in B-complex vitamins. It is much easyer to digest than seeds or nuts. Because it is highly concentrated it should be used in moderation. Add 1 tbs to a salad or prepare it in the Amino Acid Broth. When using it, be sure to combine it properly.

CARROT COCOA

Juice the following proportions:
1 oz. dandelion greens (or 1/2 oz. root)
1 oz. Beet root

10 oz. Carrot

If the taste is too bitter add extra carrot juice. Excellent blood builder, liver and kidney cleanser.

MENUS FOR A FAMINE

Breakfast: 8 oz. Rejuvilac, followed 30 minutes later by 3 oz of green juice (weeds, grasses, sprouts, indoor greens).
Lunch : Same as breakfast. Add 2 tbs of fermented seed sauce.
Supper: 1 pound of sprout salad (mung alfalfa, lentils, fenugreek, sunflower & B buckwheat)
    1/2 cup of sesame-sunflower jogurt. May delute with rejuvilac. For extra nutrition blend or add the juice
    (pulp Optional) of comfrey, indoor greens, weeds and sprouts. Season with kelp. (see page 314)

Don't waste anything The pulp, after extraction of juice from sprouts, indoor greens (hard shells removed) should be composted or else converted to a raw vegetarian loaf. The grains in   can be made into chapattii - sun baked bread. The rinse and soak water of sprouts should be used to water comfrey, indoor greens. Urine and fecal matter may be composted. When in season dry fruits, vegetables, weeds and other wild food. Soak them before using.

LIVE ORGANICALLY ON 24 CENTS A DAY

At wholesale prices you were able to purchase in Nov. 1974 the following items for survival. 2 pounds of lentils ($.80), 6 pounds mung ($3.60), 1 pound alfalfa ($1.80), 1 pound fenugreek ($.60). This will produce about 40 pounds of sprout mixture at the cost of 17 cents per pound. 1 pound buckwheat or unhulled sunflower cost about $.30 which produce 8 pounds of greens at the cost of 4 cents per pound. During a day, a person may eat the following amounts: 1 pound of sprout salad at cost $.17; 1 pound of sunflower-buckwheat mixture @ $.04; 5 oz grass juice @ $.03; 16 oz. Rejuvilac @ .02; 1/8 pound of sesame - sunflower @ $ 10 ; 1/3 oz kelp @ $.01. Total Cost for one day $.37 The cost may be further reduced if sprout salad is replaced with sunflower-buckwheat indoor greens. Reducing cost to 24 cents per day. Frequent use of weeds and fasting can reduce cost to ten cents per day. (see page 96)

VIKTORAS CITY SURVIVAL DELICIOUS DRINK

1 cup sprout mixture
1 cup chopped sunflower greens
1 cup chopped buckwheat greens
2 tbs homemade sauerkraut

1/2 cucumber (optional)
1 cup leftover salad or grated tubbers (optional)
1 cup greens or weeds to tatste (optional)

Grow sprouts long enough (at least 4 days) until starchy taste is gone. The hulls from indoor greens do not have to be removed for juicing. If sauerkraut not available may use Biotta sauerkraut (or beet) juice obtainable at health food store. Or may use instead sorrel or sour grass, or 2 tbs of fermented seed sauce mixed into the drink before serving.

VIKTORAS SURVIVAL SALAD

Mixture of favorite sprouts, half cup seed yogurt, sauerkraut and kelp to taste. If have chewing problem, run sprouts through a juicer with a little rejuvilac. Instead blender, may use the manual grain mill.

RAW SPROUT LOAF

The pulp from juicing sprouts plus hulled indoor greens can be mixed with finely grinded cellery, onion, garlic. Season to taste with vegetable powder, dulce or kelp, brewer's yeast. May add a little oil and hot pepper. Form into loaf. Expose to sun for at least 1 hour. Serve with fermented seed sauce.

INTESTINAL GARDENS

Their lips blossomed with the glowing flowers of youth. Fragrance of budding orchards charged the air; every word they spoke filled the atmosphere with joy of life. Such lovers were the sons and daughters of nature formed from the essence of ripe fruit.

The same fruit fed their beautiful, healthy intestinal flora, first implanted by mother's milk.

Many of today's lovers are not so fortunate. The advertisement media lure us "back to nature" if we buy scented "breath fresheners." They fail to tell us why we need these palliatives.

Bad breath is a sign that the original health-promoting intestinal inhabitants have been crowded out by putrefactive bacteria. These destructive bacteria grow in intestinal soil made too rich in nitrogen from a faulty diet. However, friendly bacteria can be persuaded to return to the intestinal tract if given a diet which permits them to thrive there.

Breast milk contains lactose, a form of sugar which aids utilization of protein and the absorption of calcium. This sugar acts as a bifidus factor. In breast fed baby's intestine we find practically pure Lactobacillus Bifidus. Lactobacillus Bifidus acts as protection against invading organisms. L. Bifidus culture is implanted through mother's breast milk during the first 48 hours of baby's life. This culture is good for a lifetime. However, because of bad eating habits, the L. Bifidus is lost to putrefactive bacteria, which generate poisons and offensive odors that leak into the bloodstream; through the years, they injure every gland, organ and tissue of the body.

According to Metchnikoff of the Pasteur Institute, "The presence of a large number of lactic acid bacilli will interfere with the development of putrefactive bacteria."

Ann Wigmore states:" In a healthy person, the enzymes are manufactured by the body. However, when the glands, nerves, muscles, and even blood of an elderly person becomes overdrawn, the body becomes weaker and weaker. The skin wrinkles, the hair thins and turns gray. During my many years with sick folks, I had the great privilege to observe what enzymes can do in health building. I was born sickly and had poor digestion all my life. Yet, I can keep healthy and full of energy, applying the catalyst enzymes in extra form by drinking rejuvelac, the fermented soak water of wheat. I drink six glasses every day. Life begins with catalysts and continues only through them."

Today doctors are discovering that many diseases and old age are traceable to enzyme deficiency in the food eaten, in the human cells and in the digestive tract. The peoples noted for longevity — Georgians (Ural Mts), Hunzas (Himalayan Mts), and Ecuadorians (Andes Mts) — consume a great deal of nature's predigested foods such as sprouts and fruit, also foods partially digested by bacteria such as yogurt, sour pickles, sour beets, sauerkraut and fermented green vegetables. These people are noted for their good digestion. Other factors considered, the consumption of predigested food still plays a major role in their excellent health.

Dr. Kuhl, a German researcher, has this to say regarding fermented foods: "The natural lactic acid and fermentive enzymes which are produced during the fermentation process have a beneficial effect on the metabolism and a curative effect on disease. Lactic acid destroys harmful intestinal bacteria and contributes to the better digestion and assimilation of nutrients. Fermented foods can be considered predigested foods. They are easily metabolized even by persons with weak digestive organs. Fermented foods cleanse the intestinal tract and provide a proper environment for the body's own vitamin production within the intestines. They also help a person with constipation problems." Furthermore, Dr. Kuhl, as the originator of the lactic acid fermentation diet for cancer, requires that 50 to 75 percent of the diet to be made up of lactic acid fermented foods. (Kuhl, "Checkmate For Cancer," Viadrina Vertag, A. Trowitzch, Brounlage, Harzburger Str. 6, West Germany).

The following letter was received by Ann Wigmore from an independent researcher: "You have opened a Pandora's Box with that Rejuvelac. Its potentials are tremendous. That Rejuvelac sounded like a nutty idea to me and I didn't even want to get into it but you kept hounding me on it so I figured I had better see what gave, I had no idea how even to start but start I did. I used a 2:1 ratio of water to wheat as you recommended and kept it on the top of my hot water heater where the temperature maintained an even 70 degrees F. Each day I poured off the Rejuvelac and ran a series of tests on it. After the second day, there was a slight sour odor which I couldn't quite identify. But after the third day, the odor was unmistakable. It is similar to the odor of milk turning into yogurt (lactobacilli) or the odor of beer (beer yeasts called Saccharomyces cerevisiae). I ran a bacteria culture on it and it was loaded with lactobacilli and yeasts.

"So very much depends upon the temperature at which you make the rejuvelac. The type of bacteria and yeasts depends so much upon the temperature. Too high or too low temperatures might well produce undesirable microflora. As a starter, temperatures should be maintained between 68 deg and 77 deg F.

"There is so much literature on fermentation of grains that I don't know where to start. Dr. Kuhl of Germany has done extensive work with fermenting wheat berries and has designed many of his treatments around the fermentation products. I have much of his literature and the fermentation chamber designed by E.L. David of England to be sure of getting the desired type of fermentation. You could well spend the rest of your life working on the fermentation products of wheat.

"The rejuvelac is undoubtedly rich in protein, carbohydrates, dextrines, saccharines, phosphate, lactobacilli, saccharomyces and Aspergillus oryzae. Amylases are derived from aspergillus oryzae and they have the faculty of breaking down large molecules of glucose, starch and glycogens. That is the reason Rejuvelac is so beneficial to your digestion. Rejuvelac is related to beer, although there is no alcoholic content. It is rich in the B vitamins. It is related to Brewers Yeast and is high in protein.

"Very roughly: Most beer is made from barley. The barley is sprouted to produce amylase which has the property of saccharifying the starch to sugar. The sprouts are then dried. It is then known as malt. When ready to use, the malt is ground up and placed in spring water and fermentation starts. The starch is converted to sugar by the amylase and the sugar to alcohol. After reaching the desired stage, the mix is boiled to stop the enzymatic action and then filtered.

"At what stage your rejuvelac would go to alcohol, I don't know. You play around with it and I am sure you will find out.

"Another idea is to save a little of your 'old' rejuvelac to inoculate the starting rejuvelac. The fermentation would get off to a faster and a cleaner start. You would eventually develop your 'own strain' of fermenting yeast. The Brew Masters all have their own strains of yeast."

"For example, I have made yogurt for years and have developed my own strain of yogurt bacteria. I always save a little yogurt to inoculate my fresh milk with. I would guess you could reduce the 3 day rejuvelac down to two days and have a better product.

"I might add that the 3 day rejuvelac was superior to the 4,5, and 6, and 7 day. The 'spent' wheat could be dried and ground and used as Brewers Yeast." (Harvey Lisle, RD1, Norwalk, Ohio, 44857.)

Most literature on yogurt deals with cow's, goat's or mare's milk and the changes brought about the lactobacillus bulgaricus (or acidophilus) and streptococcus thermophilicus. It has been observed that acidophilus bacilli create an acid medium in the intestine, destroying and unfriendly, disease-producing putrefactive bacteria which are associated with protein. Protein feeds the putrefactive germs but does not nourish the acidophilus bacteria. The good flora subsist, generally, on carbohydrates.

There are, however, many friendly bacteria which predigest RAW protein into amino acids, while creating lactic acids, enzymes and many vitamins, especially vitamin K and members of the B-complex family such as Vitamin B-12, riboflavin, niacin, biotin and folic acid.

Ferments made from seed milk have many advantages over animal milk products. If the seed is organically grown they are free from the pollutants that are often associated with dairy products. DDT, strontium 90, iodine 131, antibiotics, stilbesterol and the toxic by-products of pasteurization.

To make non-dairy ferment, yogurt or cheese, the following seed may be used: unhulled sesame, mixture of unhulled sesame and sunflower, almond, cashew, soaked soybean, sprouted soybean and hulled millet.

To make fermented water or rejuvelac, the following seed may be used: wheat, hulled millet, oat, sweet brown rice, rye, rice, barley, unhulled raw buckwheat. The drink can be made from whole, finely ground or sprouted seed. If seed are sprouted you should blend them when making the rejuvelac.

Seed ferments are lower in concentration of protein and are much easier to digest than the dry seed. They are delicious with sprouts, vegetables and sub-acid fruits (tomatoes, apples). Ferment them only until the mixture tastes slightly tart. Do not permit it to become too sour. If the temperature is too warm, fermentation can turn to putrefaction. If the ferment tastes very sour or smells rotten, don't eat it. Keep the temperature between 68 and 100 degrees F. A 25 watt light bulb or an insulated candle in an enclosed box can provide the desired temperature. Good ferment may be kept a whole week in a refrigerator. If the whey separates out, mix it with a fork.

In making fermented seed preparations it is very crucial that a temperature between 70-100deg. F. is maintained. To get a faster and tastier product, use ½ to 1 cup of previously made seed ferment in the new preparation. Keep a lid on to prevent the entry of other bacteria. In the first batch, it is a good practice to use rejuvelac as a starter.

FERMENTED FOODS
REJUVELAC AND FERMENTED DRINKS
Acid Forming

1 cup wheat (or other seed)   2 cups water

Grains: Organic hard or soft wheat, rye, barley, triticale, oat, millet, rice mixture of grain. Use only the highest quality seed. Avoid old, cracked or rancid grain.

Washing: Place grain in strainer and rinse thoroughly in a basin of water until free of dirt, dust, and chaff. Organic waste will cause the rejuvilac to spoil more quickly.

Water: Distilled water is best. If not available, add a dozen grass blades to purify the water. With distilled water, healthy rejuvilac production for at least 6 weeks from same batch of seeds can be obtained.

Container: Glass is best. Never use plastic jar or cover. Use cloth to cover the jar.

Spice: Most delicious effects are obtained with dill (fresh or dried), garlic, pickling herb mixture, hops. Strain.

Spoilage: Can happen because of excessive soaking or heat, bad seeds, contained water. A good ferment will taste slightly lemonish and have a sweet sour fragrance. If it doesn't feel right, do not drink it.

Temperature: 60–90 deg. F. is acceptable. Best around 70 deg. F.

Usage: As a morning drink, substitute for lemon, starter for seed yogurt, mixture for grass or green juice. If poor quality wheat is used, pour off to compost or water plants with the first 2 soakings, especially if liquid has a yellowish–brown color, it is acid, rich in enzymes and can be used as digestive aid to nuts, seeds and cooked protein, such as beans.

Method 1: Soak seed for 24 hours (in summer, only 16). Pour water into container. Use wheat for sprouting or planting. Let "soak water" ferment in warm place for 36 to 72 hours; then refrigerate. Shake the jar before pouring off the rejuvelac.

Method 2: After 2 to 3 days of soaking the seed, you may start drinking the ferment. After each drink, refill the jar with water to previous level. This makes a delicious drink, similar to whey. Its high enzyme activity acts as a digestive aid. It may be used in all sauce preparations. If produced from high quality wheat with distilled water, rejuvelac can be active for at least 5 weeks.

  If not used continuously, keep refrigerated; periodically, pour off all the water and replace it with fresh distilled water. If Rejuvelac has an offensive odor or bad taste due to spoilage, pour off all the fluid. Rinse. Refill with water and start again. If it continues to smell, compost the whole thing.

Method 3: Grind the wheat (millet or rye). Use method 2. Will give a strong lemon–like flavor. Millet produces a most delicious sweet–sour, lemon–like drink. Discontinue production after 5 days. Use the wheat in making Essene Bread or Chapati or Sun Bread. (see recipe books available from Omangod Press)

Method 4: Sprout wheat for 48 hours. Blend (optional). Let it set for at least 48 hours. Drink only the clear water. After 5 days, use wheat in bread making or compost. This is the most successful method. Limit yourself to one cup. When sipped with a transition diet of cooked foods or nuts, it is a great enzyme booster. True joy.

SEED YOGURT

1 cup sunflower seeds   2 cups of warm water
  (dry, soaked, or sprouted less than 1 day)

Blending: Place seeds and ½ water in blender. (One of the best for the money is an Osterizer, with a glass top; the popular stainless steel total blender juicer has a weak coupling and will not last long with seed sauces). As mixture thickens, add remaining liquid gradually. The final product should have the consistency of very heavy cream or pancake batter. Be sure the seeds are thoroughly liquified. A good practice is to have seeds ground in mill before blending.

Fermentation: Pour into glass or pyrex container, filling to about ¾ level. Cover with towel or lid. Place it in a warm area (75 – 95 deg. F.) in sun or on top of radiator. (Other methods: Warm to 100 deg, not painful to finger, pour into non–plastic thermos bottle, close but do not lock; install a 15 watt bulb with socket forced through the cover of small (approx. 12"x 8"x 12") closed cardboard box; this will keep an even temperature of about 80 deg.

Whey & Ferments: When a liquid whey settles out in the bottom of the fermentation container, one can mix in the liquid (generally after 4 hours) for even fermentation with a more sour taste. If it is fermented too long, the whey may be removed by pressing an opening with a spoon in the solid yogurt and pouring out the whey through it. The whey would give the yogurt much too strong a taste. Science has established that whey has similar qualities to yogurt and when used regularly will correct internal sluggishness, gas, bowel putrefaction and constipation. It particularly helps in the absorption of minerals into the system, especially calcium. Seed whey has these same properties. The yogurt may be kept up to 3 days in refrigerator. WARNING: If the yogurt smells or tastes foul or too acidic, compost it. Some of the reasons for spoilage: bad water, old seeds with rancid oil visible, bad rejuvelac, wrong temperature. Inspite of the fact that it is a predigested food, one should not overeat. Rejuvelac, yogurts, and other fermented foods should be avoided if a person has a very acid urine, (less than 6.5 ph). Under such a conditon, build up the alkalinity with vegetable and green juices, and use the ferments and acid fruit in moderation.

Without Electricity: Adjust manual grain mill to finest grind possible. Mix ground seed with rejuvelac to a creamy paste. Pour into dish or jar. Cover. Ferment.

Variations: May add sesame seeds or nuts for variety of flavors. Commercial Tofu may be blended with Rejuvelac and allowed to ferment for 8 to 12 hours. Protein becomes easy to digest and the taste is superb.

Sourness Control: (1) Do not mix in the whey; which is very sour. Just scoop off the yogurt or make a hole on side of yogurt jar and pour off the whey. (2) Soak seeds overnight and ferment for 4 to 6 hours. (3) Sprout seeds for 24 hours and fermented for 2 to 4 hours. Most mild. Drain whey through cheese cloth or sprout bag* for 4-8 hours to get rid of lactic acid.

Usage: Salad and sprout dressing, very delicious with kelp and other spices. Makes a perfect meal with subacid fruit, apple, papaya. For a very heavy meal, if digestion is good, may mix with super ripe banana. Source of complete protein and Vitamin B−12. Can be used to slow cleansing reation.

*21st Century Products, P.O. 702, Fairfield, Iowa 52556

Best Cheese From Viktoras

1 cup Sunflower Seeds
(sprouted 0-8 hours)

½ cup soaked sesame seeds
2 cups water

Blend all in same way as seed yogurt. Let sit for 8−12 hours at 75−85 deg. F. Until it reaches desired tartness. Refrigerate for a few hours. Strain off the whey through cheese cloth, either by squeezing the bag or by letting it hang for 2−4 hours. The dryer the better. Will keep for a week, refrigerated.

Variation: Add while blending: 2 small beets, 2 cloves, garlic.

SALTLESS SAUERKRAUT

To make a big supply for a family: one bushel of white (or mixture of white and red) cabbage; two ounces of Juniper berries. Make the sauerkraut in a large 5 gallon earthenware crock, glazed inside. Obtain also a heavy lid and several large clean stones or bricks.

First, rinse and clean the container, lid and other accessories. Wash the cabbage leaves and cut them into very thin shreds, or grate them. Lay the first layer at the bottom of the crock and crush the cabbage with a heavy unbreakable bottle, until the juice runs out and froth is formed. Each layer should be pressed down so that the cabbage will be saturated with its own juice.

Sprinkle a few juniper berries on top and put in the second layer of cabbage, repeating the process until the container is nearly full. Lay a few cabbage leaves on top and cover with a plate. Put the lid on top and weight it with a heavy washed stone. The juice of the cabbage should cover all the cabbage layers. Place the crock in a warm place (70 to 80 deg. F) so that fermentation starts as quickly as possible. Cover the crock with a clean cloth to protect from dust. After a few days, and then every two to three days, remove all scum. Each time wash the lid and the stone in hot water. When the scum no longer rises, the process of fermentation is finished. The sauerkraut will be ready to eat in three to four weeks. Store it in glass jars in refrigerator. Immediately start your next batch. You may add to the cabbage sliced beets, carrots, cauliflower, wakame, onions, green tomatoes, peppers, cucumbers. Serve the fermented vegetables with sprouts or blend them with seed to make delicious salad dressings. Some persons claim they can get a quick batch of sauerkraut by placing several cups of ground wheat (barley or rye) on the bottom of the crock and then covering with large cabbage leaves to prevent the seed from mixing with the vegetables. This increases the rate of fermentation and gives a much more sour taste.

INSTANT SAUERKRAUT

Juice cabbage. Mix juice with pulp. Add other optional ingredients, spices, or herbs. Press down and cover with cabbage leaf and cloth. Keep at 70 to 85 degree temperature. Ready to eat in 2 to 3 days. Refrigerate. Use 2 Tbsp. sauerkraut to start next batch.

Viktoras 3 Day Sweet Beet

Peel beets, cut away damaged sections. Juice the beets, mix pulp and juice or use the grater (pg 277). Place all in a quart size (or larger) glass jar. Press down, leave about 2'' free from top. Add water to the one inch level. Put a loose cover or lid on top to prevent evaporation. Place in warm location 60 or 75 degrees F. Daily mix thoroughly the contents of the jar from top to bottom. Let it ferment 2-4 days. Refrigerate. Use it with sprout salads. Plain shredded beets are also an excellent addition to any sprout salads. The beet is far less acid then the cabbage kraut.

Perfect Dressing

2 cups sunflower

2 cups water

Have sunflowers soaked overnight. In addition, they may be sprouted for 4-8 hours. Use warm water for blending. Reduce the mixture to a cream with high blend for about 2-3 minutes. May add other favorite vegetables to flavor, such as parsley, cellery, pepper. Pour over sprout salad, shredded zucchini and dulce leaves for a perfect meal. I use this daily in preferece to fermentations. Other seeds or nuts may be used, but avoid the fat laden ones, such as cashews,…hard on the digestion.

SUN AND SOIL

6 oz. carrots

3 oz. yellow or red delicious apples

3 oz. sugar beets

If beets and carrots are inorganic, peel them. Cut off the ends. The least contaminated are the Canadian ones. Large carrots tend to be much sweeter than small ones. According to some authorities, when vegetables or fruit are juiced, most of the pesticides (which are oil derivatives and not watersoluble) are excreted with the pulp. When juicing, it is o.k. to mix some of the fruit and vegetables, since no fermentation problem ever develops because there is no pulp and no need for starch or protein digestion.

MELLOW MILK

WATERMELON RIND – Chlorophyl rich drink from the fruit family. A very rich source of alkalizing minerals. Be sure to wash the watermelon before juicing. Cut up the rind and juice. The flesh and seeds may be juiced an hour later. Not overly sweet, just right for summer months. Great kidney cleanser.

MELON SHAKES – Excellent choice is the honeydew, pick the soft, heavy, slightly yellow melon. Peel the skin. Juice the seeds and flesh. One of the most delicious drinks in the world. Cantaloupe is another very tasty melon for juicing.

PROGRAMMING OF HAPPINESS

Reprinted from HANDBOOK TO HIGHER CONSCIOUSNESS by Ken Keyes, Jr., Copyright
Vision Books, St Mary, Kentucky 40063

Love Everyone Unconditionally—Including Yourself.

> *The Way to Become
> a Living Lover:*

Use the Twelve Pathways to take you to the Higher Consciousness Planes of Unconditional Love and Oneness.

THE TWELVE PATHWAYS:

Liberating My Conscious-awareness

1. I am freeing myself from security, sensation, and power addictions that make me try to forcefully control situations in my life, and thus destroy my serenity and keep me from loving myself and others.

2. I am discovering how my consciousness-dominating addictions create my illusory version of the changing world of people and situations around me.

3. I welcome the opportunity (even if painful) that my minute-to-minute experience offers me to become aware of the addictions I must reprogram to be liberated from my robot-like emotional patterns.

Being Here Now

4. I always remember that I have everything I need to enjoy my here and now unless I am letting my consciousness be dominated by demands and expectations based on the dead past or the imagined future.

5. I take full responsibility here and now for everything I experience for it is my own programming and actions that create the reactions of everyone around me.

6. I accept myself completely here and now and consciously experience everything I feel, think, say, and do (including my emotion-backed addictions) as a necessary part of my growth into higher consciousness.

Interacting With Others

7. I open myself genuinely to all people by being willing to fully communicate my deepest feelings since hiding in any degree keeps me stuck in my illusion of separateness from other people.

8. I feel with loving compassion the problems of others without getting caught up emotionally in their predicaments which are offering them messages they need for their growth.

9. I act freely when I am tuned in, centered, and loving, but if possible I avoid acting when I am emotionally upset and depriving myself of the wisdom that flows from love and expanded consciousness.

Realizing Cosmic Consciousness

10. I am continually calming the restless scanning of my rational mind in order to perceive the finer energies that enable me to unitively merge with everything around me.

11. I am constantly aware of which of The Seven Centers of Consciousness I am using, and I feel my energy, perceptiveness, love, and inner peace growing as I open all of the Centers of Consciousness.

12. I am perceiving everyone, including myself, as an awakening being who is here to claim his or her birthright of the higher consciousness planes of unconditional love and oneness.

> *The Scale for
> Knowing Your Level
> of Consciousness
> at Each Moment:*

The Seven Centers of Consciousness:

(1) The Security Center
(2) The Sensation Center
(3) The Power Center
(4) The Love Center
(5) The Cornucopia Center
(6) The Self-awareness Center
(7) The Cosmic Consciousness Center

> *The Five Methods for
> Working on Yourself:*

(1) Memorize the Twelve Pathways and apply them to your problems.

(2) Be aware at all times of which Center of Consciousness you are using to perceive your world.

(3) Become more consciously conscious of the cause-effect relationship between your addictions and the resulting unhappiness.

(4) Use the Catalyst ALL WAYS US LIVING LOVE as a tool for cognitive centering.

(5) Use the Consciousness Focusing Technique which can enormously accelerate the reprogramming of your addictions.

SEED OF HAPPINESS

We will set forth three types of basic programming for your biocomputer and show the way they operate to produce unhappiness, happiness, or bliss.

DEFINITIONS

First we need three definitions:

1. Unhappiness is a psychological state arising from the more or less continuous disappointment, frustration, and suffering we experience when life repeatedly gives us what we do not want to accept.

2. Happiness is a psychological state arising from more or less continuous pleasure. Pleasure comes from that which we tell ourselves we want to accept.

3. Bliss is a state of continuous happiness.

THREE TYPES OF PROGRAMMING

In the Living Love Way to Higher Consciousness, we think in terms of three types of programs for our biocomputer:

1. Addictive Programming. This type of programming is tied in with emotional responses produced in the limbic areas of our biocomputer. The use of this type of circuitry makes us experience varying degrees of emotional tension regarding our fears and desires. When our biocomputer processes the incoming sensory information and finds that it threatens the fulfillment of any one of our addictive programs, our consciousness will be dominated by feelings such as fear, anger, resentment, jealousy, or anxiety. Even when we get what we addictively want, our wanting to keep things that way automatically creates a new addiction! And we are thereby even more deeply enmeshed in an endless network of emotion-backed demands that yield continuous threat, tension, and unhappiness.

2. Preferential Programming. When we have Preferential Programming, our biocomputer does not connect the fulfillment or lack of fulfillment with the limbic areas in such a way that emotional responses of fear, anger, jealousy, resentment, etc. are produced. For example, if one has Addictive Programming regarding clear weather during a picnic, he will upset himself if it rains and his "whole day is ruined." If he has Preferential Programming for sunny skies during a picnic, and the rain comes, he just notices that his preference is not being realized. He gathers the things together and continues to enjoy the picnic in the shelter of a gazebo or the car. The flow of the here and now appreciation of life is not upset when you have Preferential Programming.

3. Bliss Programming. When a person has escaped from all of his Addictive Programs and has enjoyed the happiness-yielding Preferential Programs for a sufficient period of time, it is possible to work toward what we call Bliss Programming. Bliss Programming permits us to achieve a state of continuous happiness that is not related to any variable life realities. The nature of all life is that we "Win" some and we "lose" some. When we unitively merge with everything, winning and losing are one. Bliss Programming enables us to totally break our dependence on the actions of people or any external conditions (including our body).

THE MECHANISM OF UNHAPPINESS

Diagram 1 on the next page shows the mechanism of unhappiness that is associated with the first three Centers of Consciousness — Security, Sensation, and Power. This diagram illustrates the problem of finding happiness when our biocomputer is programmed with fears and desires that are backed up by emotional circuitry. Ninety-nine percent of the people in the world today operate their biocomputers with this type of programming that only produces unhappiness in varying degrees. Let's see why.

Let us suppose that you dislike criticism and that your biocomputer is programmed to give you feelings of resentment and anger when someone criticizes you. This may be called "Addictive Dislike Programming" in which you tell yourself, "I dislike criticism." Regardless of our likes or dislikes, the variable life reality is that sometimes we will receive criticism (Condition P — stimulus present) and sometimes we will not receive criticism (Condition N — stimulus not present).

When life gives us Condition P, in which we are criticized, the effect on our consciousness is short-term disappointment, frustration, or suffering. When Condition N occurs and we do not receive criticism, we experience neither disappointment nor pleasure. In other words, it may have no effect on our consciousness. Right now, you are not being criticized, not being beaten up physically, not being starved — and the fact that these things are not happening results in no feeling of either disappointment or pleasure since your consciousness is not preoccupied with the matter. However, if one's consciousness is preoccupied with a situation, Addictive Dislike Programming, Condition N, will bring pleasure. For example, consider the pleasure a man feels who is pardoned from the electric chair!

Now let's see what happens in those instances in which our biocomputer operates with Addictive Desire Programming. Suppose you have the programming "I desire sex." If the variable life reality offers us Condition P in which sex occurs, the effect on our consciousness is to experience a short-term pleasure. However, when we have programmed ourselves to desire sex and life gives us Condition N in which sex does not occur, we experience short-term disappointment and suffering.

If all of the above four conditions are equally probable, our life will have the following pleasure-suffering (see Table 1):

The above assumptions imply that half of our life will be spent in experiencing disappointment, frustration, and suffering, 37.5% of the time we will experience pleasure, and 12.5% will be without either suffering or pleasure. This, of course, is a theoretical model of a single addiction to help us understand the mechanism of happiness and unhappiness. Unfortunately, there is a factor that operates to keep us from experiencing pleasure even 37.5% of the time. We can call this factor "The Mosquito Effect."

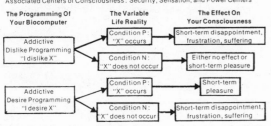

DIAGRAM 1 • THE MECHANISM OF UNHAPPINESS

Type of Programming: ADDICTIVE (Emotion-backed) PROGRAMMING
Direction of Energy Flow: Manipulating Subject-Object Relationships
Associated Centers of Consciousness: Security, Sensation, and Power Centers

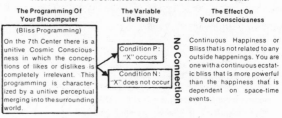

DIAGRAM 3 • THE MECHANISM OF BLISS

Type of Programming: BLISS PROGRAMMING
Direction of Energy Flow: Unitive Oneness
Associated Center of Consciousness: Cosmic Consciousness Center

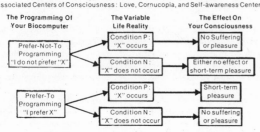

DIAGRAM 2 • THE MECHANISM OF HAPPINESS

Type of Programming: PREFERENTIAL (Non-Emotion-backed) PROGRAMMING
Direction of Energy Flow: Unconditional Acceptance or Love
Associated Centers of Consciousness: Love, Cornucopia, and Self-awareness Centers

TABLE 1	Suffering	Pleasure	No Effect
Addictive Dislike Programming, Condition P	25%		
Addictive Dislike Programming, Condition N		12.5%	12.5%
Addictive Desire Programming, Condition P		25.0%	
Addictive Desire Programming, Condition N	25%		
	50%	37.5%	12.5%

TABLE 2	Suffering	Pleasure	No Effect
Prefer-not-to Programming, Condition P			25.0%
Prefer-not-to Programming, Condition N		12.5%	12.5%
Prefer-to Programming, Condition P		25.0%	
Prefer-to Programming, Condition N			25.0%
	0%	37.5%	62.5%

If you are trying to sleep and there are ten mosquitoes whining around your head at night, you may get up and with considerable effort manage to get rid of most of them. But even though you are 90 percent effective in eliminating the mosquitoes, it only takes one mosquito whining around your head and biting you to keep you awake. Similarly, it only takes one dislike or fear or one unfulfilled desire with strong emotional programming to intermittantly or even continuously dominate your consciousness. And you have hundreds of such "mosquitoes" buzzing around your head!

When we were born into this world, we were programmed with several simple desires and fears. For example, we had Addictive Dislike Programming about loud noises that startled us, to which we would respond by crying. We had Addictive Desire Programming regarding eating from time to time. Since infancy, we have expanded the half dozen simple demands we place upon our world into literally hundreds of emotion-backed demands or addictions. Many individuals can use Addictive Desire Programming coupled with Condition N to feel frustration and suffering if they cannot afford the latest model automobile that Detroit is offering as a solution to one's security, sex, and power addictions!

Neurosis and psychosis (as well as the garden variety of anxiety, disappointment, frustration, and suffering) are all directly attributable to the very complex addictive emotional circuitry with which we have burdened ourselves. It is remarkable that human biocomputers function even as well as they do when you consider that every second we are processing millions of incoming nerve impulses to ascertain which patterns have furthering or depriving effects on the myriad of likes and dislikes with which we have blithely programmed ourselves.

Even if life gives us 90 percent of what we want and protects us from 90 percent of what we dislike or fear, the remaining 10 percent will nag our consciousness, dominate our perceptions, perpetuate the churning of our rational mind to "solve the problem" and otherwise keep us from experiencing the state of happiness. For the state of happiness is experienced only when we have almost continual feelings of pleasure. Just as one active mosquito in a room can keep us awake at night, it may take only one addiction to keep us from feeling happiness.

THE MECHANISM OF HAPPINESS

A study of Diagram 2 shows that happiness becomes an effective reality in one's life to the degree that we convert our Addictive Programming into Preferential Programming — the kind that does not activate negative emotions. For when we have upleveled our addictions to preferences, we can accept whatever life variables might present themselves without triggering the emotional feelings of disappointment, frustration, and suffering. Suppose, for example, sex is a preference rather than an emotion-backed addiction. When sex does not happen, there is no effect on happiness. But when it does happen, there is a feeling of pleasure.

Similarly, if one has Prefer-not-to Programming such as "I prefer not to have a flat tire on my car," one will not suffer frustration when life throws a flat tire at us (Condition P). We simply observe the reality of the flat tire and we immediately start doing whatever we need to do to get it changed. When we have Preferential Programming, the flat tire will give us neither pleasure nor suffering. Since our consciousness will be free of the negative feelings triggered by Addictive Programming, we will be free to enjoy whatever there is to enjoy while we're changing the tire. We may notice things in the world around us that

...d have been otherwise unobserved and thus not enjoyed. Perhaps our consciousness will permit us to appreciate the physical motions we engage in when we efficiently change a tire.

When Condition N occurs coupled with Prefer-not-to Programming, we will experience one of two possible effects depending on whether our consciousness is preoccupied with the matter. If I know air is leaking slowly from a tire and the service station is one block away, I will experience short-term pleasure if the tire takes me to the service station. However, if my consciousness is not at all concerned with the tires, the fact that the tire does not go flat has no effect on my feelings of pleasure or suffering. Hence, Prefer-not-to Programming offers an equal probability of short-term pleasure or no effect on one's feelings.

Diagram 2 shows that no frustration or suffering is possible in a life situation that has Preferential Programming. Prefer-not-to Programming (Condition P) and Prefer-to Programming (Condition N) do not produce either suffering or pleasure. When we enjoy Preferential Programming, all happenings just pass by as part of our here and now — just like birds flying across the sky. Prefer-to Programming with Condition P brings us pleasure.

If all four conditions are equally probable, two of the four will have no effect on our feelings, one of the four will bring us pleasure, and one will bring either no effect or will bring pleasure.

The Addictive Programming shown in Diagram 1 indicates that the likelihood of suffering exceeds that of pleasure if all four conditions are equally probable. With Preferential Programming, we have vastly improved the pleasure-suffering ratios. Happiness, which is more or less continuous pleasure, is now a real possibility. Based on our simplified theoretical model, here are the improved odds you get with each addiction you can uplevel to a preference (see Table 2):

Since Preferential Programming can insulate us from the "downs" in life, we are then free to enjoy only the "ups". This type of programming is characteristic of the Love Center of Consciousness and the Cornucopia Center of Consciousness. Since a mature adult in these higher consciousness levels will have many preferential circuits, the opportunities for pleasure are continuous or almost continuous. For happiness is the continuous or almost continuous experience of pleasure.

When our biocomputers instantly scan the actions and words of all of the people around us in terms of the degree of threat or assistance to realizing our Addictive Programming, real love is impossible. Real love, of course, flows from the unconditional acceptance of another person. The love that is most common in our culture is the illusion of love in which I can love you only to the extent that you do not threaten my addictions and to the extent that you help me realize my addictive desires. I am trapped in the illusion that I can love you only to the degree that you help me obtain Addictive Desire, Condition P, life situations and help me avoid both Addictive Dislike, Condition P, and Addictive Desire, Condition N, happenings! As soon as you begin to hinder rather than help me with my addictions, this conditional type of love immediately goes out the window!

Real love is possible when I reprogram my biocomputer with Preferential Programming. I can then unconditionally accept everything you do or say — regardless of whether I am willing to do or say the same things myself. For when I have Prefer-to or Prefer-not-to Programming, there is nothing you can do that enables me to make myself feel frustration or suffering. But whenever you happen to play a part in increasing the probability of Condition P when I have Prefer-to Programming, I can regard you as helping me find pleasure in life. In other words, with Preferential Programming, there is no way I can "lose" and there is definitely a way that I can "win". And the "winning" will occur more and more as my consciousness dwells in the Love Center and in the Cornucopia Center.

When you have Preferential Programming in almost all areas of your life, your programming will create a peaceful loving world for you to live in. The days are past when your Conscious-awareness was dominated by emotion-backed fears or desires. You live in the here and now. You live in a warm Ocean of loving and caring. You have gradually converted your perception of people and things around you from a subject-object basis to a cognitive framework of love and acceptance. By continually living with the programming that yields happiness, contentment, and joy, you open up the possibility for an even further step in consciousness growth.

BLISS PROGRAMMING

The ultimate state in the Living Love Way to Higher Consciousness is generated by "Bliss Programming". Bliss Programming can make it possible for your consciousness to remain in the Seventh Center (the Cosmic Consciousness Center). The primary characteristic of Bliss Programming is that the feelings of continuous happiness or bliss are not related to any outside happenings. In other words, Condition P (in which the desired or preferred thing does occur), or Condition N (in which a desired or preferred thing does not occur) are irrelevant to one's continuous happiness or bliss.

When your consciousness is in the Self-awareness Center, you witness the drama of your life from a deep calm place within. On the drama level where your body and mind are agreeing with others, disagreeing with others, earning money, making love, etc., you still have Preferential Programming. But this is all seen as "drama". It is like watching your life on a movie screen. You play your part as an actor in the great cosmic play in which your body and mind and my body and mind (as well as everybody else's) interact on this stage we call the world. But the real you is your Conscious-awareness. So you witness whatever is going on in the drama without fear or desire — without any circuitry that could make you vulnerable to emotional ups and downs. When you go to a movie, you can watch the beautiful happenings or the horrendous happenings — and just enjoy the entire show. If those things were happening to you, you would be on an up-and-down roller-coaster experience of pleasure and suffering. But when you see them on a movie screen, they're just so much interesting stuff going by for your perception and enjoyment.

In a similar fashion, when your consciousness is on the Sixth Center, you just witness the drama of your life and that of everyone else. When you are in this center on a fairly continuous basis, there arises within you a tremendous feeling of well-being and joy. You are filled to brimming with awe and gratitude in the ecstatic knowledge of the inherent goodness of life. Thus the Sixth Center of Consciousness can be regarded as an intermediate stepping stone in which your body and mind may operate as shown in Diagram 1 or 2 — but your Conscious-awareness is enjoying the entire show in a manner that is independent of the variable life realities.

The Sixth Level permits your Conscious-awareness to experience continuous happiness that is not related to anything people do or say or to any of the conditions in the environment around you. Just as the Preferential Programming described in Diagram 2 frees you from the tyranny of the subject-object way of relating your happiness to any variable life realities. When your consciousness has lived for a period of time in a state of continuous happiness (even though your body and mind interact in the drama on Preferential Programming), you may be ready to make the break-through to the highest state of consciousness.

The Seventh Level of Consciousness (the Cosmic Consciousness Center) transcends this dualistic split in which your body and mind operate according to one type of programming and your Conscious-awareness uses another. In this state your consciousness has been continuously removed from subject-object paranoia. You now begin to perceive all people and things in a unitive framework. Your perceptions and your consciousness reach out toward experiencing yourself and everything around you as an identity. Your biocomputer expands its perceptual framework so that every person and every object in your world is felt as if from within. The distinctions between inside and outside (although intellectually clear) are merged in your feelings. All is subject. There is no outside — there is no inside. There is just "us" happening. Us people, us trees, us automobiles, us rocks, us books — everything is experienced in a unitive oneness.

It should be clear that this oneness transcends love or unconditional acceptance. There is no longer anybody or anything to accept. Do you unconditionally accept your arm? It just is. It is the ultimate in love. It is not the act of loving someone outside of you. Both the outside and inside are a part of your being — as one consciousness.

When one's biocomputer functions in the unitive Seventh Level of Cosmic Consciousness, it is capable of utilizing fantastic powers that are not available in the lower levels of consciousness. When our consciousness merges the outside and inside (and everything is untuitively experienced in a unitive way), our biocomputers enable us to perceive the unspoken thoughts of people. For when our consciousness has merged with theirs, there arises an ability to directly perceive their consciousness as one's own.

THE DIRECTION OF ENERGY FLOW
In the Living Love System we have three cognitive frameworks for perceiving and responding to people and things outside of us:

1. In a **Subject-object Manner** that is characteristic of the Security, Sensation, and Power Centers of Consciousness.

2. In an **Unconditionally Accepting Manner** in which we experience the beauty of unconditional love associated with the Love Center, the Cornucopia Center, and the Self-awareness Center.

3. In a **Unitive Perceptual Manner** in which one feels no difference between one's self and all of the people and things outside. The capacity for rational discrimination is completely intact. On the rational level one can still perceive people and objects in their aspect of "separateness." But on the feeling level, there is a complete unitive merging into a oneness. This cognitive framework is associated with the Cosmic Consciousness Center.

The direction of energy flow toward the world is associated with the manner in which we work toward happiness. On the lower three levels of consciousness, we feel uncritically sure that the way to happiness lies in improving our odds in the middle column entitled "The Variable Life Reality". We put a torrent of energy into subject-object manipulation. We concentrate on preventing that which we addictively dislike, and we try to manipulate and control the people and things in the world to bring about the conditions we addictively desire. But the results are never "enough".

When you realize that no amount of powerful striving is sufficient to bring about happiness through subject-object control of the people and things in the world, you are ready to redirect your energy to the reprogramming of your biocomputer. Your energy flow then helps you become more loving and accepting. You realize that this method of producing happiness is within your conscious ability to achieve. However, it is not necessary to completely withdraw from the drama of manipulating the variable realities in your life. You will even have two of the Twelve Pathways to guide you on the "outside trip".

Two of the Twelve Pathways tell you exactly how to interact with the outside world around you — and the remaining ten Pathways tell you exactly how to work on the inside world which is yourself. The Seventh Pathway tells you to openly communicate with everyone so that you no longer feel and think of yourself as separate. The Ninth Pathway says to do anything you want to do provided you are tuned in, centered, and loving. Your actions will always be optimal if your head is in the right place. So ACT FREELY — but don't be addicted to the results. By following these two Pathways, you will be enormously more effective in changing the people and situations around you than when you put all your addictive energy into modifying the external conditions of your life. But this increased power to optimize your environment comes to you ONLY TO THE DEGREE THAT YOU EFFECTIVELY CHANGE YOURSELF USING THE REMAINING TEN PATHWAYS.

Some of the conventional methods of consciousness growth may require years or decades for substantial results. The Living Love Methods offer the possibility of rapidly reprogramming your biocomputer so that some of the pleasure and joy of Centers

Four and five may sometimes be experienced in a period of mo nths. It all depends on how much energy you are ready to use to eliminating frustration and suffering in your life. How inten sely do you want to reprogram your biocomputer to produce pleasure and happiness? How soon will you realize that the only thing you don't have is the direct experience that there isnothing you need that you don't have?

The sixth and seventh levels of consciousness require a fine tu ning of your biocomputer that may take a much longer period of time. The sixth level is far easier to experience than the seve nth. The Cosmic Consciousness Center represents an ultimate breakthrough that happens when there is a high degree of perfe ction of the Sixth Center.

You should keep your aims realistic and enjoy taking one step at a time. Once a major part of your consciousness resides in the Love Center, you will experience a happiness and beauty in your life that is "enough". Even if you do not progress beyond this Center, you will have a wisdom and effectiveness in your life that at will exceed that of most of the people in the world. The consciousness game is the greatest and most genuine of all life g ames - that one should not get hung up on the spiritual score board. Just enjoy the eternally beautiful here and now moment t hat your life continually offers you. At the end of your journey toward awakening, the only thing you will find is your real self.

THE PURPOSE OF YOUR LIFE

A first step in your growth toward higher consciousness is to se e clearly the enormous expenditure of fruitless energy that you are now putting into living out your addictive programming. Eve ry addiction you have programmed into your head will separate you and make you suffer to a greater or lesser degree. Your feeli ngs of disappointment, irritability, anger, jealousy or fear are giving you urgent messages: "Here is an addiction that you must reprogram into a preference in order to live an effective and joyous life."

The remarkable thing about growing into higher consciousnes s is that it is only the release from the emotion backed inner addiction that is required - you do not necessarily need to chang e your actions. If you are addicted to over-eating chocolate cream puffs, the problem lies not in the act of putting chocolate cream puffs in your mouth - the problem lies wholly in the circuitry of your biocomputer that makes you a slave to this inne r desire. When you use the five Living Love Methods for reprogramming your addictions, the outer behavior will then tak e care of itself. You may from time to time eat chocolate cream puffs, but you are freed from an inner addiction that dominates y our consciousness. You will not keep a fresh supply in the house. You will no longer let a large part of your calories be wasted on s uch relatively "empty" food with unfortunate consequences to your health. When you uplevel this addiction to a preferance, yo u may still enjoy a cream puff from time to time - but you can also enjoy life if you do not eat cream puffs. And so the energy th at was previously drained into an addiction can now flow into channels that add to your happiness and joy.

When you reprogram an addiction, you may find that you have no further interest in the external actions that you have been engaging in. Or when you reprogram an addiction and uplevel it to a preference, you may find that there will be no change in your external actions. For example, if you uplevel an addiction fo r not washing dishes to a preference you may find that you are now able to consciously wash dishes. Your addictive programmi ng will no longer operate to make you unhappy when you are doing this necessary job.

The Living Love Way to Higher Consciousness does not teach you to repress the emotional programming that seperates you from other people (for this causes psychosomatic diseases) or to express this duality and alienation (which is the traditional method of psychology and psychiatry). To get into higher consciousness, you must eliminate the causeof all feelings of duality, isolation, and separation that keep you from loving yourself and everyone and everything around you. The Twelve Pathways, the Seven Centers of Consciousness, and the Five Methods enable you to **eliminate the cause of your unhappiness**.

You begin to realize that a direct and rapid way to find happiness is available through using your negative emotional feelings to show you which parts of your biocomputer need reprogramming in order to enjoy every moment of your life. In the past, you have used the majority of your energy trying to control, dominate and change the people and situations in your life. Now this energy can be channeled into the Five Methods to get free of the addictive programming that can bring you down.

And then a most remarkable thing happens. When you reprogram your addictions, you will find that you can love everyone unconditionally - including yourself. As long as people were **objects to be manipulated** to help you achieve your addictions, real love (unconditional acceptance of another person) was impossible. You now find that you can love in a profoundly beautiful way that you never knew existed before.

This new dimension of love produces a miracle in your life. For it now makes you open to new experiences, new people and new activities. When you begin to live in the Fourth Level of Consciousness, you no longer experience any person or any situation as a threat. You find that you now have everything you need to be happy.

You will continually marvel at the way that the people and situations in your life are harmoniously functioning to meet your real needs. And your consciousness may go back to the day when you first discovered the Living Love book that helped to show you the way to bring about this miracle in your life. But did you discover it? Wasn't it the people and conditions of your life that offered it to you - because of your openess? Trace the major things that have happened to you since the day you first began your conscious growth toward becoming a more receptive, effective, and wiser being. You will find that you have interacted with the people and conditions of your life to help you make wiser and wiser choices that have accelerated your continuing growth into higher consciousness.

It feels so unbelievably great to be liberated from the consciousness-dominating barrage of desires, demands, expectations, inflexible patterns, models of how the world should treat you — addictions of every kind. Anyone watching you might see you doing more or less the same things you used to do, but there is a **NEW YOU** doing them. You still go the grocery store to buy food, but you do it with a biocomputer that now permits you to enjoy every minute of the experience. No matter how many items you can't find, or no matter how long you have to wait in line, you can no longer make yourself feel frustrated, disappointed, or create suffering of any sort.

Your trip to a grocery store becomes a turned-on experience. And your smiles, your helpfulness, and your vibrations of love affect those around you. Your new non-addictive being changes the path of your daily doings from a tiresome drudgery into an energy-producing delightful panorama that passes before your eyes. You find that you have discovered that all of the people in the grocery store are awakening beings who are there to help you in your journey toward higher consciousness. And you have the deep satisfaction of knowing that by living a high consciousness life, you are also doing the most (without any striving) to help other beings in their growth toward higher consciousness.

A beautiful thing about higher consciousness is that what is best for you is best for everyone else. When you begin to live on the Fourth or higher Levels, your radiant inner being creatively changes the feelings and actions of the people and the vibrations of the situations that you come in contact with. You give them the greatest gift of all — you tune in to them at the beautiful place that is behind their lower-consciousness games. You flow harmoniously with them at the place on the Fourth Level where they are pure love. And this can even be done with nothing more than a loving eye-to-eye contact or smile. By relating to that place in them where they are love, you temporarily put their consciousness into a higher place. This way of being, more than anything you could ever achieve externally in life, becomes the source of that feeling of conscious satisfaction about the "rightness" and the meaningfulness of your life.

A wonderful thing about the Living Love Way is that you can do it "alone" if need be. You can regard others as actors on the Cosmic stage who are here to make you aware of your addictions. They are helping you by creating situations in which your emotions reveal the hiding places of your addictions. Regardless of whether they know of the inner work that you are doing, everything they do or say helps you grow into higher consciousness. Even though they may be driven by addictive programming that makes them irritated or hostile, **you can use all of their actions, emotional expressions, and words to help you become free of your addictions.** And as you reprogram your biocomputer and liberate yourself, they will begin to notice the extraordinary joy, freedom and love that radiates from you irrespective of what they do or say. This transformation will be so unexpected and amazing to them that they will want to know what is happening inside of you. And when they ask, you can then joyously share the keys that you discovered for unlocking happiness.

You can show them how it is all found inside — independent of the changing world of people, objects and situations. And if they are ready to hear, they will be amazed at the simplicity of the method for growing into higher consciousness. It simply means upleveling all their addictions into preferences. It will take them a while to **really understand the awesome vastness of their addictions.** But the results in increased happiness and ability to love will arrive so rapidly that they will know they have at last found the answer to "making it" in life. And by helping themselves, they have now helped you grow even more rapidly toward the higher levels of consciousness. You will have been given the opportunity to explain it, and you will have discovered additional insights you need for your growth. Their vibrations of growing love and expanded consciousness are helping you live in a more beautiful world. They help you liberate even more energy for your own journey.

And so, hand in hand, we journey down the river of our lives toward the vast ocean of Oneness that is our source and our destiny. At last we have the profound joy of knowing:

THE PURPOSE OF OUR LIVES
IS TO FREE OUR CONSCIOUS-AWARENESS
FROM ALL ADDICTIVE TRAPS SO THAT WE
MAY BECOME
ONE WITH THE OCEAN OF LIVING LOVE

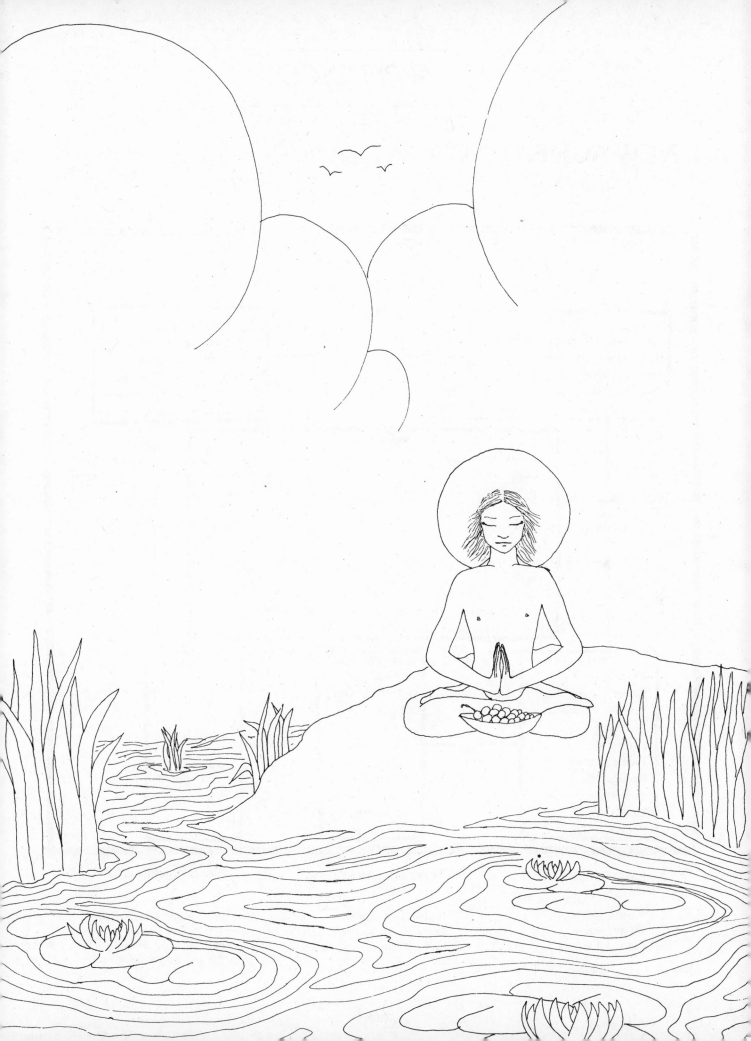

APPENDICES

I. NEW AGE EATING AT A GLANCE

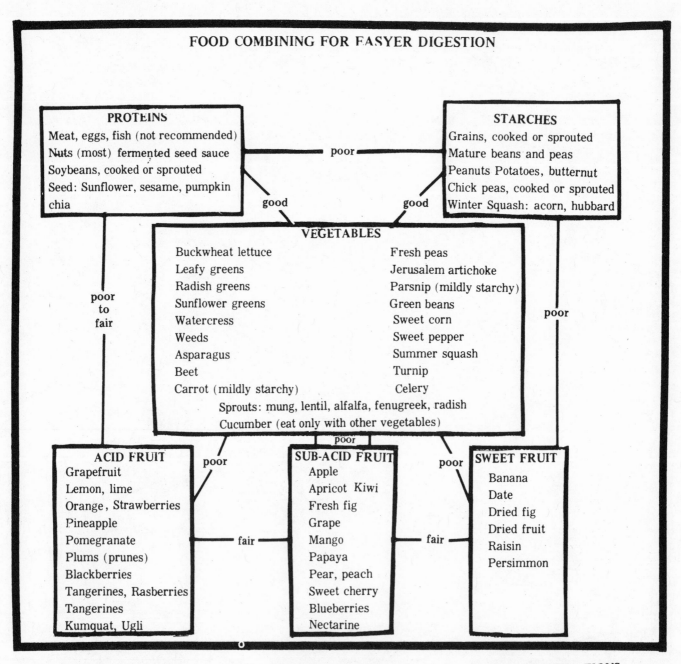

FOOD COMBINING FOR EASYER DIGESTION

PROTEINS
Meat, eggs, fish (not recommended)
Nuts (most) fermented seed sauce
Soybeans, cooked or sprouted
Seed: Sunflower, sesame, pumpkin
chia

poor

STARCHES
Grains, cooked or sprouted
Mature beans and peas
Peanuts Potatoes, butternut
Chick peas, cooked or sprouted
Winter Squash: acorn, hubbard

good   good

VEGETABLES

Buckwheat lettuce   Fresh peas
Leafy greens   Jerusalem artichoke
Radish greens   Parsnip (mildly starchy)
Sunflower greens   Green beans
Watercress   Sweet corn
Weeds   Sweet pepper
Asparagus   Summer squash
Beet   Turnip
Carrot (mildly starchy)   Celery
Sprouts: mung, lentil, alfalfa, fenugreek, radish
Cucumber (eat only with other vegetables)

poor
to
fair

poor

poor

ACID FRUIT
Grapefruit
Lemon, lime
Orange, Strawberries
Pineapple
Pomegranate
Plums (prunes)
Blackberries
Tangerines, Rasberries
Tangerines
Kumquat, Ugli

poor   poor

SUB-ACID FRUIT
Apple
Apricot Kiwi
Fresh fig
Grape
Mango
Papaya
Pear, peach
Sweet cherry
Blueberries
Nectarine

fair   fair

SWEET FRUIT
Banana
Date
Dried fig
Dried fruit
Raisin
Persimmon

BAD COMBINATIONS

Protein and starch
Oil and starch
Fruit and starch

POOR COMBINATIONS

Protein and acid fruit
Leafy greens and acid fruit
Leafy greens and subacid fruit

GOOD COMBINATIONS

Protein and leafy greens
Starch and vegetables
Oil and leafy greens
Oil and acid subacid fruit

EATING FOR HAPPINESS

DO NOT MIX more than four foods , from more than two classifications, at any one meal.
Use ONE PROTEIN food OR ONE STARCH food per meal.
OIL slows digestion. Combines best with fruit and green vegetables;combines poorly with starch and protein.
TOMATO combines best with avocado and green vegetables.
MELON (all kinds) should always be eaten alone.
AVOCADO combines best with acid fruit, sprouts and vegetables. Use in mideration.
WHEATGRASS should always be taken on an empty stomach. May mix with carrot and green vegetable and sprout juices.
SEED CHEESE goes well with ripe sub-acid fruit, banana, leafy greens, sprouts, or alone.
Use HONEY AND MOLASSES on an empty stomach to prevent fermentation.
PEANUTS are high in protein, fat and starch and therefore difficult to digest.
Try eating one kind of FRUIT at a time or combining them according to type of seed: stone fruit (peach, nectarine, apricot, cherry), citrus fruit, core fruit (apples, pears) dried fruit, melon fruit. Papaya goes well with all sub-acid fruit as well as banana.

WHAT TO EAT

Organic live food is your best medicare, your ticket to prolonged youth. Eat natural food which appeals to you most. Advance your diet according to the dictates of your body and the type of work you do.
Avoid all animal, processed, or cooked food, strong condiments and spices. Do not use the teeth to crush hard food. If hard to masticate, it is forbidden.
Grow your own food in your garden: vegetables, fruit, sprouts, 7 day greens. In a natural environment, eventually eat fruit only.
Be thrifty; eat what your own area can provide organically grown.
Eat no more than 16 ounces at a single meal. Never eat a large meal just before doing hard work. Before a difficult physical or mental task, center your energy; fast on juice or water.

WHEN TO EAT

Eat only when hungry, after the previous meal is digested. No snacks between meals. Some individuals have within the digestive tract three or more meals in a semi–digested, putrefactive state.
A day will not be wasted on a small (or no) breakfast.
Eat the biggest meal at noon when sun activity is strongest. Solar vibrations aid digestion. Eat a small meal before sunset for a longer night of fasting.
Never eat when in pain, emotionally upset, extremely tired or immediately after hard work.
Rest or relax after a meal for 45 minutes. For those with a delicate digestion, lie down for at least 10 minutes before a meal.
After retiring for the night, do not eat or drink.

HOW TO EAT

Begin with a name of God. Be grateful, ask for control in appetite. Bring a tranquil mind to meals. Do not argue or rush. Enjoy the music of birds and brook, the silence of the sky. Enjoy your food.
Eat slowly and chew each mouthful thoroughly reducing it to fluid before swallowing. Breathe long and deep with each mouthful.
Do not drink (or eat) cold or hot (beyond 104 degrees) substances.
No liquids with meals. Drink at least thirty minutes before or three hours after a meal.
Eat one food at a meal, or combine food correctly for best digestion. Eat juicy foods prior to concentrated foods. Eat raw foods before cooked foods. Stop eating before you feel full.

CHEMISTRY OF FOODS

ACID ASH: All grain (except millet), all meat, butter, cream, eggs, cheese, animal fats, sea foods, most nuts, dry peas, dry beans, most oils, lentils, peanuts, hulled sesame.
MUCUS-INDUCING FOODS: All acid ash foods. All dairy products. Sprouted grains, chick peas, lentils, seeds, nuts, potato, yam. Slightly: Squash (Acorn, Butternut, Hubbard).
ALKALINE ASH: Most dried fruit, indoor greens, all grasses, dandelion, soybean sprouts, cucumber, almond, unhulled sesame, avocado, carrot, onion, tomato, peach, plum celery, fruit and most vegetables, olive oil, sprouts from most legumes.
ACID pH FRUIT: Currant, grapegruit, kumquat, lemon, lime, loganberry, loquat, orange, pineapple, pomegranate, strawberry, tamarind, tangerine, tangelo, tomato. When ripe, all fruits produce alkaline effect in the bloodstream. Overacid condition can be generated in the stomach regions, affecting your whole body, from the intake of ascorbic acid (vitamin C),

Nicotinic Acid, or any of the acidy vitamins, just as well as from eating unripe tomatoes, citrus or pineapple. Symptoms: dizziness, fainting, pressure on the eyes, headache, burning sensation in stomach, bleeding of the gums.

SUB-ACID FRUIT: Apple, apricot, blackberry, cactus fruit, cherimoya, cherry, elderberry, gooseberry, grape, guava, huckleberry, jujube, mango, nectarine, papaya, papaw, peach, pear, persimmon, plum, kiwi, rasberry, sapodilla, sapote.

SWEET FRUIT: Banana, breadfruit, date, dried(date, apple, apricot, banana, fig, grape, peach, pear, plum), fig, plantain.

MELON: Banana, cantaloupe, casaba, christmas, crenshaw, honeydew, persain, watermelon.

ACID FRUIT: Most berries, pineapple and pomegranate leave the bloodstream more acid. When badly combined, or eaten in large quantity most food can leave the body more acid.

ALKALINE FRUIT: Citrus, tomatoes, most sweet fruit and those fruit listed in sub-acid column leave the body more alkaline. Unripe, depleted soil sub-acid fruit are really acid.

SOAKED DRIED FRUIT such as figs, apples, apricots, peaches, dates and pears leave the body more alkaline. However, too much or too frequent or badly combined can cause fermentation and acidity in the bloodstream.

COLORED VEGETABLES: Beets, carrots, red cabbage, cauliflower, corn, eggplant, kohlrabi, parsnip, rutabaga, squashes, turnips, slightly mucus inducing.

COOKED VEGETABLES: During transition to raw foods all starchy foods can be cooked. Eventually, lightly steam or bake the vegetables listed as fruit, green or colored. To slow down a rapid cleansing reaction slightly cooked vegetables may be used. Under such circumstances, you might want to blend together some raw and some cooked vegetables.

DRINK YOURSELF TO A HEALTH ATTACK

Make juices pulp free by pouring them through a fine strainer or cheese cloth. For best digestion, sip slowly.

"Juice Prescriptions"

ACNE: Carrot alone; Carrot 10 oz. Spinach 6 oz. (Big carrots have the best flavor).
ADENOIDS: (same as acne)
ALBUMINURIA: Carrot 10, Beet 3, Cucumber 3 oz.
ALLERGIES: Carrot 8, Celery 6 oz.
ANEMIA: Carrot 8, Beet 2, Celery 6 oz.
ANGINA PECTORIS: Carrot 6, Beet 5, Cucumber 5 oz.
ARTHRITIS: Carrot 8, Celery 8 oz; Grapefruit alone.
ASTHMA: Carrot 8, Celery 8 oz; Grapefruit alone.
BLOOD PRESSURE (high): Carrot 8 oz. pod of garlic.
BRIGHTS DISEASE: Carrot 8, Celery 6, Parsley 2 oz.
CANCER: Carrot, quart daily. Carrot 12, Cabbage 4 oz.
COLITIS: Carrot 8, Apple 8 oz.
CONSTIPATION: Carrot 8, Celery 4, Apple 4 oz.
CORONARY THROMBOSIS: Carrot 8, Garlic 2 oz.
DERMATITIS: Carrot 6, Beet 5, Cucumber 5 oz.
DIABETES: Carrot 6, Celery 5, Endive 2, Parsley 2 oz.
DIARRHEA: Carrot 6, Celery 5, Apple 5 oz.
FEVER: Choice of Apple, Pineapple, Grape, Orange.
GALLSTONES: Carrot 6, Beet 5, Cucumber 5 oz.
HAY FEVER: Carrot 8, Celery 8 oz.
HERNIA: Carrot 6, Celery 6, Spinach 2, Parsley 2 oz.
INFLUENZA: Carrot 8, Celery 8 oz.
NEPHROSIS: Carrot 8, Celery 6, Parsley 2 oz.
NERVOUS DISORDERS: Carrot 8, Celery 6, Parsley 2 oz.
PEPTIC ULCERS: Cabbage 16, Celery 16, Cabbage alone.
RHEUMATISM: Carrot 8, Celery 8oz.
SCURVY: Orange 8, Grapegruit 8 oz.
TUMORS: Carrot 12, Beet 3 oz.

Special Properties of Juices

APPLE: Healer of intestinal inflammation, digestant
BEET: Cancer-tumor healer, blood-builder
CUCUMBER: Alkalinizer, mineralizer
CABBAGE: Vitamin U, healer of ulcers
CARROT: Best balanced in vitamins and minerals.
CELERY: Nature's nerve tonic, alkalinizer.
DANDELION: Organic magnesium, for teeth, tonic, diuretic, kidney—liver cleanser or blood builder.
ENDIVE: Alkalinizer, rich in minerals and vitamins.

KALE: Vitamins A,B,C, rich in calcium.
LEMON: Richest in bio—flavonoids.
PARSLEY: Helps glands, nerves, blood coagulation, eyes.
TOMATO: Fruit richest in minerals.
ORANGE: Rich in calcuim, Phosphorus, Vitamins C and A.
WATERMELON: Alkalinizer, kidney activatior and cleanser.

For additional study on the healing properties of live juices, consult Walker, Lust, Kirschner, Wigmore and Lovewisdom.

ASTROLOGY AND DIET

Different signs need different amounts of sun and food colors. It does not mean one needs only the named color in food, but more of it than the other signs.
ARIES — red food; medium sun.
TAURUS — yellow food; medium to a lot of sun.
GEMINI — yellow, blue food; lot of sun.
CANCER — green food; lot of sun.
LEO — yellow, orange food; lot of sun.
VIRGO — yellow, green, blue, violet food; lot of sun.
LIBRA — red, yellow, green food; medium sun.
SCORPIO — orange food; little to medium sun.
SAGITTARIUS — red, yellow, green food; little sun.
CAPRICORN — green food; little sun.
AQUARIUS — blue, white food; little sun.
PISCES — green, juicy food; little to medium sun.

THE COLOR IN YOUR DIET

Body:

RED FOOD - speeds up your circulation when your hands and feet get cold, or for mucus and phlegm in your throat. Acts as a catalyst for ionization and breaks up the ferric salt crystals. Egocentric, brings your consciousness back into yourself. Promotes growth. Physical, alkaline, heat, yang, fire, life. Tomatoes, cherries, yam, eggplant, red cabbage, watermelon, strawberry, cranberry, radish, soybean, whole wheat and rye.

ORANGE FOOD - anti-spasmatic, for pains and cramps of any kind. rebuilds lung cell membrane tissues. Good for lungs in polluted areas. It may help to heal malignant growths as well as tumors. Provides new ideas for mental concepts. Strengthens the etheric body, the energy around you.. Provides elasticity for skin and bones. Gives you joy, gaiety, and warmth. Stimulates milk production for breast feeding. Vitality. Orange, carrot, calcium, sesame, pumpkin, dates, walnuts, apricot.

Nerves:

YELLOW FOOD - motor stimulant, it gets you going faster than coffee. Provides positive magnetic currents. Makes you happy. Strenthens the nerves and aids the brain. Good for digestion and constipation. Apple, peach, banana, papaya, mango, corn, butter, yellow squash, grapefruit. Lemon, lime, and pineapple are considered half yellow, half green.

GREEN FOOD - a cleanser and bactericide. A natural tranquilizer, it mellows one out. Controls the metabolism, the growth and destruction of the body. Dilates the capillaries and provides a sensation of warmth. For headcold and gray hair. Neutral. Wisdom. Millet, brown rice, green vegetables, weeds, grasses, brewer's yeast, B-complex vitamins, and avocadoes.

Head:

BLUE FOOD - for mental work. For headaches, stiff neck, sore throats. Builds antibodies to fight infections. Spiritual, yin, acid, cool. Makes you consciousness oriented. Blueberry, plum, grapes, potatoe, celery, parsnip, asparagus, nuts, peanut.

NATURAL LAWS OF HEALTH

There is no disease. There is only a polluted body. The road to health is detoxification of the bloodstream with pure air, water, fasting, live food and spiritual discipline.

Germs cannot harm you. They can only multiply rapidly in a congested devitalized body. They are the scavengers that feed on dead food and mucus. In a detoxified bloodstream, germs that enter through a cut, digestive or respiratory tract are quickly eleminated through the body's defense mechanisms. However, chemicals or medication introduced into a detoxified body can be deadly.

The discomforts of a healing crisis lead to health. The aches and pains of unattended disease lead to death. Each crisis of elimination will make you stronger. Do not expect robust health in a month. It may take years to become younger and healthier. For best health, use your sense of humor. Do not argue. Smile and say "yes". Chant OM. Be a wise fool. Questions are answered in the soul, not with arguments

Only you can change the condition of your health by changing your habits. There are no instant cures. Do not wear sunglasses; they disturb the endocrine system. Choose clothing colors with care. Avoid television due to the radiation hazard. Radiation pollution from electronic sources – x–ray, radio, TV stations, motors – can cause cell mutation and speed the aging process.

Don't keep persistent company with smokers. They will pollute your lungs.
Adopt a natural life–style.
The younger you start, the longer you will know youth and health.
During therapy, to conserve your energy, practice chastity.

If you have all the essential organs, live foods will eventually rebuild them. If you use drugs, you will be able to gradually take smaller dosages and, as your health improves, eventually eliminate the use of medication.

If organs have stopped functioning, have been removed, or were defective at birth and you require the use of a hormone, digestive or enzyme supplement, consider withdrawal from this medication only under a doctor's guidance.

There are stages in every disease in which an irreversible process has been reached. However there have always been exceptions. One never knows until one tries.

If you cannot give up your addiction to cooked food, at least give your children raw food.

Maintain health through diet, yoga, walking, exercise and meditation. Do not subject yourself or your children to any vaccination or medication. In case of accident or broken bones, seek natural methods such as zone therapy and the aid of a doctor to correct the condition and obtain relief.

Fast on distilled water at least 36 hours a week. Such a fast will eliminate DDT and other toxins from food and environment.
Fast at least twice a year, especially during seasonal changes, for at least 7 days. Dry fast (no water) for 12 to 36 hours once a month. For headache or indigestion, dry fast (no more than 36 hours) until nature invites you to dine. Have one day of silence each week.

Initially, let a chiropractor check your vertebral alignment at least twice a month, especially after any shock to the body.
Zone Thereapy, reflexology, acupuncture and iridology are useful for diagnosis and to improve health.
Become an example of health and you will gain followers.

SPIRITUAL FRONTIERS

The spiritual healing powers in an individual are magnified hundreds of times on a frugal live food diet. It would be interesting to see whether the teachers who take on the karma of others would be free from disease on a live food diet if all their students also switched to live food. In a pure body there is no place for disease.

Do not let any negative thoughts linger in your mind. Maintain faith, a desire for health and good reasons for living. Review in the evening your desire for health and good reasons for living. Review in the evening your daily activities. Keep a diary. Be critical, discriminating, loving; every day try to improve.

Detoxify your body to the level possible in a chosen environment. Personal pollution is much worse than external pollution. For spiritual discipline you need a flexible, healthy body, its vital force centered in the upper chakras.

Cultivate the virtues of non–injury to and love for all living things, truthfulness and selfless service.

Study the works of esoteric teachers. If need be, find a living teacher for guidance. (Nature will provide you with teachers anyway).

Work to take care of your needs. Learn to differentiate between need and desire. Do not waste.

Do not create uselessly. Do no more than is needed for yourself and others. The fun house is inside you; the admission price is devotion to truth and simplicity. Wealth consists of minimal needs – let us detach ourselves.

The ultimate adventure of this age is the inner trip to universal consciousness which destroys the illusion of time and space and brings compassion.

Perfection is found on the road of discrimination – by the self; deny the unnecessary. If you desire perfection, think perfection – it will come into being.

Air, then thoughts, then sun, then water, then frugal diet is Nature's path to endless health.

DETOXIFICATION EXPERIENCE AFTER 500 ACID TRIPS

"Peace be with you,

Here are some notes I have made based on my experiences that might be of interest or even of use for spirits walking around clothed in material bodies. My path toward greater enlightenment has taken me from a suburban American upbringing to getting high on drugs and, more recently, to learning how to stay high naturally.

I became a "vegetarian" during the height of my drug-taking days. At that time, about 5 years ago, I was experimenting quite a bit with LSD, mescaline and psylicibin (over 500 trips) and daily pot smoking. A friend suggested to me the possibility of doing without meat, and shortly, due to his and other stronger influences, I was on a "vegetarian" diet. The reasons had nothing to do with health; for the most part they had to do with becoming a non-killer of animals. At the same time, in order to feed animals that were kept where I lived, I often purchased other dead animal products. I ate a great deal of eggs, cheese, butter and ice cream.

The first two or three years of vegetarianism featured no meat, hardly any fish and a great deal of junk foods, such as sundaes, cookies, cakes, pies and pizzas. I got sick, about as often as I ever had, including my usual colds per year. I had a chronic cough from smoking literally pounds of grass.

Learning to bake breads was a new fun challenge, but I'd be so stoned that I'd eat half of the loaf almost before I could pop it out of the oven. My taste buds, however, were becoming more sensitive to the natural flavors so that eating things raw or barely sauteed was getting more interesting.

About fourteen months ago, just for the fun of it, a friend and I decided to eat all of our food raw. The notion that foods need not be cooked because the sun bakes everything to perfection felt good to me.

Just feeling, listening, as the body received and adapted to cleaner, more alive food made me feel new every moment. Shortly, I deleted all dairy products from my diet. I ate easier to digest fruits, some nuts and vegetables — all raw. Smoking grass, too, felt different. Instead of stoning me and leaving me feeling high, it zapped my nervous system. It stoned me, but as for feeling high, well, I didn't — only wasted and brought down from clearer, higher sensations. I tried not smoking and it agreed with me fine.

After two or three months of eating raw foods (about the same time we stopped smoking dope) my friend and I both developed sores on our bodies. These sores seemed amazing but fascinating and we listened about poisons that were being released. The sores went away in time, but the changes both physical and spiritual continued.

Inconsistencies with practices and beliefs have resulted in my learning some interesting lessons. For a while, several months ago, I was being treated regularly by the dentist for what I felt to be problems stemming from previous wrong living and eating. What didn't occur to me until after several visits was that no physical weakness can be patched up and made better from without, including teeth and gums. Only better maintenance from within can really produce lasting results.

So, in response to these same dental problems, I thought it would be useful to experiment with cleansing and building my temple. Some kind of a fast was what I had in mind.

The fast itself consisted of taking only liquids, both fruit and vegetable juices. My friend and I underwent a regimen of enemas each morning followed by a wheatgrass juice implant. We both followed this one month. Although we each saw and listened to many changes as our bodies eliminated their stored up poisons, neither of us experienced intense crises. All the same, there is no doubt that this fast, as Arnold Ehret has said: "put us on Nature's operating table." I feel that the constant use of wheatgrass juice in rectal implants deserves much credit for making so much toxic elimination comfortably possible. I took them twice daily using 16 oz. of pure wheatgrass juice each time. In order to have enough juice for our daily implants, we planted three trays a day and harvested on the eighth day. We also grew substantial amounts of sprouts: alfalfa, mung bean and fenugreek. We juiced the sprouts in a juice extractor and I found this drink strength giving. Sometimes we juiced organic apples, or oranges, organically grown, or watermelon from Mexico.

Having been introduced to Bernard Jensen's book on iris diagnosis, I was watchful for changes in the eyes, which hold a record of all past and present bodily disorders. All of the most favorable signs — disappearance of spots, markings, greater clarity and overall color changes — manifested themselves throughout this period of housecleaning. And of course my weakest gum areas and teeth all greatly improved (no pain, redness or swelling).

This past month, following the wheatgrass juice therapy, we have reduced the number of enemas and wheatgrass drinks but have been drinking most of our food. In place of the wheatgrass juice, we have been drinking the juice of buckwheat lettuce and sunflower greens. This green juice added to our sprout juice is remarkably palatable, unlike the wheatgrass juice, while similarly strengthening. In the last two weeks we have resorted less and less to electronic means of juicing and more upon the God-given juicer: our mouths.

This time of cleaning out has been and is (for it is still happening) a fine and enlightening experience. I can't say if it is advisable for you to fast, but I do know that if we all listen to our innermost being, that pure and unchanging total consciousness — we will be on the highest road to truth and loving ways.

The physical changes are remarkable and fascinating but they are only the tools which lead to all other awakenings. The opening up of new frequencies of feelings and listening has inevitably signified the passing of the old. This happens every moment, and, by my remembering and centering on this, I am free to enjoy each moment of the eternal now.

Love what you do, for you and it are one.

JEFF

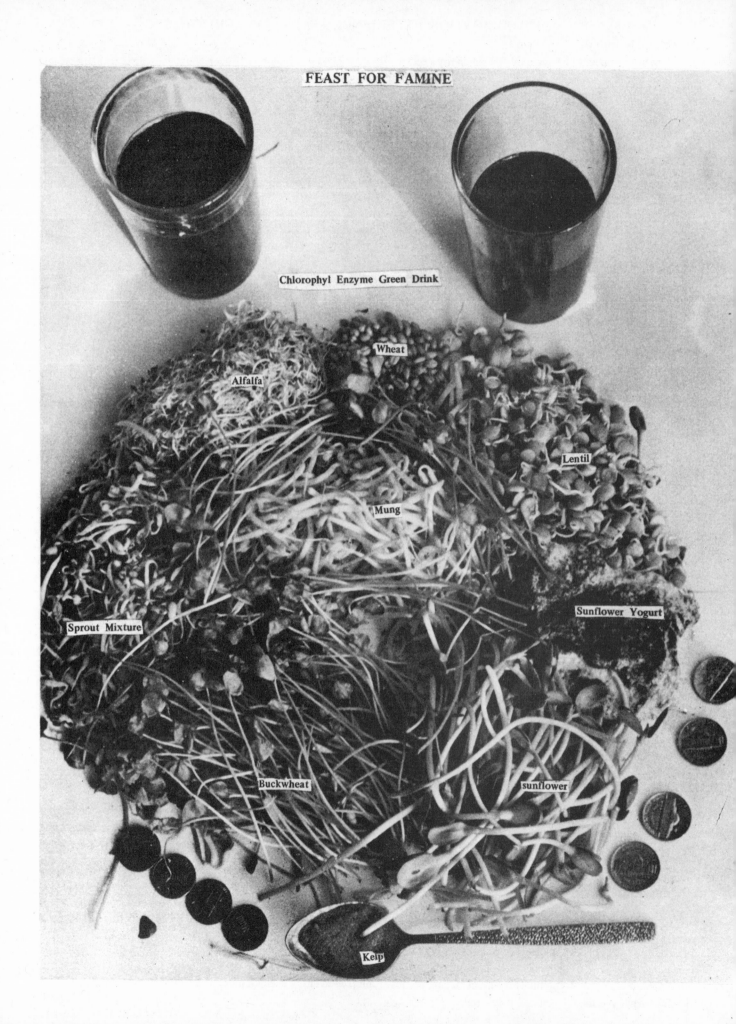

FEAST FOR FAMINE

Chlorophyl Enzyme Green Drink

Wheat

Alfalfa

Lentil

Mung

Sprout Mixture

Sunflower Yogurt

Buckwheat

sunflower

Kelp

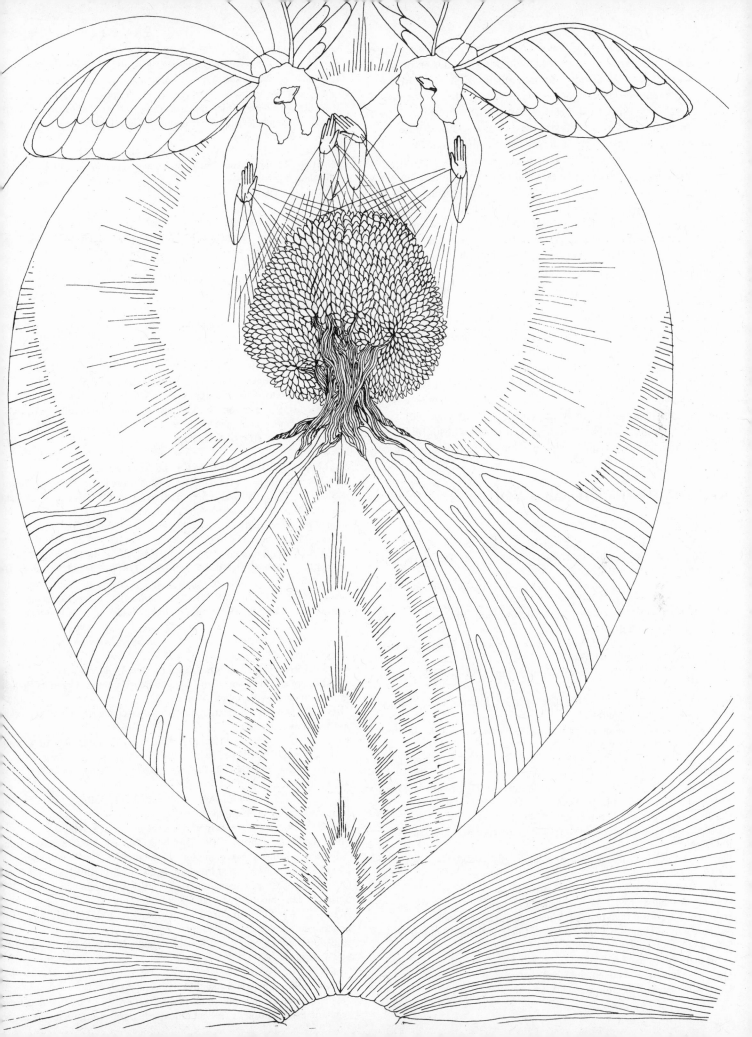

Go placidly amid the noise & 'haste, and remember what peace there may be in silence. As far as possible without surrender he on good terms with all persons. Speak your ttuth quietly & clearly; and listen to others, even tbe du~ & ignora~; the' too have their story. Avoid loud & aggressive persons, they are vexations to the spirit. If you compare yourself with others, you may become vain & bitter; for always there will be greater & lesser persons than yourself. Enjoy your achievements as well as your plans. Keep interested in your own career, however humble; it is a real possession in the changing fortunes of time. Exercise caution in your business affairs', for the world is fu~ of trn'ckery. But let this not blind you to what virtue there is; many persons strive for high ideals; and everywhere life is full of heroism. Be yourself. Especially, do not feign affection. ~either be cy~i~~l about love; for in the face of all aridity & disenchantment it is perennial as the grass. Take kindly the counsel of the years, $racefuliy surrendering the things of youth. Nurture strength of spirit to shield you in sudden misfortune. But do not distress yourself with imagir~ings. Many fears are born of fatigue & loneliness. Beyond a wholesome discipline, be gentle with yourself. You are a child of t'he urn ve rse, no less than the trees & the stars; you have a right to be here. And whether or not it is clear to you, no doubt the universe is unfolding as it should. Therefore be at peace with God, whatever you conceive Him to 'be, anO ~hatev~ your labors & aspirations, in the noisy confusion of life keep peace with your soul. With all its sham. drudgery & broken dreams, it is still a beautiful world. Be careful. Strive to be happy.   Found in old Saint Paul's Church, Baltimore; Dated 1~92

RESOURCES for a Healthier YOU

YOGA
Light on Yoga, B.K.S. Iyengar. Scocken Books, New York
Kripalu Yoga: Meditation-in-Motion, Yogi Amrit Desai. Kripalu Publications, PO Box 793, Lenox, MA 01240
The Sivananda Companion to Yoga, Lucy Lidell. A Fireside Book, Published by Simon & Schuster, Inc. New York.
Yoga With a Partner, Sandra Jordan. Arco Publishing, Inc., 219 Park Ave South, New York, NY 10003
Hatha Yoga, The Hidden Language. Swami Sivananda Radha. Timeless Books, Box 160, Porthill, ID 83853.
Stretching, Bob Anderson. Shelter Publications, Inc., PO, Box 279, Bolinas, CA 94924
Yoga Journal. A bimonthly publication by the California Yoga Teachers Association. For subscription,
    write to Yoga Journal, PO Box 469018, Escondido, CA 92046-2054. Publishes yearly directory of teachers.

FITNESS
Take Charge of Your Body, Women's Health Advisor. Dr. Carolyn DeMarco M.D, R&R Book Bar, 14,800 Yonge St, #195, Aurora, ON. L4G 1N3. Canada. For single copies, call 1-800-387-4761
The Anatomy Coloring Book, Wynn Kapit / Lawrence M. Elson. Harper & Raw Publishers, Inc., N
Flex Appeal, Rachel McLish. Warner Books, PO Box 690, New York, NY 10018
Perfect Body Parts, Rachel McLish. Warner Books.
Winning Without Steroids, Gayle Olinekova
Secrets of Successful Bodybuilding Without Steroids, Jay Robb
Natural Bodybuilding and Fitness Journal; Chelo Publ Inc., 350 Fifth Ave, Suite 3323, New York, NY 10118.
Dedicated to drug free life styles.
The New Miracles of rebounding, Albert Carter,
The Golden Seven Plus One, Samuel West.

BOOK RESOURCES
Twenty First Century Publications, PO Box 702, Fairfield, IA 52556 (8 KYE-BOOK. Wholesale and retail. Catalogue available. Line of books Live food, Vegetarians, Ecology, Consciousness, Children series Specializes in books from India and Live Foods. Publishers of Vikt Kulvinskas books. Will search nationally and locate any book that might need. Catalogue.
New Leaf Distributing Company, Atlanta GA (800) 326-2665; FAX (8 326-1066. Wholesale only books, video and audio tapes, calendars, peric cals, New Age Sidelines
Nutri-Books, Denver CO Books, Video, Tapes Wholesale only.

USEFUL RESOURCES
Yoga Works, 1426 Montana Ave, Suite 12, Santa Monica, CA 90403; (8 YOGA-WRK,
clothing etc. for Yogic lifestyles.
Deva Lifewear, 110 1st Ave West, PO Box 5H, Westhope, ND 58793-02 (Natural fabrics)
The Vermonth Country Store, PO Box 3000, Manchester Ctr, VT 052 3000 (Cotton clothing, bed and bath. They have more than one catalogue
Faith Mountain Company, PO Box 199, Sperryville, VA 22740. Clothi gifts and home accessories.
Whole Life Products, 1334 Pacific Ave, Forest Grove, OR 97116
Seventh Generation, 49 Hercules Dr, Colchester, VT 05446-1672; 1-8(456-1177. Products for a healthy planet.
Real Goods, 966 Mazzoni St., Ukiah, CA 95482 (800) 762-7325 Produ for energy, and over all, independence.
Allergy Store, (800) 767-ACHOO

NATURAL LIVING JOURNALS and Resources
The Natural Hygiene M2M, c/o Ward Nicholson, 232 S. Belmont, Wichi KS 67218 (316) 682-2814; fax: (316) 682-0459. Letters and articles sh ing the lifestyles associated with raw food and natural living. Over 1 copied pages. Monthly, Membership fees vary. Call or fax.
Choice Magazine, T.H.P. 655 South Orcas, Suite 220, Seattle, WA 981 (206) 762-8403 A monthly magazine devoted to juicing and natural living
New Life, Serenity Health Organization, 218 West 72nd St., Suite 2F NYC, NY 10023. Range in topics from spirituality to deep research ir health challenges. Organize Alternative multi-state Expos Communities, 1, Box 155, Rutledge, MO 63563. Quarterly issues and yearly directory.
Remineralize the Earth, 152 South St., Northampton, MA 01060. 3 issu per year. Issues of minerals and   survival. Superior oil grows healthy, hea ing produce.
Organic Gardening, 33 E. Minor St., Emmaus, PA 18098
Natural Organic Hair and Skin Care, Audrey Hampton (Organica Press) guide to natural and synthetic ingredients.
NAVS, PO Box 94020, Palatine, IL 60094. Personal Care - guide to produc not tested on animals.
Clayton School of Natural Healing; American Holistic College of Nutriti - Home study (800) 659-8274.
Organic Times. OFPANA, 907 North Tower, 1331 Pennsylvania Ave, N.V WDC 20004
Inner Self, 915 South 21 Ave, #2A, Hlwd, FL 33020 (305-923-073(Increase well being on all levels.
Excellent articles that can help you feel the universal goodness.
Food and Water Journal, RR1 Box 68D, Walden, VT 05873. Consum Advocacy organization working for safe food and a clean environment.
FVO Farm Organic Verified Program, PO Box 3961, Bridgeport, CT 066(OCIA Organic Crop Association, 3185 TWP. Rd, Bellefontaine, OH 4333 Sprout Letter, , box 62, Ashland, OR 97520
Acres, USA PO Box 8800, Metairie, LA 70011 (504) 889-210 Economical, ecological agriculture.
Holistic Health Directory and Resource guide, New Age Pub, 42 Pleasa St., Watertown, MA 02172
Health and Beyond, 625 Smith Dr, Metairie, LA 70005. An exploration holistic health, vegetarianism and dental challenges.
Vegetarian Times, 4 High Ridge Park, Stamford, CT 06905. Mainstrea vegetarianism. At times excellent articles. In most issues, forget the recip

much processed foods, hard to digest mixes.

LLNESS, HERBS and NATURAL HEALING - books

for a New America, John Robins. May All Be fed: Diet for a New
ld.
nposition and Facts about Foods, Ford Heritage (Health Research, PO
M.H.,, CA 95245
ural Healing With Herbs; Intuitive Eating. Humbart Santillo, Excellent
a live food orientation.
ool of Natural Healing, Dr. John R. Christopher.
lers on Healing, Edited by Richard Carlson Ph.D.
rnative Health Care Resources, Directory and Guide. Brett Jason
lair. Very middle of the road.
siology of the Algae, Christian Drapeau, MSc.
Colon Health Handbook, Robert Gray
d Combining Made Easy, Herbert M. Shelton
Can Master Disease, Bernard Jensen
rnative Medicine: The Definitive Guide, Burton Gulberg Group
ty Harvest, Dr. Bernard Jensen. Link between soil, minerals and health.
at Your Doctors Won't Tell You, Jane Heimlich
ling Your Body Naturally, Gary Null
book of Natural Healing, Pizzarno & Murray
gers of Compulsory Education and How to Avoid Them Legally, Atrny
Finn

Children's Health Food Book, Ron Seaborn (great explanation of health
diet point, geared for
child within you, a must reading for every concerned parent).
nmercial Foods Exposed and How to Replace Them, Gaye Horsley
Medical Mafia, Guylaine Lanctoc, MD
-Prescription Drugs and Their Side effects, Robert Benowicz
't Drink Your Milk, Frank Oski MD
, Crime and Delinquency, Alexander Scauss
vival Guide for the New Millennium and How to Survive the Coming
h Changes, B. Kirkwood
s Dreams of the Future, Chet Snow, Ph.D.
tivating Female Sexual Energy, Mantak and Maneewan Chia
v to Counteract Environment Poisons, Clara Kroeger Foote
Smart, Diana Fairechild. 200 tips to beat the jet lag
l Health at the Computer, Martin Sussman and Dr. Ernest Loewenstein

TITUDE and INSPIRATION

da Grover, August Celebration, a Molecule of Hope for a Changing
ld.
a Seville & Nereyda Aquirre, The Nicaragua Report. Effect of Super
e Green Algae on scholastic performance. A Miracle.
rew Weil, MD, Spontaneous Healing. How to activate the natural heal-
power.
rt Wilde: Affirmations.
Keys: Handbook to Higher Consciousness.
pak Chopra MD, Quantum Healing
ise Hay: You Can Heal Your Life; Heal Your Life Workshop.
r McWilliams: You Can't Afford the Luxury of a Negative Thinking;
101.Lenard Shaw: Love and Forgiveness.
et Lerner: The Dance of Anger and the Dance of Intimacy.
s Griscom: The Healing of Emotions.
dra Ray: Loving Relationships.
n Gray, Ph.D.: What You Feel, You Can Heal.
n D. Biro, Beyond Success, the 15 Secrets of a Winning Life
r L. Hirsch, Living With Passion, 10 Simple Secrets that Guarantee Your
ess
ert Keith Wallace, The Neurophysiology of Enlightenment
istiane Northrup MD, Women's Bodies, Women's Wisdom;

ZYMATIC AND LIVE FOOD LIFESTYLES

ou are looking for true health and a lasting impact on your life, then start
)

Victor Kulvinskas M.S.: Survival Into 21st Century (Still one of the best
books on health) Don't Dine Without Enzymes; How to Enzymize Your Diet
(most practical transition to live foods), Lover's Diet, Love Your Body, Life
in the 21st Century, Sprout for the Love of Everybody.
Ann Wigmore, Hippocrates Diet
Brian Clements, Belief: All There is; Hippocrates Health Program.
Edmond Szekely: The Chemistry of Youth, Essene Gospel of Peace; Essene
Gospel of Peace Vol 4.
Gabriel Cousens: Conscious Eating (The best documented and most current
book live foods); Spiritual Nutrition and the Rainbow Diet (philosophy)
Dr. John W. Apsley ND: The Genesis Effect, Spearheading Regeneration
with Blue Green Algae
DA Lopez MD et al, Enzymes the Fountain of Life
Humbart Santillo ND: Food Enzymes, The Missing Link to Radiant Health
Edward Howell, MD Enzyme Nutrition; Food Enzyme Concept; Enzymes
for Health and Longevity.
Mark M. Braunstein: Radical Vegetarianism, The Sprout Garden.
Joe Alexander, The Blatant Raw Foodist Propaganda
Noel Johnson, The Living Proof; Dud at 70, Stud at 80. (He is in his 90's and
still running the marathons)
Gabree Amlak, The Superior Aspects of Women, A Tribute to Feminine
Nobility.
Theodore Baroody, Alkalize or Die
Ted Morter, Your Health, Your Choices.
Bernard Jensen, Tissue Cleansing Through Bowel Management.
Jacques de Langre, Ph.D., Seasalt's Hidden Power, Whole Sea Minerals,
Their Biologica
    Action on Body and Mind.
Laurence Badgley, MD, Healing AIDS Naturally - works with live foods,
enzymes, algae, holistic
Dean Ornish, MD, Dr. Dean Onrush's Program for Reversing Heart Disease;
Eat More, Weight Less.

NATURAL & LIVE FOODS, HERBS and VEGETARIANS GO ON the WEB, email etc.

The Natural Hygiene M2M, email: wardnik@southwind.net. Ward
Nicholson. Letters and articles sharing the lifestyles associated with raw
food and natural living. Wild humor. Over 150 copied pages. Monthly,
Membership fees vary. Call/fax..
Veg-raw Access the Internet and FTP to integrate net. The listserv veg-raw
is the resource listserv on vegetarian/vegan raw food diets. To subscribe,
send mail to majordomo@intergate.net, with the contents: subscribe veg-
raw. If have question, call Bob at 214-790-2520.
Steve Levine (415) 461-3590, Natural Life Styles and Vegetarian Directory
Vegan Action- vegan@mellersl.psych.berkeley.edu.
General Complementary Medicine Reference
(http://www.forthrt.com/~chronicl/archiv.htm) Mind/body/spirit, herbs, chiropractic resources, Ayurveda, Vegetarianism, Feng Shui, healing, alternative cancer therapies, . Created and maintained by Synergistic Medicine
Center, Chapel Hill, NC.
Herb Hall (http//www.crl.com/~robbee/herbal.html/) Herb schools, wild-
crafting resources, Michael Moore's on-line newsletter, botanical sources
and much more.
Thomas Register (http://www,thomasregister.com/) 52,000 categories for
products and service suppliers of American Manufacturers.
FDA (http:www.fda.gov/) Reulations, policies etc.
Yahoo (http://www .com/) and Infoseek (http://www2 .infoseek.com/) Two
good places to start for seeking of any kind of information.
Jeanne C. Ryer, A Pocket Tour of Health & Fitness on the Internet.
Miracle on Line Marketing, 620 N. Brand Blvd, Suite 310, Glendale, CA
91203 (800) 818-2646.
    Create and maintain internet Web site. Many other services.
U.S.-EURO-NET, 615 W. Grand Ave, Suite 1, Hot Springs, AR 71901 (501)
620-4049. Free copy of
    "How to Design and Promote Your Internet Storefront for Fun and Profit."
Complete line of
    service to play on the internet.

WELLNESS RESOURCES - request a catalogue.

(For those who are in need of a system to 'jump start their life' then go for three weeks at a centers.)

Resort to L.O.V.E. (1489 Airport Rd, Hot Springs AR 71913) Youkta and Viktoras offers women retreats during 1996; In 1997 Spring, a school will be opened with residential program. Dance, Yoga, Live foods, Hands on training in the Live Food Culinary arts by Viktoras. Cleansing and Detox programs, as well as weight loss and gain systems.Live Food Maintenance programs. Over 25 years of experience.

Love Foods, PO Box 2853, Hot Springs, AR 71914. Send $2 for info, audio and video tape on wild organic wild food, as well as other super foods that facilitate rapid healing.

Hippocrates Health Institute, 1443 Palmdale Court, West Palm Beach, FL 33411 A full educational experience with certification. The most researched and advanced systems in natural therapies. Includes a very professional staff. Makes use of live foods, wheatgrass and Super Blue Green algae as well as other food concentrates. A place for those who are seeking cleansing, holistic education and experience into meaning of true health. Offers a 3 week or longer program as well as a long term residential certification program for the health professionals. The institute was started by Dr. Ann Wigmore and Viktoras Kulvinskas M.S. over 25 years ago. It is under the directive of Brian and Anna Marie Clements.

Tree of Life Rejuvenation Center, PO 1080, Patagona, AZ 85625 (520) 394=-2520. Started by Dr. Gabriel Cousins MD. An author, Essene minister, yoga practitioner and teacher. Offers programs in fasting, Panchakarma rejuvenation, Ayurvedic approach with live food. Internship in live food and permaculture. Essene Order of Light training intensives.

Optimal Health Institute, 6970 Central Ave, Lemon Grove CA 92045. (619) 464-3346. A 3 week cleansing program

Ann Wigmore Foundation, Porto Rico (809) 868-6307, 3 week health vacation with live food

Creative Health Institute, 918 Union City Rd, Union City, MI 49094. (517) 278-6260 3 week cleansing program.

Integral Yoga Institute, 2103 Maple Ave, Fairlawn, NJ 07410 (201) 796-7585 A non-residential program offered in yoga, live food and healing. Ongoing classes and certification in many healing modalities. Director: Margabandhu.

Optimal Health, 963 Peaceful Court, Brighton, MI 48116 (810) 229-1666. Joyce Olivetto director. Offers full line of natural therapies. Also available sprouting seeds, water filters and other appliances.

IMPORTANT ORGANIZATIONS IN QUALITY OF LIFE

YES (Youth for Environmental Sanity) 706 Frederick St., Santa Cruz, CA 95065. (408) 459-9344. Empowering young people across the world, with over 1/2 million members. Founders: Ocean Robins and Ryan Elision.

Earth Save, founded by John Robins, excellent booklet on the impact of diet on health, ecology and sanity. (800) 362-3648

Relay team 2000. Created by Cell Tech to connect and educate the persons on nutrition, health, ecology and how to make a difference. Dial from your fax machine (904) 422-2122 Ext 505, request document 111. You will have it faxed back to you the current schedule. Call 501-760-2280 for membership in the wholesale purchase of super foods.

National Health Federation, PO Box 688, Monrovia, CA 91017. National organization established 35 years ago for the preservation and restoration of ones right to determine one's own health care program.

The Health Resource, 209 Katherine Drive, Conway, AR 72032. (501)-329-8700. A comprehensive report on your medical condition. Copies of articles. Works well with alternative therapies. $70 for a 20-25 page mini report.

World Research Foundation, 15300 Ventura Blvd., #405, Sherman Oaks, CA 91403. (818) 907-5483. Extensive library system, with computer linkup to over 500 data bases giving one access to important medical, scientific and environmental information from over 100 countries. Basic fee for search is .

Alternative Medicine, compiled by The Burton Goldberg Group. two inch thick. Includes extensive write up on all the modalities, as well as where to go and what else you can read. the truly holistic approaches have been excluded, no mention of live foods, wheatgrass, Super Blue Green Algae. However, it does give an excellent presentation of all the well documented

healing approaches. Retails for $60, ask your library for review or may ⌷ from (800) KYE-BOOK.

National Vaccine Information Center, 512 W. Maple Ave, Suite 206, Vie Virginia, 22180 (703) 938-0342. Clearinghouse for possible dangers as ⌷ ated with vaccination. Before you take a shot, call.

or get the vaccination education kit ((818) 357-2181.

The Alliance for Alternative Medicine, PO Box 59, Liberty Lake, WA 9⌷ (509) 255-9246. Referral for alternative treatments.

International Association for Cancer Victors and Friends, 7740 ⌷ Manchester Ave, Suite 110, Playa del Ray, CA 90293 (310) 822-5⌷ Information, books and referral.

American Association of Naturopathic Physicians, 2366 Eastlake Ave, ⌷ 322, Seattle, WA 98102

International Association of Professional Natural Hygienists, 2000 S⌷ Ocean Dr, Hallandale, FL 33009 (305) 454-2220. Therapeutic Fasting holistic model

American Colon Therapy Association, 11739 Washington Blvd., ⌷ Angeles, CA 90066 (310) 390-5424. Training and referral.

Citizens For Health, PO 368, Tacoma, WA 98401 (800) 357-2211. Free ⌷ of choice in healing systems.

American Preventative Medical Association, PO Box 211, Tacoma, ⌷ 98401.

LIVE FOOD RECIPE BOOKS:

Love Your Body; How to Enzymize Your Diet, Lover's Diet V⌷ Kulvinskas

Living With live Foods, Steven Levine, most recent chef of Hippocrate⌷

Light Eating for Survival, Marcia Acciardo

Sweet Temptations, Natural desert Book; Frances Kendall (best to eat ⌷ as a complete meal)

Eydie Mae's Natural Recipes, E. Hunsberger

Dining in the Raw, Cooking with the Buff; Rita Romano. Former che⌷ Hippocrates health Institute.

Favorite Recipes of Living Foods Children, Denise Swan

SEED SOURCES

Besides the local Coops' and Health Food Stores, one can also try ⌷ untreated seeds at seed suppliers and look in the yellow pages for "⌷ Stores"

Entry Level, small volumes:

Hippocrates Health Institute, 1443 Palmdale Court, West Palm Beach, ⌷ 33411 (407) 471-8876, Quarterly Journal. Many variety, small volume⌷ beginners.

Mountain Ark Trading CO, 120 South East Ave, Fayetteville, AR 72701 ⌷ mixes, sea weed.

The Herbarium, PO Box 246836, Sacramento, CA 95824

Walnut Acres, Penns Creek, PA 17862. Variety of seeds, plus transiti⌷ foods.

Apradisia, 28 Carmine St, NYC, NY 10014 Alfalfa, fenugreek, flax, b⌷ and yellow mustard seeds etc.

Seed Savers Exchange, 3076 N. Winn Rd., Decorah, IA 52101 Collec⌷ rare seeds, mainly heirloom variety, . The seeds are offered through ⌷ annual yearbook at a fee of $25.

Seeds of Change, PO Box 15700, Santa Fe, NM 87506-5700. Source of n⌷ hybrid, organic seeds.

Large Volume:

Jaffe Bros Inc., PO Box 636, Escandido, CA 92082 (619) 749-1⌷ Wholesale and retail organic seeds, grains, nuts, dried fruit, oil We purc⌷ from them twice a year.

Living Farms, Box 50, Troy, MN 561754 Beans, grains and seeds

Cross Seed CO, HC 69, Box 2, Bunker Hill, KS 67626 Large selection

Stockton Roller Mill, PO Box 26, St. Charles, MN 55971 (507) 932-4⌷ Large selection

Sanctuary Seeds, 2774 West 4th St., Vancouver, BC, V6K 1R1 (604) 7⌷ 4724 Large choice.

Ozark Warehouse Coop. 1601 Pump Station Rd, Fayetteville, AR 72⌷ Large selection of seeds, as well as other dried goods. Newsletter. Deli⌷

Diamond K Enterprises, RR1 Box 30, St. Charles, MN 55972 (507) 932-4308. Variety.

International Sprout Growers Association, 7300 Lincolnshire DR, Sacramento, CA 95823

Survival Supply Co.P.O. Box 1745, Shingle Springs, CA 95682. Long term 45# plastic buckets. Some items natural and organic.

EQUIPMENT

Many of the useful appliances can be purchased at health food stores and coops, as well as department stores. We selected the finest that is available through the mail. You will need a water purifier, can cost from 150 to 1000 dollars. Choose at least a solid block carbon filter, to reverse osmosis or distiller. Your cost per gallon will vary between 5 and 10 cents. Consider that you are between 65 and 80% water, it is important to have daily at least a quart of pure water.

Mail order companies or local distributors is the way to go. Do some serious research by reading a book.

Love Foods, PO Box 2853, Hot Springs, AR 71914. Wild Enzymatic Super Foods, appliances, long term storage bucket seeds, sea weed, books.

Hippocrates Health Institute, 1443 Palmdale Court, West Palm Beach, FL 33411 Juicers, dehydrators, automatic sprouter and baby green grower, water and air purifiers, books, enzymes.

Sproutamo, PO Box 203, New Lisbon, WI 53950 "Easy Sprouter"

Sprout Ease, PO 1876, Kerrville, TX 78029 (512) 866-0117. Sprout screens for jars & the tube sprouter.

Creative Craftsman, 4855 Mandarin Blvd., Loxahatchee, FL 33470 (407) 790-4647 Sprout units, video.

Karen's Fresh Fields Restaurant, 3351 N. Lincoln Ave, Chicago, IL 60657. Besides an all live food restaurant, Karen is the manufacturer of a manual wheatgrass juicer. Live food and wheatgrass via mail.

Bee Beyer's Food Dryer, 1154 Roberts Lane, Los Angeles, CA (213) 472-8961

Excaliber, 6083 Power Inn Rd, Sacramento, CA 95824 (916) 381-4254 Dehydrators.

Cuisinart Food Processor, Greenwich CT 06830 (203) 975-4600

Oster Blender, Rt. 9 Box 541, McMinnville, TN 37110 (800) 356-7837 One of the most cost effective blender, also has available a food processor attachment that works well for the road, as well as small family.

Quality Health, 922 Black Diamond Way, Lodi, CA 95240 (800) 826-4148 The Champion Juicer.

SEA VEGETABLES

(Check out the local Oriental Markets for quality low cost sea weeds, especially nori, wakame.)

Maine Seaweed CO, Box 57, Steuben, ME 04680 (207) 546-2875

Macrobiotic Company of America, 799 Old Leicester Hwy, Ashville, NC 28806 (800) 438-4730. 2 pound units of wide choice of sea vegetables, unpasteurized low salt miso. Wholesale.

Atlantic Mariculture, Box 2368, Darmouth, Nova Scotia, Canad . Seaweeds.

Medocine Sea Vegetables, Box 372, Navarro, CA 05463 (707) 895-3741

HERBS AND SEASONINGS

The Grain and Salt Society, Box DD, Magalia, CA 95954 (916) 873-0294. Celtic Salt.

Carothers' Research Laboratories, PO Box 3307, Flint, MI 48502 (810) 235-2055. Raw Olive Oil

Frontier Herbs, Box 299, Norway, IA 52318 (800) 669-3275

HerbPharm, Williams, OR 97544 (800) 848-4372. Organic, wild crafted whenever available. Apprentice program. Research.

Dragon River Herbals, PO Box 9040, Santa Fe, NM 87504

Great Lakes Herb Co., PO Box 6713, Minneapolis, MN 55406

Herb Research Foundation, 1007 Pearl St, Suite 200, Boulder, CO 80302 (303) 449-2265

American Herb Association, PO Box 1673, Nevada City, CA 95959, (916) 265-9552. Send $4 for a listing of more than 50 mail order herb sources.

Blessed Herbs, 109 Barre Plains Rd, Oakham, MA 01068 (800) 489-4372

Pacific Botanicals, c/o Catalog Request, 4350 Fish Hatchery Rd, Grants Pass, OR 97527. Organic herb growers.

FRESH ORGANIC FOOD SOURCES

National Organic Directory 1996. Guide to organic info resources. Community Allience with Family Framers (CAFF), Davis, CA 95617. (916) 756-8518 * (800) 852-3832 * (916) $34.95

Eden Acres Organic Network, 12100 Lima Center Rd, Clint (517) 456-4288. Offers an international directory of Organic fo Andy Firk (305-) Organic food growers. Listings available t Albert's Organics, Los Angeles, CA (213) 234-4595; (800) 89 Bandwagon Brokerage Inc. Produce, Los Angeles, CA (21 Wholesale fresh produce.

Glasser Farms Fruits, Miami FL (305) 238-7747. Fresh and d vegetables.

Organically Fresh, Teeca Plaza, 4814 NW 2nd Ave, Boca Rat((407) 998-3379 Low price, organic produce.

Corganics, North Carolina (800) 987-4924.

Diamond Organics, (800) 922-2396 Fresh produce and baby gr catalogue.

For wholesale Super Blue Green Algae and other su contact the person who introduced you to this

Rev. Viktoras Kulvinskas Ph.D., N
PO 1556
Mt. Ida, AR
71957
Viktoras4u.com
viktorasretreats@gmail.com

Viktoras Kulvinskas Experience with Super Blue Green Algae™ 1982 to 1999

Dear Reader, please note, that this is my personal experience. It is not intended to imply that any of the food products mentioned in this story are therapeutic, healing or curative. There is no attempt to prescribe or diagnose or cure. It is a story that gives life to the old saying "Let food be your medicine and medicine be your food" of Hippocrates.

It would not be an exaggeration to say that Super Blue Green Algae™ saved my life. It is my hope that my story will inspire you to give algae a chance to work miracles in your life, too.

In the early 1980's, I created a residential healing community called the All Life Sanctuary, located in Woodstock Valley, Connecticut. A long time friend of mine, Showshawme, lived there for about a year. We experimented with live food, communal living and few whole food supplements - aspergilus plant based food enzymes as well as spirulina.

Showshawme left us for Hawaii, where he continued to experiment with various whole green foods and green supplement products. Some of the products that he was using included fresh and powdered wheatgrass, barley grass, spirulina, and chlorella, and eventually, the species of algae known as aphanizomenon flos aquae, commonly known as Cell Tech's Super Blue Green Algae™.

By 1982, the money I was making from the "Survival Into 21st Century". I had spend in supporting the All Life Sanctuary community. My health also was suffering from malnutrition - years of cleansing programs as well as cooked food binges. I sold the farm and I walked away with few thousand dollars. I ended up drifting through northern New York state. During that period I created a successful healing resort in the Catskill's as well as set up life food restaurants at new age expos. However, I was emotionally isolated and empty, ravaged by manic depression with lack of direction or passion for life. In 1985I returned to live with my parents in Connecticut.

Showshawme likewise was back in Hartford. He was fired up by Super Blue Green Algae™ and was trying to turn on others to this wonder food. He tried to get me involved in using algae and then selling to others. But something in me resisted and wasn't ready. I avoided making any commitment to Showshawme despite his persistence.

At that time I believed that advocating the live food system and selling health products just didn't mix. Eventually I came to realize that Super Blue Green Algae™ was essentially in the same category as other water-grown foods (i.e. nori, dulce, kelp, Hiziki, etc.) which I was already suggesting that people include in their diet. What's more, Super Blue Green Algae™ was enzymatically active, grown wild in the full spectrum, mineral rich, alkaline sweet waters of Klamath Lake in Oregon.

As I was to discover, Super Blue Green Algae™ was almost a complete food in itself that could be eaten in increasing quantities as one

becomes more and more detoxified and was able to handle the p[ow]erful energies of this Super Food.

At the time I was putting up all these objections to Showshaw[me's] plea to give the Super Blue Green Algae™ a try, I was secretly [on] a heavy bulimic trip, glutting myself on junk food vegetarian fe[ast] and then regurgitating to relieve myself.

Eating large quantities of food and then purging ones' self thro[ugh] self-induced vomiting is called bulimia. My bulimia evolved a[s] outcome of a twenty-year long history of migraine headac[he] which were as frequent as twice a week, starting at six years of a[ge] though infrequent, and by eighteen, the migraines were wee[kly] which I found I could usually be relieved by vomiting the stom[ach] acid rot. I was totally debilitated by age 28.

When I went on a vegetarian live food diet at Hippocrates He[alth] Institute in the late 1960's, I became migraine free. However, [the] detoxification that simultaneously occurred with this diet a[lso] brought up to the surface a lot of emotional and mental pain tha[t] apparently still needed to work out. I was a walking emotional-ti[me bomb]

A major source of much of this emotional pain had its origin in [a] childhood filled with violence of World War II, as well as commu[ni]cation problems and the explosive imagination that lived thro[ugh] fairy stories filled with the battle between good and evil. I ne[ver] could deal with darkness of night and the imagination that surfa[ced] the terror of the fairy tales. Throughout my youth I had a long [his]tory of both manic depression and catatonic schizophrenia; I [was] also a pretty wild teenager and lived quite irresponsibly. By sev[en]teen, the ongoing emotional stress had brought on a bleeding ulc[er]

I found that eating was the way to reduce stress and experience te[m]porary oblivion from memories and conflicts that seemed to be s[o] facing. As an escape, I used food to suppress this psychological b[ag]gage. Even when I was eating only live food, I would eat huge me[als] that would leave me feeling bloated and fatigued. I found from ex[pe]rience that if all this food stayed in my stomach, it would ferment [and] bring on headaches as well as sciatic pain. So for relief, I vomite[d]

Eventually, vomiting became a daily practice. I fell into eating m[ore] and more cooked and junk food. The problem became more [dis]abling, both physically and psychologically, for I was living a d[ouble] life. In public, I would give health talks and lifestyle consultatio[ns.] In private, I was a junk food eater and bulimic. The hypocrisy o[f it] all was destroying further me from the inside out.

One positive practice that really saved me from much of the harm[ful] effects of this negative cycle, was the daily intake plant-ba[sed] digestive enzymes along with the food that I ate. Because of t[his] practice, unlike most bulimic, my immune and digestive system w[as] able to maintain much of its overall power and functionality. O[ne] area I suffered greatly, was due to the ongoing acid condition, I w[as] loosing a great deal of calcium from teeth and bone. One cannot co[n]tinually mistreat the body with disrespect and get away with [it.] During this period, I became re-addicted to coffee, which I consum[ed] daily.

As a cumulative result of abusing my body in all these ways, cel[lu]lar acidosis became rampant and my migraine attacks again beca[me] more and more frequent. At times, the acidity in my body became

t of balance that I had several near-death experiences. In fact, I
is roused from an unconscious state many times by my friends as
ll as mother and father, who just happened to appear at these crit-
l life-threatening moments in time to then save or rescue me.

, at this precarious time in my life, Showshawme visited me from
waii, bringing with him tales of miracle healing from folks that
ed Super Blue Green Algae™. At first, I listened to these stories
th skepticism, for I knew that these stories did not constitute strict
entific studies but were only anecdotal.

wever, I could not deny that I was losing my memory-concentra-
n and that I was a full blown, closet bulimic. Part of me listened
ently to Showshawme's accounts, while the other part, my ego,
isted the notion that I needed help.

nally I decided to give Super Blue Green Algae™ a try.
owshawme had me sign the distributor form and order the algae.
took care of all the details, for I never would have taken the ini-
tive and follow through by myself. When the algae arrived, he
lled me daily to find out if I was using it. It took a whole week
fore I broke down and took some.

om the time I began taking algae that auspicious week, renewed
ental clarity and a concern for my personal well-being re-entered
y life. I gradually moved from food addiction toward living a more
sponsible life-positive lifestyle. I have never regressed back to
limia. My life has been getting better and better ever since. Super
ue Green Algae™ has taken on a central place in my growth.

have experimented using Super Blue Green Algae™ in various
ounts through different periods of my life. All my experiences
ve been positive. As one example, I have given some of my best
ture presentations while ingesting only the Omega Sun algae and
ter. I have eaten as much as a single bottle of the Super Blue
een Omega Sun Algae (cell wall removed, with higher concentra-
n of small chain amino acids and alkaline minerals to impact the
ental functions) during a ten hour raw food intensive workshop I
is giving.

this one memorable workshop, I attribute the profound connection
ad with this audience directly to the intuitive-clarity-heightening
ects of the Omega Sun. I was also told that I was incredibly funny
d that I was answering the participants' questions before they were
rbally asked. I remember one woman at this particular workshop
ite vividly.

e told me in the past her attention span was usually no longer than
minutes at a time. Ordinarily, she continuously needed to take
eaks. However, because of impact of my spontaneous and dramat-
style of delivery, as well as relevance of the material, she stayed
the full eight hours presentation without needing her customary
eaks. She became a user of the Omega Sun herself, even before I
ished half of the workshop.

wadays, I still love food as always. I eat mostly raw live foods and
a weekly basis my diet would be considered to be at least 98%
e/raw. However, I do not have an addictive relationship to main-
ning this diet nor do I feel deprived on this functional nutritional
ogram. I feel comfortable, as I see fit, to enjoy sweet cooked pota-
s and sprouted bread. I occasionally eat beans and take extra

enzymes when I eat these cooked foods.

Generally, on my favorite program, I enjoy a breakfast of green juice
and wheatgrass, with other fluids taken in as I need it during the day.
In the afternoon I have two to four small meals, depending on my
schedule, which center around sprouted grain/soaked seed, sea
weeds, greens and soaked nut/seeds. Between meals, when hungry, I
take Super Blue Green Algae™, mixed in water. I mix this nourishment around in my mouth with my saliva, and allow maximum time
for absorption, before I swallow.

Presently, I am free from food cravings thanks to the Omega Sun balancing effect. For me, it works best not to eat any solid meal before
3 PM. I rest for an hour during the day and sleep three to five hours
during the night.

Super Blue Green Algae™ has been a great teacher in my life, helping to lead my consciousness into LIFE and away from destructive
directions of my past. My productivity and creativity has blossomed
over the last few years, and I am grateful for the balancing and ener-
gizing contribution of Super Blue Green Algae™ toward the
progress I have made.

I am presently sixty. I feel more vital and happier than I have ever
been in my life. I feel that I have not reached the peak of my productivity. I presently operate four health-oriented businesses and jug-
gle several other projects at any one time. I am also about half of the
year on the road giving workshops, participating at conferences and
sharing the live food lifestyles with a Super Blue Green Algae™
twist.

After being friends and co-workers, I married Youkta, who is a life
time yoga and dance instructor, creative artist, as well as a body
builder. Due to her influence, I am a devoted weight lifter, where I
am doing 405# 3 set, ten reps, as well as progressing on all my body
parts. On the live food program, that I fully describe in Lover's Diet,
I have been able to gain 1 pound a week of lean muscle mass. I also
do 6 hours of yoga weekly at classes that Youkta conducts.

I have opened myself to the path of limitless growth. I am challenged
by my occasional minor imbalances in my energy levels which I
attribute to my tendency to overwork, but now I am finally in control
of my life.

In my present life, I am now able to relate to other people from a
place where I have no fear. I am able to feel comfortable under conditions which would have been very stressful in the past. I now look
at these stressors as challenges and opportunities for growth with
expanded horizons, wrapped with the gift of joy & love in the making. I do not give energy or thought or feeling to places that seems to
present areas of fear, darkness and discomfort. For what you give
attention to, you attract. I resist nothing and only attracted and
focused on place of goodness and joy.

My vision of what it means to live a life of service to the world community has expanded immeasurably. My concentration keeps
improving. My mental powers and psychic abilities that I had as a
youth have returned. I feel I am as a child, being reborn into an ever
more perfect form. I cannot imagine being able to maintain this level
of functioning without my daily use of Super Blue Green Algae™.

It is said that the mind is like a parachute - it works best when it is open. It is my hope that you open your mind, like I did, to the possibility that Super Blue Green Algae™ can be helpful, or even key, for your optimal physical, mental, emotional and spiritual evolution. Give it a try, won't you? It is unconditionally guaranteed and you have nothing to lose and much to gain.

I appreciate you for you having taken the time to read my story. I hope it will help you and many others. Love in Service.

What is so special about the Super Blue Green Algae.

The SBG Algae has a 15 year history of successful usage by well over a million people who have tried it. It is enzymatic, wild crafted, with a highest concentration of pre-digested protein (over 60%), pro-carotene and the right form of Vitamin B-12.

It is unique in the way it goes through a collar dispersion. It gives one a clear indication of impact on the person. Dissolve in a glass jar (3.5' diameter and 10 inch high) 2 caps of the Super Blue Green Algae™. Let it sit for 1 hour, stir a few times so that all the powder is dissolved. Place a Tenson (available from most lamp or department stores) floodlight directly above the glass canister. When looked at the glass container, you will see 25% from the top a radiant purple/magenta color; the lower portion is sky blue with some green on the bottom. The only other enzymatic algae, is the spirulina from Hawaii. It shows up totally green. The grass powders, likewise show up strictly green.

From the color therapy perspective, as well as from spiritual studies, you know that purple/magenta enhance intuitive and spiritual consciousness; where as the blue effects the intellectual, and green the physical.

There is no food that has the 3 color dispersion pattern like the Super Blue Green Algae™. Because of the high presence of the blue, I was not surprised to discover that it has a the most dramatic effect on academic performance. It has effected me greatly. Also, there is the classic study, published as the Nicaragua Report, which was initiated in Carmela Noguera School of Nandaime, Nicaragua where 2000 primary school children who had one of the worst school record in the country were fed 1 cap of the SBG Algae™ twice a day. After one school year, they achieved first place academically among all primary schools in Nicaragua in 1993. (for copy of report, send $2 to Viktoras).

Similar observations has been reported in USA. However, because the parents give to their children not only the SBG Algae™ but also all the other super foods from Cell tech, the results of outstanding nature, is in general achieved in a matter of two months (for such results, ask for the ADD and ADHD Report from Viktoras).

Another exciting feature about the Cell Tech SBG Algae™ is the energy dispersion pattern that shows up through the color Opto-Crystallization. "The patterns of SBG Algae™ parallel that of a thriving beech tree standing at full growth - a miracle of photosynthesis and natural energy. The patterns of Chlorella and Spirulina, however are relatively flat and unsophisticated, indicating a far less energetic vibrational field.

Some years ago, I discovered the kitchen enzyme test on the Super

Blue Green Algae™ Alpha Sun (the whole algae) , which follow Cell Tech is the only harvester from the Klamath Lake that has a d ing process that operates on low enough temperature, so that enzymes are intact. The other companies degrade the algae, weath it is in the dehydration of the storing, so that there is no enzy activity level indicated. When enzymes are destroyed, you also d organize all the proteins, amino acids, you loose a great deal of t vitamins as well as the organic structure of minerals. Of course t Kirlian energy field is gone. Kinesiology (or muscle) Test indica that all the other blue green algae tested has a weakening effect the hundredths of vegetarians that I have tested.

I am also including summary on some of the research that has be performed by universities and independent labs on the miracles the Super Blue Green Algae.

A STUDY OF PROTEALITIC ENZYME ACTIVITY OF BLUE GREEN ALGAE

The study demonstrates that the Cell Tech's Super Blue Green Algae is enzymaticly superior over the other Klamath Lake h. vested algae as well as over other tested spirulina and chlorella alg products found in the health food stores.
,,Viktoras Kulvinskas MS; (1996 - 1998) 2 pages Revised and u dated as of Feb. 1998.

Over the years, I have been seeking out foods of high quality. Eve algae company claims there product is the best. However, one of key ingredients of quality, as well as a measure of life, is the pre ence of enzyme activity in an algae, matter fact, any food. As a resu I have been concerned in finding a simple test that can be perform at home to indicate enzyme activity. Simple tests for an enzyme su plement, which will demonstrate amylase and protease activity a described in my booklet "Don't Dine Without Enzymes" on page The following contains a description of such experiments.

According to Dr. Howell, author of "Enzyme Nutrition" and "Fo Enzymes for Health and Longevity", there is a direct relationsh between the complex macro-molecules in food and the presence precise enzymes to break them down. Hence a raw high starch fo has a high amylase, a starch digesting enzyme, presence. Grai (high in starch) after sprouting, have a surplus enough enzymes digest cooked rice into a sweet tasting cream. For documentatio and introduction to the wonder of sprouted wheat and other grair see my book "Sprout for the Love of Everybody".

Considering that Super Blue Green™ Algae is over 62‰ prote one would anticipate it to have a high protealitic enzyme concentr tion. The sprouted wheat gluten test discovery goes back 5 yea where during a long journey, I attempt to flavor my sprouted whe meal with Super Blue Green™ Algae Alpha Sun™.

The wheat was sprouted for at least two days. I chewing a handf of wheat sprouts and after a few minutes (at least 3) I was left wi a glob of gluten gum (similar to the wheat-gluten-setian-protein ve etarian steaks you can buy at health food store) in my mouth.

However, to my surprise, when I had chewed the sprouted whe with one gram (4 caps) of Super Blue Green™ Algae Alpha Sun (as well as Omega Sun™) powder, the gluten liquefied and disa peared into a simpler form of protein. This proved that not on er Blue Green™ Algae was enzymatically active, but it also had e than enough extra enzymes to act on other protein structures, h as gluten, whereby Super Blue Green™ algae's naturally urring enzymes were able to digest the gluten.

ther tests with the other two companies algae products that are vested from the Klamath Lake, I found them to be inactive on the en. They either had only enough activity to act on itself, but none ct on other foods; OR, they had NO enzyme activity. The differ- e is in the superior and more conscious methods of the Cell Tech ne harvest and preparation for the market. Low temperature and lity care makes all the difference.

SECOND test, I call the Viktory over Jello test.

demonstrate enzyme activity, I tried many different combinations r a period of time. Eventually I gave up until it came to me in a am to try an equal weight of Super Blue Green™ Alpha Sun™ ae and jello. It worked. I am going to describe the exact test. I d Knox Unflavored Gelatin - which is available in most grocery es.

lit the package of powder in half , which was 3.5 grams (as mea- ed on a metric scale). Then I brought water to boil, filled a cup h 4 oz water and added the Gelatin. I used a wooden chopstick each sample. Then I let it sit for few minutes, stirred as neces- y, until the gelatin was fully dissolved. Then I added another 4 water and stirred it and let the liquid cool to about 105 deg F.

xt, I mixed in 3.5 (14 caps) grams of the Super Blue Green™ pha Sun™ Algae powder and stirred it vigorously, until it fully solved. I put the liquid mix inside a food dehydrator- to provide sistent warmth for enzymatic activity. The temperature was set 100 deg F, however, the inside thermometer read about 110 deg let it sit for 1 hour. I stirred the mix every 15 minutes. Then I ked it again and transferred it to refrigerator, at about 40 deg F.

ours later, the mix was still liquid. By now, one would anticipate ave the jello turn solid.

comparison, next I ran 2 other algae samples from other com- ies that harvest on Klamath Lake; also, I included other algae ducts like Chlorella, Spirulina (Hawaian), Spirulina (Japanese) well as plain Gelatin.

e test was run simultaneously for the samples mentioned under ntical conditions. After 3 hours, Cell Tech Super Blue Green™ ha Sun™ Algae. and the were the only ones that stayed liquid, other 'jello algae' mixes turned solid. The Cell Tech Omega n™ jello mix was totally liquid (1998). All the other companies' cept for the Spirulina(Hawaian)) algae jello mixtures were solid d did not pour at all.

oticed, after being such an enzymatic perfectionist in the mar- place, that our competitors decided to do something about it, i.e. e of the harvesters added enzymes to their enzymeless algae. For plicity, I will call this product 'BRAND X'. Cell Tech's Super e Green™ Alpha Sun™ Algae needs no addition of enzymes, ce the enzymes are not destroyed in their freeze drying process.

ecided to run the jello test on their new and improved 'BRAND

X', using the Alpha Sun™ as a control. I prepared jello in the usual fashion. The 'BRAND X' even with the enzymes added, turned to solid jello. However, the Alpha Sun™ stayed liquid.

I redid the gluten test with 1 gram (2 caps) powder of 'Brand X', it did not dissolve the gluten - it just turned it into green gum. Then I used 1 gram (4 caps) powder of Alpha Sun™, it dissolved the gluten to a simpler form which was absorbed within my mouth. Hence, the Cell Tech Alpha Sun™ has surplus enzymes to dissolve gluten bonds and 'Brand X' does not.

The 'BRAND X' is still a dead algae product. The amount of enzymes they added was probably enough to digest the heat treated protein of the 'BRAND X', but it had no surplus of enzymes to also digest the collagen of jello. You cannot resurrect the dead. The 'BRAND X' has gone through a processing by the harvesters that destroy the enzymes. The adding of enzymes does not resurrect the loss of organic minerals (thus bio-availability) - the heat has broken the amino bonds to the minerals and made the minerals inorganic, with reduced absorption; furthermore, the loss occurred in a wide range of vitamins which are heat sensitive; not to mention, the loss of electro-magnetic life force vibrational energies which contribute to the subtle life energy fields. It's time to stop the lies that other competitors' of algae products, like 'BRAND X' are as good as the Cell Tech's Super Blue Green™ algae.

COMMENTS: The surplus enzymes that were in the Cell Tech Super Blue Green™ Algae acted on the gelatin and broke the gelatin pro- tein into a much simpler form, thus preventing the formation of the solid jello. However, the other companies algae products failed to have surplus enzymes and as a result, they were not able to have any enzymatic influence on the gelatin, hence the liquid mix turned solid.

CONCLUSION: - Based on the two tests, the Super Blue Green‰ Algae samples have a much higher enzyme activity than any of the other algae products tested. That is, the other algae are either totally enzymatically inactive, or at least have a far lower enzyme activity than the Super Blue Green™ Algae. The Cell Tech Super Blue Green™ Algae were the only one's of the samples tested that had any detectable enzymatic activity on the protein structures of gelatin and gluten. Don't be fooled by other companies claims to have special cold flash drying processes etc..

Once again Cell Tech comes out light years ahead in quality algae products over any competing algae products.

Special acknowledgment for review and editing by Showshawme of Transformational Research.

VIKTORAS LIFE TODAY

As I sit gazing out at the acres of natural beauty that surround me on my Hot Springs, Arkansas homestead (which we've named the "All Life Sanctuary,") I feel wonderfully blessed beyond words to express...And my thoughts drift back to a time when I WASN'T pros- perous, WASN'T healthy and strong (even though I was younger), WASN'T in control of my time, WASN'T able share from the depths of my heart with loved ones, WASN'T able to create the kind of life that I had always dreamed of...

In reflecting upon these challenging times—compared to the fantastic experience I have today—I realize that my life wouldn't be the same without "the algae," or "Super Blue-Green Algae (AFA-algae), or "Aphanizomenon flos-aquae (AFA)"—whatever name YOU use to refer to that most powerful, pristine and primal of all healing green gifts of MotherNature.

For me, it was AFA-algae that gave my body, and too easily frazzled mind, the nutrients and energy they needed to heal.

It was AFA-algae that gave me a sense of renewed purpose over 15years ago when I came to a critical crossroads in my life as a natural healer and health educator.

It was AFA-algae, through Cell Tech, that gave me the income I needed— simply by spreading the good word about AFA-algae to others—which enabled me to create the All Life Sanctuary—not only AROUND me but IN my very being as well.

Because AFA-algae has done so much for me and the thousands of people I've told about the algae whose lives have been transformed, nowadays, even more than before, I tell a whole lot of people about AFA-algae—the person seated next to me while flying on an airplane, someone in line at the bank, my dentist. In these matters, I let my intuition be my guide in creating these "magical moments" when I become the instrument for positive change.

And perhaps you've experienced similar "magical moments" when sharing AFA-algae with others. Do you sometimes notice that at the moment they finally "get it," you see a special glimmer in their eye— that's the very instant when the artificial resistance of their limited programming begins to melt by the power of the truth you're sharing.

And THEN what happens? Based on the efforts you made— which sometimes takes some courage on your part to initiate— the person actually tries the algae, because of you.

And THEN what happens? Most often they get profound, life-changing results, they feel better.

And THEN what happens? They tell others.

THEN the circle comes back to you and your loved ones again and again, in ever-increasing, concentric circles of love and prosperity.

As I write this OPEN LETTER to you I realize that what I want more of in MY life NOW is that YOU have more of what YOU want in YOUR life NOW—whatever that might be for you.

For I believe the way it works on a deeper unseen level is that when you finally get more of the wholesome things that you want in life, your awareness naturally begins to think and feel more for the welfare of others as well. I guess that's why I'm writing this OPEN LETTER.

So I sincerely encourage you to increase your efforts to create the reality you really deserve in your life. For me, it takes the form of simply spreading the truth of my conviction about the benefits of AFA-algae. This may be more of your life-path than you presently know at this moment in time.

So it can really be this simple: EAT the algae. Feel the algae. Spread the algae. Another image just bubbled up in my awareness: Just as algae is nourished and naturally supported as it floats atop the flowing waters of Klamath Lake, let eating, feeling and spreading the algae support you as you go with the flow of life—your needs WILL be met.

Breakthrough Studies on the SBG Algae™

We've come a long way since the 1960's when I first started out in the natural health field. Back then, I had SOME scientific research to support the natural way of eating I was advocating, but sometimes not enough to convince everybody all of the time.

Well, I'm so excited to share that now, on the cusp of the New Millennium, more and more solid scientific research on AFA-algae is finally being performed. What this means is that what we've known about AFA-algae by virtue of our own experience—how the algae

boosts our health—as well as from the healing testimonials of ot has now been demonstrated by way of controlled experiments an in the domain of SCIENTIFIC FACT.

This also means that we can now speak to medical doctors others with a scientific bent with more confidence, to share this b tiful algae with them, AND SIGN THEM UP as product distribu

IT IS IMPORTANT TO MENTION TO THESE HEALTH P FESSIONALS THAT THE STUDIES YOU ARE TELLING TH ABOUT WERE "DOUBLE BLIND PLACEBO CONTROLLEI STUDIES, BECAUSE THIS IS THE "GOLD STANDARD" FAR AS SCIENTIFIC STUDIES GO. FOR BASED ON TH TRAINING, THEY'LL HAVE A HARD TIME FINDING FAU WITH THIS TYPE OF THE EXPERIMENTAL DESIGN, A THE RESULTS.

I will very briefly summarize the major studies that have rec ly been published on AFA-algae that we can now speak to ot about, even medical doctors, who often have huge client-bases.

NK STUDY

This breakthrough study was conducted at Royal Vict Hospital, a Canadian hospital affiliated with prestigious Mc University. The study actually shows "HOW" AFA-algae strength the immune system. To review, the immune system is a collectio specialized cells, glands and organs that in various ways protect bodies from internal and external invaders. I say "internal" as w because when our own cells mutate and become cancerous, it becomes an invader from the point of the view of the health of whole body. And from the perspective of the immune system's j cancer cells must somehow be reduced, eliminated and/or destroy One way the immune system works is through "NK cells." NK c stands for "natural killer" cells. NK cells knows how to recogr cancerous and virally infected cells and destroy them. They do by adhering to the surface of the cell and pulling them out of cir lation, sort of like a "lock and key" effect.

The study showed that after eating 1.5 grams of AFA-algae, t in the 50 healthy people that participated in this DOUBLE BLI CROSS OVER STUDY, the activity of their NK cells increased d matically, enabling the killer cells to be more effective in scaveng for health-destroying invaders and sick cells in the body. Now, th are other substances, like green tea and ginkgo biloba, that a increase the activity of NK cells, but listen to this: only AFA-al triggered the NK cells to move FROM the bloodstream INTO T TISSUES where many "sick cells" live. After two hours, the P cells moved back into the bloodstream.

In addition, the beneficial adhesiveness of the NK cells were increased from two to three times, enabling them to more effecti ly move from the capillary walls into the tissues.

So we can now say, with science backing us up completely, th AFA-algae boosts the immune system, something we've known in itively, but we didn't know exactly HOW this accomplished it u now.

The next step in research will be to see if AFA-algae can be sho to REVERSE cancer, viral and bacterial infections in UNHEALTH people. We already know that AFA-algae a possesses the very sa specific nutrients that have been proven to help PREVENT canc such as chlorophyll, beta-carotene and phycocyanin. Wouldn't it great if a double blind, placebo controlled study found that AF algae was actually able to REVERSE cancer? Keep your ears a eyes open and I promise to also keep YOU posted.

(For those who wish to consult the original study, the title and citation of the study is as follows:

Manoukian, R., Citton, M. ,Huerta, P., Rhode, B., Drapeau, C , and Jensen, G (1998) "The Effects of the Blue Green Algae Aphanizomenon flos-aquae on Human Natural Killer Cells," found in the IBC Library

Series, Volume 1911, Chapter 3.1 entitled, "Phytoceuticals: Examining the health benefit and pharmaceutical properties of natural antioxidants and phytochemicals")

BRIEF REVIEW OF OTHER STUDIES
AFA-ALGAE INCREASED RED BLOOD CELLS, REDUCES CHOLESTEROL, IN HEALTHYSUBJECTS

Another double-blind placebo-controlled study was conducted on 50 healthy subjects at the Royal Victoria Hospital and found that AFA-algae may increase the production of oxygen-carrying red blood cells. Researchers hypothesize that this may be a result of the high B12 found in AFA-algae. Another beneficial effect was observed: that AFA-algae reduces cholesterol in the healthy subjects that participated in this study. A new study is underway to see if AFA-algae reduces cholesterol in UNHEALTHY people, people who already have elevated cholesterol.

AFA-ALGAE ELIMINATES ABNORMALINTESTINAL PERMEABILITY

One of the most under-recognized, under-diagnosed and difficult to treat root-causes of many disease processes is what is called the "leaky gut syndrome." This is when there is abnormal intestinal permeability and the some of the contents in the intestines leaks out into the bloodstream and thereafter finds its way to parts of the body it shouldn't be.

What leaks out of our intestines are not only poisons to be eliminated, but undigested food in the form of large macro-molecules. When these macro-molecules cross over into the bloodstream, they stimulate a natural immune response that can cause symptoms ranging from mild and severe allergies to migraine headaches. A study conducted at the University of New Mexico found that eating AFA-algae for one month reversed this abnormal intestinal permeability or "leaky gut syndrome.

MENTAL ALERTNESS AND AFA-ALGAE

Another study done at the University of New Mexico showed that eating AFA-algae beneficially stimulated specific areas of the brain to produce increased integration of cognitive functions and an improved ability to process information. This was measured by way of highly sophisticated tests using an electroencephalegram (EEG). (Gee, so the increased clarity we feel when we use AFA-algae isn't our imagination!)

AFA-ALGAE MAY REVERSE ESSENTIAL FATTY ACID DEFICIENCIES

An as yet unpublished study being conducted at Boston University has found preliminary data which suggests
that AFA-algae may reverse symptoms caused by essential fatty acid deficiencies (EFA). Cardiovascular disease, the diseases responsible for the most deaths per year in North America, have been associated with EFA deficiencies, as have certain forms of cancer, arthritis and depression. Almost 50% of all the lipid (fat) content in AFA-algae is in the form of the "omega-3" essential fatty acids.

THE FUTURE IS BRIGHT

An exciting ongoing research study will be underway shortly at the University of Illinois which will attempt to scientifically docu-

ment that AFA-algae DOES in fact reverse and cure life-t diseases such as cancer, arthritis, heart disease etc. The st effect elevate the testimonial, anecdotal reports of cure familiar with to the level of scientific fact.

INTENTIONAL (WHAT TO DO NOW!)

Based on all these studies and the more open-minded society, there hasn't been a better time to get more involv AFA-algae and Cell Tech products. As mentioned in "Tl Optimal Health Report (Apprise Publishing), "the day ma ing when blue-green algae will be as much a part of mc supplemental arsenal as vitamin C." Cell Tech is taking an in speeding us to this day.

So next time you read an unfavorable article on AFA-a written by ill-informed writers with vested interests who r not be well-intentioned—(people who don't know the "w and perhaps have only read poorly researched and biase tion out of context,) please know that Cell Tech is cove bases, from research and development, product quality company policy decisions that effect the environmer design, marketing plan, etc.

Cell Tech is working for you, even when you sleep, r demonstrating their over-the-top integrity, leadership sense of social responsibility.

Again, I look forward to hearing from you. I can be cc phone, fax, email. Maybe we'll meet (again?) some day.

For wholesale Super Blue Green Algae and other su
contact the person who introduced you to this !

Rev. Viktoras Kulvinskas Ph.D.,
PO 1556
Mt. Ida, AR
71957
Viktoras4u.com
viktorasretreats@gmail.com

Special Greetings to the World of Dance and Life Honoring Movement
from Vihara Youkta!

Our lives have evolved, and with this evolution comes necessary change. We've decided to leave our ninety acre woodland home in the pristine Ouachita Mountains of Arkansas, and begin a new journey o sharing our knowledge and experience of good health and well being in a magical jungle of Costa Rica We acquired a beautiful piece of land there twenty years ago. Knowing the management of both properties would be too stressful and time consuming to handle, we determined the best idea was to move on and to establish our school sanctuary: Vihara Youkta Sanctuary (School of Movement).

Our site overlooks the tiny village of Montezuma, with a panoramic view of the Pacific Ocean border by a river of cascading waterfalls. We are entertained by an array of friendly wildlife. The temperatur maintains in the 80's all year round.

We believe this mystical place will provide the perfect setting for studying, practicing, and enjoying tl programs provided. We hope to offer a vast dimension in the joys of movement via the many differen forms of dance, yoga, et cetera.

Our projected plans are for the doors to Vihara Youkta Sanctuary (School of Movement) to open by tl year 2008. As this time approaches, we will send an informative newsletter with specifics.

Please take note, if you are an instructor, or know of one who would like to present a seminar or a workshop, we can provide a perfect environment and services guaranteed to inspire a successful learnin experience for all participants.

Because we, ourselves, live an alternative dietary lifestyle, we shall also offer support and insight into helping interested guests' with transition into their own personal and appropriate nutritional lifestyles with emphasis on what is necessary to reach and maintain optimal health at any age.

We are looking forward to the day we welcome you to our Sanctuary! Until then, should you have an questions or comments, please send them to: youkta@youkta.org. Thank you.

Love in Service!
Vihara Youkta
www.youkta.org

Eternal Dance
Daughters of Wind and Moon
Spirit , Skinned over Water
Wings of Scarves
Rainbow of crystal
Cascadence of Heart rhythm
Hips, delight the toes immersed in bosom
Perfume Magic with Auric lights
Resurrect primitive Urges ,
Tell Ancient Stories in the flicker
Drum Thundered passion
Chakra Ambrosial Divine Spine Wine
Raising the Spirit
Tidal wave of applause and Encore
So Good, cannot Get enough.
Viktoras 2005

Winter Soul Journey Solstice
Dance - be yourself
To be free in Self
Revisit past feelings
Dance to fill space with joy
Dance within a whirl of memorie
Dance for no Reason
Celebrate the Seasons
Back to life beginning
You are born anev
Viktoras 2004

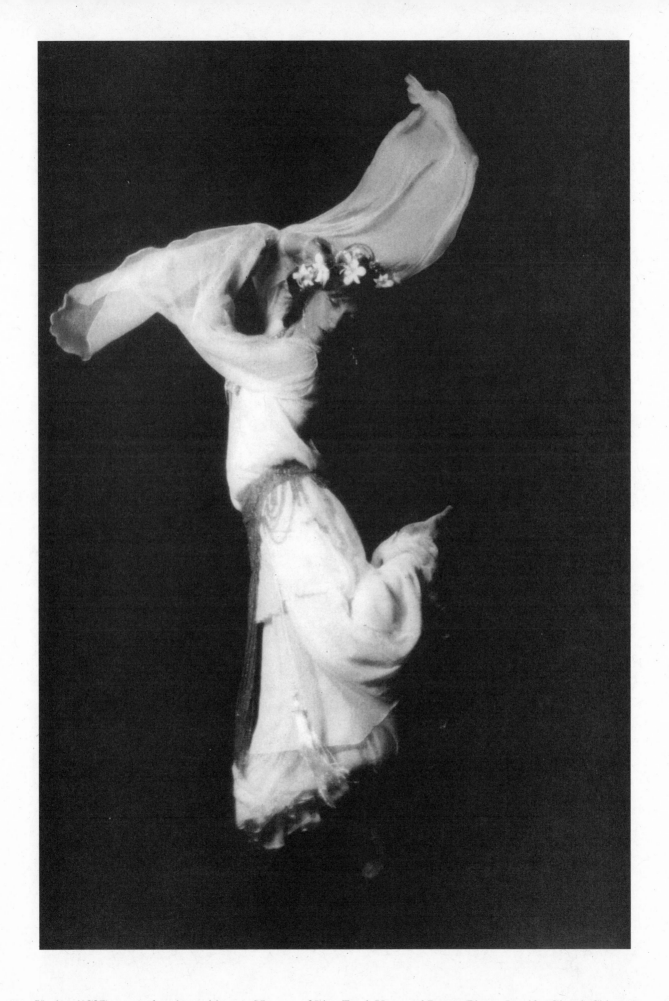

Youkta (1997), a grandmother, with over 25 years of Live Food, Yoga and Dance (Photo: Jennifer Girard, Chicago)

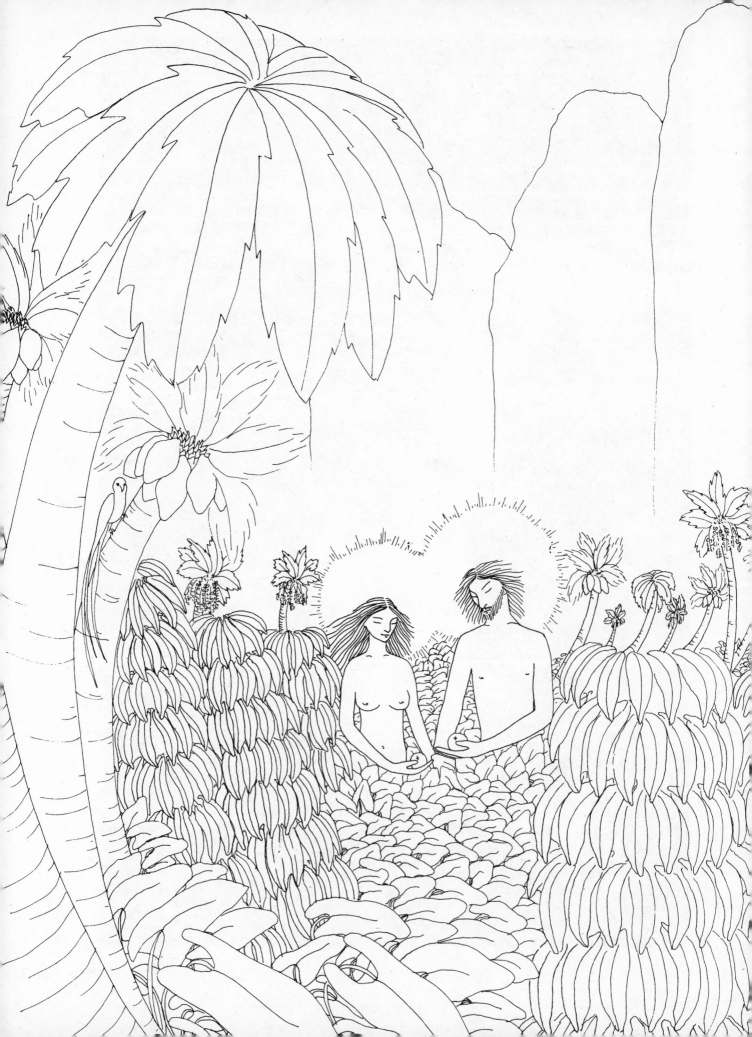

IV. BIBLIOGRAPHY

1. WICKENDEN, L., Our Daily Poison, The Devin-Adair Co., NYC.
2. WINTER, R., Poison In Your Food, Crown Publishers Inc., NYC.
3. STONE, D.; LAMSON E.; CHANG, YS; PICKERING, K.W.; SCIENCE 164, 568 (1969).
4. LEGATOR M.S.; PALMERKA, M.J.; BALK, N., Science 165: 1140 (1969)
5. COHEN, N.M.; MARINELLO, M.J.; BALK, N.; Science 155: 1417 (1967).
6. OSTERTAG, W.; Mutation Res, 3: 249 (1966).
7. New York Times, Jan. 8, 1970.
8. Science News, 7/26/1969 p. 84.
9. Science News Letter 89: 136, Feb. 26, 1966.
10. New York Times, Feb. 19, 1955.
11. CLARK, L., Stay Young Longer, Pyramid Pub. NYC. p. 80
12. Knight G.F. Modern Nutrition, Ap., Sep., Dec., 1952
13. Nature, Vol. 224 Dec. 27, 1969, p. 1249.
14. New York Times, March 25, 1967, p. 25
15. Boston Globe, Jan. 26, 1970, p. 2.
16. DOLMAN C.E., 1957 "Epidemiology of Meat Borne Disease", Meat Hygiene, W.H.O., Monogram 33.
17. J.A.M.A. May 16, 1953.
18. National Health Federation Bulletin, Sep. 1969.
19. Consumer Bulletin, May 1962.
20. Agricultural Research, USDA, March 1968.
21. LIJINSKY and SHUBIK, Industrial Medicine and Surgery, Feb. 1965, p. 152.
22. MANNELLI, Ann. Fac. Econ. Commer. Univ. Studi. Messina. 4: 467, 1966.
23. HARRISON R, Animal Machines, Ballantine Books, NYC.
24. National Provisioner, Ap 20, 1963.
25. Boston Globe, Oct. 22, 1969.
26. HOUSER, Journal of Environment Health, Oct. 66.
27. Newsweek, Nov. 24, 1969, p. 74.
28. WHITE, J., TOAL, J.N., MILLAR, F.K., and BROOKS, R.H. (Laboratory of Physiology, National Cancer Institute) J. Nat. Cancer Inst. 24, 197-209, 1960.
29. ELVEHJEM C.C. "Amino Acid Supplementation of Cereal" Cereal Science Today, p. 162-64, 1956.
30. BIELER, H., M.D., Food Is Your Best Medicine, Random House, NYC.
31. KALIKOWSKI, B.; ARMATA, J.; GARWICZ, S.; "Low Protein and Purine Free Diet in Acute Leukemia in Children. Polish Medical Journal 5 (3): 558, 1966. Also, The Lancet, Mr. 27, 1965.
32. LINTZEL, W.; Deutsche Med. Wochenschrift, LXXX, 1955 p. 1047.
33. Proc. Nat. Food and Nutr., USDA Handbook no. 56, 1952 p. 86.
34. SPENCER R.P. The Intestinal Tract. Charles Thomas Pub. Springfield, Ill. 1960.
35. WEST P.M.; HILLARD J., "Proteolytic Inhibitors of Human Serum In Health and Disease." Proc. Soc. Expte. Bid. Med. 71: 169, 1949.
36. ZICHGRAF, G., Munch. Med. Wach. 79: 998, 1932 and SAUNDERS, C.W., Proc. Soc. Exp. Biol. N.Y., 23: 788, 1925.
37. KOHLER, G.O., et al, Journal of Nutrition, 15, 445, 1938, also J. Nutr 14: 131, 1937.
38. ANNAND, J.C., "Trombosis, Further Evidence Against Heated Animal Produce" J. Coll. Gen. Pract. 7: 386, 1964.
39. COWDRY, E.W. "Trends in Cancer Research," Cancer Research, 11: 603-607, 1951.
40. BLOND, KASPER, THE LIVER AND CANCER, Bristol: John Wright & Son LTD 1960; Distributed by: Cancer Victims and Friends.
41. ABRAHAMSON, E.M., M.D., Body Mind and Sugar, Holt, Rinehart & Winston Pub., NYC.
42. J.A.M.A. Vol. 176, 1961 p. 806.
43. Journal of American Medical Assoc. 10/10/66; p. 137-146
44. TRAP J., A Gift of Love, West Publishing Corp. Pty. LTD, Barrack St., Sydney, 1971.
45. GERSON, Max, M.D. A CANCER THERAPY — FIFTY CASE HISTORIES, Distributed by Cancer Book House 2043 N. Berendo St., L.A., Cal. (Publ.: Whittier Beeks, NYC.)
46. MURPHY, Clinical Medicine, Aug., 1944.
47. BUCKLEY, Cancer, July, 1927.
48. SEEGER, Hippocrates (German Medical Journal) Vol. 13, 1951.
49. TIDSKRIFT, For. Halsa., No. 2, 2-1972, Stockholm, Sweden.
50. DAHI, "Hold That Salt", Consumer Bulletin, Sep. 1959.
51. RATCLIFF, "Body Fluids   A Major Medical Problem" Colliers, Nov. 26, 1954.
52. INGELFINGER, F.J. For want of an enzyme. Nutrition Today. Sep. 1968.
53. McCOY, T.A., Neoplasia and Nutrition. In World Review of Nutrition and Dietetics. Ed. Bourne G.H., Vol. 1, 1959, Phil, Lippincott.

54. BOGERT, J. Nutrition and Physical Fitness. W.B. Sounders Co., London, pg. 372.

55. ENGEL, R.W. and COPELAND, D.H. "Protective Action of Stock Diets Against Cancer by 2-Acetylamino fluorine" Cancer Research, V12: 211-215, 1952.

56. LOCKE, D.M. Enzymes — The Agents of Life. Crown Publishers Inc., New York.

57. GERALD, R.W. editor — R.J. Block, N. Jollife, C. McCay, S.E. Smith and Soskin. Food For Life. University of Chicago Press. 1965.

58. SUMNER, J.B. The Secret of Life — Enzymes. National Enzyme Co., Chicago.

59. TANNENBAUM A., Nutrition and Cancer In Physiopathology in Cancer. Ed. Homburger F. Second Edition 1959.

60. TANNENBAUM A., Relation of Body Weight to Cancer, Arch Path, 30: #2, 509-517, Aug. 1940.

61. HILLEMANN HOWARD H., M.A., Ph.D. "Comparison of Cancer Incidence and Subsequent Mortality in Deficient, Whole and Supplemented Diet Fed Golden Hamsters." Dept. of Zoology, Oregon State College. International Record of Medicine and G.P. Clinics, Aug. 1953, p. 316.

62. BEADLE, B.W. et al. J Biol Chem 149: 339, 1943.

63. CHELDELIN, V.H., A.M. WOODS and R.J. WILLIAMS. J. Nutr. 26: 477, 1943.

64. ELVEHJEM, C.A., and P.L. PAVCEK. Mod Hospital. 61: 110, 1943.

65. FARRER, K.T.H. Australian Chem Inst J. Proc. 8: 113, 1941.

66. FRITZ, J.C. et al. Poultry Sci, 21: 361, 1942.

67. HARRIS, P.L., et al. J. Nutr. 40: 367, 1950.

68. HELLER, C.A.; C.M. McCAY and C.B. LYON. J. Nutr. 36: 377, 1943.

69. HARRIS, R.S. Vitamins Hormones. 20: 603, 1962.

70. Information Bulletin 112, Human Nutrition Research Branch, U.S. Dept. of Agriculture, 1954.

71. BENERJEE D.K. and J.B. CHATTERJEA. Vitamin B12 Content of some articles of Indian diet and effect of cooking on it. Bri J Nutr. 17: 385, 1963.

72. BOCTOR, A.M. and A.E. HARPER. Measurement of Available Lysine in heated and unheated foodstuffs by chemical and biological methods. J. Nutr. 94: 289, 1968.

73. POTTENGER, F.M. Jr. The effect of heated processed Foods and metabolized Vitamin D milk on the dento-facial structure of experimental animals. Am j Orthodontics and Oral Surg. Aug. 1946.

74. TANNENBAUM A., Cancer Res., 5: 609 (1945).

75. HENDERSON, J.F. and LEPAGE, G.A.; Cancer Research Oct. 1959, p. 887.

76. CORI C.F. and CORI G.T., J. Biol. Chem. 65: 11-22, 1925.

77. TERTULLIAN, De Jejunics: Adversus Psychios.

78. MILLET H., J. Biol. Chem., 78: 281-88, 1928.

79. Editorial, President Status of Heat Processing Damage to Protein Foods." Nutrition Review 8 (7) 193, 1950.

80. BEARD, F.T.; PIERCE. J.C.; HANKINS. O.G.; GINGERS, I.D., WASHTER, J.P.; DOTY. D.M.; SCHWEIGERT, B.S., "Effects of Aging and Cooking on the Distribution of Certain Amino Acids and Nitrogen in Beef Muscle" Journal Paper No. 83. American Meat Institute Foundation, Dec. 5, 1953 p. 410.

81. EVANS and BUTTS; Inactivation of Amino Acids; Science 109: 569, 1949.

82. OLSEN E.M., Canadian J. of Biochemistry, 45: 1673; 1967.

83. KYUSHU, Memoirs of Medical Science, Vol. 2, No. 1-2.

84. Boston Evening Globe, Nov. 15, 1972.

85. Der Wendepunkt, Mr. 6, 171, 1966.

86. HUGHES J.H. and LATNER A.L. "Chlorophyl and hemoglobin regeneration after hemorrhage."J. Physiology 86: 388, 1936.

87. AIN, A., Pfugers Arch., 225: 728, 1930.

88. PUTEK and MINOT, "Bile Pigment and Hemoglobin Regeneration," Am. J. Med. Science 188: 206, 1934.

89. MILLER, L.M., "Chlorophyl for Healing" Sc. News Letter Mr. 15, 1941, p. 171.

90. PATEK A.J., "Chlorophyl and Regeneration of Blood," Archives of Internal Medicine 57: 76, 1936.

91. SAUNDERS, C.W., Proc. Soc. Exp. Biol., N.Y. 23: 788, 1925.

92. BINET, L. and STRUMZA, M.W., Sang. 8: 1041, 1934.

93. BURGI, C. VON TRACZEWSKY, Biochem Z. 98: 256, 1919.

94. AOKI S., Sei-I-Kwai Med. J. 50: 1, 1931; Chem Abst., 26: 3847, 1932.

95. ZICHGRAF, G. Munch Med Woch. 79: 998, 1932.

96. ROTHEMUND P., McNARY, R.R.; IMMAN, O.L.; J. Am. Chem. Soc. 56: 2400, 1934.

97. HAVEN F.L., J. Biol. Chem., 118: 111-121, 1937.

98. BOWERS W.S., "Chlorophyl in Wound Healing and Suppurative Disease", Am. J. Surg. 73: 37, 1947.

99. FILLERUP D.L. et al, J. Biol. Chem., 233: 98-101, 1958.

100. BOEHME, E.J. "The Treatment of Chronic Leg Ulcers With Special Reference to Ointment Containing Water Soluble Chlorophyl", Lahey Clin. Bull., 4:242, 1946.

101. BERTRAM, R.O.; WEINSTOCK, B.S. "A Clinical Evaluation of Chlorophyl, Benzocaine and Urea Ointment in Treatment of Minor Infections of the Foot," J. Am. Podiat. Assoc., 19:366, 1959

102. OFFENKRANTZ, W.G., "Water Soluble Chlorophyl in the Treatment of Peptic Ulcer of Long Duration." Rev. Gastroenterology, 17: 359, 1950.

103. CARPENTER, E.B., "Clinical Experiences With Chlorophyl Preparations with Particular Reference to Chronic Osteomyelitis and Chronic Ulcer" Am. J. Surgery, 77: 167, 1949.

104. CARLESON; GARSYEN; "Septofyllin (chlorophyl preparation) Especially in Chronic Leg Ulcer," Nord. Med., 47: 412, 1952.

105. JUUL-MOLLER; MIKKELSEN, "Treatment of Hypertension and Crural Ulder with Chorophyllin," Ugesk. Laeger, 114: 1726, 1952.

106. RAFSKY, KRIEGER, "Treatment of Intestinal Diseases with Solutions of Water Soluble Chlorophyl," Rev. Gastroentology, 15: 549, 1948.

107. PALOSCIA; POLLOTTEN; "Chlorophyl Therapy" Lotta. Contra. Tuberc. 22: 738, 1952.

108. "Results of Chlorophyl Therapy," Bull Assoc. Franc Poletude due Cancer, 24: 15, 1935.

109. PLAGNIEL, "Remarkable Tonic Power of Chlorophyl Pigment ir Asthenic Toxemia of Cancer," J. de Med. de Paris, 53: 664, 1933.

110. "Chlorophyl Therapy for Cancer," Progress. Med., Ap. 6, 1935, pg. 583.

111. FOWLER, "Placebos, Anti-sludging Drugs and Disorders of the Ear," Ann. Otol; 70: 839, 1961.

112. SMITH, "Remarks Upon the History, Chemistry, Toxicity and Antibacterial Properties of Watersoluble Chlorophyl Derivatives as Therapeutic Agents," Am. J. Med. Soc. 207:649, 1944.

113. MILLER; JACKSON; COLLIER; "The Inhibition of Clotting by Chlorophyllin," Am. J. Surgery, 95: 967, 1958.

114. LOVRON, LARTIGUE, "The Influence of Diet on the Biological Effects Produced by Whole Body X-irradiation," Experientia, 6: 25, 1950.

115. DUPLAN, "Influence of Dietary Regimen on Radiosensitivity of the Guinea Pig," Compt. Rend. Acad. Sc. 236: 424, 1953.

116. SPECTOR; COLLOWAY; "Reduction of X-radiation Mortality by Cabbage and Broccoli," Proc. Soc. Exptl. Biol. Med. 100: 405, 1959.

117. COLLOWAY; CALHOUN; MUNSON; Quartermaster Food and Container Institute for the Armed Forces Report. N.R. 12-61, 1961.

118. DESNOO, Am. J. Obstet. Gynec. 34: 911, 1937.

119. GUYTON, A., Physiology of the Body; W.B. Saunders Co., Philadelphia, 1964.

120. ANDERSON, Am. J. Obstet. Gynec, 40: 517, 1940.

121. DE ALVAREZ, Am. J. Obstet. Gynec. 39: 476, 1940.

122. FLODIN, N.W., Agr. and Food Chem. 1, 222 (1953)

123. EVANS, Journal of Metabolic Research, Mr. 1922.

124. Am. J. Obst. and Gyne, May 1951.

125. BIELER, H.G., M.D., Natural Way to Sexual Health, Charles Pub., Los Angeles, 1972. p. 172.

126. RHODES P., Prof. Of Obstetrics & Gynecol. Univ. London, Repro Physiol For Med Students, J. & A. Churchill LT 9, London 1969, p. 48-55.

127. LEATHEM, J.H., R ECENT Progr. in Hormone Research, 14, 141 (1958).

128. BALL, et. al; Am J. Physiol. 150, 511 (1947).

129. SCHUTZE M.D. J. Nutr. 56, 25 (1955).

130. KAHLER H. and ROBERTSON W.V.B., J. Nat. Cancer Inst., 3: 495-501, 1943.

131. ISRAEL, S. LEON, M.D. Diagnosis & Treatment of Menstrual Disorders & Sterility, Fift. Edition, Hoeber Pub., N.Y. 1967.

132. SMITH, "The Effect of Wartime Starvation in Holland Upon Pregnancy and its Product", Am. J. Obstet. & Gynec., 53: 599, 1947.

133. MILLIS, Med. J. Malaya, 6: 157, 1952.

134. SCHROYER, Diseases of Women.

135. REYNOLDS, J.A.M.A., 135: 552 (1947)

136. MACH and LUBIN, J. Pharmacol & Exper Thera 22: 413 (1924)

137. FRANK, The Female Sex Hormone.

138. CROSSEN, M.D. Disease of Women, C.W. Mosky Co., St. Louis 1953.

139. STARR, GEORGE, The Emancipation of Woman

140. Family News, Vol. 2, No. 7, July 1955, Page Foundation, St. Petersburg, Fla.

141. KERVRAN, L., Biological Transmutations, Swan House Pub. Co., P.O. Box 638, Binghamton, N.Y. 1972.

142. EL MEHAIRY, M.M., Brit. J. Cancer 4:95 — 102, 1950.

143. MIDER, G.B., Cancer Research, 11:821 — 29, 1951.

144. MIDER, G.B.; TESLUR, H.; and MORTON J.J. Acta Unio. Internat. contra cancrum 6:409 — 20, 1948.

145. HENDERSON J.F.; and LEPAGE G.A., Cancer Research October 1959, p. 887-902.

146. LEPUGE G.A., et al, "Observations on the Inhibition of Development of Spontaneous Leukemia in Mice by Under feeding." Cancer Research, July 1944. p. 401.

148. WHITE, J., et al, J. Nat. Cancer Inst. 24: 197-209, 1960.

149. MARSHALL, et al, AMA Arch. Neurol and Psych. 69: 760, 1953.

150. Parade, Boston Sunday Globe, Oct. 21, 1973.

151. CHEN P, Soybeans, Chemical Elements Pub., Mass.

152. Proceedings of the Nutrition Society, seventy first Scientific Meeting, London School of Hygiene and Tropical Medicine, Jan. 5 1952, Vitamin B-12, page 295.

153. Voisin A., Soil, Grass and Cancer, Crosby Lockwood and Son LTD, 26 Old Brompton Rd., S.W.7. 1959.

154. Boston Globe, Oct. 2, 1973. "Diet Linked to Prevention of Cancer".

155. Journal of Clinical Nutrition, August 1972, "Length of Life and Caloric Intake".

156. Prevention, Oct. 1973, p. 31, "Eat Less To Live More."

157. U.S. Public Health Service No. 149.

158. BEGG R.W., Adv. Cancer Res., 5: 1-54, 1958.

159. USDA Official Report, Feb. 8, 1966.

160. National Geographic, Jan. 1973.

161. New York Times, Oct. 20, 1971.

162. Science News, Dec. 19, 1970.

163. Science News, Aug. 21, 1971.

164. American Schizophrenia Association, 56 West 45th St., NYC, 212-972-0705.

165. HAVEN F.L., and BLOOR W.R., Adv. Cancer Res., 4: 237-314, 1956.

166. HOTEMA, H. Man's Higher Consciousness, Health Research, 1962.

167. KOHLER G.O.; C.A. ELVEHJEM; E.B. HART; Growth Stimulation Properties of Grass Juice; Science 83: 445, 1936.

168. O. SCHNABEL, C.F., "Grass The Forgiveness of Nature." ACRES, U.S.A. Box 1456, Kansas City, Mo. March, April, May, July, August 1973.

169. HAVEN, BLOOR, RANDALL, Cancer Res., 9: 511-14, 1949.

170. Nautilus Magazine, quoted by R. Collier, Law of the Higher Potential, Cullier Pub., Tarrytown, N.Y.

171. MIDER, TESLUK, MORTON, Acta Unio internat. contra cancrum, 6: 409-20, 1948.

172. STEWART, BEGG, Cancer Res., 13: 560-65, 1953.

173. LISLE, HARVEY, RDI, Norwalk, Ohio, 44851.

174. HAY, W., How To Always Be Well, Groton Press. 1961.

175. ELWOOD, CATHARYN, Feel Like A Million, Devin-Adair.

176. Nutritional Evaluation of Sprouts and Grasses, and how to help them grow, V. Kulvinskas $2, Omangod Press, 211 Garden St., Wethersfield, Conn. 06109.

177. Cancer News Journal, Jan./Feb. 1972 and Aug. 1970. Association of Cancer Victims and Friends, Solana Beach, Cal.

178. Life, Southwest Bakes in Ruinous Drought, June 4, 1971.

179. Garden Research, 736 Darling St., Ogden, Utah 84403.

180. Walnut Acres, Penns Creek, Penn.

181. Minigardens for Vegetables, Home and Garden Bulletin No. 163 from Department of Agriculture, Washington D.C.

182. JENSEN B., The Science and Practice of Iridology, Jensen Product, P.O. Box J, Escondido, Cal.

183. GROLLMAN S., The Human Body, MacMillan Co., London, pg. 38.

184. HAVEN F.L. and BLOOR W.R., Adv. Cancer Res., 4: 237 — 314, 1956.

185. London Sunday Chronicle, June 17, 1951.

186. Life Natural, Ganeshnagar, Padukottai, S. Ry, India. Nov. 1960.

187. DHANJLSHAW D. PATELL, F.R.C., Rosicrucian Digest, June 1959.

188. HOTEMA, Live 1400 Years, Health Research.

189. India's Message, Jan. 1932.

190. Bombay Press, Aug. 20, 1953.

191. Aberree, May 1960.

192. PARAMAHANSA YOGANANDA, Autobiography of a Yogi.

193. OTT, JOHN N., Health and Light, Devin-Adair Co. Pub., 1 Park Ave., Old Greenwich, Conn.

194. J. Reprod. Med., Vol. 3, No. 2, Aug. 1969.

195. LAKHOVOSKY, G., The Secret of Life; Health Research.

196. KERVRAN L., Biological Transmutation, Tao Pub., Boston.

197. JONES H. B. et al, Am. J. Cancer, 40: 243-50, 1940.

198. LOVEWISDOM, JOHNNY, Ecuador, South America.

199. Runners World, July 1973.

200. DR. H.H. SHELDON, University of New York, as quoted by Prof. Hotema, "Man's Higher Consciousness," Health Research Press.

201. SIR AUROBINDO, The Supramental Manifestation; Crescent Moon Ranch, Sedona, Arizona

202. GILLMAN, J. AND GILBERT C., S. Afr. J. med. Sci., 21:89, 1956

203. ACTA Medicine Scandinavia 192:231-9, Sept. 1972.

204. SZEPSENWOL, J.; J. Proc. Exp. Biol. and Med., 1957, V96, 332 and P.S.E.B.M. Feb. 20, 1963, V112, P1073

205. WHITE F.R. and White J.; J. Nat. Cancer Inst., 4:413 (1944)

206. DUNNING W.F., Curtis M.R. and Moun M.E., Cancer Res., 10:454 (1950); 10:319 (1950)

207. BABSON A.L., Cancer Res., 14:89, 1954

208. ROUS P., J. Exper. Med 20: 433, 1914

209. SWEET J.E., Corson-White E.P.P., Saxon G.J., J. Biol. Chem-15:181, 1913

210. GREENE C.H., Sandiford K., Ross, H., J. Biol. Chem., 58:845, 1923

211. AVERBACH, V.H. and Waisman H.A., Cancer Res., 18:536, 1958

212. KELLY, J.J., Waisman H.A., Blood 12:635, 1957

213. SAXTON Jr., J.A., Boon M.C., Furth J., Cancer Res, Vol. 4, July 1944, p. 408

214. MADDEN, F.C., British Med. J., Aug. 3, 1902

215. DAILY NEWS, May 7, 1973, p 25

216. WARBURG, Otto, The Prime Cause and Prevention of Cancer, Publ by Konrad Triltsch, Wurzburg, Germany; 1969; Dist by Cancer Victims and Friends.

217. SCIENCE NEWS, Aug 21, 1971, p 123

218. LORINCZ, A., Nebraska State Medical Journal, Dec. 1965.

219. CANCER CONTROL JOURNAL, 2043   N. Berendo St., L.A., Cal. July/Aug 1973 and Cancer News Journal, 5726 La Jolla Blvd., La Jolla, Cal Sep/Dec 1970.

220. ANNAND, J.C., L. Coll. Gen. Pract., 2:365, 1959

221. YARUSHALMY T. Hilleboe, H.E., N.Y. State T. Med. 53:2343, 1957

222. GROEN, Tijong, Kaminga, Willebrands. Voeding, 13:556, 1952

223. MORSE, E.M., Overlay, V.A., J. Nutr. 72:317, 1960

224. OLIVER M.F., Lancet, 1:653, 1962

225. MCDONALD L., Edgill M. Lancet, 1:996, 1958

226. CHEN, P.S., Soybean, Chemical Elements Publ, 1956

227. NATURAL LIVING (1560 Broadway, NYC) 1973.

228. KOCH, W.F., Ph. D., M.D. Neoplastic and Viral Parasitism, Distr: Cancer Victims and Friends.

229. BEGG, Dickenson, Cancer Res., 11:409-12, 1951

230. WHITE, Ellen, "Counsels on Diet and Food," Review and Herald Publ Assoc., Takoma Park, Wash. D.C.

231. Von Haller, Albert; The Vitamin Hunters, The Chilton Co., Publishers 1962 p. 140

232. TOMPLINS, Peter, The Secret Life of Plants, Harper & Row Pub., NYC, 1972

233. American Vegan Society, Box H, Malaga, N.J.

234. BASS, Stanley, 3119 Coney Island Ave., Brooklyn, NYC

235. CANCER NEWS JOURNAL, May/Aug. 1970 p. 15

236. LOVEWISDOM, Johnny, Order of Paradise

237. Scientific Tables, published by Geige Pharmaceutical Division of Geige Chemical Corp., Ardsley, N.Y., Pages 501-514.

238. ORR, M.A. and B.K. WATT, Amino Acid Content Of Food. Superintendent of Documents, U.S. Government Printing Office, Wash. D.C.

239. WADE C., Vegetarianism; Herald of Health, LXXII, Ap. 1967, p. 14.

240. ALTMAN, P. and D. DITTER, Metabolism; Federation of Am. Soc. For Exp. Biol. Publ., Bethesda, Maryland.

241. DE LA TORRE, T., Psycho-Physiopathy, Vol. 3, Imprento Tormo, San Jose, Costa Rica. 1957.

242. BERNARD, Raymond, Ph.D.; Nutritional Sex Control and Rejuvenation; Health Research Publ., Mokelumne Hill, Cal.

243. BENEDICT, Francis, "Human Vitality and Efficiency Under Prolonged Restricted Diet." Publ. 280, Carnegie Institute, Wash., D.C., 1919.

244. SMITH, G.L., "Studies in the Experimental Analysis of Sex." Quart. Jour. Micr. Sci. IV, 1910, p. 225.

245. Ellis. William. N.D.   . P.O. Box 220 . R.D. 6, Tarentum, Pa. Asparagus Therapy in cancer and warts.

246. Mayer, Jean, Post Graduate Medicine, 32: 394, 1962.

247. Schlenker, E D . Am J. Clin. Nut. , Oct 1973

248. McCay, C M , Prolonging the Life Span. Sci. Monthly, vol 139, p 405, 1934.

249. McCay, C M , Nutrition, aging and Longevity. Trans & Studies Coll. Physicians Phila. Penn. 4 Ser. vol 10. 1942.

250. McCay, C M Life Span In Rats, Arch. Bio. Chem. vol 2, p 469, 1943.

251. ANNAND, J.C. Further Evidence in the Case Aginst Heated Milk Protein, Atherosclerosis, 15:129, 1972.

252. VANECEK, K. and Zapletal A., Sensibilization of Guinea Pigs with Cow's Milk as a Model of Sudden Death in Infants and Children. Acta. Univ. Carol. Med. , 13:207-213, 1967.

253. LOTZOF L., Dairy Produce and Coronary Artery Disease, Med. J. Aust., 1:1317, 30 Jun 73.

254. DOHAN F.C., Relapsed Schizophrenics Earlyer Discharge from the Hospital After Cereal Free, Milk Free Diet,Am. J. Psy., 130:685, Jun 1973.

255. MURRAY A.B., Infant Feeding and Respiratory Allergy, Lancet, l:497, 6 Mr. 71.

256. TOMMORI, J., Milk Sensitivity in Asthmatic Children, Acta Allergol (kbh), 28:107, Jul 73.

257. FREIR S. and B. Kletter, Milk Allergy in Infants and Young Children, Clin. Pediat. (phil), 9:449, Aug 70.

258. BEER, Allan E. and Judy Head, Southwestern Medical School, Dallas, 1974. Observed that feeding infants mothers' milk may be the solution to the "crib deaths", which is a disease of bottle fed babies. "No infant is totally safe without the protection of his mothers milk."

259. MOON, Yogamundi, Pathological Calcification ($1.75, G. Ohsawa Macrobiotic Foundation,   1471 10th Ave, S. F., Cal.). Bibliography has 623 references to medical journals. Story of vitamin D and milk.

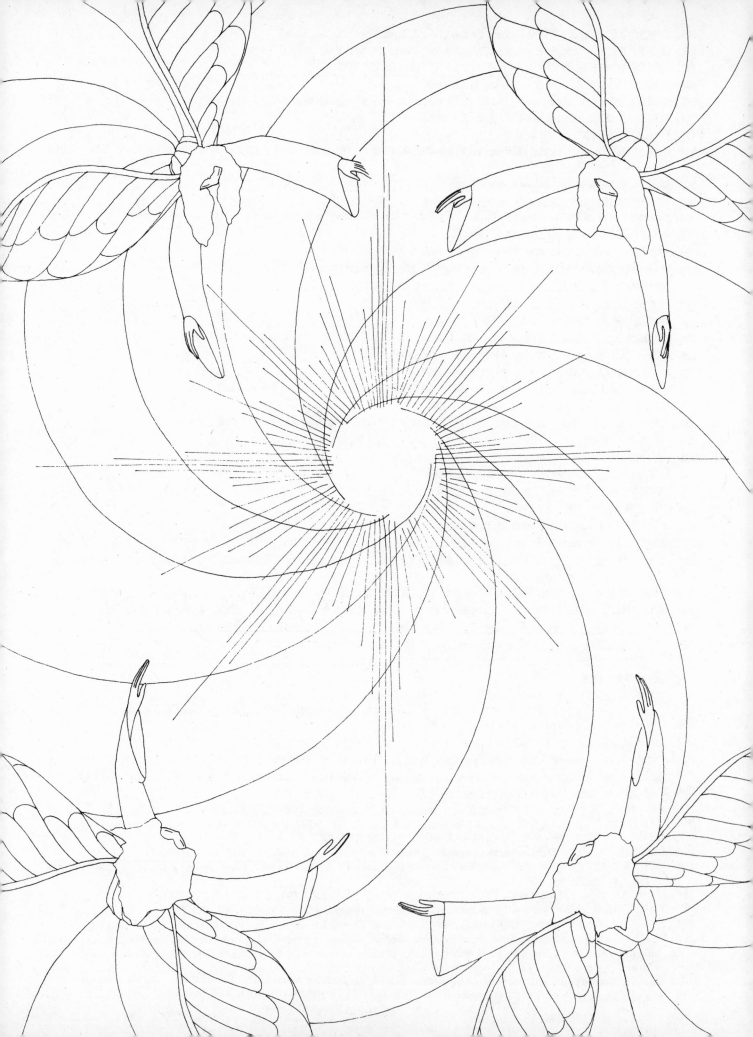

V. INDEX

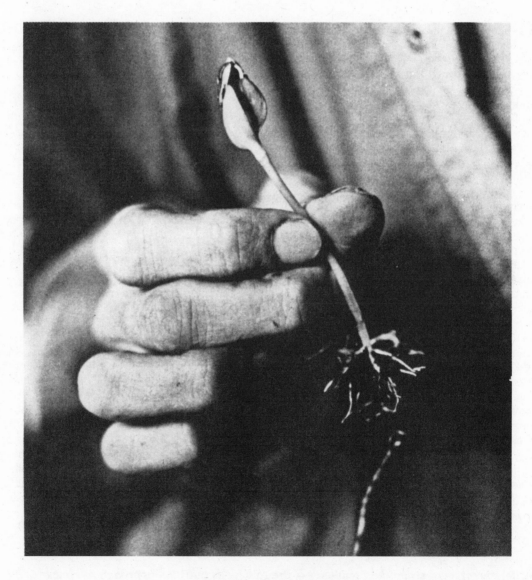

6 Day Sunflower Sprout

VI. RESEARCH UPDATE

WHEATGRASS JUICE STOPS CANCER

Many years ago I met Dr. Chiu-Nan Lai at one of my weekly seminars at the Hippocrates Health Institute. She was then a biology graduate student at the Massachusetts Institute of Technology. We talked about the need for research to prove the therapeutic value of wheatgrass juice and live foods to the scientific community.

In 1978 it was a great joy to reestablish aquaintance with Dr. Lai and to discover that wheatgrass juice is being tested by researchers on rats and bacteria to bear out the results obtained at Hippocrates.

She has discovered that extracts of wheatgrass, alfalfa sprouts, carrot and parsley display a powerful action against chemical mutagenics in bacteria tests. Presently, the extracts are being examined for cancer-preventing potential in mice, according to the American Chemical Society

The following study was reported by Dr. Chiu-Nan Lai in the "Report to the Physicians of Texas Newsletter", July-August, 1978.

Recent experiments with wheat plants here at M. D. Anderson Hospital have shown that extracts of wheat sprouts exhibit antagonistic activity toward known carcinogens in vitro, as measured by the Ames test. The test, which measures the production of histidine-independent revertants in specially constructed mutants of Salmonella typhimurium, is a direct mutagenesis assay with apparent good predictive value for carcinogenesis.

Untreated wheat from Arrow Mill, Texas was soaked overnight in water, spread over a container that allowed drainage, and allowed to sprout. The sprouts were harvested when 4 to 5 inches tall (approximately 7 to 14 days). Extracts were prepared from the roots and leaves of the plants by first pounding them with a pestle in a mortar over ice and mechanically pressing out the juice. The undiluted juice was then centrifuged for thirty minutes at $30,000 \times g$ at 4 degrees C. The clear liquid was sterilized by filtration through Millipore filters.

Several potent carcinogens that require metabolic activation, as well as some that do not, were tested for mutagenicity by the Ames test. The compound 2-acetylaminofluorene (2-AAF) and its derivatives N-hydroxy-2-acetylaminofluorene (N-OH-AAf) and N-hydroxy-aminofluorene (2-AF) with and without wheat extracts were preincubated with the bacteria at 37 degrees C for 30 minutes before placing with top agar. Others, such as benz (a) pyrene (BP) and 3- methylcholanthrene (3-MC) were tested by direct plate incorporation. Additionally, BP was tested for levels of metabolite production in the presence and absense of wheat extract by high-pressure liquid chromatography.

Results from the mutagenic assay were surprising. Extracts from both leaves and roots of wheat sprouts selectively inhibited the mutagenic effects of compounds that require metabolite activation. No inhibition was observed for those carcinogens not ordinarily requiring metabolic activation (2-nitrofluorene, ethyl-methansulfonate, and N-methyl-N-nitro-N-nitrosoguanidine). The extracts were most active in altering the metabolic pathway of 2-AAF, and less active in inhibiting its derivativesN-OH-AAFand 2-AF. These results agree with the in vitro inhibitory action of selenium in a similar mutagenic assay.

Alteration of the formation of BP metabolites was observed in the high-pressure liquid chromatography profile. The wheat extracts selectively reduced formation of metabolites of carcinogens, especially dihydrodiols. Hydroxides also were reduced somewhat. Hydroxides were also reduced somewhat. Extracts from roots were more effective than extracts from leaves in suppressing dihydrodiol formation.

These results are of interest for two main reasons: 1) the inhibition of metabolic activation of potent carcinogens is quite high for low levels of extract, and 2) wheat sprout extract is non-toxic, whereas most known inhibitors of carcinogens are toxic at high levels of concentration. Trace elements such as arsenic, iodine, platinum, copper, and particularly selenium in a certain oxidation state, have known antineoplastic effects.

The inhibition of carcinogen metabolism by wheat extract, however, cannot be explained by the action of selenium or any other metals. Analysis for selenium in wheat extract performed in our laboratory yielded less than 0.5 ppm in the leaf extract. . . Finally, wheat sprouts were not unique in inhibiting carcinogenic activity in the in vitro assay. Extracts from carrots and parsley also inhibited carcinogenic activity, but were not as potent as wheat sprout extract.

The following exerpt, suggesting the credibility of the raw foods nutrition approach to cancer and reporting the success of Dr. Lai's research, appeared in the May, 1979 issue of Science Digest.

Some vegetarians and health food devotees would have you believe that raw grains represent no less than salvation for humankind. Medicine, for the most part, has lifted its collective eyebrow and yawned. Now, we hear hints that there may be something in the theory after all.

In a provocative report at the meeting of the American Chemical Association, Drs. Chiu-Nan Lai, Betty J. Dabney and Charles R. Shaw of the University of Texas

(Houston) suggested that a few of these items may have distinct cancer—preventive properties.

When Dr. Lai and her colleagues applied extracts of wheat sprouts to certain known chemical mutagens, the activity of the chemicals diminished radically, by 99% in some instances. Mung beans and lentil sprouts performed similarly, while extracts of carrots and parsley didn't do very well.

The key appears to be chlorophyll, which, it seems, is an effective inhibitor of certain mutagenic chemicals — those, in particular, that are activated by enzymes in the body. Only wheat sprouts grown for a week or two, until four or five inches high, showed any inhibitory properties. Heating the extract lessened the potency. An analysis showed that carrots and parsley have less chlorophyl than the sprouts.

The researchers reached their conclusions by using a standard test to measure the ability of the chemicals to mutate bacterial cells — an accepted signal of possible carcinogenic (cancer-causing) potential. Next step: extract in mice treated with proved cancer—causing agent.

Dr. Chiu-Nan Lai's results were also reported in a 1979 issue of "Let's Live" magazine:

NATURAL EXTRACT MAY FIGHT CANCER

Extracts of wheat sprouts, mung beans, and lentils display a powerful action against chemical mutagens in bacterial tests and are being examined for cancer preventing ability in mice, according to the American Chemical Society.

If animal studies bear out results obtained so far on bacteria, "it would lend support to the dietary goals recommended by the McGovern subcommittee - that is, less meat, fat, and more vegetables, fruits and whole grains in the American diet," reported Dr. Chiu-Nan Lai of the University of Texas System Cancer Center, Houston.

"Chlorophyll, the major active constituent of wheat extract, is responsible for converting sunlight into chemical energy in green plants. By itself, chlorophyll is a potent inhibitor of the chemical mutagens, requiring only small amounts to produce an effect," said Dr. Lai.

Applying the extract to potent chemical mutagens diminished activity in the Ames test for mutagens by up to 99 percent. (The popular Ames test measures the ability of chemicals to mutate bacterial cells - an indication of possible carcinogenicity, the authors said.)

The results are of interest for two reasons: the inhibition of activation of carcinogens is quite strong at a reasonably low level of extract, and the wheat sprout extract is non-toxic even at high levels," according to the authors.

The usefulness of the extract is limited, however, to those chemicals which require activation by body enzymes before they can exert a mutagenic effect.

This article, indicating that the raw food diet significantly reduces the size and number of cancerous growths, appeared in the National Financial weekly "Barron's" on June 11, 1979

OF MICE AND MEN

By James Grant

Menlo Park, Calif. — Sixteen years ago, Authur B. Robinson earned an "A—" from Dr. Linus Pauling in a chemistry course at the California Institute of Technology by coming up with a plausible answer to the question: "What is the electronic structure of the tripositive gadolinium ion?" Six years ago, the eminent chemist and his former student helped to found what today is known as the Linus Pauling Institute of Science and Medicine.

Twice Pauling has won the Nobel Prize, first in chemistry, in 1954, then in Peace in 1962. In 1975, he was presented by President Ford with the National Medal of Science, it being reported at the time that President Nixon had withheld the same honor on account of Pauling's politics.

Robinson, who received his Ph.D. in chemistry from the University of California at La Jolla in 1967, and who was immediately invited to join the faculty there, began the experiments at the Institute in 1976. The work was still under way in June 1978, when his trouble with Pauling began. Robinson says that he designed and managed the tests, and in part conceived them, although he drew heavily on the research of several other scientists, among them Homer Black, Ewan Cameron (now at the Institute), Malcolm Dole and Pauling himself, as well as on the suggestions of Eydie Mae Hunsberger and Arnold Hunsberger, nonscientists who have a special interest in diet and cancer. (Mrs. Hunsberger is the author of the book, "How I Conquered Cancer Naturally")

In keeping with the spirit of the Robinson—Institute dispute, which is one of disbelief on both sides, Pauling says that he, not Robinson, designed and managed the work and that the results are too tentative for anyone's comment. Robinson, of course, says that HE designed the tests. The purpose was to see whether a diet in which the Hunsbergers laid great store would work for cancerous laboratory mice. Thus, Robinson says, he induced squamous cell carcinoma, a kind of skin cancer, on the backs of 900 hairless mice. He fed one group the usual run of mouse food; a second, nothing but raw fruits and vegetables; a third, the same vegetarian diet heavily laced with vitamin C, and so on, in variations for 12 more groups.

He found that a pure diet of raw fruit and vegetables significantly reduced the size and number of cancerous sores in the mice; and that a conventional diet supplemented by very high doses of vitamin C (the human equivalent of 50 grams a day) had roughly the same beneficial effect. When the two regimens were combined – heavy vitamin C together with raw fruit and vegetables – the results were "just fantastic."

Dr. Arthur B. Robinson responded with the following editorial which emphasizes the symbiotic relationship between diet and cancer in the September 3, 1979 issue of "Barron's":

In James Grant's article of June 11, "Of Mice and Men", he refers to a three year series of experiments on squamous cell carcinoma (skin cancer) and nutrition in mice that I designed and directed at the Pauling Institute. . .

Cancer was induced by daily ultraviolet radiation of hairless mice that lived throughout the experiments on the designated diets. At dosages comparable to 10 grams of vitamin C per day for humans, the cancer incidence was increased about twofold, whereas at dosages comparable to 100 grams per day, it was decreased about fivefold. A diet restricted to apples, pears, carrots, tomatoes, wheatgrass, sunflower seeds and bananas decreased the cancer by about the same amount as the very high vitamin C dosages, whereas addition of protein to this diet seemed to eliminate its benefits. When used together, the raw fruits and vegetables and vitamin C caused a remarkable 35-fold decrease in cancer incidence.

The incidence of severe lesions in these experiments was caused to vary over a 70-fold range by nutritional measures alone. Regardless of the specific nutrition or the specific cancer assay system used, this result supports the view that optimum nutrition should be given a high priority in cancer research.

The Sunday Times, London, reported the following research results in January, 1977, in an article entitled "New Clues to Cancer" by Oliver Gillie, medical correspondent:

A number of surveys have found that people who eat plenty of fresh vegetables - such as lettuce or celery - are less likely to get stomach cancer. The importance of vegetables in the diet for cancer prevention has also been demonstrated in animals and has led to the discovery of a new class of substances which protect against cancer.

Dr. Leo Wattenburg, working at the University of Minnesota School of Medicine discovered that rats fed a balanced, highly purified diet containing all known vitamins and nutrients were not able to make certain enzymes (biological catalysts) in the liver which inactivate cancer-causing chemicals. However, when the rats were fed a crude diet containing alfalfa, they were able to produce the enzymes. And when alfalfa alone was added to the purified diet this caused the enzymes to be made.

Other experiments showed that this enzyme increased protection against cancer even when cancer-carrying chemicals were added to their diet. Dr. Wattenburg found that cabbage, brussel sprouts, turnips, broccoli, cauliflower, spinach, dill, and celery caused the enzymes to be made but varied in effectiveness according to their freshness and the soil in which they were grown.

Dr. Wattenburg identified the actual chemicals in the vegetables which cause the protective enzymes to be formed. They belong to a well-known family of organic chemicals called indoles. He also found that citrus fruits contain chemicals called flavones which have the same effect as indoles. Beans and seeds are rich in plant proteins called lectins which have been found to protect animals against cancer in laboratory experiments.

The national weekly, "The Globe", printed the following article on the triumph of Eydie Mae Hunsberger over cancer through her dedicated application of the wheatgrass therapy and a raw foods diet.

HOW I BEAT CANCER
by Bruce MacDonald

You can lick your cancer if you eat the right foods says a woman who believes she did just that.

The secret, says Eydie Mae Hunsberger lies in eating only "live, natural" foods and avoiding all animal products and sugar.

Eydie, who was told six years ago that she was dying of breast cancer, tells you how she did it in her new book, "How I Conquered Cancer Naturally", published by Harvest House.

"The therapeutic diet I used was very strict. I used no cooked foods at all," the 52 year old housewife told GLOBE this week from her suburban San Diego, California home. "In attempting to regain my health I absolutely limited myself to the diet. It's unwise to cheat where cancer or any other disease is concerned. These diseases are unforgiving of even the smallest infractions of the diet rules."

Eydie prefers to call her diet "non-animal" rather than vegetarian because it involves a strict schedule that rules out a number of vegetable food products. . . like sugar, honey, dried fruit and most spices.

"At first my husband Arn and I were concerned that we wouldn't be getting all the vitamins, minerals and proteins our bodies require", she pointed out. "Well meaning professionals and friends warned us about anemia if our diets were not supplemented with animal products or store-bought vitamins."

But she and her husband, who joined her in the diet, have no second thoughts about their decision. In fact, Eydie reports her total protein level read a perfect 7 at her last blood analysis. And, she says, she now suffers less from headaches, flu and colds - and generally feels better than she ever has before. Eydie says she maintains her protein level by eating avocado, various seeds and sprouts, and keeps her overall health in tip-top shape by eating wheatgrass.

"If you've ever noticed, a sick animal will go out and start eating grasses," she said. "I found the animals go to the wheatgrass first." In her book, Eydie explains how you can grow this grass right in your own basement using small trays and wet peat moss. "I can assure you I have no desire to return to my body-destroying, slow-death diet," she said. "It's marvelous how the tastebuds become more sensitive and delicate to the differences in the many varieties of such things as, say, peaches

Eydie Mae Hunsberger is a healthy 52 year old today. But it was a different story in February, 1973. Her doctors told her she had breast cancer and advised a radical mastectomy and cobalt treatments. Afterwards they were planning another radical on the other side, followed by removal of the ovaries, the adrenal gland and the pituitary gland.

"Without these treatments they told me I might live another year . . .and with them may be another five . I didn't want to spend those years in a hospital being taken apart", she recalled. "I said I wanted to live three good years. But before I died I wanted to think I had tried something. At that point I had nothing to lose so I might as well go into nutrition". And the result was her "live foods" diet and a victory over cancer.

LEUCOCYTOSIS OF DIGESTION CAUSED BY COOKING

A study by Paul Kauchakoff, M. D., of the University of Clinical Chemistry, Lausanne, Switzerland states "After over 300 experiments on 10 individuals of different age and sex, we have come to the following conclusion: 1) The augmentation of the number of white corpuscles and the alteration of the correlation of the percentage between them which takes place after every consumption of food, and which was considered until now as a physiological phenomenon, is, in reality, a pathological one. It is called forth by the introduction into the system of foodstuff altered by means of high temperatures, and by complicated treatments of ordinary products produced by Nature; and 2) After the consumption of fresh raw foodstuff, produced by Nature, our blood formula does not change in any lapse of time nor in consequence of any combination"

The critical temperature is not the same for all raw foodstuff. It varies within a range of 10 degrees. The lowest critical temperature for water is 191; for milk, 191; for cereal, tomatoes, cabbage and banana, 192; for pear and meat, 193; for butter, 196, for apple and orange, 197, for potatoe, 200; for carrot, strawberry and fig, 206 degrees fahrenheit (Proceedings: The First International Congress of Macrobiology, Paris, 1930).

HIGH PROTEIN DIET CAUSES AGING

I. M. Spector of the Institute of Traumatology in Russia reported: "In terms of lifespan, there is a negative correlation between the longevity of animals and their protein turnover rate." Thus, the faster the turnover, the shorter the life. Or, the more protein an animal eats, the shorter is the lifespan. (Animal Longevity and Protein Turnover Rate; "Nature", 249:66, May 3, 1974) From previous studies (see chapter on Longevity in text) we know that the conclusions follow for humans as well as for other animals.

KIDNEY AND HIGH PROTEIN DIET

"The kidneys of adult rats responded in even one week to a high protein level in the diet. After removing one kidney from rats, the other was found to be 5% enlarged after 3 days and 45% enlarged after 150 days. This increase is proportional to the protein level in the diet." (Smith and Moise, Journal of Experimental Medicine, Vol. 46, no. 24, 1927) Considering that most forms of death are due to an overacid condition of the body, a low level protein diet, when properly chosen, would be conducive to a healthy kidney which would prevent acidity.

CHELATED MINERALS

The health field is giving more recognition to the value of minerals in the bloodstream. It is being recognized that inorganic minerals are poorly absorbed. A good example is iron. A normal (unhealthy) individual requires daily 18 mg. of iron, which is commonly administered in the form of ferrous sulfate. It required the 18 mg. dose level because of poor absorption through the intestinal tract which results in the absorption of only 4% of the dose into the bloodstream.

The alternative is to use nature's method of mineral transport. In this case the mineral is hooked up to an amino acid, sometimes, also, a vitamin. Today's literature calls these arrangements chelated minerals. However, this is just another name for many of the enzymes.

Cooking inactivates enzymes as well as chelated minerals by breaking up the arrangement as well as causing changes to the amino acid. Hence you lose the amino acid as well as the transport potential of the mineral.

Raw foods are your best, cheapest source of chelated minerals. Such minerals enter the bloodstream in volume and quickly produce dramatic healing results.

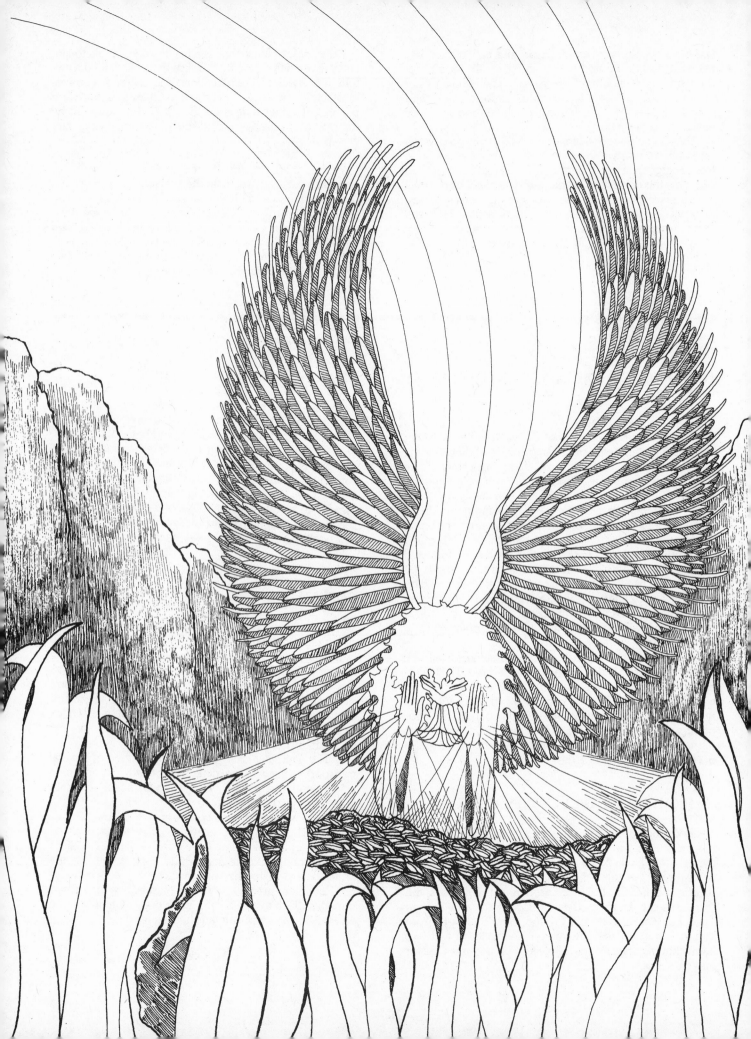

MEAT CAN MAKE YOU UNCONSCIOUS

Dr. Ernest Hartman, Boston sleep researcher, showed in his experiments that tryptophan, an essential amino acid, where flesh and dairy products have the highest concentration - up to twenty times higher than in fruit - is the dietary factor that produces drowsiness after a meal.

(Archives of General Psychiatry, September, 1974, vol. 31, no. 3, p. 394) This is why meat eaters feel drowsy after the heavy protein meal and need the stimulation of coffee. Excess of tryptophan poisons the bloodstream and starts making one unconscious.

FUNDS RAISED BY NINE HEALTH AGENCIES

[And Amounts Allocated to Research]

AGENCY	FUNDS RAISED	ALLOCATED TO RESEARCH
National Foundation for Infantile Paralysis	$18,669,229	$2,479,617
National Tuberculosis Association	18,655,524	Unknown
American Cancer Society	13,211,069	3,300,000
American Heart Association	2,502,176	250,000
Arthritis and Rheumatism Foundation	222,606	None
National Committee for Mental Hygiene	217,624	45,237
National Multiple Sclerosis Society	147,967	62,368
American Diabetes Association	91,366	300
National Association to Control Epilepsy	33,373	8,482

SPROUT A COMPLETE PROTEIN

There are two ways to establish whether a food item supplies a complete protein. First through biological studies using animals (or by observing cultural diet patterns of humans) who eat a controlled diet. If adequate protein is present, then the researchers expect a normal growth rate, absence of classical protein deficiency disease, longevity pattern of that species and healthy reproduction for at least several generations. Second, through chemical analysis.

By the first method, Dr. Francis Pottenger Jr. (175) had found "sprouted grain to be a complete protein in an animal test, completely servicing the reproduction program through generations (p. 40)...he had found sprouted legumes and grains to contribute enough first quality protein to be classed as complete (p. 295)." Likewise, Dr. C.F. Schnabel (168) showed grass is adequate in providing all needed nutrients, including protein, in animal experiments.

To establish by the second method one has to take the indirect approach because of lack of nutritional data on sprouts.

From the study of germination process, Drs. Mayer and Poljakoff—Mayber (Germination of Seed, Pergamon Press, 1963) of the Botony Dept. Hebrew University, Jerusalem, observed: "Nitrogen (protein) appears to be very carefully conserved. In place of the protein broken down there appears free amino acids and amides." That is, in germination, the amino acids are freed (not destroyed) from their protein structure. Hence, if a seed contains a complete protein (of lower density due to the dilluting effect of water) containing all the amino acids that were in the original seed protein.

From the following table (Amino Acid Content of Food, Orr and Watt, U.S.D.A., Wash., D.C.) we see that the listed seeds contain a complete protein. Hence the sprouts of the seeds are also complete proteins.

The table values are for raw produce. Pasteurized dairy produce, cooked eggs and meat do not have the amino acids listed in the table when they are served in the cooked form. With out any other considerations, if one is to choose a food item that would supply a complete protein source, one would choose raw sprouted seeds.

	chick peas	lentil	mung	soy	wheat	buck wheat	sun flower	soy sprout	buck spr (a)	su t spr (a)	mear	human milk	date	egg	sesame
tryptophan	0.170	0.216	0.180	0.526	0.173	.17	0.343	0.017	.03	.06	0.220	.103 .058	.06	.211	.33
threonine	0.739	0.896	0.765	1.504	0.403	.46	0.911	0.159	.09	.15	0.830	.284 .257	.06	.637	.71
isoleusine	1.195	1.316	1.351	2.054	0.607	.44	1.276	0.225	.09	.21	0.984	.344 .240	.07	.850	.95
leucine	1.538	1.760	2.202	2.946	0.939	.68	1.736	0.265	.15	.30	1.540	.567 .475	.08	1.126	1.7
lysine	1.434	1.528	1.667	2.414	0.384	.69	0.868	0.211	.16	.12	1.642	.413 .353	.07	.819	.58
methionine	0.276	0.180	0.265	0.513	0.214	.21	0.443	0.045	.04	.07	0.466	.128 .051	.03	.401	.64
phenylalanine	1.012	1.104	1.167	1.889	0.691	.44	1.220	0.186	.09	.20	0.773	.272 .142	.06	.739	1.5
valine	1.025	1.360	1.440	2.005	0.648	.61	1.354	.225	.12	.21	1.044	.391 .283	.09	.950	.89
argine	1.551	1.908	1.370	2.763	0.670	.93	2.370	.43	.19	.30	1.212	.253 .172	.05	.840	1.9
histidine	0.559	0.548	0.543	0.911	0.286	.26	0.586		.05	.09	0.653	.138 .061	.05	.307	.44
total protein	28%	25%	24.4%	35%	14%	12%	23%	6%	2	4%	19%	1.4% .8%	2.2%	13%	19%

VII. TESTIMONIALS

SHATTERED DISK, PARALYSIS AND SURGERY ARE FOLLOWED BY WHEAT GRASS JUICE FAST, SPROUT DIET AND COMPLETE RECOVERY WITH LOVE.

Dear Viktoras,

I just completed a 43−day fast in the desert. I've been eating sprouts and wheatgrass for 21 days and helping some interested people in the course of transition from meat/grain diets to raw/fruit ones. I had written to Viktoras over a year ago telling him of my paralysis and totally non−functioning elimination system, etc. He wrote back to me suggesting a few avenues, all of which cost money. I had none. He suggested I fast at home, which I did then for 50 days or more, and told me I'd soon be healing in a river of love. True, true, Brothers and Sisters! Last Sept. 2, I had spinal surgery to remove bone chips from inside my spinal column, which were severing my motor nerve and causing great trauma to the sensory nerves. The 4th lumbar vertabra was shaved down, since a bony tumor or deposit had collected there and was blocking off all functions in this area. The shattered disc was removed, which took the pressure off the sciatic nerve and straightened my spine, which was slanting crazily anteriorly toward the right in the sacral caudal region.

I was advised after surgery of all the things I could never do again. I lived in a hospital bed for about 2 more months doing the most shallow breathing excercises, mental hatha yoga and meditation. By February I was on my way to the Anza Borrega desert, where I walked, with an angel brother who helped me, for 3 days to an isolated spot and fasted. I walked out strong and supple after 43 days of camping above the ½−mile long staircase of the enchanted tiger, by the river of love.

Today I began a new 50−day fast and I am well, perfectly so. Thanks for your real and gentle encouragement, Viktoras, when it was coming from nowhere else but inside me and needed reinforcement. One ashram I wrote to ask permission to fast there had told me they couldn't handle the intensity of a person fasting as I had described, among them, etc. Some were derisive around me, so...I'm able to do mayurasana again for 2 mins. and salabhasana for 60 seconds and other hatha yoga asanas, e.g., Ardhamatsyendrasana. I can grab and hold the opposite ankle comfortably indefinitely. I was told I'd never do these anymore. By now I should be able to be painfully carefully lift a few lbs. In the desert I had to carry 80 and 90 lb. rocks to put inside my tent to fasten it down in the 100 mph winds... even handstands. **Surgeons' knives can't touch chakras.**

Know what, my cats love sprouts and eat my wheatgrass pulp every days. When available they love watermelon pulp.

Maureen Madden

Dear Viktoras−−I have been reading, and re−reading the flyer of "Survival" − re−reading it because I have not read for modern times so moving a manifesto of love. It is as if you are cradling your readers in your arms, crooning to them loving words of comfort and security. I have for a long time now so pictured Spirit, holding us in loving arms, showering love upon us, whether or not we knew it. **San Francisco**

Dear Vik−−"Survival" is fantastic. I feel it's one of the most important books I've ever read. A true manual and guide for the New Age. It has so much in it that is of value to me that I'm reading only a few pages each day. This book will be my dietary bible. I hope to continue my purification and one day, hopefully soon, live in a warmer climate where I can detoxify further and go on a fruitarian diet.

Dear Viktor−−What a holy, holy book you have written. The world says thank you. Words fail us, but it is so beautifully done−−the Bible for the Aquarian Age. Truely, you have created something the earth has been crying for. **Bosley and Ea Hiss.**

Dear Viktoras−−My admiration of your spiritual depth is boundless. Your writing is pure poetry.

Viktoras−−"Survival" is wonderful! Thank you!! Shalom... **Joe and Cathy, Ferraro's Pure Carrot Juice, Monrovia, California.**

Dear Viktoras−−"Survival" is a masterpiece! A collection of much needed information for the whole world. It really falls into the category of "The Bible of Human Survival." I do hope that you can get it reviewed, televised, etc., etc, promoted nationwide, not only in the realm of nutriton, but as a text for all humans, whether young or old. This much − needed publication should be sent to every library in the nation, and made available in all bookstores. This no longer must be kept as a fad but as a necessity of human knowledge and enlightenment. **The brothers of St. Francis of Assisi, Ravena, New York.**

Dear Viktoras−−I am absolutely thrilled with "Survival"−− which I will circulate at my newly−formed SOUTHERN CALIFORNIA VEGETARIANS. God Bless you! **Blanche Leonard, Santa Monica, California.**

Dear Viktoras − "Survival" is great! I find myself just sort of awestruck by the completeness of it all and the feeling of all the work that went into it. It's really almost perfect as far as content goes. For years I have longed for such a compilation of knowledge, practicality, details, clear account of the cleansing process in all aspects, plus the record of what the scientific community is doing in research to back up the intuitions for those people who can't yet let go of the need for "proof." ...Love, **Mary Sacks.**

Dear Victor − Cleansing from last Christmas spree is making me see how much God loves through his Son, if we will only let him come. Want to let you know your splended book "Survival Into The 21st Century" and The Bible are my guide lights for survival after February's bout with penicillin and pneumonia! Can still read and write, never could remember well, nor spell. Thanks for being you and helping me become Be−er−through Jesus Christ. Love you, **Mary D. Latane (86 YEAR MONTH), Baltimore, MD**

Dear Omangod People − As I make my way around Geneva I meet people talking of "Survival Into The 21st Century" and of going on wheatgrass juice fast. So I borrowed copy for the weekend. OH WOW! And it fits just into the line I am searching these days. I was just on my own realizing how powerful psycho therapy food eating could be and guy comes along talking of eating food according to energy and vibrations higher and your book falls in my hands. Please send copy. AIR MAIL. **Spyros Root, Switzerland**

A TRIBUTE TO VIKTOR Kulvinskas was enxtended from a group of American Chiropractors attending the Stoner Clinic in Las Vegas recently. Stephen Kashuba, D.O. from Mt. Carmel, reviewed Viktor's "Survival..." book for a half hour to the 130 attending the seminar on kiniseology. The after−the−meeting response from 90 per cent of the group was tremendously positive & quite a few planned to order the book (it's $8.00−−like 6 books in 1). Says Kashuba, "Much of the material I have somewhere in my research papers at home−−but Viktor put them all together for me." (Note: The Stoner Chiropractic Research Foundation, P.O. Box 15208, Las Vegas, NV 89109. Offers a 4−day course for approx. $285, plus lodging, 4 times a year, next one in May. Incidentally, Viktor's book contains current research from Harvard Medical Library and MIT which is not yet available through outside sources).

Dear Vik--I write from Washington State Penitentiary. Recently, I requested your book and you sent it no charge with the others; "Love Your Body", "Unity Consciousness", "Instant Apt. Farming", "The Sacred Science of Love Wisdom." On behalf of myself and the group here at our Prison Ashram I want to say THANKS! We have begun sprouting (most of us are vegetarian or semi vegetarian). Your timing was good as it arrived midst a six day fast for me; hence I was really open to it. It has since been in continual circulation and high demand with a waiting list. It's really, really, really a great book that offers a lot for us on the path here. I am so excited about this book that I super want to share it with my people on the outside for Christmas. There are 4 families which at $8 each is out of my reach as a convict making 25 cents a day. Have a good day. **Ron.**

Dear Vik--Want you to know that Survival arrived today bringing sunlight into this

subzero weather. Thank You. **Kate B., Woodstock, Illinois.**

Dearest Viktor--We are deeply touched and grateful for the time, love, effort and spirit of truth that has gone into your book Survival Into the 21st Century. Thank you so much. It is truly the answer to many prayers. With love, **Virginia R., Jamul, California.**

Dear Viktoras--Can't resist commenting again on "Survival." The more I read, the more I am awed by the magnitude of the compilation necessary to produce that book. I am just SO grateful for it. Love, **Joyce.**

Dear Viktoras--Your book shines with the light of a strong love. I'm so happy to have it as an aid, an ally, in my study of nutrition, healing, and of nature. Hopefully your sales in the midwest will be enhanced by my friends who see the copies you sent, and want their own copy...This just can't wait! Two days after starting to chew wheatgrass, a sore from my friend's radiation treatment in his mouth disappeared! Nice to have immediate results to help build his confidence in the healing properties of chlorophyll. His proper attitude and increased sprout intake has enabled him to have the first unassisted bowel movement in months...The Walker Community Video group im Minneapolis is interested in making a 30 minute video tape for the instruction and general education on the art of indoor gardening. If I have your permission, I'd like to use a lot of the material from Survival...**Phillip B., Northfield, Minn.**

Viktor--Book is fascinating! Wonderful collection! Congratulations for the tremendous effort! Love you brother - you are a gift to us all. All our faith in you. Love, **Ed and Ro, Alameda, California.**

Dear Viktoras--I thout I woud rit you a little letter. I'm Dawn Butler, Donald's twin sister--the one how rot you a letter the farst time. My Mother reads a lot of your books. We are fruit giys. We just love fruit. I'me 10 years old, but I'm not very tall. I work on the farme with my Mother and father. We love it. We have sower grass and wheat grass and wild radish. My father isn't into this. I feel for him though. Vik, you are a inportant man. We were siprised to get a letter from you. You are so bizzy. We have other brothers and sisters in Michigin. They are not into this ether, but I'm thankfull we are. And you are too. We are in home school and our Mother teaches us. We don't eat nuts becuse it's too much and it clogs us all up. Well, Vik, you're a good man. I'll go now. I love you. **Dawn Butler.**

Hi Brother--Thanks for "Survival." It's time for things to be more accepted in the South. Still a lot of educating needs to happen--and it will. In our publication we might do articles on cancer, meat, and menstruation as spoken of in your book--trying to interest a lot of folks...so many people are ready to learn of the benefits of raw food. **D.D., Well-Being, San Diego, Calif.**

Viktoras--your name's symbolic effect is more evident after reading your book. Your book is a bible. 3,000 things occur to me to do after reading it. One, the most important, is to get it out in paragraph seed form through public service announcements. I'm going to write Mildred in Summertown, Tennessee, today about doing the same thing. They have video tape facilities there and can change the world there with their 500 vegans. **Donald C., Washington, D.C.**

Dear Viktoras--Don has been security guarding and every night he reads your book. He has started sprouting. I've been trying to go the complete fruitarian route--without sprouts...**Washington, D.C. (American Vegetarians)**

Dear Viktoras--I've read Survival through 3 times now. It's great--in every way. What else can I say?...I finally made it through. I'm gaining weight on oranges and sapotes. I think back on avocados like dope or cigarettes. Now I'm off to the high desert near Yuma for the best tangelos I've ever tasted...In 2-½ years my eyes went from dark brown to mostly green. Time will tell what my true colors are. Much love and good luck. **Steve D., Santa Barbara, California.**

Dear Viktor--"Survival" is a classic gem and should be placed alongside the Bible in every home as a complete guide to better health, inspirational living, and a new world order. In fact, I would say that this book could well replace all the books found in the Library of Congress! **Sam D., Pittsburgh.**

Dear Viktoras--I was very impressed with your book, and I've been spreading the word about it to everyone. I was especially pleasantly surprised to see Just's and Eugene's photos. We were also at the gathering, but when you were there, we were working at the Orange Grove Health Ranch in Arcadia...spent the summer in Texas, then to the Kona Coast in Hawaii...I'm writing a paper entitled, "Fruit is the best food there is."...Here are some sayings I'd like to share with you: "Elimination is a waste of time." "Death is a forced fast." "Life is one big elimination." "Be where you are, not where you think you should be." "We don't need two-ply toilet paper anymore." "Copulation brings population." Here are some others by some of my favorite writers: "Lay down your stones, bring it home." "Let my life be your love song." "I think the best is yet to come, cause where I'm from is also where I'm going." "Don't you see, that the purpose of living is to love and be loved, again and again." **Burk S., Escondido, California**

Greetings from your Millennial A.T.A. Base: Am thankful to see that you have gone to such an extent into your work "Survival."It is "warming to the heart." You have many of the answers that it will take in order to survive. Continue to seek your awareness--there is no end. Sincerely, **Duncan P., New Age Center, Weslaco, Texas.**

Viktoras--To the beautiful things you're doing! You're unreal, you're beautiful in body, mind and soul. I've felt I've known you for always. I would truly like to belong to the book club. Words I read from you are living breathing life--they make me burst with excitement, knowing there are others like me! Love and peace, **Vivian A., Phoenix, Ariz.**

Viktor--Love you for coming to help the people of our earth. "Survival" should be lots of fun with you making those wonderful blueprints for how-to. It's fantastic. It's poetic. Thanks for the book, your guidance and inspiration. **Divine Light Mission, Denver, Co.**

Dear Viktoras--I have found "Survival" a most inspiring incentive in my life and by far the most sensible and rational approach to changing one's diet and one's outlook on life. Would you believe--I had to go all the way to Mexico to find that book? Picked it up at the vegetarian restaurant in Cuernavaca!

Dear dear Viktoras--You are the reincarnations of many beautiful souls! How else could one write of love as you do. As I read your "Survival", breathing came slower. I was floating. You are pure.......**Omeonta, N.Y.**

Dear Viktor--Mr. and Mrs. Irons are very much impressed with your book "Survival" Will you quote a price on a minimum of 10 books? Please let me know and we will place the order -with check- from this office. Many thanks. **C.W. Dahlin**

Dear Viktor--"Survival" is the greatest! I'm working on reviews of it for the paper (Vegetarian World)...prospective card or poster publishers...symposium on longevity...interviews for East/West and New Age journals...new age book stores...college bookstores..major New Age spokesmen like Airola, Roszak (who just got into the natural diet), Tom Laughlin (Billy Jack movies), etc. Love and thanks, **Scott, VEGETARIAN WORLD, Los Angeles, California.**

Dear Viktoras--Was greatly impressed as well as pleased with the information and format of "Survival." Many thanks for bringing this book into being for the service of man. **Michael M., Mesa, Arizona.**

Dear Viktoras--I have read "Survival" cover to cover and now want all of my friends and relatives to learn about the right way to live also. Thank you. **Barbara B., N. Miami**

Dear Viktoras--Thanks for your love and light. Your new book is really beautiful...if you need any assistance in the future, call or write. All love in the light. **Elliott McL., Banyen Bookshop, Vancouver, B.C.**

Dear Viktor--Your "Survival" is most stimulating, encyclopedic and a bold attempt at a whole integrated look at Man and the Universe. Keep up the good work. I'm recommending it to patients. **Stanley Bass, D.C., Brooklyn, N.Y.**

Viktoras--The book is beautiful. My love opened and flowed out to you. **Norma Lusk**

Viktoras--Thank you for sending me "Survival." It is a marvelous masterpiece by a witty, clever fellow. I'm happy the Great Spirit gave us Friend Viktoras, the Mathematician and Piscean Poet. Peace, **John G., Green Bay, Wisc.**

Dear Viktoras--An enormous THANKS from our entire community for your generosity in sharing with us your unique contribution for everyone's welfare. congratulations for the excellent performance! I thank God for gifting you with such unique potential. Your book is receiving wide Franciscan circulation. May you sense the vibrations of pride in your performance! Gratefully. **Sister Felice, St. Francis Catholic Convent.**

WEIGHT G(r)AIN

Many raw foodist complain about the weight issue. Easy to lose but hard to gain. First, need to understand that what we are looking for in weight gain is increase in muscle mass. Some of the gain will be from nzymatic raw fat, making for males about 15% and 20% for female - though most can do well at much lower percent.

My wife http://www.youkta.org initiated her search for a calorie rich, with balanced protein, diet that one can maintain without stuffing self with dozens of bananas, bunches of avocado, loads of unsoaked nuts and in general eating a large volume of food.

Vihara Youkta discovered that successful athletes and body builders center on grains and high protein. She converted to sprouted grains, soaked seeds and soaked nuts, as well as super foods. Eventually, after just adding such foods to our diet, we evolved recipies that made it very acceptable and tasty for all palates.

This presentation, is a summary - practical search of success as a raw food explorers in the body building camp. Eventually, I joined Youkta both in diet and also in weight training both by self, with Youkta and with a trainer. The back cover photos, gives some indication of our success.

The first step to weight gain, is have more energy to digest the higher concentrated foods and to take on more strenuous resistance training (max out on weight),balanced by adequate recovery time.

The way one builds energy, is through more than adequate rest, strenuous/max resistance workouts (20 to 40 min, allowing oneself complete recovery after each workout - ie - pain free), , following carefully the eating guidelines and eating small meals only when stomach is empty, emotional peace and good happy relation with self, finances and others. Adequate intake of warm water, in timely fashion; as well as alkalizing super foods (like blue green algae and grasses) - take before and after workout; as well as enzymes after workout as well as taken with all meals.

Four weeks ago, I ended up reflecting, how successful body builders gain and maintain there superior stature. Well, they do identical, as do babies, that is:
1. Sleep, and nap at least 12 to 16 hours per day. Limits calorie expenditure and allows for maximum muscle growth.
2. Strenuous challenging activities. when awake.
3. Many small, predigested concentrated meals - 5 to 8 meals per 24 hours.

I thought I would try it for a week -- I gained about 4 pounds - and I still have maintained it weeks later. My strength also increased - I increased bench press from 80 pounds to 115; deadlift from 120 to 160 pounds etc. That is, I did 3 serious workouts that week. And I did Isometric and flexing and stretching exercises the rest of the week. I cat napped - when-ever felt like, and fell asleep for 1 to 2 hours. I slept about a total of 14 hours per day.

My meals were mostly - almond milk made with few figs; well strained and then blended with 1 banana. I was using about 1 cup of soaked almonds with 2 cups of water. I took 4 enzymes and 2 bacteria pills and 3 times per day, I took also 4 caps of Omega algae. I had about 4 to 6 such meals and then I also had sprouted grains/with soaked seed pate (and or breakfast cereal) made with oil and sea vegetables. I also had 1 blended avocado/greens/apple (papaya) thick soup with dulce

Now lets get back to the science of weight gain.

WEIGHT GAIN SYSTEM

To gain weight of lean muscle mass at a rate faster than it is torn down, one needs to push exercise to levels of resistance training, where the present muscle mass is inadequate to meet the physical stress demands which of course stimulates the body to build more muscle, to handle the increased demands.

For new muscle to grow one has to have:
<u>Nutritionally:</u> adequate calorie increase, usually with more protein and calories with adequate hydration to expel the metabolic waste products
<u>Rest:</u> recovery time, via way of rest and spacing of the resistance training Rest includes cat naps.
<u>Body building:</u> the intensity of training, without overload/injury with adequate recovery time.

<u>The following components are important.</u>
1. Weight Training. Should entail one day every 1 to 2 weeks, where one pushes oneself to limits, jet guided by wisdom and damage prevention. Stress ,of this intense level, especially in the beginner, could benefit from a massage, the following day, as well as if there is any feeling of mis-alignment, a visit to the chiropractor. If there are joint issues or hand sensitivity to the weight levels, Glucosamine complex might be advised, until the symptoms are corrected, followed by a maintenance level. On the day on intense workout, there is increase in tissue breakdown as well as an increase in lactic acid hence (1). 4 enzymes and 4 blue green algae after the workout (2) taking liquids for several hours is desirable, as

well as increased sweating and possibly 30-60 min salt bath (at night) thus reducing the aches and pains that do show up. During the day, one should have a hyper sensitivity about sleep, ie if feel any degree of sleepiness, one should lay down until it passes. Definitely, more sleep is desired on that night. The following day. A massage would be greatly benefited. One should have the rest of the week-long trainings be light and maintenance. In weight training, one should not over do the aerobics, which will place more calorie demands on the system, though the jogging is beneficial for circulation.

2. WELL FUNCTIONING INTESTINAL TRACT

Difficulty will arise if there is

A. Toxic stomach (such as a lots of brown in the first oval around the pupil of the iris. Or the Kirlian photo, show weak stomach.). Concentrated effort has to applied in planning the meals only when hunger/empty-stomach, using at least 2 times a year a psyllium/Bentonite (Dr Jensen or VE Irons Cleansing System) for 3 to 7 days at a time; strenuous yogic breath of fire; crunches, trampoline, cayenne with all juices, weekly juice day with high amount of cayenne. This might seem like gong backwards on the weight gain. One needs to follow up the fast with carefully orchestrated re-building eating programs.

B. Mucus residue within small intestine where they interfere with the flow of calories, fats, aminos, enzymes and minerals and the absorption into the blood and lymph, to provide the nutrition for muscle building. Jensen's Detox will help

C. If large colon is being disturbed by a significant volume of parasites, warms and pathogens. A good indicator is failure in weight gain, gas and loose stool on an ongoing basis. To determine, it is recommended a stool analysis, if shows presence, depending on what it is' there are available rigorous programs of colema, proper herbs and Soil-Bases Organisms/probiotic oral intake to correct the situation. It could be foundation for bio-availability and absorption of nutrients and the removal of a high drain of key nutrients, because the nutrients were being eaten by the parasites.

D. Emotional stress- can have high calorie demand, which prevents weight gain. Also, tension, lead to indigestion, sourness of meals eaten.

E. Failure to comply with good eating practices, which maximize bio-availability of food

    1. Not following food combining

    2. Not chewing food thoroughly- or using food processor/blender when in hurry or not desiring to spend lot time chewing.

    3. Eating when stomach is not empty and or when not hungry. Snacking on a non-empty stomach.

    4. Being tired In such cases, best if <u>stomach is empty</u> some juice followed, if wish, with rest. If <u>stomach not empty</u>, some tea such as mixture of dandelion, comfrey, cascara Sagrata, burdock, red clover. OR just a Senna with psyllium complex. We liked the gentle results from New Season Cleanse (1-800-800-1300, for wholesale ID 472483). Take enzymes and take a nap..

    5. Eating when you are cold or overheated, since then the digestion is poor

    6. Eating cold food (with meal or as a dessert) slows the digestion, and will interfere with digestion.

    7. Drinking more than 1/2 cup of warm tea or warm water with meal.

    8. Indulging in alcohol with starchy meals.

    9. Failing to have adequate amount of enzymes within the meals

    10. Eating close to bedtime. <u>Please note:</u> It is OK to take a cat nap after a meal, matter fact DESIRABLE. It is siesta. All forces will be concentrated on digestion. Also, there is the light to stimulate digestion. Going to sleep after a meal at night, might act as sedative, however, it can be causing poor digestion and restless night. Since the first stage of sleep, all energy is concentrated on finishing the digestion. Then the next phase is detox of the waste build up during the waking hours. Beneficial hormonal action of the night s lost. One feels sleepy or not fully rested. In emergency situation, a small 40 watt bulb light, by the bed, will assist tremendously in digestion.

    11. Emotional discussions, with anger and/or discussion of stressful subjects.

    12. Spinal mis-alignment

    13. Inadequate calories on daily basis.

    14. Hormones low

14. Not detoxed far enough, so that the membranes of GI, lymph, cell, blood vessels are creating obstruction to the flow of nutrients.

For the rest of details, please visit, the program and recipies, at

Viktoras4u.com   viktorasretreats@gmail.com

WHAT ARE ENZYMES?

The word "enzyme" comes from the Greek word enzymes, which means "to ferment" or "cause a change."

The medical dictionary defines an enzyme as "a protein produced in a cell capable of greatly accelerating, by its catalytic action, the chemical reaction of a substance (the substrate) for which it is specific."

According to Dr. Howell, enzymes are the body's workers, operating on a biological and chemical level, perhaps even the radiological level. Every organ, fluid and chemical, are important to the 'dance of life' and we would run into problems, with deficiency, in any vitamin, mineral, hormone, amino acid, essential fats and other substances However, it is enzymes that perform the work and utilize these substances in restoring, repairing and maintaining 'the dance of life.'

Attempts to produce synthetic enzymes have failed. Science has identified over 50,000 unique enzyme systems. They suspect that there may be hundreds of thousands, even millions of different types of enzymes.

An enzyme is a specialized protein structure which carries with it an energetic charge. Enzymes speed up chemical reactions that normally take place very slowly or not at all. It is the energy behind the protein structure that makes enzymes different from other protein-based substances. It is this energetic "life principle" that animates all living forms and "runs the whole show" we call life.

The father of modern enzyme therapy, Dr. Edward Howell, once said that enzymes emit a "kind of radiation" that can be picked up on Kirlian photo- graphs.

Howell can be singled out from other researchers because he stressed that food enzymes (as found in raw foods) are not merely expendable, protein-based chemical catalysts that move along chemical reactions... He forcefully argued that enzymes are none other than units of life-energy that use various protein molecules as their carriers.

Enzymes are much more sensitive to destruction by heat or cold than vitamins and minerals. Food cooked over 118 degrees for more than a half an hour will kill all naturally-occurring enzymes. In the event that dry heat is used, the critical temperature for enzyme destruction is about 150 F

Enzymes are the "true workers" in and out of our cells. As Dr. Richard Gerber M.D. states, "The enzymes catalyze specific reactions of chemicals either to create structure through molecular assemblies or to provide the electrochemical fire to run the cellular engines and ultimately keep the entire system working."

VIKTORAS DISCOVERS HOWELL'S MANUSCRIPTS

Viktoras was perhaps the first person to popularize the long out-of-print writings of the enzyme researcher Dr. Edward Howell. He discovered the original manuscript ("The Status of Food Enzymes in Digestion and Metabolism") at the Harvard Medical Library and immediately recognized it as the missing science that explain the magic of Raw Live Food. After several years of tracking down Dr Howell, who was then a very elderly person, though still doing research. Viktoras persuaded Dr. Howell to allow him to publish his manuscripts. The book was renamed "Food Enzymes for Health and Longevity", was edited, with undated writings by Viktoras. Viktoras published 10,000 copies at great personal expense and risk. The book did not sell well, thought it impacted the professional community, with a dramatic increase in enzyme awareness.

The publication of this first of many of Howell' works resurrected from obscurity fifty years of priceless research regarding the crucial role of enzymes for high level wellness and extended lifespan. Viktoras' premiere publication of Howell's book stimulated a whirlwind of interest which is still growing today. In fact, as a direct result of the resurgence of interest in enzymes, digestive enzyme supplement companies based on Howell's original formula have become a multi-million dollar industries.

VIKTORAS STARTS ENZYME FORMULATIONS

Realizing, like Dr. Howell, that not everybody is ready or willing to eat a sufficient quantity of living foods to make a positive impact on health, I pioneered enzyme supplementation and enzyme systems I initiated research, development and marketing of whole food enzymatic nutritional supplements. Over 60 formulas were released for multi-national companies. It is my contention that whole food supplements such as algae, wheatgrass, vegetarian enzyme/herbal formulations can greatly minimize the effects of cooked foods, environmental toxins and inherited constitutional weaknesses.

HOW ARE FOOD ENZYMES GROWN

A few more words about aspergillus oryzae enzymes. This booklet would not have been written, nor perhaps would I be as alive and healthy as I am today, if it were not for the amazing properties of these "angel-hair-in-appearance" microscopic plants and the enzymes they create.. Over 65 years ago, Dr. Howell began to cultivate one special species of the many aspergillus plants that existed in the plant kingdom. He picked the "oryzae" strain because there were no harmful aflatoxins (a type of poison) associated with this plant. Since then many other safe species have been discovered.. More importantly, however, this strain contained a rich store of the very same enzymes that the human body used to digest food.

The Aspergilus is fed in a specialized environment of controlled pressure, temperature and humidity. Depending on what type of food is fed, the aspergilus excretes surplus specific enzymes to digest this food. After the digestive process is completed, the aspergilus is removed as a film, the remaining enzymes are harvested and are tested for safety and potency. Then, they are dried for future use in formulas.

For the first time in recorded history, Howell gave the powdered enzymes from these little plants directly to human patients. He found that the enzymes created by aspergillus oryzae was a key to treating a whole host of seemingly unrelated ailments. Because of the success of his clinical work, he dedicated his life to working out a theoretical and experimental platform to explain how the seeming these miracles had been accomplished. The "Food Enzyme Concept" in human nutrition was the product of this great man's life-work.

DO WE REALLY NEED PLANT ENZYMES?

Some medical authorities make the claim that since your body can make its own enzymes, it is unnecessary to take supplemental food enzymes. They believe that the body develops a dependence on external enzyme sources and stops producing its own enzymes. As you'll read, this position is unfounded. Throughout the millions of years of evolution that led up to the present, humans subsisted on an enzyme-rich diet and still continued to make enzymes.

The ideal as far as ease of digestion is concerned is that the enzymes present in the food itself do as much work as possible before your body's own enzymes "kick in" to finish the job with its own secretions. The specific enzyme secreted by the body (and the amount) is dictated by what nutrient (protein, starch, fat) needs to be digested after the food enzymes have done their work. Consistently eating an external source (exogenous source) of enzymes conserves your own body's digestive secretion of enzymes.

RAW FOODIST NEED EXTRA ENZYMES

Everyone would benefit from extra enzymes. The studies on longevity, show that cultures, which were noted for low infant mortality, low disease patterns and outstanding longevity, had in common only one dietary factor, ie consuming enzymatic beverages that were being created by friendly bacteria action -- like unpasteurized tamari and miso which are high in enzymes and high in aspergilus bacteria; souerkrout, yogurt, unpasteurized beer and Rejuvilac etc.

There are over 3500 enzyme complexes, which play key roles in digestion, immune action and metabolism.

When you eat cooked food or breath in pollutants, the enzymes are used by the immune system to clean up the internal pollution. If you live in a city, you are ingesting cooked air-born oils, fragments of cat/dog/rat protein hair - which is challenging the immune system. If toy are an athlete, every workout involves tissue breakdown and creation of an inflamatory state, hence you need the anti-inflamatory support of extra enzymes.

Why do athletes age, as a rule, faster than average population. Because athletics can be a major stress. The superior athletes, especially the Olympic competitors, most are using enzymes to reduce recovery time and to minimize the injuries.

For support of immune system and metabolic activity, always take extra enzymes between meals.and during fasting. To support digestion and get more energy out of the food, take enzymes with meals.

FOOD ENZYMES IN PREDIGESTION:

Clearly by design, we see that wild animals rely on exogenous (external , food based) enzymes in the food supply to accomplish dietary predigestion. Are our bodies so different that our own digestive abilities override this most basic need? The answer is absolutely not, not without sacrificing health and longevity.

Human digestive physiology allows time for exogenous enzymes to act on foods consumed in the upper or gastric portion of the stomach. Masticated foods remain in this portion of the stomach for an hour or more while hydrochloric acid is concentrating in the lower or Gaylord portion of the stomach.

This may seem a short time for any significant predigestive activity to occur, but food enzymes are very fast and efficient. This can be observed by bruising an apple and noticing how quickly the enzymes begin working, by evidence of discoloration of the breached area.

This experiment is best performed on tree picked fruit, as irradiation (which is very damaging to enzymes) has been approved as a method of extending the shelf life of fresh raw foods. Unfortunately, this technological advancement also expedites the nearly complete removal of exogenous enzyme sources from the average diet.

ENZYME Work FAST to CHANGE FOOD

Experiment One- If you chew a slice of bread long enough, the starch will be converted to the sweet-tasting form of sugar called maltose by the action of ptyalin enzymes in the mouth.

Experiment Two - In a cup of body temperature water, add 1 Tsp of oil. Open a cap of good quality enzyme, sprinkle on the oil spill and watch the oil disperse and disappear. By taking enzymes between meals, many of the enzymes get through the intestinal track and end up dissolving blood vessel deposits, excess cholesterol deposits in blood vessels disappears. In obese individual, the weight loss is accelerated.

Experiment Three - Prepare Jello as is directed as per the instructions except pour the Jello-to-be liquid into two separate containers. One container will be "the experiment" and the other container will be "the control". (Don't you feel like a real scientist by now?!) Let both the containers that are filled with "unjelled" Jello to cool down to body temperature. In the experimental container, mix in the powder from one capsule of aspergillus plant enzymes. Refrigerate both containers. The container with the enzymes will not solidify into Jello because the gelatin protein has been digested by the action of the protease protein enzymes in the capsule. The last step in the experiment is to throw out the Jello because it is a junk food!

Experiment Four. Take one cup of cooked rice and blend it with just enough warm water to make it into a cream. Let the batch cool down to about 110 degrees Fahrenheit. Open one capsule of aspergillus plant enzymes, pour the powder into the batch and blend. Let it sit for about 20 minutes. You will discover that the rice will turn to sweet custard. This is the action of the amylase enzymes in the capsule on the starch in the rice. The amylase enzymes transform the starch into several forms of simple sugar. In your body, taking food enzyme capsules with a meal of cooked rice will produce the same results in your stomach.

Rot in the Absence of Enzymes

The human body is an incredibly resilient organism using enzymes to control every known biochemical process. Every cell in the body produces enzymes, which are used to power physical movement, regulate organ function, and power the immune system. Even thinking and breathing are processes that depend on enzymatic activity. Digestion of food is also dependent on enzymes. In fact, an enzyme is the only known compound capable of the hydrolysis of food. Digestion of foodstuffs in the absence of naturally occurring enzymes negates the process of predigestion forcing the body to produce pancreatic enzymes to digest 100% of the nutritional factors of that food.

This is the beginning of degeneration of the organism. As the body must provide digestive enzymes to sustain some level of dietary integrity it must sacrifice metabolic enzymes to do so. This fact was best proven by Dr. Paul Kutchacoff in his studies entitled" The Effects of Food Cooking on the Blood

Formulas of Man". In this work, Dr. Kutchacoff found that shortly after ingestion of cooked foods the white blood cell count was sharply increased while ingestion of raw foods showed no such increase. This fact would suggest that the body is isolating the enzymes of the immune system to assist in the digestion of enzyme void foods. This concept of robbing the metabolic enzyme pool for digestion becomes very dangerous when we sacrifice the integrity of the immune system, especially when we suffer such a high rate of immune related diseases. Unfortunately the body's attempt to complete digestion by this means proves most inadequate. This is because exposure to pancreatic enzymes is only possible after the food leaves the stomach, which means that digestion is beginning at the point where the system should be assimilating the nutritional factors for utilization. The result is poorly digested or undigested foods, some of which may pass into the system in an attempt to be utilized, but most of which will simply move into the colon and begin the putrefactive process before being excreted.

The Putrefactive Process Initiate Disease:

Consumption of enzyme deficient foods and the bypassing of natural predigestion marks the beginning of the putrefactive process and promotes conditions conducive to degenerative disease. Materials that remain undigested, or are partially digested, bypass the uptake sites in the small intestine and collect in the colon. The limited enzyme' contribution by the pancreas is soon exhausted and any possible assimilation is completed, leaving the undigested foodstuff to undergo the process of bacterial breakdown or putrefaction.

Unlike fermentative bacteria, which are beneficial, putrefactive enteric bacteria produce extremely toxic by-products. These toxins, especially those related to protein putrefaction, are drawn from the colon during the compressing stages and filtered through the eliminative organs creating even greater strain on an already overtaxed system. The first line of defense is the liver, which, if functioning properly, can remove many of these harmful toxins only to empty directly back into the intestine for removal by excretion, if the system is moving regularly. Some of these toxic compounds are not removed by the liver and are released into the general circulation where they travel throughout the body. Those, which do not accumulate in, weakened tissue, arteries, etc., are then filtered through the kidneys and excreted via the urine. This process is known as intestinal toxemia and has been associated with degeneration and disease.

The Cooked Protein Connection
to Long-term Degeneration

Although protein is the most difficult dietary constituent to digest and is a major contributor to intestinal toxemia, it is also a most important nutritional factor to consider. Proteins are the building blocks of the body and are necessary to transport vitamins and minerals to the bloodstream. The liver uses protein to regulate blood sugar levels through the process of gluconeogenesis. The body uses proteins to make hormones and most importantly, to make enzymes. This fact marks the protein connection to long-term degeneration.

As the weakened pancreas fails to deliver dietary amino acids/proteins for use in these areas, the body is unable to secure the raw materials to produce the enzymes needed to digest protein. The effects of this process can be observed by considering the health problems that are occurring in our society at present. An endless list of hormonal imbalances such as PMS, blood sugar problems such as hypoglycemia, can be associated to protein deficiencies. A body that can not deliver sufficient quantity and quality proteins through dietary means must use raw materials from inner sources. These materials must come from the breakdown of the organism itself. This process is known as catabolism. The body literally must consume itself in order to continue to function. Long-term survival dictates that only the least amount of materials necessary be taken for this purpose. Years of slow deterioration of the quality proteins in the body set up conditions conducive to serious disease and poor quality of life.

ENZYME LOGIC IN DOLLARS & SENSE

Let's play a little with the concept of enzymes by using our day-to-day experience of banking as a metaphor.

Your body's enzymes can be likened to cash reserves in your own life-force bank account. Each time you eat enzymeless food, you tax your system by making a withdrawal from this enzyme bank.

Meal by meal you decrease your enzyme net worth, which can be equated with your life potential. Since at least half of all enzyme capital in the body is assigned to digesting foods, eating life-less cooked foods in effect puts a continual hold on 50% of your budget. Your individual budget limit is determined by your genetic inheritance.

If one's enzyme capital is frozen in this way, your ability to allocate funds to improve the quality of your life is then on hold to the tune of 50% of your net worth! You'll then have limited enzyme resources with which to make much-needed home improvements (cleansing and rebuilding organs and tissues) and protecting your enzyme life savings ,via a strong immune system.

To complicate matters, your bills are coming due, and guess what, your account is low in funds! You're desperate, so you borrow (take stimulants such as coffee to keep going) because your credit rating (overall health) is bad due to years and years of withdrawals. You now wish that you had made more enzyme deposits in your life force bank account, so that you wouldn't be finding yourself in arreaers, experiencing energy deficiencies.

You get the point. Now that you know how health finances work, before life hands you a big bill that you can't afford to pay, start investing in your future health by taking plant-based enzymes today! It could be the best investment, with a return of new youthful energy and freedom from the mid-age crises.

ENZYMES AND AGING

Dr. James B. Sumner, Nobel Prize recipient and Professor of Bio-chemistry at Cornell University wrote in his book, The Secret of Life - Enzymes that the "getting old feeling" after forty is due to reduced enzyme levels throughout the body. Young cells contain a hundreds times more enzymes than old cells. Old cells are filled with metabolic waste and toxins.

In Today's Health (September 1960), which is published by the American Medical Association, Dr. Ratcliff states that "many research men believe that the aging process is the result of the slowing down and disorganization of enzyme activity. Might it eventually be possible to restore youthful patterns of activity by supplying those enzymes that are deficient.?"

Ratcliff goes on to say that "researchers are convinced that virtually all disease can be traced to missing or faulty enzymes...To date, an estimated forty-four diseases have been related to enzyme disturbances."

Enzymes can make the difference between a long life of vibrant health and the half-dead, half-alive limbo state experienced by all too many of us. In the final analysis, the nutritional value of a food cannot be judged by the amount of calories, vitamins and minerals it possesses but rather by the life-force or enzyme potential present in the food. It is a fact that without enzymes, essential vitamins and minerals cannot work.

The miracle of life would be impossible without enzymes. Enzymes are at the heart of all the body's activities, from digesting the food we eat to blinking our eyes. It has been said that the human body is nothing but a series of thousands of enzymatic reactions. Without enzymes, the body would be nothing but inorganic matter.

The length and quality of life is directly proportional to the amount of available enzymes in the body. The level of amylase in human saliva is approximately 30 times more abundant in the average 25 year old than the average 81 year old. In contrast, whales and dolphins, who live in the perfectly balanced aquatic environment and eat entirely on raw foods (like the rest of the two million species of this planet) have no difference in cell enzyme composition in young and old. (Murray M.D., Sea Energy Agriculture)

Enzyme pioneer Dr. Howell has stated, "The fact that the enzyme content of organisms is depleted with increasing old-age is forcibly presented when fluids or tissues are examined at different ages. After full mature growth has been attained there is a slow and gradual decrease in the enzyme content of organisms. When the enzyme content becomes so low that metabolism cannot proceed at a proper level, death overtakes the organism." More simply put, what Dr. Howell is saying is that with increasing age, when our enzymes run out, our physical body dies.

Not only do we run out of enzymes, but as an organism grows older, more metabolic errors occur which affect the quality of the synthesis of enzymes. According to Dr. David Greenberg, chairman of the Department of Biochemistry at the University of California at San Francisco, "Enzymes are becoming increasingly important in medical research because an ever-growing number of diseases can be traced to some defect in the enzyme process."

Just a few of the highly respected researchers who feel that ill health is linked to enzyme deficiency are Dr. Franz Bergel of London; Dr. Holman from the University of Wales, Dr. Potter, professor at the University of Wisconsin; Dr. Manner from Loyola University; and Dr.Salter from Yale Medical School.

ENZYMES THROUGHOUT HISTORY

In the 1890's, the forerunners of the modern science of nutrition discovered building-block substances in food. They named these building-blocks proteins.

At the turn of the 20th century, a new word was

coined to refer to a class of food-based, bio-active, organically-bound chemical substances found to be essential for human health. These substances were called vitamins.

And about a decade or so later, the importance of organic minerals in food was recognized to be equally essential to health.

In the 1990's, one hundred years after the birth of modern scientific nutrition, we find ourselves at an exciting juncture: A missing link in our understanding of the life-giving properties of food is being illuminated by the increasing acceptance of the critical role of food-based enzymes for health and longevity predict that in the near future, the impact of enzymes on health will be more profound than was vitamins, minerals and proteins in the past.

When it comes to a discussion of the history of nutrition as it relates to enzymes, let's begin with what is our first food, milk. Numerous medical studies and current public health statistics confirm what our pre-historic ancestors knew, that infants who were breast-fed on human-mother's milk had less health problems than those infants who were raised on pasteurized cow-mother's milk. Aside from the self-evident fact that human mother's milk is ideally suited for human infants and cow's milk is ideally suited for calves, it is significant that the former is unheated and therefore enzyme-rich and the latter is heated and therefore enzyme-poor.

No one knows exactly when primitive cultures began using enzymatic fermentation to help to digest their food, but we do know it was probably a trial-and-error affair. Who knows, one of your very distant hairy cousins could have been the one to discover that the liquid run-off of yesterday's crushed berries tasted mighty good the next day- and also kept spirits really high for the whole tribe- for reasons that they just couldn't figure out!

Today, both traditional and modern societies have inherited several pre-historic food-processing technologies which involve the transformation of food using enzymes. These advances have lasted to this day because they possessed survival value- they improved digestibility, storage ability and even improved the taste of foodstuffs.

Among the more well-known foods and beverages that we continue to supply (and demand) are alcoholic beverages; the fermentation of soy products such as miso, tamari and tempeh; sauerkraut; bread-making with the aid of yeast plants; and the natural fermentation of the milks of various species of animal with the help of lactobacillus bacteria.

From the above list of foods, soy product ferments are of special interest to our discussion of modern day plant-based enzyme supplementation. Thousands of years ago, Asian cultures discovered a certain species of fungus, (named aspergillus oryzae in western nomemclature), that could pre-digest soybeans if special growing conditions were met. In the 1930's, enzyme pioneer Dr. Edward Howell took this age-old discovery of the East to the West. He went on to pioneer the use of plant enzymes for human nutrition and therapy.

Over thirty years ago, I discovered The Status of Food Enzymes in Digestion and Metabolism. Dr. Howell graciously gave me permission to reprint the book with Viktoras' fifty-page update under the new title, Food Enzymes for Health and Longevity.

About a decade later, Howell's classic was again republished in a simplified and popularized version by Avery

Press and renamed Enzyme Nutrition. With this last release, the long-ignored discoveries of Dr. Howell spread to many health practitioners and seekers of health around the world.

Today, every nutritional company has their own enzyme formula.

DR. HOWELL'S FOOD ENZYME CONCEPT

Dr. Edward Howell was the first nutritional scientist to develop a large experimental and theoretical body of work aimed at answering the complex and critically important question, "What is the connection between food or supplement-based enzyme intake, health, disease and longevity?"

Howell devoted his entire adult-life to conducting numerous animal and human experiments in his attempt to strengthen the theory that food enzyme deficiencies promote disease and premature aging whereas enzyme-rich diets promote good health and longevity. To this end, his book, The Status of Food Enzymes in Digestion and Metabolism cited over 400 research papers, which in his day represented the cutting edge of science at the time of its publication. Modern researchers have yet to fully comprehend the implications of this great work. As Dr. Howell once said, " To say that the body can easily digest and assimilate cooked foods may some day prove to be the most grievous oversight yet committed by science."

Dr. Howell theorized that on a largely cooked, low-enzyme diet, the digestive system borrows enzymes from the body's general metabolic enzyme pool to help digest enzyme-less cooked food. Howell emphasized that the consequences of this adaptive measure was great in that diverting enzymes from one system to another eventually weakened the functioning of these other systems and the body in general.

For example, he argued that the immune system was compromised due to gradual enzyme deficiency and that this set the stage for numerous health problems such as allergies, cancer and diabetes. If he were alive today, Howell would undoubtedly include AIDS to this list.

In treating his patients, Dr. Howell initially prescribed raw food diets but soon found this to be impractical as far as the will-power required to stay on such a regime. However by 1932, he had already developed a plant-based enzyme supplement designed to replace the enzymes lost in a typical cooked food diet.

Dr. Howell discovered that enzyme supplements from plant sources were uniquely effective. Below are just a few of some of Howell's basic concepts. For a more complete discussion, please consult the book Enzymes for Health and Longevity:

1. Food enzymes are essential nutrients.

2. Being more fragile to the effects of heat than vitamins and minerals, food enzymes are destroyed by the high temperature of cooking.

3. When food is chewed and swallowed in its raw natural state, enzymes immediately go to work   in the upper cardiac portion of the stomach.

4. Eating a low enzyme, cooked food diet the size of the pancreas increase, a sign that this organ being overworked. He further hypothesized that this condition is a precursor to various forms of dysfunction such as hypoglycemia, diabetes and metabolic imbalances.

5.A deficiency of food enzymes in the diet gives rise to "digestive leukocytosis", (excess white cells in the digestive system and blood) which is not the case when raw, high-enzyme foods are eaten.

TYPES OF ENZYMES

The previously mentioned kitchen experiments give you an idea of how digestive enzymes do their work. However, in the human body, there are more types of enzymes than just digestive enzymes. In fact, there are thousands of different enzymes, so many that one cannot separate enzyme activity with the process of life itself. From moving a muscle to blinking an eye, no biological work can be accomplished independent of enzymes.
(I hope you're beginning to believe me by now!)

Enzymes can be grouped in three main categories. The first category are digestive enzymes, which the digestive system collects, manufactures and secretes to break down food. Examples of digestive enzymes are protease, which digests protein; amylase, which digests starch; and lipase, which digests fat. Each enzyme almost always has only one specific function which it carries out. For example, the enzyme protease only digests protein. The enzyme amylase only digests starches.

The second type of enzymes are metabolic enzymes, which are present in every cell, tissue and organ and act as biochemical catalysts in the second-to-second functioning of living cells. The metabolic antioxidant enzyme Superoxide Dismutase (SOD), which is present in all cells, reduces free radical damage, thus retards the aging process. Raw foods, especially sprouts and algae, are rich in SOD.

The third type of enzymes are food enzymes , which come from raw, uncooked foods. The process of enzymatic digestion begins when you masticate your food in your mouth. When you chew, you not only mix the enzyme ptyalin from your salivary glands into the food but allow the food-based enzymes present in the food to be released onto itself. This occurs from the moment that you rupture the cell walls of the food with your teeth.

Most fresh, well-grown produce has at least enough enzymes to digest the specific amount of protein, starch or fat found in the food itself. As a general rule, the higher the caloric content of an uncooked food, the more enzymes "Nature" will have put in the food to handle the exact amount of nutrients present. Nature is so considerate and thoughtful, don't you think?

So, foods high in protein will have a high amount of protease or protein-digesting enzyme. Examples are blue green algae and sunflower seeds. Foods such as whole oats have a high amount of amylase or starch-digesting enzymes. Foods such as avocados and nuts has naturally-occurring lipase or fat-digesting enzymes. Nature is so balanced- I wish I could balance my checkbook as easily!

RECYCLING and SPECIFICITY OF ENZYMES

The editor of the Scottish Medical Journal (1966) wrote that "probably nearly half of our daily production of protein in the body are enzymes." In ways, our bodies are like big enzyme factories.

There is strong evidence that the body seeks to conserve its digestive enzymes. In the prestigious scientific journal

Science, Liebow and Rothman (1975) describe an experiment in which it was found that pancreatic enzymes given by mouth can be absorbed intact from the gut, transported through bloodstream and then be re-secreted into the duodenum by the pancreas. If only my home's heating system would be as efficient!

There is an antagonistic relationship between the demands of the digestive system for a continual supply of enzymes and the need of the organs, glands and immune system for enzymes with which to do its work. The competition for enzyme resources can easily be relieved by the consumption of food-soured enzymes.

Dr. Guyton's authoritative Textbook of Medical Physiology (1986) states that the pancreas, stomach and possibly other organs secrete specific digestive enzymes according to the type and quantity of food present.

The ingestion of plant enzymes may have a saving effect on the body's own digestive enzymes, possibly aiding cell and organ regeneration by digesting the foods which normally would have required the body's own pancreatic enzymes.

ENZYMES WORK!

This section is brief because Dr. Howell's powerful words say it all:

"There is no other mechanism in the body except enzyme action to protect the body from any hazard. It is ambiguous to say that "nature cures" when we must know that the only machinery in the body to do anything is enzyme action. Hormones do not work. Vitamins cannot do any work. Minerals were not made to do any work. Proteins cannot work. Nature does not work. Only enzymes are made for work. So it is enzymes that 'heal'. Therefore, the ability of the body to make any of the numerous enzymes needed for good health and long life must be kept at a high level by the methods incorporated in the Food Enzyme Concept."

PLANT VERSUS ANIMAL ENZYMES

Animal-based enzymes work very powerfully on food when the optimal acid-alkaline (pH) environment that these animal-based enzymes require are present. What animal enzyme manufacturers and those that prescribe these products do not tell you is that the optimal conditions that are necessary for animal-based enzymes to work optimally do not correspond to the actual "in vivo" (in the body) conditions of the human gastro-intestinal track. Outside of this narrow, optimal range, animal enzymes do not work as well as aspergillus plant-based enzymes.

Pepsin, which only digests protein, is taken from pig carcasses and works if and only if the acid environment stomach reaches a pH of 3 or less. This is not always the case, especially in people who would need supplemental pepsin in the first place.

Pancreatin, which is taken from the cow carcasses, works best in the neutral or slightly alkaline environment of the duodenum at a pH of between 7.8 and 8.3. These conditions are also not always present.

In contrast, plant-based aspergillus oryzae enzymes, function well in the wide pH range actually found in the human gastro-intestinal track.

Aspergillus oryzae plant enzymes are active in the stomach during the first 30 to 60 minutes of the meal. When the acidity of the lower (pyloric) stomach climbs, the aspergillus enzymes are temporarily inactivated. However, when the food passes into the alkaline environment of the duodenum, aspergillus becomes re-activated again.

Aspergillus can be taken by capsule, dissolved in water or some other beverage, or sprinkled on the food on your plate. When aspergillus is sprinkled on food, its mild, chalky taste does not alter the desired taste of your food. Animal-based enzymes, however, have a pungent taste and foul smell and cannot be sprinkled on food without destroying the taste of the food. Animal-based enzymes can only be taken in capsules or tablets.

DO PLANT ENZYMES SURVIVE GUT ACIDS

Less than one fifth of all medical schools in the United States teach even the elementary aspects of nutrition. Of those that do teach it, the true role of food enzymes are rarely if ever taught. According to the prevailing accepted dictum, enzymes found in foods are destroyed by the hydrochloric acid of the stomach and are of virtually no use in the digestive economy. However, Dr. Howell has shown that as soon as a particular food is masticated in the mouth, the enzymes begin to digest the food. This has been confirmed by Finnish Nobel Prize winner Artturi Virtanen.

When the food reaches the first part of the stomach, (upper cardiac stomach) the food enzymes are still actively working. It takes up to 30 minutes for the hydrochloric acid level to rise to the critical level where the acidity of the hydrochloric acid could inactivate the food enzymes in the food. Until this level is reached, enzymes are still working. What is more, not all foods stimulate hydrochloric acid production appreciably. Foods like fruit, sprouts, grasses and many raw vegetables do not cause hydrochloric acid production to increase rapidly or in any great quantity. In this environment enzymes present in food have a longer time to do their work. According to Howell, even though saliva enzymes shut off in the presence of acid, food enzymes are not markedly disturbed.

CO-ENZYMES MAKE SUPER-ENZYMES

Organic minerals and vitamins are sometimes bound to enzymes which are integrated into the enzyme structure and referred to as co-enzymes. According to Dr. Maynard Murray, M.D., every naturally-occurring organic mineral found in the body should be considered essential for optimal health. Minerals are essential for the working of enzymes and enzymes are essential for the working of minerals.

A few examples: If a certain enzyme is lacking an essential co-factor mineral such as zinc, then the enzyme cannot successfully activate the Vitamin A to do its work.

If a co-factor of Vitamin C lacks the proline hydroxylase enzyme, this will lead to impaired collagen synthesis which will profoundly affect muscle recovery and wound healing. Co-enzymes give the enzymes the high energy power to do their work.

Medical researcher Dr.Hagivara M.D. concludes: "Modern science has made it clear that all chemical changes within the cells of man are performed by the action of enzymes. It has been found that minerals have much to do with the activities of enzymes. In that sense, minerals can be said to be enzymes for the enzymes."

Super Blue Green Alpha Sun Algae™ has the highest

total mineral concentration of all greens as well as the widest range of co-enzyme minerals and vitamins. When "married" to aspergillus enzymes, the partnership creates a synergy of nutritional wealth that far exceeds their separate potencies. I find, Enzyme E12 as the best,

HOW SAFE ARE ENZYMES

Enzymes are safe, when properly used, and have no undesirable side-effects: "It was impossible to determine the lethal dose since the animals survived outrageously large quantities without damage. Guinea pigs and rats, for example, were fed a daily dose of enzyme mixture for 6 months which would have corresponded to approximately 250 tablets per day for a 60kg man." (Enzymes, The Fountain of Life)

Contraindications for hemophiliacs, ulcer patient, pregnancy, patients on blood thinners, those on immune suppressant drugs as well as time release drugs.

Such individuals still can sprinkle enzymes on their warm food and initiate the pre-digestive activity.

I personally have taken enzymes over a period of 30 years, 5 to 10 times the recommended dose on a daily basis. with each meal -purely for the health benefit, as related to digestion, immune system, cardiovascular system, improved energy.

We have use enzymes with all our clients at the Hippocrates Health Institute (www.hipocratesinst.org), including diabetics, for over ten years, with exceptional results.

To get a general education on enzymes, an excellent book is "Enzymes, the Fountain of Life (Williams MD, Miehlke MD, Lopez MD 1994) or a more recent text ALTERNATIVE MEDICINE GUIDE: The Enzyme Cure -- How Plant Enzymes Can Help You Relieve...Problems Goldberg, Burton et al.

GENETIC ENZYME INSUFFICIENCIES:

A great deal of evidence has surfaced to support the fact that enzyme potential is passed on to future generations. A most convincing work was completed by Dr. Henry Pottenger, who carried out a very comprehensive study of dietary effects on cat physiology. Dr. Pottenger scientifically grouped cats and regulated their diets: one group being fed only raw (enzyme rich) foods, another group only cooked (enzyme void) foods. What resulted can be seen as conclusive evidence that enzyme potential is passed on to future generations. While the raw food animals remained stable and healthy, the cooked food animals rapidly deteriorated and carried the deterioration into the genetic structure of their offspring. Pottenger's cooked food cats suffered many of the same diseases that are seen in human population today. Later generations even lost the ability to perpetuate the species, while the raw food animals displayed vigorous vitality with each new generation. The practice of researching family background for genetic disease traits is well accepted by the medical establishment. This concept also applies to traits of vitality and longevity as Pottenger's cat studies suggest. The link between enzyme potential and vibrant health stands on firm scientific ground and without doubt can be passed on in the organ reserve of the offspring.

ENZYME DEFICIENCY DISEASES

If one were to analyze the bloodstream of newborns and elderly persons, there would not be very much difference in the comparative blood levels of most vitamins and minerals in the infant and the old person. Amazingly however, there is over one hundred times more enzymes present in the bloodstream of a newborn than that of an elderly person! This is to me is a mind-boggling fact that almost makes the enzymes floating in my own bloodstream take a deep breath and ponder this startling fact!

If this is true, can we then not look at premature old age, or for that matter, the aging process itself, as a biological condition with a major characteristic being a pronounced enzyme deficiency? According to Dr. Humbart Santillo, "enzyme deficiencies account for more disease than all other diseases combined." At this point I ask to reader to follow the trail of my deductive reasoning "down a theoretical river"... but I will not ask you to jump in with me unless you want to!

OK, here we go: In my own experience working as a nutritional consultant, as well as my ever- increasing understanding of the medical literature, most forms of cancer are preceded by many years of indigestion. Chronic severe indigestion leads to functional pancreatic breakdown and the inability to handle protein digestion. One of the effects of the pancreas not working efficiently is that the bloodstream is flooded with incompletely metabolized proteins. This condition has been strongly linked to the development of allergies and cancer. Dr. Howell had great success reversing allergies by enzyme supplementation. Dr. William Kelly has successfully used supplemental pancreatic enzymes to reverse even so-called "terminal cancer."

The excess intake of cooked fats leads to the exhaustion of the body's ability to manufacture sufficient amounts of lipase, or fat, enzymes. This in turn can lead to obesity, adult onset diabetes and cardiovascular disease. Eskimos can eat up to a pound of lipase-rich raw blubber a day each and every day and not have any signs or symptoms of cardiovascular disease. However, when Eskimos began to cook their fats like Westerners, they began to suffer from the same degenerative diseases of Western cultures.

The National Digestive Disease Information Clearinghouse in Bethesda, Maryland published these 1993 statistics for the U.S., as follows: 116,609 digestive system cancer deaths; 20 million cases of gallstones; 66 million reports of "heartburn" each month; 20 million cases of irritable bowel syndrome; 191,311 total deaths due to digestive diseases; 22.3 million work-loss days due to chronic indigestion; 9 million work-loss days due to acute indigestion; 4.5 million hospitalizations due to indigestion; 13% of total hospitalizations due to digestive disorders; 5.8 million digestive system surgeries and 7% of the total number of surgeries performed were digestive system related.

Indigestion brings in its odorous trail a host of symptoms and discomforts such as heartburn, gas, bloatedness, nausea, burping, bad breath, body odors, headaches, abdominal pain, insomnia, nightmares, allergies, fatigue, constipation, diarrhea, irritable bowel syndrome, diverticulosis, cramps, spasms, skin problems, acne, pimples, food allergies, antacid dependency, post-meal mental fatigue, lack of concentration, memory loss and nervousness.

I wish I could say that the situation was getting better. Though some people are healing themselves with enzymes and other natural methods, the number of people getting sick far outstrip those that are getting healthier. With all our medical sophistication, much of what passes as health care is only a reaction to disease processes that have been set in motion long ago by our nutrition and lifestyle habits.

The diseases that become manifest are but the end-result of our own actions. "Big Business" food manufacturers are feeding the causes of these largely unnecessary diseases by providing us with increasing amounts of unhealthy dead and dying processed foods. And an uneducated public continues to swallow it all down, victims of their own lack of knowledge of what is really going on. The cost of all this is astronomical- not only in terms of money but in the unmeasured cost to the reduced quality of human life.

So if you already have health problems, I advise that you consult a qualified, nutritionally-oriented health professional. It may be equally wise that you consider plant enzyme supplementation whether or not your practitioner is aware of its benefits. It has been my experience working with thousands of individuals that most people benefit immediately by consuming plant food enzymes along with modifications in their dietary intake in the direction of natural foods.

CAN CHILDREN USE PLANT ENZYMES?

Most children have strong digestive systems. However, the fact that they can digest less-than- optimal cooked foods does not automatically make these foods ideal for the future unfoldment of their maximum health potential. Sure, kids will digest the foods served them and still be full of youthful energy, but the same health principles hold for children as they do for adults, namely, that the process of aging is accelerated when enzyme reserves are squandered by the burden of digesting excessive amounts of cooked food.

So the answer is "yes", children can and should use plant enzymes, especially if the child has a weak constitution and/or a history of health problems. Wise parents can avoid future health problems such as allergies and frequent colds by keeping their digestion as strong as possible- with the use of plant enzyme supplementation and as much uncooked food you can get down them!

PLANT ENZYMES AND MEDICATION

For those people who are under medical care who are also taking oral medications of any kind, to avoid any inactivation of the enzymes by your medications, it is suggested that you do the following: Sprinkle plant enzyme powder on the food itself instead of taking the capsules or powder directly into your body. Make sure, however, that the food has cooled down a bit or else the enzyme powder will be damaged by the high heat of your food. In this way, the pre-digestive action of the enzymes will work directly on the food and not have to come in contact with the drugs that may be in your stomach.

PLANT ENZYMES ENDORSEMENT
BY MEDICAL RESEARCHERS

"For I tell you truly, live only by the fire of life, and prepare not your foods with the fire of death, which kills your foods, your bodies, and your souls also."
Jesus, Essene Gospel of Peace Book 1

A new breed of medical researchers have rejected the still taught but erroneous belief that food enzymes and enzyme supplements are destroyed by stomach acids before they confer useful biological work to the organism. These pioneers under-

stand that enzyme supplements are a critical part of disease prevention and for this reason alone are important elements to be included in the daily diet.

In the textbook Enzymes in Health and Disease, co-edited by Dr. David Greenberg Ph.D., Chairman of the Department of Biochemistry at the University of California School of Medicine at San Francisco, this editor suggests that for optimal health, longevity and the reduction of many of the diseases of old age, the use of proteolytic (protein-digesting) enzymes should begin about the age of forty and should optimally continue for the rest of the life-span.

In a similar vein, Dr. Max Wolf, M.D., in his book Enzyme Therapy , strongly endorses the use of the plant-based enzymes. Dr. Wolf states: "Indigestion due to greasy foods is common... Plant-based enzymes are helpful for weak digestion common in old age, or for digestive disturbances. Enzymes are helpful with large rich meals or hard to digest foods. Preparations fortified with plant lipase, prevent post-prandial (after eating) discomfort or gallbladder attacks."
If the food we eat is rich in enzymes, vitamins and minerals, it will add to our lives. If it is deficient in any of these elements, this will take away from the total life-force available to us. Vitamins, minerals and hormones cannot work without the presence of enzymes. According to Dr. Henning Karstrom, Swedish raw food therapy authority, " Even though one may get all the 50 plus known nutrients in one's diet- i.e. vitamins, minerals, essential amino acids, fatty acids, etc. one's health will still suffer unless you also include large quantities of uncooked and unprocessed foods."

Dr. Peter R. Rothchild M.D., a world-renown researcher who was nominated for a Nobel Prize in Physics in 1986 writes: "Evidence of the effectiveness of enzymes taken orally is beginning to overcome skeptics. Much of the evidence comes from many studies performed in West Germany, Switzerland, Australia, Italy and Mexico. Many of these studies show proteolitic enzymes, when taken orally, demonstrate benefits against circulating immune complexes, rheumatic disorders and auto-immune diseases. More recently, studies conducted with antioxidant enzymes are beginning to objectively confirm clinical success in veterinary and medical practices."

GET A LIFE! GO RAW!!!

Enzymes are without a doubt the most important and most overlooked elements in nutrition today. A deficiency of but one enzyme may cause the malfunctioning of an entire metabolic chain reaction in the body, thereby preventing some vital function from unfolding.

And what is more vital than the unfolding of life itself?: In the September 1991 issue of Time, the article entitled "Curing Infertility." reports the work of researchers who have pinpointed why some sperm cannot penetrate the ovum. Want to guess? Yes, you're right? A missing enzyme in the sperm. Talk of "getting a life with enzymes" is empty saying!!

The solution to the infertility problem that the researchers are using is to inject these weak sperms into the egg by way of a syringe. This strategy may work for the short-term goal of fertilization but does not address the problem of what set up the enzyme deficiency in the first place. This booklet has addressed itself to the mechanisms by which enzyme deficiencies come about.

ENZYME FASTING AND HEALING

When you fast or go on a liquid diet of raw fruit and vegetable juices, your digestive system no longer has to produce enzymes. According to what Dr. Howell's refers to as the "law of adaptive secretion," the enzymes that are no longer invested into digesting food can now be utilized by the general metabolic pool. These enzymes are now free to repair and rejuvenate the tissues and organs that need attention in other parts of the body.

Many a seriously ill person has surprised family, friends and doctors by healing themselves of so-called incurable diseases when they adopted a total life-enhancing regime that included a high enzyme diet, sufficient rest, appropriate exercise, positive mental attitude and a conducive social and physical environment.

For a person who is "run-down" and toxic, it is not impossible to adopt such a program at home, but for those that are sick, the supervision of a competent health professional is strongly advised. One can also travel to the health centers that specialize in educating and/or healing people who are dedicated to regaining their health. A few places in Europe include the Bircher-Benner Clinic in Switzerland, Joseph Issel's Ringberg Clinic in West Germany and Dr. Essen's Vita Nova in Sweden. In the United States, Hippocrates Health Institute of West Palm Beach, Florida provides a beautiful residential setting where one can "learn by doing."

ENZYMIZED ESKIMOS

Most health practitioners would agree that a diet consisting of up to ten pounds of meat and animal fat each day is harmful. However, primitive Greenland Eskimos who followed this diet for generations did not suffer from high blood pressure, high cholesterol, heart trouble or kidney stones! How is this possible? Greenland Eskimos eat their food raw and/or slightly fermented! The word "Eskimo" when translated, means, "he who eats it raw."

Dr. William A. Thomas of the MacMillan Arctic Expedition of 1926 wrote: "Eskimos live on an exclusively meat and fish diet, all usually and preferably eaten in the raw. .. There was no unusual prevalence of renal and vascular disease. However, the Eskimos that began living mostly on cooked foods, their health changed... Cancer and heart disease appeared and their longevity was reduced 50%.

OBESITY and Excess Fat

The excess intake of cooked fats leads to the exhaustion of the body's ability to manufacture sufficient amounts of lipase, or fat, enzymes. This in turn can lead to obesity, adult onset diabetes and cardiovascular disease. Eskimos can eat up to a pound of lipase-rich raw blubber a day each and every day and not have any signs or symptoms of cardiovascular disease. However, when Eskimos began to cook their fats like Westerners, they began to suffer from the same degenerative diseases of Western cultures.

Dr. David Galton of Tufts University, School of Medicine, examined eleven individuals weighting around 235 pounds and found lipase enzyme deficiency in the fatty tissue, as well as the fatty tumors. Without the fat splitting enzyme lipase, fat builds up throughout ones body.

Even the small-town local paper in Hot Springs, Arkansas ran a piece entitled "Can Enzyme Regimens End Obesity?"

The article was an account of a National Dietary Research Council experiment in which the researchers had the test subjects consume at least six large meals per day along with an enzyme complex supplement that was thought might help the body overcome it's resistance to weight loss. Of the 50 people who participated in the study, the women lost an average of one pound a day. The men lost an average of two pounds a day.

ENZYMES SPEED INJURY RECOVERY

For athletes, the time lost due to injuries such as strains, sprains, muscle strains and bruises, is of critical importance.

Leo Marty, director of Sport Medicine at Portland State University conducted a double-blind controlled study of 64 football players. Use of oral enzyme mixture reduced the time loss from playing compared to the placebo by about 50%. (Am. Chiropractor, Sept/Oct 1981, 32-3)

Karate, where the participants try to hit hard as possible, with frequent injuries. Dr. J. M. Zuschlag used a double-blind investigation on 10 karate fighters (of both sexes) who were treated with enzyme mix before fighting, 5 tablets, three times daily. Another group of 10, received same placebo dosages. The hematomas of the enzyme group disappeared in under 7 days, for the placebo group, it took almost 16 days. The swelling for the enzyme group subsided after 4 days, while the controls took almost 10 days. Restrictions, as a result of pain and injury, disappeared in 5 days of the experimental group, whereas those in control group, took over 12 days (Mucos-Pharma GMBH, 1988, 1-5).

F.J. Sweeney, studied 100 professional athletes plus college athletes and their injuries. He obtained marked results in 87% of the athletes and moderate results in 10% of the cases, particularly in the reduction of edema, associated pain and return of full activity of the injured area. ("Treatment of Athletic Injuries with an Oral Proteolithic Enzyme", Medical Times, 1963).

ENZYMES INCREASE IMMUNE 1300%

Athletic activities are leads to high tissue breakdown, with circulation of tissue protein fragments. The immune system support in clean up of the post workout tissue loss. Dr. Leskovar has shown that the immune system is greatly enhanced by oral enzyme intake, whereby "the macrophages activity increase by 700% and the natural killer cell activity by 1300%". Hence the intake of enzymes before workout for minimizing the injury and accelerating the recovery. and enzyme intake after a workout to speed the recovery time.

Athlete's just like the rest of the population have problems in maintaining low fat levels. Enzymes can help greatly in this challenge.

As the enzyme levels decrease with aging, so does the capacity to build up one amino acids from the digested protein With aging we Protease and lipase becomes low.

What about increased longevity for athletic career? Another factor affecting athletic performance is the process of aging. As we grow older, many of our nutritional requirements increase, and our glands and organs do not function as well as when we were younger. Often organs and glands begin to atrophy. This is why we generally become more susceptible to degenerative and infectious diseases as we age. Enzymes are connected to every working organ in our body and run our life's processes.

ENZYMES For Beautiful Skin and Face

I recall a remark that was made by a beautician friend of mine, "What you eat and do not digest, you end up wearing on your face, packed around your waist and have it smeared all over your skin.

It is more and more recognized in the industry that true beauty is 'from inside out'. Skin is an eliminative organ. Body dumps through skin what was not evacuated through normal channels.

In general ., over 4000 people die every day in America from heart disease or cancer related deaths. Once enzyme balance is lost, it can be difficult to regain, unless one goes on special enzyme diets and supplementation of enzymes.

It is much better, as a preventative to start early to consume protective foods and supplements for maintaining and improving the quality of life.

Enzymes are the only nutrients that do work and supply the body with energy. Lack of adequate enzyme levels can impair the function of the body, making it susceptible to acute problems like colds flue and headaches; and of course, eventually more chronic conditions like cancer, obesity, cardiovascular challenges and many other complications.

Large pores has a lot to do with lack of adequate amount of amino acids due to low protealitic enzyme activity. Person gets fat if they do not have adequate lipase enzymes to digest the fat. Bags under eye appear if kidney is overworked due to excess of circulatory waste and inadequate protealitic enzymes. . Allergies develop if deficient in protealitic enzymes. No energy to exercise if have low amylase enzymes to digest complex carbohydrates and sugars. Body is exhausted after exercise, partially due to lack of protealitic enzymes to recycle the post-exercise generated worn out tissue etc.

HOW DOES FACE SHOW ENZYME DEFICIENCY?

1. Fatty face, with a swollen neck - lack of protealitic and fat split enzymes 2. When acute, swollen lower lip - looks like just had an implant of silicon. 3. Crease in the center of tongue. 4. Crease in the earlobes - indicate chronic blood vessel congestion.5. Liver marks on face, hands and skin. Liver tries to take on digestion function, when the pancreas is over-worked by enzymeless cooked foods. As liver get overworked, the skin acts as back up for dumping incompletely metabolized waste through skin, hence the liver spots.

6. Circle under eye - overworked kidney indicator.
7. Pimples, acme and other skin blemishes associated with fat
8. Warts - associated with inadequate protealitic enzymes.

TO MAINTAIN A HEALTHY LOOKING SKIN:

Alkaline fluids (such as fresh vegetable juices), salads and ripe fresh fruit. Aloe drinks - fresh (blend flesh of the aloe with orange juice, bananas).

Pure water - few glasses upon arise and 1/2 cup every hour -that is sip water all day long. Stay away from all pasteurized milk products - instead use from health food store the grain milks or at home make milks from soaked overnight nuts and seeds (blend in fruit and spice). Stop all heat treated fats; add extra virgin olive oil to the foods before served. Breath deeply and exercise. Laugh a lot and always have an inner smile. Meditate and have a good attitude - it will make you look young. Exercise your face and practice yoga.

AVIAN FLU, PLAGUES AND ENZYMES

In the past, the major environmental challenge has been toxic microbes. the Bubonic Plague in 1350, killed over 50% of the people of Europe (25 million); In 1918 a global influenza wiped out over 11 million people, with hundredths of thousands dying in USA. Today, germs, are the 5th leading cause o death. According to government, over 100 thousand patients die in hospitals due to infections. The Readers Digest (11/99) did an extensive article, on the "Coming Soon: The Next Grea Flu Epidemic and how to prepare for these killer viruses".

Over the years scientist wondered why some people survived and others died under the germ attack.

Finally thanks to advances of science, technology it has become clear that most people succumb to ailment and acceler ated aging due to weakened immune system.

The immune system function is to fight off all foreign invaders in the body, such as viruses, carcinogens, radiation, bacteria and all foreign chemicals. It relies almost totally on enzymes to do its job.

A weakened immune system has a diminished volume of enzymes due to high stress on the system by all the chemicals and microbes, as well as due to diets lacking in enzymes and the high stress life.

FLUE, Plague protection - strong Immune system -

TRY: enzymes, probiotics, natural cellular defense and blue green algae - as well as a smile, laughter and avoidance of fear.

Enzymes: By ingesting enzymes, the natural killer cells increase by as much as 1300% and macrophages by 700%' - Dr Leskovar

Korean dish 'may cure bird flu' By David Chazan http://news.bbc.co.uk/2/hi/asia-pacific/4347443.stm

Sauerkraut could fight bird flu, say scientists By Jasper Copping Filed: 13/11/2005 Telegraph.co.uk Probiotics and Flu http://www.birdflubeacon.com/HowCanIBoostMyImmunityTo BirdFlu.htm

ENZYMATIC FRIENDLY BACTERIA

In a healthy GI tract there can be over 3 pound of friendly bacteria - aver 200 trillion -which is about 20 times more than the total number of body cells. The friendly bacteria inside our GI track can be a major daily creator of surplus enzymes, just as much as the dietary intake of food borne enzymes.. Ingesting anti-biotic (from food or drugs), chlorinated water, alcohol, coffee etc., reduces radically the friendly bacteria in the GI tract.

If you cook or pasteurize, you destroy the enzymes, at temperatures as low as 120 deg Fahrenheit. So you must obtain enzymes from raw foods, or unpasteurized fermentation products (like kraut) or from supplements of enzymes and or friendly bacteria.. Sad to say, most of the dietary intake is either cooked or processed, so most people get very little enzymes in their diet.

For the best in enzymes and probiotics, blue green algae visit for guidance

Viktoras4u.com

viktorasretreats@gmail.com

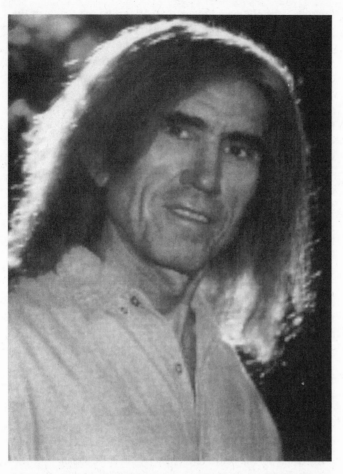

Viktoras 1998 (Joe Correia, Photograher)

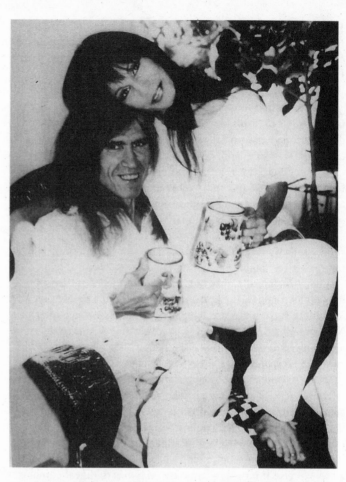

Viktoras and Youkta 1997 (Photo:Jennifer Girard)

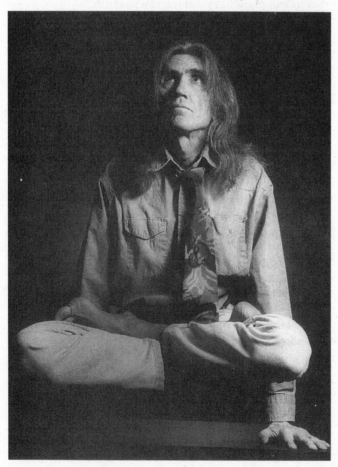

Viktoras 1997 (Photo:Jennifer Girard)

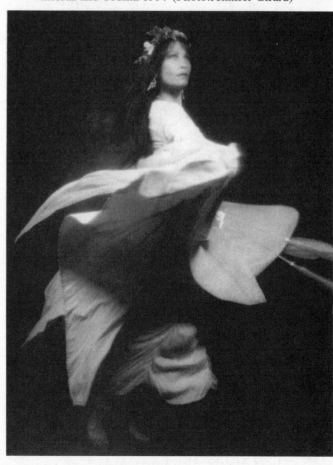

Youkta 1997 (Photo:Jennifer Girard)

Viktoras Kulvinskas

Born in Lithuania, during World War ii, under a Piscean sky, he received his M.S. Degree in pure mathematics from the University of Connecticut, where he later taught mathematics. For six years he was computer consultant for Harvard University, the Massachusetts Institute of Technology, the Smithsonian Astrophysical Observatory, the Apollo Project, etc. He is a member of the Physics honor society Sigma Pi Sigma. He also co-founded, with Dr. Ann Wigmore, the Hippocrates Health Institute in Boston, where he was the Director of Research. As a nutritionist, he was the personal health consultant to comedian/activist Dick Gregory during his 900 mile run for peace. He is an independent Senior Double Diamond Super Blue Green Algae distributor and lectures at Cell tech functions.

Viktoras is the author of five books, and has contributed articles to many New Age journals, among them, "Vegetarian Voice", "Vegetarian Times", "Vegetarian World", "Health Street Journal", and "Alternatives". Besides his best seller Survival Into 21st Century, he has authored Sprout for the Love of Everybody, Love Your Body", New Age Directory, Life Extension Recipes and Program, Life in the 21st Century, Don't Dine Without Enzymes. This year he will be releasing three new books.

Viktoras travels extensively, and has given seminars for the World Symposium on Humanity in Canada and Australia. He has lectured for over 10,000 hours at such events as the New Earth Exposition, the Whole Earth Festival, the World Vegetarian Congress, the Cancer Victims and Friends Convention, the National Health Federation Convention, and others.

Viktoras invites you to write him and share your comments with him. Soon to be released are new books, indoor garden and food preparation videos, newsletters, Internet home pages, retreat and lecture schedules, news on the Arkansas Women's Festival of the Healing Arts, update on resources to appliances, seed sources and other helpful connections. Feel free to write

VIKTORAS CONTRIBUTIONS TO THE LIVING FOOD
by Eliot Rosen

Viktoras Kulvinskas entered in the natural health movement in 1967 shortly after, he became part of Dr. Ann Wigmore's Boston-based Rising Sun Christianity. Within two years, jointly they started the Hippocrates Health Institute. Before Viktoras came to Rising Sun Christianity, cooked foods was still served and the center did not offer any coherent program organized around a set of guiding health principles. Much of what was taught and practiced was primitive, underdeveloped and not very well thought out. There was no living foods program to speak of. However, divine guidance played a role, and the system had some degree of success.

The crux of Viktoras greatness at this juncture was that through his diamond sharp intellect and intuitive genius he saw the tremendous potential in living foods. He saw something others did not fully see, and asked the kind of questions others had never before asked. Viktoras' contribution as founding visionary has never sufficiently been recognized, in part because of Viktoras' unassuming humility.

Nevertheless, in profound and subtle ways he brought to bear ingenious solutions to perplexing theoretical and practical problems in the development of the living food protocol. His contributions include advances in food-growing systems, the creation of entirely new foods and food preparation methods, as well as his highly original seminal literary works. In the final analysis, he was the key player in transforming what was mere latent potential into the innovative directions that the living food movement has taken.

Below are but a few of his pioneering contributions.

1) His book Survival into the 21st Century was this generation's most impressive scientifically referenced assemblage of documented evidence for the value of uncooked nourishment in the human dietary. To this day Survival continues to be regarded as the " Living Foods Bible" by respected leaders in the health field. Released at a time when to be a vegetarian meant eating cooked rice and beans, Viktoras possessed the intellect and research skills to pull together a coherent empirical rebuttal to the unsubstantiated belief that cooking foods was a harmless practice.

In Survival Viktoras powerfully championed what is nothing less than a new paradigm in nutrition: that a high enzyme, low protein, low starch, high liquid, pre-digested uncooked vegetarian diet consisting of fruits, vegetables, sprouted seeds and grains, grasses, weeds, algae and sea weeds was the key to preserving youthfulness, reversing the aging process and extending the lifespan. He is responsible for creating never-before formulated theoretical models for cancer, arthritis, menstruation and life extension that has withstood the scrutiny of critical scientific analysis.

It is not an exaggeration to say that a whole new generation of live food doctors and living food practitioners were inspired by Viktoras' cutting edge nutritional thinking. He is often quoted as an authority on health issues by other health authors such as Fit for Life's Harvey and Marilyn Diamond. Marylin in her 1997 book, Fitonics, quotes Viktoras in many locations, and thanks him in acknowledgments, for his contribution to her enzyme education. Dr. Smokey Santillo, Dr. Gabriel Cousens and a host of others too numerous to mention. express their gratefulness. He is quoted so often, many think he must be dead.

2) Viktoras was perhaps the first person to popularize the long out-of-print works of enzyme researcher Dr. Edward Howell. The book, Enzymes for Health and Longevity, was edited and published by Viktoras at great personal expense and risk. The publication of this first of many of Howell' works resurrected from obscurity fifty years of priceless research regarding the crucial role of enzymes for high level wellness and extended lifespan. Viktoras' premiere publication of Howell's book stimulated a whirlwind of interest which is still growing today. In fact, as a direct result of the resurgence of interest in enzymes, digestive enzyme supplement companies based on Howell's original formula have become a multi-million dollar industries. All of us owe a great debt to Viktoras for having the original foresight to recognize the importance of this great man's work.

3) Realizing that not everybody is ready or willing to eat a sufficient quantity of living foods to make a positive impact on health level, Viktoras has added another pioneering dimension to his life work by continuing the research, development and marketing of whole food nutritional supplements. It is his contention that whole food supplements such as algae, wheatgrass, vegetarian enzyme/herbal formulations can greatly minimize the effects of cooked foods, environmental toxins and inherited constitutional weaknesses.

To conclude, let it be said that Viktoras' contribution to the design and operationalization of the present Health Center is undoutably of inestimable value in increasing the speed at which investors get a return on their investment.

Extensive write-up on Viktoras can be found in "The Heart of Greatness - Ordinary People Creating Extraordinary Success" (1997) and "Wheatgrass , Natural Finest Medicine" (1998) - the complete guide to using grasses to rejuvenate your health - by Steve Meyorowitch.

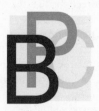
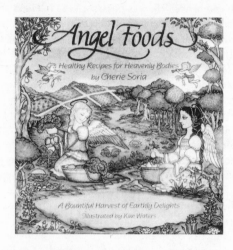
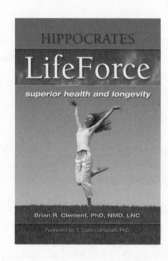
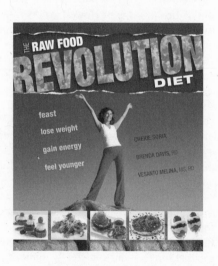